Advances in Peptide and Peptidomimetic Design Inspiring Basic Science and Drug Discovery

Advances in Peptide and Peptidomimetic Design Inspiring Basic Science and Drug Discovery

A Themed Issue Honoring Professor Victor J. Hruby on the Occasion of His 80th Birthday

Special Issue Editors

Henry I. Mosberg
Carrie Haskell-Luevano
Tomi K. Sawyer

MDPI • Basel • Beijing • Wuhan • Barcelona • Belgrade • Manchester • Tokyo • Cluj • Tianjin

Special Issue Editors
Henry I. Mosberg
College of Pharmacy,
University of Michigan
USA

Carrie Haskell-Luevano
College of Pharmacy,
University of Minnesota
USA

Tomi K. Sawyer
Maestro Therapeutics
USA

Editorial Office
MDPI
St. Alban-Anlage 66
4052 Basel, Switzerland

This is a reprint of articles from the Special Issue published online in the open access journal *Molecules* (ISSN 1420-3049) (available at: https://www.mdpi.com/journal/molecules/special_issues/Peptide_Peptidomimetic).

For citation purposes, cite each article independently as indicated on the article page online and as indicated below:

LastName, A.A.; LastName, B.B.; LastName, C.C. Article Title. *Journal Name* **Year**, *Article Number*, Page Range.

ISBN 978-3-03928-288-3 (Pbk)
ISBN 978-3-03928-289-0 (PDF)

Contents

About the Special Issue Editors ix

Preface to "Advances in Peptide and Peptidomimetic Design Inspiring Basic Science and Drug Discovery" xi

Katherine N. Schlasner, Mark D. Ericson, Skye R. Doering, Katie T. Freeman, Mary Weinrich and Carrie Haskell-Luevano
Structure–Activity Relationships of the Tetrapeptide Ac-His-Arg-(*p*I)DPhe-Tic-NH_2 at the Mouse Melanocortin Receptors: Modification at the (*p*I)DPhe Position Leads to mMC3R Versus mMC4R Selective Ligands
Reprinted from: *Molecules* **2019**, *24*, 1463, doi:10.3390/molecules24081463 1

Xue Zhi Zhao, Kohei Tsuji, David Hymel and Terrence R. Burke Jr.
Development of Highly Selective 1,2,3-Triazole- containing Peptidic Polo-like Kinase 1 Polo-box Domain-binding Inhibitors
Reprinted from: *Molecules* **2019**, *24*, 1488, doi:10.3390/molecules24081488 15

Jascha T. Manschwetus, George N. Bendzunas, Ameya J. Limaye, Matthias J. Knape, Friedrich W. Herberg and Eileen J. Kennedy
A Stapled Peptide Mimic of the Pseudosubstrate Inhibitor PKI Inhibits Protein Kinase A
Reprinted from: *Molecules* **2019**, *24*, 1567, doi:10.3390/molecules24081567 31

Héloise Boullet, Fayçal Bentot, Arnaud Hequet, Carine Ganem-Elbaz, Chérine Bechara, Emeline Pacreau, Pierre Launay, Sandrine Sagan, Claude Jolivalt, Claire Lacombe, Roba Moumné and Philippe Karoyan
Small AntiMicrobial Peptide with In Vivo Activity Against Sepsis
Reprinted from: *Molecules* **2019**, *24*, 1702, doi:10.3390/molecules24091702 45

Bartlomiej Fedorczyk, Piotr F. J. Lipiński, Anna K. Puszko, Dagmara Tymecka, Beata Wilenska, Wioleta Dudka, Gerard Y. Perret, Rafal Wieczorek and Aleksandra Misicka
Triazolopeptides Inhibiting the Interaction between Neuropilin-1 and Vascular Endothelial Growth Factor-165
Reprinted from: *Molecules* **2019**, *24*, 1756, doi:10.3390/molecules24091756 81

Shabnam Jafari, Yann Thillier, Yousif H. Ajena, Diedra Shorty, Jiannan Li, Jonathan S. Huynh, Bethany Ming-Choi Pan, Tingrui Pan, Kit S. Lam and Ruiwu Liu
Rapid Discovery of Illuminating Peptides for Instant Detection of Opioids in Blood and Body Fluids
Reprinted from: *Molecules* **2019**, *24*, 1813, doi:10.3390/molecules24091813 101

Michael A. McMechen, Evan L. Willis, Preston C. Gourville and Caroline Proulx
Aza-Amino Acids Disrupt β-Sheet Secondary Structures
Reprinted from: *Molecules* **2019**, *24*, 1919, doi:10.3390/molecules24101919 117

Yanwen Zhong, Xuanyi Li, Hequan Yao and Kejiang Lin
The Characteristics of PD-L1 Inhibitors, from Peptides to Small Molecules
Reprinted from: *Molecules* **2019**, *24*, 1940, doi:10.3390/molecules24101940 129

Nalini Schaduangrat, Chanin Nantasenamat, Virapong Prachayasittikul and Watshara Shoombuatong
ACPred: A Computational Tool for the Prediction and Analysis of Anticancer Peptides
Reprinted from: *Molecules* **2019**, *24*, 1973, doi:10.3390/molecules24101973 147

Bethany Algayer, Ann O'Brien, Aaron Momose, Dennis J. Murphy, William Procopio, David M. Tellers and Thomas J. Tucker
Novel pH Selective, Highly Lytic Peptides Based on a Chimeric Influenza Hemagglutinin Peptide/Cell Penetrating Peptide Motif
Reprinted from: *Molecules* **2019**, *24*, 2079, doi:10.3390/molecules24112079 . . . . **175**

Anthony W. Partridge, Hung Yi Kristal Kaan, Yu-Chi Juang, Ahmad Sadruddin, Shuhui Lim, Christopher J. Brown, Simon Ng, Dawn Thean, Fernando Ferrer, Charles Johannes, Tsz Ying Yuen, Srinivasaraghavan Kannan, Pietro Aronica, Yaw Sing Tan, Mohan R. Pradhan, Chandra S. Verma, Jerome Hochman, Shiying Chen, Hui Wan, Sookhee Ha, Brad Sherborne, David P. Lane and Tomi K. Sawyer
Incorporation of Putative Helix-Breaking Amino Acids in the Design of Novel Stapled Peptides: Exploring Biophysical and Cellular Permeability Properties
Reprinted from: *Molecules* **2019**, *24*, 2292, doi:10.3390/molecules24122292 . . . . **199**

Bamaprasad Dutta, Jiayi Huang, Janet To and James P. Tam
LIR Motif-Containing Hyperdisulfide β-Ginkgotide is Cytoprotective, Adaptogenic, and Scaffold-Ready
Reprinted from: *Molecules* **2019**, *24*, 2417, doi:10.3390/molecules24132417 . . . . **221**

Tae-Kyung Lee, Preethi Ravindranathan, Rajni Sonavane, Ganesh V. Raj and Jung-Mo Ahn
A Structure—Activity Relationship Study of Bis-Benzamides as Inhibitors of Androgen Receptor—Coactivator Interaction
Reprinted from: *Molecules* **2019**, *24*, 2783, doi:10.3390/molecules24152783 . . . . **235**

Cornelius Domhan, Philipp Uhl, Christian Kleist, Stefan Zimmermann, Florian Umstätter, Karin Leotta, Walter Mier and Michael Wink
Replacement of L-Amino Acids by D-Amino Acids in the Antimicrobial Peptide Ranalexin and Its Consequences for Antimicrobial Activity and Biodistribution
Reprinted from: *Molecules* **2019**, *24*, 2987, doi:10.3390/molecules24162987 . . . . **253**

Yang Zhou, Abid H. Banday, Victor J. Hruby and Minying Cai
Development of *N*-Acetylated Dipalmitoyl-*S*-Glyceryl Cysteine Analogs as Efficient TLR2/TLR6 Agonists
Reprinted from: *Molecules* **2019**, *24*, 3512, doi:10.3390/molecules24193512 . . . . **265**

Julien Poupart, Xin Hou, Sylvain Chemtob and William D. Lubell
Application of *N*-Dodecyl L-Peptide to Enhance Serum Stability while Maintaining Inhibitory Effects on Myometrial Contractions Ex Vivo
Reprinted from: *Molecules* **2019**, *24*, 4141, doi:10.3390/molecules24224141 . . . . **275**

Deanna Montgomery, Jessica P. Anand, Mason A. Baber, Jack J. Twarozynski, Joshua G. Hartman, Lennon J. Delong, John R. Traynor and Henry I. Mosberg
Structure–Activity Relationships of 7-Substituted Dimethyltyrosine-Tetrahydroisoquinoline Opioid Peptidomimetics
Reprinted from: *Molecules* **2019**, *24*, 4302, doi:10.3390/molecules24234302 . . . . **293**

David J. Diller, Jon Swanson, Alexander S. Bayden, Chris J. Brown, Dawn Thean, David P. Lane, Anthony W. Partridge, Tomi K. Sawyer and Joseph Audie
Rigorous Computational and Experimental Investigations on MDM2/MDMX-Targeted Linear and Macrocyclic Peptides
Reprinted from: *Molecules* **2019**, *24*, 4586, doi:10.3390/molecules24244586 . . . . **317**

Shubh Sharma, Alastair S. Garfield, Bhavik Shah, Patrick Kleyn, Ilia Ichetovkin, Ida Hatoum Moeller, William R. Mowrey and Lex H.T. Van der Ploeg
Current Mechanistic and Pharmacodynamic Understanding of Melanocortin-4 Receptor Activation
Reprinted from: *Molecules* **2019**, *24*, 1892, doi:10.3390/molecules24101892 . . . . **345**

Rongjun He, Brian Finan, John P. Mayer and Richard D. DiMarchi
Peptide Conjugates with Small Molecules Designed to Enhance Efficacy and Safety
Reprinted from: *Molecules* **2019**, *24*, 1855, doi:10.3390/molecules24101855 . . . . **359**

About the Special Issue Editors

Henry I. Mosberg earned a BS degree in Chemistry from the University of Illinois-Chicago and a Ph.D. in Physical Chemistry from the University of Illinois, Urbana-Champaign. He joined Victor Hruby's lab in 1978, first as a postdoctoral fellow and, later, as an Assistant Research Professor. Originally hired to perform biophysical studies on conformationally restricted peptides, he soon became interested in peptide drug design and embarked on a project to develop receptor-selective, conformationally constrained opioid peptides. This proved to be very successful, led to independent funding from NIH, and paved the way to a tenure track appointment, in 1983, at the University of Michigan, where he remains today as the Tom D. Rowe Professor of Medicinal Chemistry. Dr. Mosberg's research interests remain primarily focused on opioid peptides and peptidomimetics, in particular, bifunctional opioids with improved side effect profiles. He has also been involved in the development of peptide and peptidomimetic inhibitors of RGS proteins and of thrombin, and agents for the treatment of rheumatoid arthritis. He is a Fellow of the American Association for the Advancement of Science and of the American Association of Pharmaceutical Scientists.

Carrie Haskell-Luevano earned her BS degree in Chemistry from the California State University of Fresno (1990) and her Ph.D. degree in Chemistry (1995) at the University of Arizona under the mentorship of Dr. Victor J. Hruby. Subsequently, and with an NRSA NIH postdoctoral fellowship in hand, Dr. Haskell-Luevano joined the laboratory of Drs. Ira Gantz and "Tachi" Yamada at the University of Michigan for postdoctoral training in G-protein Coupled Receptor pharmacology and molecular biology. Concurrently, she was awarded "visiting scientist" status at Parke-Davis Warner Lambert (ex-Pfizer location in Ann Arbor) under the direction of Dr. Christine Humblet within the Basic Structure and Drug Design Department. Subsequent to her training in both these environments, Dr. Haskell-Luevano continued her postdoctoral training at the Vollum Institute in Portland Oregon (OHSU) under the direction of Dr. Roger Cone in neuroscience and molecular pharmacology. During her training at the Vollum, she was awarded the prestigious Burroughs Welcome Career Award in the Biomedical Sciences (only 25 granted that year in the US and Canada) that enabled her to finish up her postdoctoral studies and start an independent research program at the University of Florida Department of Medicinal Chemistry in the College of Pharmacy (1998). At the University of Florida, Dr. Haskell-Luevano was promoted through the ranks of Assistant, Associate, and Full Professor. In 2011, Dr. Haskell-Luevano was recruited to join the University of Minnesota Department of Medicinal Chemistry as a Professor and the inaugural Philip S. Portoghese Endowed Chair in Chemical Neuroscience and a University of Minnesota Institute for Translational Neuroscience Science Scholar. She currently serves as Associate Department Head and Associate Editor of the ACS *Journal of Medicinal Chemistry*. Dr. Haskell-Luevano's research focuses on the neuroendocrine regulation of food intake and energy homeostasis; specifically, the melanocortin pathway, involving multiple endogenous agonists, antagonists, and GPCRs. Her research approaches utilize a variety of multidisciplinary techniques including peptide, small molecule, and combinatorial chemistry synthesis and assays, chemical biology, neuromolecular pharmacology, working with knock out mice, and neuroscience. Dr. Haskell-Luevano's research has been continuously and generously supported by NIH (NIDDK) resulting in over 130 published peer-reviewed manuscripts, reviews, book chapters, and conference proceedings. Multiple patents have been issued based upon the discovery of novel ligands towards metabolic disorder, obesity, and anorexia/cachexia therapeutic applications.

Tomi K. Sawyer earned a BS degree in Chemistry from Minnesota State University Moorhead and a Ph.D. in Organic Chemistry from the University of Arizona with Prof. Victor J. Hruby. He is now Founding Chief Drug Hunter and President of Maestro Therapeutics, an emerging R&D enterprise dedicated to transforming and accelerating peptide modality therapeutics. Most recently, Tomi was a Distinguished Scientist, in Global Chemistry at Merck & Company (NYSE: MRK), where he led a Peptide Drug Hunter Network of more than 100+ scientists actively engaged in peptide drug discovery, core capabilities, and a knowledge engine. This effort advanced new cell permeability screening tools and design rules for macrocyclic peptides, including those generated by super-diverse mRNA-display libraries in a strategic R&D collaboration with PeptiDream. Prior to joining Merck & Company in 2014, Tomi was the Founding Chief Scientific Officer at Aileron Therapeutics from 2007 to 2013 and Senior Vice-President of Drug Discovery at Ariad Pharmaceuticals (recently acquired by Takeda) from 1997 to 2006. He is credited with building a stapled peptide technology platform at Aileron Therapeutics and a multi-targeted R&D collaboration with Roche Pharma. Tomi has recently launched the Peptide Drug Hunter Consortium, a non-profit global network to empower the advancement of peptide preclinical research and clinical development at the interface of academia, biotech/pharma, and investors, as well as contract organizations and vendors engaged in peptide science. He is well known for his contributions to GPCR, kinase, protease, and protein–protein interaction drug discovery. Tomi has three marketed drugs, including Scenesse® (a peptide superagonist of MC1R for the treatment of the orphan skin disease known as erythropoietic protophyria and related indications), Iclusig® (a small-molecule inhibitor of Bcr-Abl kinase for the treatment of clinically-resistance of chronic myelogenous leukemia), and Ridaforolimus (a natural product macrocycle mTOR antagonist for the treatment of coronary artery disease via an EluNIR® stent system). Some other examples of his drug discovery campaigns include peptidomimetic renin inhibitors (Ditekiren and U-84700), the first reported peptidomimetic HIV protease and nonpeptide inhibitors (U-81749 and PD-107067), the first reported peptidomimetic and nonpeptide Src SH2 antagonists (AP21774 and AP22408), the first reported small-molecule dual Src/Bcr-Abl kinase inhibitor (AP23464), and the first stapled peptide dual MDM2/MDMX antagonist (ALRN-6924) to advance into clinical trials. Tomi is credited with more than 600 scientific publications, patents, and presentations. He holds Adjunct Professorship and Scientific Advisory Board appointments at the University of Massachusetts, the University of Arizona, and the Northeastern University Center for Drug Discovery. At his undergraduate alma mater, Minnesota State University Moorhead, Tomi is a Distinguished Alumni Scholar and has served as a member of the MSUM Alumni Foundation Board. At his graduate alma mater, the University of Arizona, he is a Distinguished Alumni Entrepreneur and has affiliations with the College of Science, College of Medicine, College of Pharmacy, and Tech Launch Arizona. He has been honored with a DuVigneaud Award (American Peptide Society), a Distinguished Alumni Award (Minnesota State University Moorhead), and a Professional Achievement Award (University of Arizona). He is a member of numerous editorial boards (including Peptide Science), and he was the Founding Editor-in-Chief of *Chemical Biology and Drug Design*. Tomi is past-President of the American Peptide Society and co-Chair of the Eighteenth American Peptide Symposium.

Preface to "Advances in Peptide and Peptidomimetic Design Inspiring Basic Science and Drug Discovery"

Fueled by a wide-ranging, probing curiosity complemented by an energetic, engaging personality and a highly collaborative approach to science, Prof. Victor J. Hruby's research accomplishments have spanned a staggering breadth of scientific endeavors resulting in well over 1300 publications, numerous patents, and a worldwide reputation as a preeminent scholar. Victor was born in Valley City, North Dakota and received his B.S. and M.S. degrees with A. William Johnson at the University of North Dakota. He went on to Cornell University for graduate studies with A. T. Blomquist. After receiving his Ph.D., Dr. Hruby joined the Cornell University Medical College as an Instructor, working with Prof. Vincent duVigneaud, Nobel Laureate. He moved to the University of Arizona in 1968 as an Assistant Professor and rose through the academic ranks to be Regents Professor in the Department of Chemistry and Biochemistry in 1989. He is now Emeritus Regents Professor and has remained very active in both mentoring and collaborative work at the University of Arizona and throughout the world. Prof. Hruby's many accomplishments include the following: (i) the rational design of novel, extensively used and highly cited ligands for opioid, melanocortin, oxytocin, glucagon, and neurokinin receptors; (ii) the development and application of approaches for incorporating conformational constraints into peptides to improve selectivity and bioavailability and to aid elucidation of bioactive conformations; and (iii) key contributions to combinatorial chemistry, and the application of biophysical methods (e.g., NMR, X-ray crystallography, fluorescence, plasmon waveguide resonance spectroscopy) to the determination of biomolecular structure and mechanism. Molecules is highly pleased to host a Special Issue honoring Prof. Victor J. Hruby on the occasion of his 80th birthday for his outstanding achievements to advance peptide and peptidomimetic design, as well as inspiring both basic science and drug discovery. There are twenty articles included in this Special Issue of Molecules that reflect the innovative spirit and passion for science of Prof. Hruby.

Henry I. Mosberg, Carrie Haskell-Luevano, Tomi K. Sawyer
Special Issue Editors

molecules

Article

Structure–Activity Relationships of the Tetrapeptide Ac-His-Arg-(*p*I)DPhe-Tic-NH$_2$ at the Mouse Melanocortin Receptors: Modification at the (*p*I)DPhe Position Leads to mMC3R Versus mMC4R Selective Ligands

Katherine N. Schlasner, Mark D. Ericson, Skye R. Doering, Katie T. Freeman, Mary Weinrich and Carrie Haskell-Luevano *

Department of Medicinal Chemistry & Institute for Translational Neuroscience, University of Minnesota, Minneapolis, MN 55455, USA; schlasner@gmail.com (K.N.S.); erics063@umn.edu (M.D.E.); skye.doering@gmail.com (S.R.D.); freem236@umn.edu (K.T.F.); maryweinrich@mail.usf.edu (M.W.)

* Correspondence: chaskell@umn.edu; Tel.: 612-626-9262; Fax: 612-626-3114

Received: 28 February 2019; Accepted: 4 April 2019; Published: 13 April 2019

Abstract: The five melanocortin receptors (MC1R–MC5R) are involved in numerous biological pathways, including steroidogenesis, pigmentation, and food intake. In particular, MC3R and MC4R knockout mice suggest that the MC3R and MC4R regulate energy homeostasis in a non-redundant manner. While MC4R-selective agonists have been utilized as appetite modulating agents, the lack of MC3R-selective agonists has impeded progress in modulating this receptor in vivo. In this study, the (*p*I)DPhe position of the tetrapeptide Ac-His-Arg-(*p*I)DPhe-Tic-NH$_2$ (an MC3R agonist/MC4R antagonist ligand) was investigated with a library of 12 compounds. The compounds in this library were found to have higher agonist efficacy and potency at the mouse (m) MC3R compared to the MC4R, indicating that the Arg-DPhe motif preferentially activates the mMC3R over the mMC4R. This observation may be used in the design of new MC3R-selective ligands, leading to novel probe and therapeutic lead compounds that will be useful for treating metabolic disorders.

Keywords: MC3R; MC4R; mixed pharmacology; tetrapeptides; melanocortins

1. Introduction

The melanocortin system consists of five receptors (MC1R–MC5R) [1–8] belonging to the class A family of G protein-coupled receptors (GPCRs). The melanocortin receptors are involved in numerous physiological functions and primarily signal through the $G_{\alpha s}$ pathway, increasing production of cyclic adenosine monophosphate (cAMP) upon receptor activation [9]. The MC1R is involved in the regulation of skin pigmentation [2,3]. The MC2R, implicated in steroidogenesis [3], is only activated by the adrenocorticotropic hormone (ACTH) and not other endogenous melanocortin ligands [10]. The MC3R and MC4R have been demonstrated to regulate appetite and energy homeostasis [4–6,11–14]. While the function of the MC5R has not been clearly elucidated in humans, this receptor has been linked to exocrine gland function in mice [1,7,8,15]. The melanocortin receptors are stimulated by endogenous agonists derived from the proopiomelanocortin (POMC) gene transcript [16], and include the α-, β-, and γ-melanocortin stimulating hormones (MSH) and ACTH, as previously reviewed [17,18]. Common to the endogenous agonists is a His-Phe-Arg-Trp tetrapeptide sequence, the minimum sequence when the N-terminal is acetylated and the C-terminal is amidated to produce a functional response in the frog (*Rana pipiens*) and lizard (*Anolis carolinensis*) skin bioassays [19,20]. The melanocortin system also contains two naturally occurring antagonists, agouti-signaling protein (ASP) and agouti-related protein (AGRP), which possess an Arg-Phe-Phe tripeptide motif hypothesized to be important for antagonist activity [21,22].

Studies in mice have indicated the important roles of the MC4R and MC3R in maintaining energy homeostasis. Knock-out (KO) MC4R mice are hyperphagic and obese compared to wildtype littermates [13]. While the MC3R may play a subtle role in regulating food intake [23], MC3R KO mice exhibit increased fat mass, reduced lean mass, and maintain a similar body weight compared to wildtype littermates [11,12]. Double MC3R/MC4R KO mice are significantly heavier than MC4R KO mice, suggesting non-redundant roles for the MC3R and MC4R in energy homeostasis [12,24–26]. Central administration of non-selective melanocortin agonists has been shown to decrease food intake in rodents [14,23,27], while the administration of MC3R/MC4R antagonists increases food intake [14,23,28]. Targeting the MC3R and MC4R may therefore lead to the development of treatments for metabolic disorders such as obesity, anorexia, and cachexia. Similar to MC4R KO mice, select human MC4R single nucleotide polymorphisms result in a hyperphagic and increased weight phenotype, as previously reviewed [29]. MC4R-selective ligands have been reported to reduce body weight, although these compounds possess side effects including increased blood pressure [30], erectile activity [31–33], and skin darkening [34,35]. While the skin darkening is most likely due to the stimulation of the MC1R, the increases in blood pressure [36] and erectile activity [37,38] are postulated to be MC4-mediated. In the case of blood pressure, the lack of reported adverse cardiovascular side effects of the MC4R-selective setmelanotide [34] indicates that this may be ligand-dependent. Though polymorphisms in the MC3R may predispose an individual to obesity, the role of the MC3R has not been clearly elucidated [39]. While selective probes and therapeutic compounds have been developed for the MC4R, there remains a need for MC3R-selective compounds to clarify the role of this receptor in energy homeostasis and as potential lead ligands in the development of novel weight management therapeutics that bypass the reported side effects of MC4R-selective ligands.

To identify novel scaffolds with agonist selectivity for the MC3R over the MC4R, our laboratory performed a tetrapeptide mixture-based positional scan [40]. From this study, a new scaffold tetrapeptide (Ac-His-Arg-(*p*I)DPhe-Tic-NH_2) was identified that possessed nanomolar agonist potency at the MC3R (EC_{50} = 40 nM) and was an antagonist at the MC4R (pA_2 = 7.0) [40]. Compared to the endogenous tetrapeptide melanocortin sequence (His-Phe-Arg-Trp), the new scaffold switched the Phe and Arg positions and incorporated a Tic residue in place of the Trp. A follow-up study utilized the most potent MC3R substitutions at each position within the tetrapeptide from the mixture-based positional scan, retaining the switched Phe and Arg positions (Arg or Gln were utilized in the second position, while (*p*I)DPhe or (*p*Cl)DPhe were substituted at the third position) [41]. A 100-fold selective MC3R versus MC4R agonist compound was identified (Ac-Val-Gln-(*p*I)DPhe-DTic-NH_2) that did not possess antagonist potency at the MC4R and only partially stimulated the MC4R (less than 50% efficacy of NDP-MSH) [41]. Switching the Arg and Phe positions within the melanocortin tetrapeptide sequence may therefore lead to MC3R-selective ligands that may be further developed into probe and therapeutic lead compounds.

In previous studies examining the traditional melanocortin tetrapeptide sequence, the substitution of (*p*I)DPhe for Phe, yielding the ligand Ac-His-(*p*I)DPhe-Arg-Trp-NH_2, resulted in a full agonist at the MC4R and a partial agonist with antagonist activity at the MC3R [42,43]. This contrasts to the observed MC3R agonism and partial agonism with antagonist activity at the MC4R for the scaffold Ac-His-Arg-(*p*I)DPhe-Tic-NH_2, where switching to the Arg-(*p*I)DPhe motif and substituting Tic results in opposite MC3R–MC4R activities. Further examination of the DPhe *para*-position within the Ac-His-(*p*I)DPhe-Arg-Trp-NH_2 scaffold demonstrated that this position influenced the efficacy at the MC3R. Full MC3R agonist activity was observed when DPhe, DTyr, (*p*Me)DPhe, (*p*CN)DPhe, (*p*F)DPhe, and (*p*Cl)DPhe were incorporated, while (*p*I)DPhe, (*p*Br)DPhe, (*p*CF_3)DPhe, and (3,4-diCl)DPhe resulted in up to 50% receptor activation and micromolar to sub-micromolar antagonist potencies at the MC3R [42]. All of these substitutions maintained full MC4R efficacy [42].

Since switching the Phe and Arg positions results in MC3R agonism and MC4R partial agonism/antagonism for the Ac-His-Arg-(*p*I)DPhe-Tic-NH_2 scaffold, it was hypothesized that further substitutions at the *para*-position might result in decreasing MC4R efficacy while retaining MC3R agonism. Therefore, a library of 12 peptides was synthesized based upon the scaffold Ac-His-Arg-(*p*X)DPhe-Tic-NH_2 (substitutions for (*p*X)DPhe can be found in Figure 1) and assayed at the mouse MC1R, MC3R, MC4R, and MC5R, in order to understand how the *para*-position within this scaffold influences melanocortin receptor selectivity, potency, and efficacy.

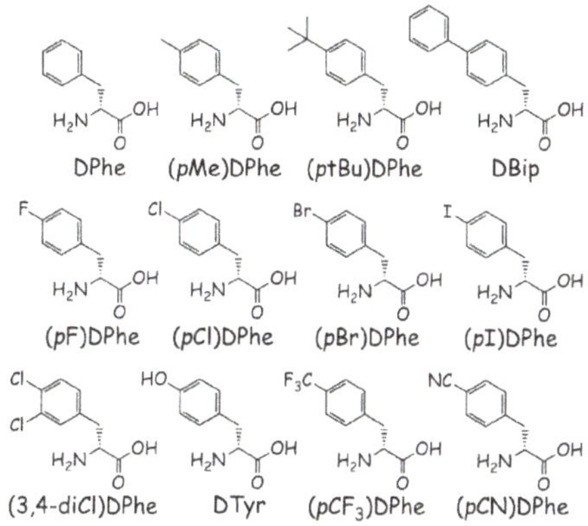

Figure 1. Structures and abbreviations of the amino acids used to replace the third amino acid in the peptide template Ac-His-Arg-Xxx-Tic-NH_2.

2. Results

Peptide Synthesis and Pharmacological Evaluation

Peptides were synthesized manually with microwave irradiation using standard Fmoc synthesis techniques [44,45] and purified using semi-preparative reverse-phase high-pressure liquid-chromatography (RP-HPLC). Peptide molecular mass was confirmed through ESI-MS (University of Minnesota Mass Spectrometry Laboratory), and each peptide was assessed for purity (>95%) using analytical RP-HPLC in two different solvent systems (acetonitrile and methanol; Table 1). Agonist pharmacology was measured at the mMC3R, mMC4R, and mMC5R using a colorimetric β-galactosidase assay that measures cAMP production [46]. Agonist pharmacology was assessed at the mMC1R using the Amplified Luminescent Proximity Homogenous Assay Screen (AlphaScreen, PerkinElmer), as previously described [47–49]. The MC2R is only stimulated by ACTH, and was not examined in this study. For both assays, HEK293 cells stably expressing the mMCRs were used. For agonist assays, the peptide ligands NDP-MSH [50] and Ac-His-DPhe-Arg-Trp-NH_2 [51] were used as positive controls. Ligands were considered full agonists if they stimulated the receptor to >90% of the maximal signal of NDP-MSH and were considered inactive if they did not stimulate the receptor to at least 20% of the signal of NDP-MSH at a 100 μM concentration. Compounds that did not possess at least 50% of the maximal NDP-MSH signal were assessed for antagonist pharmacology using a Schild assay design [52], with NDP-MSH as the agonist. Compounds that were within 3-fold potency range were considered equipotent and within the inherent experimental error of the assays.

Similar to prior reports [49,51], the Ac-His-DPhe-Arg-Trp-NH_2 peptide (**KNS2-153**) possessed agonist potencies of 10, 190, 12, and 5 nM at the mMC1R, mMC3R, mMC4R, and mMC5R, respectively (Figure 2, Tables 2 and 3). The lead ligand for the current series (**KNS2-22-4**) switched the Arg and DPhe positions, utilized a (*p*I)DPhe in the place of DPhe, and substituted a Tic residue in the place of Trp compared to **KNS2-153**. These alterations resulted in a ligand that maintained full agonist efficacy at the mMC1R, mMC3R, and mMC5R (EC_{50} = 0.7, 13, and 5 nM, respectively; Tables 2 and 3), and partial agonist efficacy at the mMC4R (40% of the NDP-MSH signal, EC_{50} = 150 nM; Figure 3). An antagonist pA_2 value of 7.3 was observed for **KNS2-22-4** at the mMC4R (Figure 3). In prior studies, this compound was observed to possess nanomolar agonist potency at the MC3R (30–40 nM), partial agonist stimulation of the MC4R, and sub-micromolar antagonist potency at the MC4R (pA_2 of 6.6–7) [40,41], similar to the results in the present study.

Table 1. Analytical data for peptides synthesized in this study [a].

Peptide	Sequence	Retention Time (min)		M (Calculated)	M + H (Observed)	Purity (%)
		System 1	System 2			
KNS2-153	Ac-His-DPhe-Arg-Trp-NH_2	10.1	15.6	685.3	686.4	>98
KNS2-22-4	Ac-His-Arg-**(*p*I)DPhe**-Tic-NH_2	14.9	23.6	784.2	785.3	>97
KNS2-22-3	Ac-His-Arg-**(*p*Br)DPhe**-Tic-NH_2	14.9	23.2	736.3, 738.3 [b]	737.3, 739.3 [b]	>98
KNS2-22-1	Ac-His-Arg-**(*p*Cl)DPhe**-Tic-NH_2	14.6	22.7	692.3	693.5	>97
KNS2-22-2	Ac-His-Arg-**(*p*F)DPhe**-Tic-NH_2	13.5	20.8	676.3	677.5	>95
KNS3-10	Ac-His-Arg-**DPhe**-Tic-NH_2	12.8	20.1	658.3	659.5	>99
KNS2-23-4	Ac-His-Arg-**(3,4-diCl)DPhe**-Tic-NH_2	15.6	24.2	726.3	727.4	>97
KNS2-23-7	Ac-His-Arg-**(*p*Me)DPhe**-Tic-NH_2	14.3	22.3	672.4	673.5	>97
KNS2-23-6	Ac-His-Arg-**(*p*CF_3)DPhe**-Tic-NH_2	15.0	23.4	726.7	727.5	>98
KNS2-23-3	Ac-His-Arg-**(*p*tBu)DPhe**-Tic-NH_2	17.5	26.5	714.4	715.4	>95
KNS2-23-1	Ac-His-Arg-**DBip**-Tic-NH_2	16.7	25.9	734.3	735.5	>96
KNS2-23-9	Ac-His-Arg-**DTyr**-Tic-NH_2	10.5	15.0	674.3	675.4	>96
KNS2-23-8	Ac-His-Arg-**(*p*CN)DPhe**-Tic-NH_2	11.5	17.2	683.3	684.3	>97

[a] HPLC retention time (min) for peptides in solvent system 1 (10% acetonitrile in 0.1% trifluoroacetic acid/water and a gradient to 90% acetonitrile over 35 min) or solvent system 2 (10% methanol in 0.1% trifluoroacetic acid/water and a gradient to 90% methanol over 35 min). An analytical Vydac C18 column (Vydac 218TP104) was used with a flow rate of 1.5 mL/min. The peptide purity was determined by HPLC at a wavelength of 214 nm. [b] Two peaks were observed for the (*p*Br)DPhe amino acid due to the approximately equal natural abundance of ^{79}Br and ^{81}Br.

Table 2. Tetrapeptide pharmacology at the mouse melanocortin-1 receptor using the AlphaScreen cyclic adenosine monophosphate (cAMP) assay [a].

Peptide	Sequence	mMC1R EC_{50} (nM)
NDP-MSH	Ac-Ser-Tyr-Ser-Nle-Glu-His-DPhe-Arg-Trp-Gly-Lys-Pro-Val-NH_2	0.009 ± 0.002
KNS2-153	Ac-His-DPhe-Arg-Trp-NH_2	10 ± 3
KNS2-22-4	Ac-His-Arg-**(*p*I)DPhe**-Tic-NH_2	0.7 ± 0.2
KNS2-22-3	Ac-His-Arg-**(*p*Br)DPhe**-Tic-NH_2	0.7 ± 0.3
KNS2-22-1	Ac-His-Arg-**(*p*Cl)DPhe**-Tic-NH_2	0.8 ± 0.2
KNS2-22-2	Ac-His-Arg-**(*p*F)DPhe**-Tic-NH_2	1.8 ± 0.7
KNS3-10	Ac-His-Arg-**DPhe**-Tic-NH_2	4.6 ± 0.4
KNS2-23-4	Ac-His-Arg-**(3,4-diCl)DPhe**-Tic-NH_2	5 ± 2
KNS2-23-7	Ac-His-Arg-**(*p*Me)DPhe**-Tic-NH_2	1.0 ± 0.3
KNS2-23-6	Ac-His-Arg-**(*p*CF_3)DPhe**-Tic-NH_2	5 ± 1
KNS2-23-3	Ac-His-Arg-**(*p*tBu)DPhe**-Tic-NH_2	9 ± 3
KNS2-23-1	Ac-His-Arg-**DBip**-Tic-NH_2	0.6 ± 0.1
KNS2-23-9	Ac-His-Arg-**DTyr**-Tic-NH_2	40 ± 10
KNS-2-23-8	Ac-His-Arg-(*p*CN)DPhe-Tic-NH_2	27 ± 6

[a] The indicated error represents the standard error of the mean determined from at least three independent experiments performed in duplicate replicates.

Table 3. Tetrapeptide pharmacology at the mouse melanocortin-3, -4, and -5 receptors using the β-Galactosidase cAMP assay [a].

Peptide	Sequence	mMC3R EC_{50} (nM)	mMC4R		mMC5R EC_{50} (nM)
			EC_{50} (nM)	pA_2	
NDP-MSH	Ac-Ser-Tyr-Ser-Nle-Glu-His-DPhe-Arg-Trp-Gly-Lys-Pro-Val-NH_2	0.52 ± 0.05	0.32 ± 0.02	-	3.4 ± 0.7
KNS2-153	Ac-His-DPhe-Arg-Trp-NH_2	190 ± 40	12 ± 3	-	5 ± 2
KNS2-22-4	Ac-His-Arg-**(*p*I)DPhe**-Tic-NH_2	13 ± 2	Partial Agonist 150 ± 40 (40% NDP)	7.3 ± 0.8	5 ± 1
KNS2-22-3	Ac-His-Arg-**(*p*Br)DPhe**-Tic-NH_2	90 ± 20	Partial Agonist 290 ± 50 (55% NDP)	-	9.7 ± 0.5
KNS2-22-1	Ac-His-Arg-**(*p*Cl)DPhe**-Tic-NH_2	120 ± 20	Partial Agonist 280 ± 60 (70% NDP)	-	18 ± 6
KNS2-22-2	Ac-His-Arg-**(*p*F)DPhe**-Tic-NH_2	450 ± 70	Partial Agonist 560 ± 60 (70% NDP)	-	70 ± 40
KNS3-10	Ac-His-Arg-**DPhe**-Tic-NH_2	Partial Agonist 900 ± 200 (85% NDP)	3000 ± 2000	-	Partial Agonist 200 ± 30 (65% NDP)
KNS2-23-4	Ac-His-Arg-**(3,4-diCl)DPhe**-Tic-NH_2	400 ± 100	>100,000	6.15 ± 0.05	70 ± 7
KNS2-23-7	Ac-His-Arg-**(*p*Me)DPhe**-Tic-NH_2	110 ± 20	Partial Agonist 700 ± 200 (50% NDP)	-	17 ± 4
KNS2-23-6	Ac-His-Arg-**(*p*CF_3)DPhe**-Tic-NH_2	90 ± 30	Partial Agonist 600 ± 300 (20% NDP)	6.5 ± 0.2	13 ± 4
KNS2-23-3	Ac-His-Arg-**(*pt*Bu)DPhe**-Tic-NH_2	Partial Agonist 13 ± 4 (85% NDP)	>100,000	6.8 ± 0.3	3.4 ± 0.3
KNS2-23-1	Ac-His-Arg-**DBip**-Tic-NH_2	14 ± 2	Partial Agonist 1400 ± 700 (45% NDP)	5.9 ± 0.2	7.6 ± 0.7
KNS2-23-9	Ac-His-Arg-**DTyr**-Tic-NH_2	Partial Agonist 4200 ± 800 (85% NDP)	>100,000	<5.5	1000 ± 500
KNS2-23-8	Ac-His-Arg-**(*p*CN)DPhe**-Tic-NH_2	Partial Agonist 4000 ± 1000 (75% NDP)	40% @ 100 μM	<5.5	500 ± 100

[a] The indicated error represents the standard error of the mean determined from at least three experiments performed in duplicate replicates. The value of >100,000 nM indicates that the compound was assayed but no agonist activity was observed up to a concentration of 100 μM. A percentage denotes the percent maximal stimulatory response observed at 100 μM, but not enough stimulation was observed to determine an EC_{50} value. Partial agonist indicates a partial agonist with the percent maximal stimulation (relative to NDP-MSH) and the apparent EC_{50} value. Antagonist pA_2 values were determined using a Schild analysis [52] and the agonist NDP-MSH. The value of <5.5 indicates that no antagonist potency was observed in the highest antagonist concentration range assayed (10,000, 5000, 1000, and 500 nM). A dash (-) indicates that the compound was not assayed as an antagonist at the mMC4R.

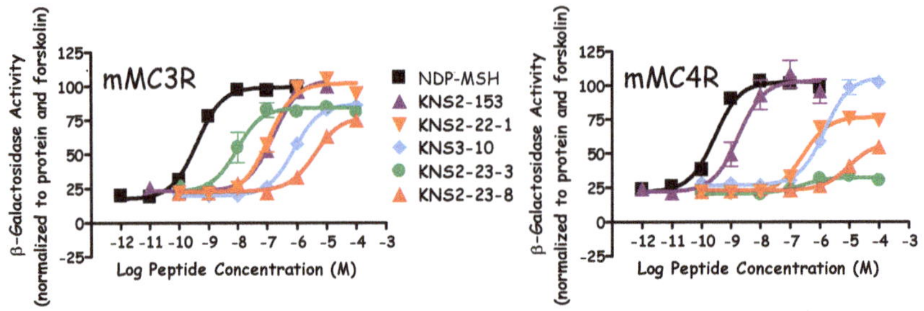

Figure 2. Illustration of the agonist pharmacology of NDP-MSH, **KNS2-153**, **KNS2-22-1**, **KNS3-10**, **KNS2-23-3**, and **KNS2-23-8** at the mMC3R and mMC4R.

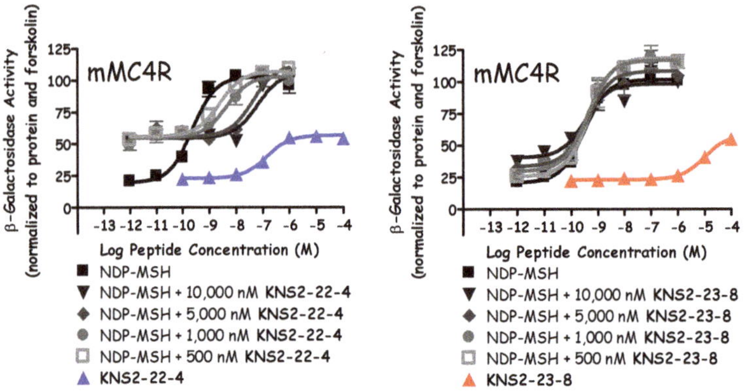

Figure 3. Illustration of the antagonist pharmacology of **KNS2-22-4** and **KNS2-23-8** at the mMC4R.

Replacing (*p*I)DPhe with (*p*Br)DPhe (**KNS2-22-3**) resulted in similar potencies at the melanocortin receptors assayed compared to **KNS2-22-4**, although higher efficacy was observed at the mMC4R (55% maximal NDP-MSH signal). The (*p*Cl)DPhe-substituted **KNS2-22-1** maintained similar potencies compared to **KNS2-22-4** at the mMC1R and mMC5R, but was 9-fold less potent at the mMC3R (120 nM, Figure 2) and possessed an increased partial agonist response relative to NDP-MSH (70%, EC_{50} = 280 nM) at the mMC4R (Figure 2) compared to **KNS2-22-4**. The Ac-His-Arg-(*p*Cl)DPhe-Tic-NH_2 (**KNS2-22-1**) tetrapeptide was previously reported to possess agonist pharmacology at the mMC3R (110 nM) and partial agonist activity at the mMC4R (EC_{50} = 140 nM), similar to the values observed in the present study [41]. While similar potency relative to **KNS2-22-4** was observed for the (*p*F)DPhe-substituted **KNS2-22-2** at the mMC1R, this substitution decreased potency at the mMC3R and mMC5R (30- and 14-fold as compared to **KNS2-22-4**, respectively). Similar to **KNS2-22-1**, a 70% partial agonist response at the mMC4R (EC_{50} = 560 nM) was observed for **KNS2-22-2**.

The DPhe-substituted **KNS3-10** possessed decreased agonist potency compared to **KNS2-22-4** at the mMC1R (6-fold), mMC3R (70-fold), and mMC5R (5-fold). This substitution resulted in a partial agonist response at the mMC3R and mMC5R (85% and 65% maximal NDP-MSH signal, respectively), and was the only compound in the series to possess full agonist efficacy at the mMC4R (EC_{50} = 3 μM; Figure 2). The only di-substituted ring examined, (3,4-diCl)DPhe (**KNS2-23-4**), possessed decreased potency at the mMC1R (7-fold), mMC3R (30-fold), and mMC5R (14-fold) compared to **KNS2-22-4**, and did not result in stimulation of the mMC4R at concentrations up to 100 μM. This substitution resulted in micromolar antagonist potency at the mMC4R (pA_2 = 6.2).

Replacing (*p*I)DPhe with (*p*Me)DPhe (**KNS2-23-7**) resulted in similar agonist potencies at the mMC1R and mMC5R compared to **KNS2-22-4**, an 8-fold decreased potency at the mMC3R, and stimulated the mMC4R up to 50% of the maximal NDP-MSH signal (EC_{50} = 700 nM). Substituting a *p*-trifluoromethyl group (**KNS2-23-6**) retained similar potency at the mMC5R compared to **KNS2-22-4**, but decreased potency at the mMC1R and mMC3R (7-fold for both). This substitution resulted in 20% stimulation of the mMC4R (relative to NDP-MSH), with an agonist potency of 600 nM and an antagonist pA_2 value of 6.5. The incorporation of (*p*tBu)DPhe resulted in tetrapeptide **KNS2-23-3**, with decreased potency at the mMC1R (13-fold) compared to **KNS2-22-4**, similar potency at the mMC3R and mMC5R, and produced a partial agonist response (85% relative to NDP-MSH) at the mMC3R. This substitution resulted in minimal agonist activity (<20%) at the mMC4R (Figure 2), but resulted in the second highest antagonist potency observed at the mMC4R (pA_2 = 6.8). When another aromatic ring was extended from the *para*-position (DBip, **KNS2-23-1**), similar potencies at the mMC1R, mMC3R, and mMC5R were observed compared to **KNS2-22-4**, with decreased agonist (1.4 μM) and antagonist (pA_2 = 5.9) potencies at the mMC4R.

The least potent compounds possessed a hydroxyl (**KNS2-23-9**) or nitrile (**KNS2-23-8**) group at the *para*-position. The substitution of DTyr (**KNS2-23-9**) resulted in potencies of 40 nM, 4300 nM, and 1000 nM at the mMC1R, mMC3R, and mMC5R, respectively, and did not possess agonist or antagonist activity at the mMC4R in the concentrations assayed. An 85% partial agonist response was observed at the mMC3R. Similar agonist potencies of 27 nM, 4000 nM, and 500 nM at the mMC1R, mMC3R, and mMC5R were observed for **KNS2-23-8**, with partial efficacy at the mMC3R (75%). At 100 μM concentrations, this ligand was able to partially stimulate the mMC4R (40% of the maximal NDP-MSH signal; Figures 2 and 3) and did not result in antagonist activity (Figure 3).

3. Discussion

Previous results exploring the DPhe *para*-position in the Ac-His-DPhe-Arg-Trp-NH_2 scaffold resulted in full MC4R agonists with different MC3R agonist and antagonist activities [42]. Select substitutions resulted in full MC3R agonist efficacy, while others resulted in partial receptor activation at 100 μM concentrations and micromolar to sub-micromolar antagonist potencies [42]. Thus, a DPhe-Arg motif resulted in full agonism at the MC4R and full to partial agonism at the MC3R accompanied by antagonist activity (dependent on the DPhe *para*-position). Due to the MC3R agonism and MC4R antagonism observed in the Ac-His-Arg-(*p*I)DPhe-Tic-NH_2 ligand [40,41], it was hypothesized that different substitutions at the DPhe *para*-position within this scaffold (possessing an Arg-DPhe motif and a Tic residue in position 4) may modulate MC4R agonist efficacy. The results in Table 3 demonstrate that the efficacy at the mMC4R was modulated by various *para*-substitutions. Full agonism was observed for the ligand Ac-His-Arg-DPhe-Tic-NH_2 (**KNS3-10**) at the mMC4R (Figure 2), and an additional four substitutions resulted in over 50% agonist efficacy at the mMC4R ((*p*Br)DPhe, (*p*Cl)DPhe, (*p*F)DPhe, and (*p*Me)DPhe). Modest agonist efficacy (20–50%) was observed for four ligands (possessing the (*p*I)DPhe, (*p*CF_3)DPhe, DBip, and (*p*CN)DPhe substitutions), and three substitutions ((3,4-diCl)DPhe, (*p*tBu)DPhe, and DTyr) resulted in compounds that did not produce >20% response of the maximal NDP-MSH signal at up to 100 μM concentrations at the mMC4R. A partial agonist response at the mMC3R was also observed for four of the ligands. Thus, the *para*-substitution at the DPhe position within the Ac-His-Arg-(*p*I)DPhe-Tic-NH_2 scaffold modulates agonist efficacy at both the mMC3R and mMC4R, with the Arg-DPhe motif in general resulting in a more efficacious response at the mMC3R.

Several compounds from this study may be useful lead ligands in the development of MC3R/MC4R-selective compounds. One compound (**KNS2-23-9**) possessed micromolar mMC3R agonist potency and did not possess agonist or antagonist activity at the mMC4R. An additional three compounds were at least 100-fold selective agonists for the mMC3R over the mMC4R (**KNS2-23-4**, **KNS2-23-3**, and **KNS2-23-1**), though these three ligands possessed micromolar to sub-micromolar mMC4R antagonist potencies. Further optimization to increase MC3R potency and efficacy, and to minimize MC4R pharmacology, may be required to develop selective MC3R ligands that can elucidate the roles of the MC3R. The use of MC3R KO and MC4R KO mice may also be used with the present ligands to begin to clarify the roles of the different melanocortin receptors in vivo. Alternatively, three compounds (**KNS2-22-4**, **KNS2-23-6**, and **KNS2-23-3**) possessed mMC3R agonist potencies of less than 100 nM and were sub-micromolar potent mMC4R antagonists. Further optimization of this dual pharmacology (increased MC3R agonism with increased MC4R antagonism) might result in novel tool compounds that can characterize the in vivo role of the MC3R and MC4R in the regulation of food intake.

While these substitutions had an effect on efficacy at the mMC3R and mMC4R, all compounds assayed were full agonists at the mMC1R, and only one compound was not a full agonist at the mMC5R (**KNS3-10**, stimulating the mMC5R to 65% of the maximal NDP-MSH response). It therefore appears that the Arg-DPhe position switch may only lead to mMC3R over mMC4R selectivity. Potency trends at the mMC1R and mMC5R were similar to that at the mMC3R. The two compounds that were micromolar potent mMC3R agonists (**KNS2-23-9** and **KNS2-23-8**) were also the least potent mMC1R (40 and 27 nM, respectively) and mMC5R (1000 and 500 nM, respectively) agonists. While no compound was significantly more potent than the Ac-His-DPhe-Arg-Trp-NH_2 ligand at the mMC5R, five ligands resulted in at least a 10-fold potency increase at the mMC1R (**KNS2-22-4**, **KNS2-22-3**, **KNS2-22-1**, **KNS2-23-7**, and **KNS2-23-1**).

Another report investigated the *para*-position within the Ac-His-DPhe-Arg-Trp-NH_2 scaffold for MC1R selectivity [53]. In addition to *p*F, *p*Cl, *p*Br, and *p*CF_3 substitutions, Arg was replaced with a neutral Nle residue due to hypothesized interactions with the Arg and basic residues in the MC3R and MC4R [53]. As a general trend, these substitutions increased binding affinity at the MC1R compared to the other melanocortin receptors, as well as increased agonist selectivity for the MC1R [53]. Intraperitoneal (i.p.) injection of the *p*CF_3 substituted ligand resulted in in vivo pigmentation effects when administered to *Anolis carolinesis* lizards [53]. Our results indicate that switching the Phe-Arg positions and substituting Tic for Trp may also increase MC1R potency. When combined with the Nle substitution at the Arg position, these substitution patterns may result in increased MC1R selectivity and/or potency.

4. Materials and Methods

4.1. Reagents

4-(2′,4′-Dimethoxyphenyl-Fmoc-aminomethyl)phenoxyacetyl-MBHA resin (rink-amide-MBHA (100–200 mesh), 0.66 equivalents/g substitution), 2-(1H-benzotriazol-1-yl)1,1,3,3,-tetramethyluronium hexafluorophosphate (HBTU), and the amino acids Fmoc-His(Trt), Fmoc-Arg(Pbf), Fmoc-DPhe, Fmoc-Trp(Boc), Fmoc-(*p*F)DPhe, and Fmoc-(*p*Cl)DPhe were purchased from Peptides International (Louisville, KY, USA). Fmoc-(*p*Br)DPhe, Fmoc-(3,4-diCl)DPhe, Fmoc-(*p*CN)DPhe, Fmoc-(*p*Me)DPhe, and Fmoc-(*pt*Bu)DPhe were purchased from BACHEM (San Carlos, CA, USA). Fmoc-(*p*I)DPhe was purchased from Alfa Aesar (Tewksbury, MA, USA). Fmoc-(*p*CF_3)DPhe was purchased from Chem Cruz (Dallas, TX, USA). Fmoc-D-4,4′-biphenylalanine (Fmoc-Bip) and Fmoc-1,2,3,4-tetrahydroisoquinoline-3-carboxylic acid (Fmoc-Tic) were purchased from Synth Tech (Albony, OR, USA). Fmoc-DTyr(But) was acquired from Advanced Chemtech (Louisville, KY, USA). Triisopropylsilane (TIS), dimethyl sulfoxide (DMSO), *N*,*N*-diisopropylethylamine (DIEA), 1,2-ethanedithiol (EDT), piperidine, pyridine, and trifluoroacetic acid (TFA) were purchased from Sigma-Aldrich (St. Louis, MO, USA). Acetonitrile (MeCN), *N*,*N*-dimethylformamide (DMF), dichloromethane (DCM), methanol (MeOH), and acetic anhydride were purchased from Fisher Scientific. All reagents were ACS grade or higher and were used without further purification.

4.2. Peptide Synthesis

Peptides were synthesized on a CEM Discover SPS manual microwave synthesizer using standard fluorenyl-9-methyloxycarbonyl (Fmoc) methodology [44,45]. The rink-amide resin was added to a fritted polypropylene reaction vessel (25 mL CEM reaction vessel). The resin was allowed to swell in DCM for 1 h. Deprotection of the Fmoc group consisted of two steps: (1) 20% piperidine in DMF at rt for two minutes, followed by (2) 20% piperidine in DMF using microwave irradiation for 4 min at 75 °C with 30 W. The resin was washed with DMF, and the presence of a free amine was assessed using the ninhydrin [54] or chloranil [55] (for the Tic residue) tests. Coupling reactions were carried out with 3.1 equivalents (eq) of the incoming Fmoc-protected amino acid, 3 eq HBTU, and 5 eq DIEA using microwave irradiation (5 min, 75 °C, 30 W). A lower temperature (50 °C) was utilized for His. For Arg coupling, higher equivalents of Arg (5.1 eq), HBTU (5 eq), and DIEA (7 eq) were used with a longer (10 min) microwave irradiation time. Following resin washing with DMF, the completeness of the coupling reactions was assessed with the ninhydrin or chloranil tests, and amino acids were recoupled if necessary. Following the coupling of the N-terminal His residue, the final Fmoc group was removed and the N-terminal was acetylated with 3:1 acetic anhydride:pyridine for 30 min at rt. Peptides were side-chain deprotected and cleaved from the resin for 2 h using a 91:3:3:3 TFA:thioanisole:TIS:H_2O solution, except for **KNS2-23-9** (Ac-His-Arg-DTyr-Tic-NH_2), which was cleaved in a 91:3:3:3 TFA:EDT:TIS:H_2O solution. After cleavage, peptides were precipitated in ice-cold diethyl ether, and pelleted using a Sorvall Legend XTR centrifuge using a swinging bucket rotor (4000 rpm for 4 min at 4 °C). The peptide was washed with diethyl ether and pelleted at least three times before drying overnight in a desiccator.

The peptides were purified by RP-HPLC on a semipreparative C18 reverse-phase column (Vydac 2181010, 10 × 250 mm) using a Shimadzu UV detector (Shimadzu, Kyoto, Japan). The collected fractions were concentrated on a rotary evaporator and lyophilized. The purified compounds were characterized analytically by RP-HPLC on an analytical C18 reverse-phase column (Vydac 218104; Hichrom, Theale, UK) using two solvent systems—methanol and acetonitrile. Peptides were determined to be greater than 95% pure as assessed by peak area at 214 nm, and the correct average molecular mass was confirmed using ESI/TOF-MS (Bruker, BioTOF II, University of Minnesota Department of Chemistry Mass Spectrometry Laboratory, Minneapolis, MN, USA).

4.3. *AlphaScreen Bioassay*

Peptide ligands were dissolved in DMSO at stock concentrations of 10^{-2} M. To assess the pharmacological activity of the tetrapeptides at the mMC1R, HEK293 cells stably expressing the mMC1R were stimulated with the ligands using the cAMP AlphaScreen assay (PerkinElmer) according to the manufacturer's instruction and as previously described [47,49,56].

Cells were grown at 37 °C with 5% CO_2 in cell media (Dulbecco's Modified Eagle's Medium (DMEM) containing 10% newborn calf serum (NCS) and 1% penicillin-streptomycin) in 10 cm plates to 70–95% confluency. Cells were dislodged with Versene (Gibco) at 37 °C, and 10,000 cells/well were plated in a 384-well plate (Optiplate) with freshly made stimulation buffer (Hank's Balanced Salt Solution (HBSS, 1×), 0.5 mM 3-isobutyl-1-methylxanthine (IBMX), 5 mM HEPES, and 0.1% bovine serum albumin (BSA), pH = 7.4) with 0.5 µg anti-cAMP acceptor beads per well. The cells were stimulated with the addition of 5 µL stimulation buffer containing peptide (a seven-point dose response curve was used starting with peptide concentrations of 10^{-4} to 10^{-7} M, determined by ligand potency) or forskolin (10^{-4} M) and incubated in the dark at rt for 2 h.

Following stimulation, biotinylated cAMP (0.62 µM) and streptavidin-coated donor beads (0.5 µg) were added to the wells in a subdued light environment with 10 µL lysis buffer (0.3% Tween-20, 5 mM HEPES, and 0.1% BSA, pH = 7.4). Plates were incubated for an additional 2 h in the dark. Post incubation, the plates were read by an EnSpire plate reader (PerkinElmer, Waltham, MA, USA).

4.4. *β-Galactosidase Assay*

The peptide ligands were assessed for pharmacological activity at the mMC3R, mMC4R, and mMC5R using a β-galactosidase assay. Briefly, HEK293 cells stably expressing the MC3R, MC4R, or MC5R were plated into a 10 cm dish and grown to 40% confluency. The HEK293 cells were transfected with 4 µg of

CRE/β-galactosidase using the calcium-phosphate method, as previously described [46]. Cells (5000 to 15,000) were plated on collagen-treated Nunclon Delta Surface 96-well plates (Thermo Fisher Scientific) and incubated at 37 °C with 5% CO_2. Plates were stimulated 48 h post-transfection with 100 µL solutions of peptide (a seven-point dose response curve with concentrations between 10^{-4} to 10^{-12} M, depending on potency) or forskolin (10^{-4} M) in assay media (DMEM containing 0.1 mg/mL BSA and 0.1 mM IBMX) for 6 h. The assay media was aspirated and 50 µL of lysis buffer (250 mM Tris-HCl, 0.1% Triton X-100, pH 8.0) was added to each well. Plates were stored at −80 °C for up to two weeks.

Thawed plates were assessed for protein content and assayed for β-galactosidase activity. Relative protein concentration was determined by adding 10 µL of cell lysate to 200 µL of a 1:5 dilution of Bio Rad G250 protein dye in a 96-well plate. Absorbance was measured using a 96-well plate reader (Molecular Devices) at λ = 595 nm. To determine β-galactosidase activity, 40 µL of 0.5% BSA in phosphate buffered saline (PBS) (37 °C) and 150 µL of the β-galactosidase substrate (60 mM Na_2HPO_4, 1 mM $MgCl_2$, 10 mM KCl, 50 mM 2-mercaptoethanol, and 660 µM 2-nitrophenyl β-D-galactosidase) were added to the remaining 40 µL of cell lysate. Plates were incubated at 37 °C and periodically read on the 96-well plate reader until the absorbance at λ = 405 nm reached approximately 1.0 relative absorbance units for the positive controls.

4.5. Data Analysis

The EC_{50} and pA_2 values represent the mean of duplicate replicates performed in at least three independent experiments. The EC_{50} and pA_2 values and their associated standard errors (SEM) were determined by fitting the data to a nonlinear least-squares analysis using the PRISM program (v4.0, GraphPad Inc., San Diego, CA, USA). The ligands were assayed as TFA salt and not corrected for peptide content.

5. Conclusions

The tetrapeptide Ac-His-Arg-(*p*I)DPhe-Tic-NH_2, possessing a switched Arg-DPhe motif and Tic at the fourth position relative to the Ac-His-DPhe-Arg-Trp-NH_2 melanocortin agonist sequence, was characterized to be an MC3R agonist/MC4R antagonist ligand following a mixture-based positional scan to identify MC3R agonist-selective ligands. Previous characterization of the DPhe *para*-position within the Ac-His-DPhe-Arg-Trp-NH_2 scaffold indicated that substitutions influenced MC3R efficacy while maintaining full MC4R agonism. It was therefore hypothesized that different substitutions at the DPhe *para*-position in the Ac-His-Arg-(*p*I)DPhe-Tic-NH_2 scaffold might modulate MC4R efficacy while maintaining MC3R agonism. A range of MC4R efficacies was observed from the library of 12 compounds, including one full agonist and three ligands that possessed no agonist activity at concentrations up to 100 µM. Efficacy at the MC3R was also modulated, though all compounds maintained at least at 75% stimulation of the MC3R relative to NDP-MSH. Thus, the inversion of the Arg and DPhe positions within the melanocortin tetrapeptide sequences appears to result in preferential MC3R agonism over MC4R, a useful design motif for the development of MC3R-selective ligands that may serve as novel probe and lead ligands in the treatment of various disorders of altered energy balance.

Author Contributions: K.N.S. and M.D.E. contributed equally to this manuscript. The research was designed by K.N.S., S.R.D., and C.H.-L. Compounds were synthesized and purified by K.N.S. and M.W. In vitro assays were performed by S.R.D. and K.T.F. Data were analyzed by K.N.S., M.D.E., and C.H.-L. The manuscript was written by M.D.E., with the assistance of K.N.S. and C.H.-L.

Funding: This work was supported by NIH Grants R01DK091906 and R01DK108893, as well as by a 2017 Wallin Neuroscience Discovery Fund Award through the University of Minnesota (C.H.-L.). Mark Ericson was a recipient of an NIH F32 Postdoctoral Fellowship (F32DK108402).

Conflicts of Interest: The authors declare no conflict of interest.

References

1. Chhajlani, V.; Muceniece, R.; Wikberg, J.E. Molecular cloning of a novel human melanocortin receptor. *Biochem. Biophys. Res. Commun.* **1993**, *195*, 866–873. [CrossRef]
2. Chhajlani, V.; Wikberg, J.E. Molecular cloning and expression of the human melanocyte stimulating hormone receptor cDNA. *FEBS Lett.* **1992**, *309*, 417–420. [CrossRef]
3. Mountjoy, K.G.; Robbins, L.S.; Mortrud, M.T.; Cone, R.D. The cloning of a family of genes that encode the melanocortin receptors. *Science* **1992**, *257*, 1248–1251. [CrossRef] [PubMed]
4. Roselli-Rehfuss, L.; Mountjoy, K.G.; Robbins, L.S.; Mortrud, M.T.; Low, M.J.; Tatro, J.B.; Entwistle, M.L.; Simerly, R.B.; Cone, R.D. Identification of a receptor for γ melanotropin and other proopiomelanocortin peptides in the hypothalamus and limbic system. *Proc. Natl. Acad. Sci. USA* **1993**, *90*, 8856–8860. [CrossRef] [PubMed]
5. Gantz, I.; Konda, Y.; Tashiro, T.; Shimoto, Y.; Miwa, H.; Munzert, G.; Watson, S.J.; DelValle, J.; Yamada, T. Molecular cloning of a novel melanocortin receptor. *J. Biol. Chem.* **1993**, *268*, 8246–8250. [PubMed]
6. Gantz, I.; Miwa, H.; Konda, Y.; Shimoto, Y.; Tashiro, T.; Watson, S.J.; DelValle, J.; Yamada, T. Molecular cloning, expression, and gene localization of a fourth melanocortin receptor. *J. Biol. Chem.* **1993**, *268*, 15174–15179. [PubMed]
7. Gantz, I.; Shimoto, Y.; Konda, Y.; Miwa, H.; Dickinson, C.J.; Yamada, T. Molecular cloning, expression, and characterization of a fifth melanocortin receptor. *Biochem. Biophys. Res. Commun.* **1994**, *200*, 1214–1220. [CrossRef] [PubMed]
8. Griffon, N.; Mignon, V.; Facchinetti, P.; Diaz, J.; Schwartz, J.C.; Sokoloff, P. Molecular cloning and characterization of the rat fifth melanocortin receptor. *Biochem. Biophys. Res. Commun.* **1994**, *200*, 1007–1014. [CrossRef]
9. Haynes, R.C. The activation of adrenal phosphorylase by the adreno-corticotropic hormone. *J. Biol. Chem.* **1958**, *233*, 1220–1222. [PubMed]
10. Schioth, H.B.; Chhajlani, V.; Muceniece, R.; Klusa, V.; Wikberg, J.E. Major pharmacological distinction of the ACTH receptor from other melanocortin receptors. *Life Sci.* **1996**, *59*, 797–801. [CrossRef]
11. Butler, A.A.; Kesterson, R.A.; Khong, K.; Cullen, M.J.; Pelleymounter, M.A.; Dekoning, J.; Baetscher, M.; Cone, R.D. A unique metabolic syndrome causes obesity in the melanocortin-3 receptor-deficient mouse. *Endocrinology* **2000**, *141*, 3518–3521. [CrossRef]
12. Chen, A.S.; Marsh, D.J.; Trumbauer, M.E.; Frazier, E.G.; Guan, X.M.; Yu, H.; Rosenblum, C.I.; Vongs, A.; Feng, Y.; Cao, L.H.; et al. Inactivation of the mouse melanocortin-3 receptor results in increased fat mass and reduced lean body mass. *Nat. Genet.* **2000**, *26*, 97–102. [CrossRef]
13. Huszar, D.; Lynch, C.A.; Fairchild-Huntress, V.; Dunmore, J.H.; Fang, Q.; Berkemeier, L.R.; Gu, W.; Kesterson, R.A.; Boston, B.A.; Cone, R.D.; et al. Targeted disruption of the melanocortin-4 receptor results in obesity in mice. *Cell* **1997**, *88*, 131–141. [CrossRef]
14. Fan, W.; Boston, B.A.; Kesterson, R.A.; Hruby, V.J.; Cone, R.D. Role of melanocortinergic neurons in feeding and the agouti obesity syndrome. *Nature* **1997**, *385*, 165–168. [CrossRef] [PubMed]
15. Chen, W.; Kelly, M.A.; Opitz-Araya, X.; Thomas, R.E.; Low, M.J.; Cone, R.D. Exocrine gland dysfunction in MC5-R-deficient mice: Evidence for coordinated regulation of exocrine gland function by melanocortin peptides. *Cell* **1997**, *91*, 789–798. [CrossRef]
16. Nakanishi, S.; Inoue, A.; Kita, T.; Nakamura, M.; Chang, A.C.; Cohen, S.N.; Numa, S. Nucleotide sequence of cloned cDNA for bovine corticotropin-β-lipotropin precursor. *Nature* **1979**, *278*, 423–427. [CrossRef] [PubMed]
17. Eipper, B.A.; Mains, R.E. Structure and biosynthesis of pro-adrenocorticotropin/endorphin and related peptides. *Endocr. Rev.* **1980**, *1*, 1–27. [CrossRef]
18. Smith, A.I.; Funder, J.W. Proopiomelanocortin processing in the pituitary, central nervous system, and peripheral tissues. *Endocr. Rev.* **1988**, *9*, 159–179. [CrossRef]
19. Hruby, V.J.; Wilkes, B.C.; Hadley, M.E.; Al-Obeidi, F.; Sawyer, T.K.; Staples, D.J.; Devaux, A.E.; Dym, O.; Castrucci, A.M.D.; Hintz, M.F.; et al. α-Melanotropin: The minimal active sequence in the frog-skin bioassay. *J. Med. Chem.* **1987**, *30*, 2126–2130. [CrossRef] [PubMed]
20. Castrucci, A.M.; Hadley, M.E.; Sawyer, T.K.; Wilkes, B.C.; Al-Obeidi, F.; Staples, D.J.; de Vaux, A.E.; Dym, O.; Hintz, M.F.; Riehm, J.P.; et al. α-Melanotropin: The minimal active sequence in the lizard skin bioassay. *Gen. Comp. Endocrinol.* **1989**, *73*, 157–163. [CrossRef]

21. Kiefer, L.L.; Veal, J.M.; Mountjoy, K.G.; Wilkinson, W.O. Melanocortin receptor binding determinants in the agouti protein. *Biochemistry* **1998**, *37*, 991–997. [CrossRef]
22. Tota, M.R.; Smith, T.S.; Mao, C.; MacNeil, T.; Mosley, R.T.; Van der Ploeg, L.H.T.; Fong, T.M. Molecular interaction of agouti protein and agouti-related protein with human melanocortin receptors. *Biochemistry* **1999**, *38*, 897–904. [CrossRef]
23. Irani, B.G.; Xiang, Z.M.; Yarandi, H.N.; Holder, J.R.; Moore, M.C.; Bauzo, R.M.; Proneth, B.; Shaw, A.M.; Millard, W.J.; Chambers, J.B.; et al. Implication of the melanocortin-3 receptor in the regulation of food intake. *Eur. J. Pharmacol.* **2011**, *660*, 80–87. [CrossRef]
24. Atalayer, D.; Robertson, K.L.; Haskell-Luevano, C.; Andreasen, A.; Rowland, N.E. Food demand and meal size in mice with single or combined disruption of melanocortin type 3 and 4 receptors. *Am. J. Physiol. Regul. Integr. Comp. Physiol.* **2010**, *298*, R1667–R1674. [CrossRef]
25. Rowland, N.E.; Fakhar, K.J.; Robertson, K.L.; Haskell-Luevano, C. Effect of serotonergic anorectics on food intake and induction of Fos in brain of mice with disruption of melanocortin 3 and/or 4 receptors. *Pharmacol. Biochem. Behav.* **2010**, *97*, 107–111. [CrossRef]
26. Rowland, N.E.; Schaub, J.W.; Robertson, K.L.; Andreasen, A.; Haskell-Luevano, C. Effect of MTII on food intake and brain c-Fos in melanocortin-3, melanocortin-4, and double MC3 and MC4 receptor knockout mice. *Peptides* **2010**, *31*, 2314–2317. [CrossRef]
27. Brown, K.S.; Gentry, R.M.; Rowland, N.E. Central injection in rats of α-melanocyte-stimulating hormone analog: Effects on food intake and brain Fos. *Regul. Pept.* **1998**, *78*, 89–94. [CrossRef]
28. Ebihara, K.; Ogawa, Y.; Katsuura, G.; Numata, Y.; Masuzaki, H.; Satoh, N.; Tamaki, M.; Yoshioka, T.; Hayase, M.; Matsuoka, N.; et al. Involvement of agouti-related protein, an endogenous antagonist of hypothalamic melanocortin receptor, in leptin action. *Diabetes* **1999**, *48*, 2028–2033. [CrossRef]
29. Hinney, A.; Volckmar, A.L.; Knoll, N. Melanocortin-4 receptor in energy homeostasis and obesity pathogenesis. *Prog. Mol. Biol. Transl. Sci.* **2013**, *114*, 147–191.
30. Greenfield, J.R.; Miller, J.W.; Keogh, J.M.; Henning, E.; Satterwhite, J.H.; Cameron, G.S.; Astruc, B.; Mayer, J.P.; Brage, S.; See, T.C.; et al. Modulation of blood pressure by central melanocortinergic pathways. *N. Engl. J. Med.* **2009**, *360*, 44–52. [CrossRef]
31. Dorr, R.T.; Lines, R.; Levine, N.; Brooks, C.; Xiang, L.; Hruby, V.J.; Hadley, M.E. Evaluation of melanotan-II, a superpotent cyclic melanotropic peptide in a pilot phase-I clinical study. *Life Sci.* **1996**, *58*, 1777–1784. [CrossRef]
32. Lansdell, M.I.; Hepworth, D.; Calabrese, A.; Brown, A.D.; Blagg, J.; Burring, D.J.; Wilson, P.; Fradet, D.; Brown, T.B.; Quinton, F.; et al. Discovery of a Selective Small-Molecule Melanocortin-4 Receptor Agonist with Efficacy in a Pilot Study of Sexual Dysfunction in Humans. *J. Med. Chem.* **2010**, *53*, 3183–3197. [CrossRef] [PubMed]
33. Hadley, M.E. Discovery that a melanocortin regulates sexual functions in male and female humans. *Peptides* **2005**, *26*, 1687–1689. [CrossRef]
34. Kuhnen, P.; Clement, K.; Wiegand, S.; Blankenstein, O.; Gottesdiener, K.; Martini, L.L.; Mai, K.; Blume-Peytavi, U.; Gruters, A.; Krude, H. Proopiomelanocortin deficiency treated with a melanocortin-4 receptor agonist. *N. Engl. J. Med.* **2016**, *375*, 240–246. [CrossRef]
35. Clement, K.; Biebermann, H.; Farooqi, I.S.; Van der Ploeg, L.; Wolters, B.; Poitou, C.; Puder, L.; Fiedorek, F.; Gottesdiener, K.; Kleinau, G.; et al. MC4R agonism promotes durable weight loss in patients with leptin receptor deficiency. *Nat. Med.* **2018**, *24*, 551–555. [CrossRef]
36. Ni, X.P.; Butler, A.A.; Cone, R.D.; Humphreys, M.H. Central receptors mediating the cardiovascular actions of melanocyte stimulating hormones. *J. Hypertens.* **2006**, *24*, 2239–2246. [CrossRef]
37. Martin, W.J.; McGowan, E.; Cashen, D.E.; Gantert, L.T.; Drisko, J.E.; Hom, G.J.; Nargund, R.; Sebhat, I.; Howard, A.D.; Van der Ploeg, L.H.T.; et al. Activation of melanocortin MC4 receptors increases erectile activity in rats ex copula. *Eur. J. Pharmacol.* **2002**, *454*, 71–79. [CrossRef]
38. Van der Ploeg, L.H.T.; Martin, W.J.; Howard, A.D.; Nargund, R.P.; Austin, C.P.; Guan, X.M.; Drisko, J.; Cashen, D.; Sebhat, I.; Patchett, A.A.; et al. A role for the melanocortin 4 receptor in sexual function. *Proc. Natl. Acad. Sci. USA* **2002**, *99*, 11381–11386. [CrossRef] [PubMed]
39. Yang, Z.; Tao, Y.X. Mutations in melanocortin-3 receptor gene and human obesity. *Prog. Mol. Biol. Transl. Sci.* **2016**, *140*, 97–129. [PubMed]

40. Doering, S.R.; Freeman, K.T.; Schnell, S.M.; Haslach, E.M.; Dirain, M.; Debevec, G.; Geer, P.; Santos, R.G.; Giulianotti, M.A.; Pinilla, C.; et al. Discovery of mixed pharmacology melanocortin-3 agonists and melanocortin-4 receptor tetrapeptide antagonist compounds (TACOs) based on the sequence Ac-Xaa(1)-Arg-(pI)DPhe-Xaa(4)-NH2. *J. Med. Chem.* **2017**, *60*, 4342–4357. [CrossRef]
41. Fleming, K.A.; Freeman, K.T.; Powers, M.D.; Santos, R.G.; Debevec, G.; Giulianotti, M.A.; Houghten, R.A.; Doering, S.R.; Pinilla, C.; Haskell-Luevano, C. Discovery of polypharmacological melanocortin-3 and -4 receptor probes and identification of a 100-fold selective nM MC3R agonist versus a μM MC4R partial agonist. *J. Med. Chem.* **2019**, *62*, 2738–2749. [CrossRef]
42. Proneth, B.; Pogozheva, I.D.; Portillo, F.P.; Mosberg, H.I.; Haskell-Luevano, C. Melanocortin tetrapeptide Ac-His-DPhe-Arg-Trp-NH(2) modified at the para position of the benzyl side chain (DPhe): Importance for mouse melanocortin-3 receptor agonist versus antagonist activity. *J. Med. Chem.* **2008**, *51*, 5585–5593. [CrossRef] [PubMed]
43. Holder, J.R.; Bauzo, R.M.; Xiang, Z.M.; Haskell-Luevano, C. Structure-activity relationships of the melanocortin tetrapeptide Ac-His-DPhe-Arg-Trp-NH2 at the mouse melanocortin receptors: Part 2 modifications at the Phe position. *J. Med. Chem.* **2002**, *45*, 3073–3081. [CrossRef] [PubMed]
44. Carpino, L.A.; Han, G.Y. 9-Fluorenylmethoxycarbonyl function, a new base-sensitive amino-protecting group. *J. Am. Chem. Soc.* **1970**, *92*, 5748–5749. [CrossRef]
45. Carpino, L.A.; Han, G.Y. The 9-fluorenylmethoxycarbonyl amino-protecting group. *J. Org. Chem.* **1972**, *37*, 3404–3409. [CrossRef]
46. Chen, W.B.; Shields, T.S.; Stork, P.J.S.; Cone, R.D. A colorimetric assay for measuring activation of G_s- and G_q-coupled signaling pathways. *Anal. Biochem.* **1995**, *226*, 349–354. [CrossRef] [PubMed]
47. Ericson, M.D.; Schnell, S.M.; Freeman, K.T.; Haskell-Luevano, C. A fragment of the *Escherichia coli* ClpB heat-shock protein is a micromolar melanocortin 1 receptor agonist. *Bioorg. Med. Chem. Lett.* **2015**, *25*, 5306–5308. [CrossRef] [PubMed]
48. Tala, S.R.; Schnell, S.M.; Haskell-Luevano, C. Microwave-assisted solid-phase synthesis of side-chain to side-chain lactam-bridge cyclic peptides. *Bioorg. Med. Chem. Lett.* **2015**, *25*, 5708–5711. [CrossRef] [PubMed]
49. Singh, A.; Tala, S.R.; Flores, V.; Freeman, K.; Haskell-Luevano, C. Synthesis and pharmacology of α/β^3-peptides based on the melanocortin agonist Ac-His-DPhe-Arg-Trp-NH_2 sequence. *ACS Med. Chem. Lett.* **2015**, *6*, 568–572. [CrossRef]
50. Sawyer, T.K.; Sanfilippo, P.J.; Hruby, V.J.; Engel, M.H.; Heward, C.B.; Burnett, J.B.; Hadley, M.E. 4-Norleucine, 7-D-phenylalanine-α-melanocyte-stimulating hormone—A highly potent α-melanotropin with ultralong biological-activity. *Proc. Natl. Acad. Sci. USA* **1980**, *77*, 5754–5758. [CrossRef]
51. Haskell-Luevano, C.; Holder, J.R.; Monck, E.K.; Bauzo, R.M. Characterization of melanocortin NDP-MSH agonist peptide fragments at the mouse central and peripheral melanocortin receptors. *J. Med. Chem.* **2001**, *44*, 2247–2252. [CrossRef]
52. Schild, H.O. pA, a new scale for the measurement of drug antagonism. *Br. J. Pharmacol. Chemother.* **1947**, *2*, 189–206. [CrossRef]
53. Haghighi, S.M.; Zhou, Y.; Dai, J.X.; Sawyer, J.R.; Hruby, V.J.; Cai, M.Y. Replacement of Arg with Nle and modified D-Phe in the core sequence of MSHs, Ac-His-D-Phe-Arg-Trp-NH_2, leads to hMC1R selectivity and pigmentation. *Eur. J. Med. Chem.* **2018**, *151*, 815–823. [CrossRef]
54. Kaiser, E.; Colescott, R.L.; Bossinger, C.D.; Cook, P.I. Color test for detection of free terminal amino groups in the solid-phase synthesis of peptides. *Anal. Biochem.* **1970**, *34*, 595–598. [CrossRef]
55. Christensen, T. Qualitative test for monitoring coupling completeness in solid-phase peptide-synthesis using chloranil. *Acta Chem. Scand. Ser. B* **1979**, *33*, 763–766. [CrossRef]
56. Lensing, C.J.; Freeman, K.T.; Schnell, S.M.; Adank, D.N.; Speth, R.C.; Haskell-Luevano, C. An in vitro and in vivo investigation of bivalent ligands that display preferential binding and functional activity for different melanocortin receptor homodimers. *J. Med. Chem.* **2016**, *59*, 3112–3128. [CrossRef] [PubMed]

Sample Availability: Samples of the compounds are available from the authors.

molecules

MDPI

Article

Development of Highly Selective 1,2,3-Triazole-containing Peptidic Polo-like Kinase 1 Polo-box Domain-binding Inhibitors

Xue Zhi Zhao *, Kohei Tsuji, David Hymel and Terrence R. Burke Jr. *

Chemical Biology Laboratory, Center for Cancer Research, National Cancer Institute, National Institutes of Health, Frederick, MD 21702, USA; kohei.tsuji@nih.gov (K.T.); hymel.david@gmail.com (D.H.)
* Correspondence: xuezhi.zhao@nih.gov (X.Z.Z.); burkete@nih.gov (T.R.B.J.); Tel.: +1-301-846-5907 (X.Z.Z.); +1-301-846-5906 (T.R.B.J.)

Academic Editors: Henry Mosberg, Tomi Sawyer and Carrie Haskell-Luevano
Received: 29 March 2019; Accepted: 14 April 2019; Published: 16 April 2019

check for updates

Abstract: Members of the polo-like kinase (Plk) family of serine/threonine protein kinases play crucial roles in cell cycle regulation and proliferation. Of the five Plks (Plk1–5), Plk1 is recognized as an anticancer drug target. Plk1 contains multiple structural components that are important for its proper biological function. These include an N-terminal catalytic domain and a C-terminal non-catalytic polo-box domain (PBD). The PBD binds to phosphothreonine (pT) and phosphoserine-containing sequences. Blocking PBD-dependent interactions offers a potential means of down-regulating Plk1 function that is distinct from targeting its ATP-binding site. Previously, we demonstrated by tethering alkylphenyl chains from the $N(\pi)$-position of the His residue in the 5-mer PLHSpT, that we were able to access a hydrophobic "cryptic" binding pocket on the surface of the PBD, and in so doing enhance binding affinities by approximately 1000-fold. More recently, we optimized these PBD-ligand interactions using an oxime ligation-based strategy. Herein, using azide-alkyne cycloaddition reactions, we explore new triazole-containing PBD-binding antagonists. Some of these ligands retain the high PBD-binding affinity of the parent peptide, while showing desirable enhanced selectivity for the PBD of Plk1 relative to the PBDs of Plk2 and Plk3.

Keywords: Plk1; selectivity; polo-box domain; peptide; triazole

1. Introduction

Members of the polo-like kinase (Plk) family play crucial roles in mammalian cell cycle regulation and proliferation [1]. Proper function of Plks 1–4 requires the coordinated phosphorylation of serine and threonine residues by *N*-terminal kinase domains (KDs) as well as engagement of protein-protein interactions (PPIs) with phosphoserine (pS)/phosphothreonine (pT)-containing sequences by means of their *C*-terminal polo-box domains (PBDs) [2]. While Plks 1–3 share significant homology, Plk4 is more distantly related [3,4]. The association of Plk1 over-expression with neoplastic transformation and tumor aggressiveness has defined it as a potentially promising anticancer molecular target [5–8]. To date, issues of collateral cytotoxicity have arisen for Plk1 kinase inhibitors. This is in part due to a lack of selectivity arising from the general homology among kinase catalytic domains. Given the uniqueness of PBDs to the Plk family, targeting PBD-mediated PPIs may allow down-regulation of Plk1 function with greater kinome selectivity than with inhibitors directed at the KD. However, Plk2 and Plk3 have roles in checkpoint-mediated cell-cycle arrest and maintenance of genetic stability, and they may serve as potential tumor suppressors [3,4,9]. Therefore, in developing PBD-binding inhibitors, it is desirable that they are selective for Plk1 versus Plk2 and Plk3. Because of the high homology among the PBDs of Plks 1–3, achieving selectivity for the PBD of Plk1 presents an important and challenging objective [7,8,10–13].

In designing Plk1 PBD-binding inhibitors, we have previously started with the polo-box interacting protein 1 (PBIP1)-derived 5-mer PLHSpT (**1**) (Figure 1) [7,14]. We found that up to 1000-fold enhancement of Plk1 PBD-binding affinity can be achieved by appending alkylphenyl groups from the His *N*(π)-position (as exemplified by **2a**) [15]. A crystal structure of PBD-bound **2a** revealed that the alkylphenyl group is situated within a hydrophobic aromatic box defined by residues Y417, Y421, Y481, L478, F482 and Y485. This may be considered as being "cryptic" in nature, since it is revealed by rotation of the Y481 side chain [15]. We have reached the pocket from parent **1** by a variety of approaches, including tethering alkylphenyl groups from the Pro residue [16], an amino-terminal *N*-alkyl Gly residue [17] and from macrocyclic variants [18,19]. The pocket can also be accessed from more extended peptides, such as the amino-terminal Phe residue of the PBIP1-derived peptide FDPPLHSpTA [20–22].

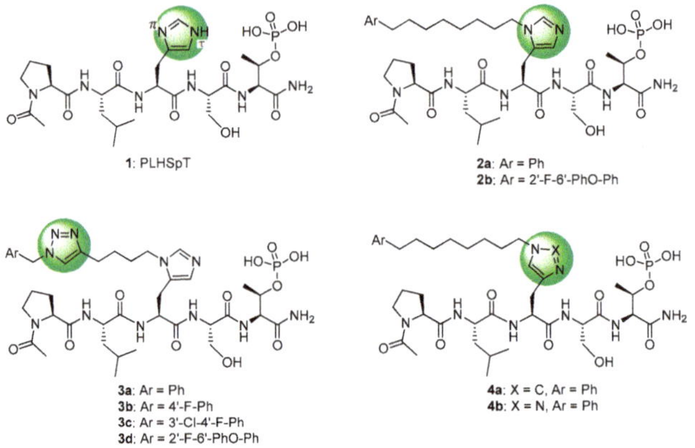

Figure 1. The polo-box interacting protein 1 (PBIP) pT78-derived peptide **1** and related derivatives discussed in the text.

The ability to engage the cryptic pocket has been a critical element of the highest affinity PBD-binding ligands reported to date. Within this context, the pT-2 position arguably represents the most efficient position from which to achieve this access, since it is the most proximal residue to the critical "SpT" recognition motif [23]. By examining a variety of non-proteinogenic amino acid residues at the pT-2 position, we found that the highest affinities were shown by those peptides having alkylation at the His-*N*(π) position, which provided approximately 50-fold higher affinity than alkylation at the isomeric His-*N*(τ)position (peptides **2a** and **4a**, respectively, Figure 1) [24]. Yet, optimizing these interactions has been made difficult due to the tediousness of preparing individual His-*N*(π)-alkyl analogs. In response to these challenges, we employed an oxime-based post-solid phase peptide diversification strategy that allowed us to screen more than 80 analogs. Ligands such as **2b** resulted, which show enhanced Plk1 PBD affinity or selectivity relative to parent **2a** [25,26].

The utility of 1,2,3-triazoles for introducing conformational constraint in peptidomimetic chemistry has been reported [27–35]. A triazole replacement of the imidazole ring in His has been used to prepare constrained His mimics [36]. More recently, triazole-based His mimetics bearing long-chain alkylphenyl groups have been examined within the context of non-peptidic Plk1 PBD inhibitors [37]. However, the best of these constructs showed Plk1 PBD-binding affinities that were 5- to 18-fold less potent than **1** (which itself exhibits 3-orders of magnitude less affinity than **2a**) [37]. Herein, we report the use of on-resin azide-alkyne cycloaddition reactions to introduce 1,2,3-triazole functionality into potent lead Plk1 PBD inhibitors based on **2a** [15] and **2b** [25,26]. The triazole rings were intended either to induce conformational constraint (**3a**–**3d**) or to serve as a His mimetic (**4b**). This work has allowed us to prepare in facile fashion, new ligands that retain the high Plk1 PBD-binding affinity of the parent peptide, while enhancing selectivity for the PBD of Plk1 relative to the PBDs of Plk2 and Plk3.

2. Results and Discussion

2.1. Synthesis

Benzylazides **9a–9d** were prepared using S_N2 reactions of sodium azide with commercially available benzyl bromides **8a–8c** and freshly prepared **8d** (Scheme 1). Bromide **8d** was synthesized in three steps from commercially available 2,6-difluorobenzylaldehyde (**5**). Displacement of one fluoro group in **5** by phenol afforded **6** [25], which was then reduced with sodium borohydride to yield alcohol **7**. Application of the Appel reaction [38] using carbon tetrabromide and triphenylphosphine afforded bromide **8d** (Scheme 1).

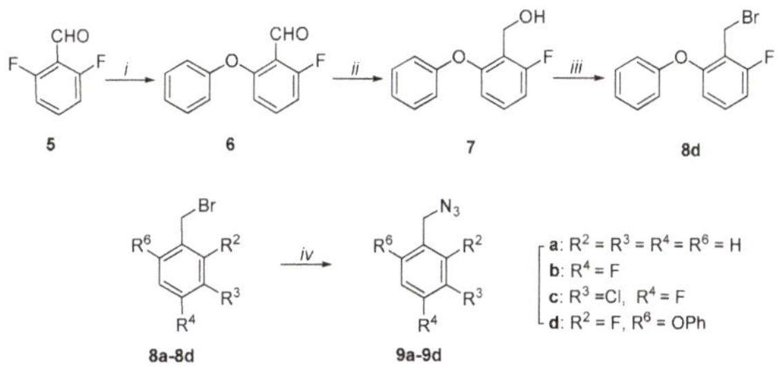

Scheme 1. Preparation of azides **9a–9d**. *Reagents and Conditions: i)* PhOH, K_2CO_3, dimethylacetamide (DMA), 165 °C; *ii)* $NaBH_4$, MeOH; *iii)* CBr_4, PPh_3, CH_3CN; *iv)* NaN_3, acetone:H_2O (5:1).

The protected $N(\pi)$-alkyne-labeled His derivative **11** was easily obtained by alkylating N^{α}-Fmoc-N^{τ}-Trt-L-His 2,4-dimethoxylbenzyl ester (**10**) [25] with hex-5-yn-1-ol according to our previously reported methodology [39]. This was then used to prepare the fully protected alkyne-containing peptide **12** on NovaSyn® TGR resin by standard Fmoc solid-phase peptide synthesis (SPPS) protocols in *N*-methylpyrrolidone (NMP) (Scheme 2). Resin **12** was subsequently subjected to Cu(I) catalyzed [3 + 2] cycloaddition reactions (on-resin CuAAC) with the related benzylazides **9a–9d** (Scheme 2). The regioselective CuAAC reaction has been an important advance that provides a reliable means for selectively assembling 1,4-disubstituted 1,2,3-triazoles [40–42]. The resins were cleaved using a cocktail solution of TFA:H_2O:triisopropylsilane (TIS) (95:2.5:2.5) to provide the triazole-containing peptides **3a–3d** following HPLC purification. Alkyne-labeled peptide **13** was prepared by cleavage of **12** directly.

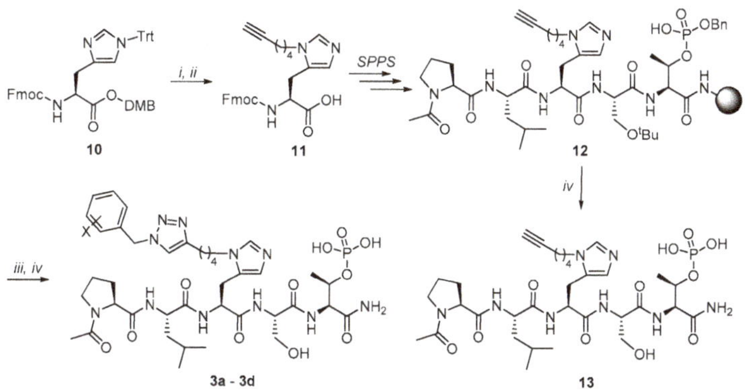

Scheme 2. Preparation of triazole-containing peptides **3a–3d** and alkyne-labeled peptide **13**. *Reagents*

and Conditions: i) CH≡C(CH_2)$_4$OH, trifluoromethanesulfonic anhydride (Tf_2O), *N,N*-diisopropylethylamine (DIEA), dichloromethane (DCM); *ii)* trifluoroacetic acid (TFA), triisopropylsilane (TIS); *iii)* Bn-N_3 (**9a–9d**), CuI, L-ascorbic acid, dimethylformamide (DMF):BuOH:Pyr (3:5:2); *iv)* TFA:H_2O:TIS (95:2.5:2.5).

Preparation of the triazole-based His mimetic containing peptide **4b** and alkyne-labeled peptide **17** are shown in Scheme 3. Protected **15** was prepared on NovaSyn® TGR resin using commercially available Fmoc-L-propargylglycine (**14**) and standard Fmoc SPPS protocols. Cleavage of resin **15** and HPLC purification yielded alkyne-containing peptide **17** directly. Alternatively, an on-resin CuAAC reaction of **15** with phenyloctylazide **16** followed by resin cleavage gave peptide **4b** after HPLC purification (Scheme 3).

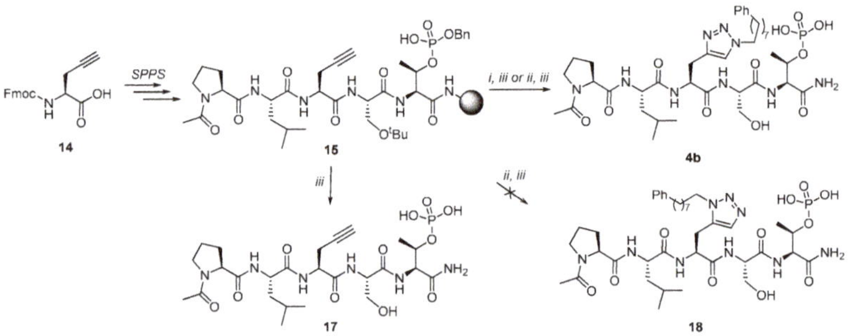

Scheme 3. Preparation of triazole-containing peptides **4b** and alkyne-labeled peptide **17**. *Reagents and Conditions: i)* Ph(CH_2)$_8$$N_3$ (**16**), CuI, L-ascorbic acid, DMF:BuOH:Pyr (3:5:2); *ii)* Cp*RuCl(PPh_3)$_2$, Ph(CH_2)$_8$$N_3$ (**16**), DMF; *iii)* TFA:H_2O:TIS (95:2.5:2.5).

It was our original intent to prepare both 1,4-substituted and 1,5-substituted triazoles as mimetics of the isomeric *N*(τ)- and *N*(π)-alkylated His analogs, respectively. As stated above, the CuAAC reaction provides a reliable means for selectively assembling 1,4-disubstituted 1,2,3-triazoles [40–42]. Accordingly, when we subjected resin-bound alkyne-containing peptide **15** to CuAAC-catalyzed cycloaddition with phenyloctylazide **16**, we obtained a peptide following resin cleavage and HPLC purification, whose structure we assigned as **4b** (Scheme 3). Alternatively, the ruthenium-catalyzed cycloaddition of azides with alkynes (RuAAC) has been reported to regioselectively yield 1,5-disubstituted 1,2,3-triazoles [43,44]. Based on this, we used the on-resin RuAAC-catalyzed [3 + 2] cycloaddition reaction of the alkyne group of resin **15** and azide **16** with the expectation of obtaining the isomeric 1,5-substituted triazole **18** (Scheme 3). However, the resulting peptide was identical in all respects with peptide **4b** (^{1}H-, ^{13}C- and ^{31}P-NMR). At this point, a search of the literature revealed that a simple method has been reported, which permits reliable establishment of triazole regio-substitution based on chemical shifts in one-dimensional ^{13}C-NMR spectra [45]. The C5 signal of 1,4-disubstituted-1*H*-1,2,3-triazoles characteristically appears at approximately $\delta = 120$ ppm, while the C4 signal of 1,5-disubstituted-1*H*-1,2,3-triazoles is usually found at $\delta = 133$ ppm. In our case, the products obtained from both CuAAC and RuAAC chemistries provided a diagnostic signal of $\delta = 123.04$ ppm, indicating that the 1,4-substituted triazole (**4b**) was obtained in both cases.

2.2. Biological Evaluation

We employed fluorescence polarization (FP) assays to evaluate binding affinities against the isolated PBDs of Plk1, Plk2 and Plk3 (Table 1, Figure S1 in Supplementary Material). Compared with the parent peptide **1** (IC_{50} = 650 nM) replacement of the His imidazole ring with an alkyne group resulted in an approximate 2-fold loss of Plk1 PBD-binding affinity (**17**, IC_{50} = 1000 nM, Table 1). Interestingly, peptide **13** (IC_{50} = 1100 nM) showed equivalent Plk1 PBD-binding affinity, in spite of the fact that it included a hex-5-yn-1-yl moiety at the His *N*(π)-position. This group would be expected to partially engage the hydrophobic channel leading to the cryptic pocket. We have previously shown that peptides **2a** and **2b** exhibit binding affinities (IC_{50} values of approximately 15 nM) that are significantly more potent than parent peptide **1** (approximately 650 nM) [25,26]. Peptides **2a** and **2b** show more than 10-fold selectivity for Plk1 relative to Plk2 and approximately 70-fold and 20-fold over Plk3, respectively (Table 1).

Table 1. Inhibitory potencies of peptides containing different linkers using a fluorescence polarization (FP) assay. Polo-like kinase (Plk), polo-box domain (PBD).

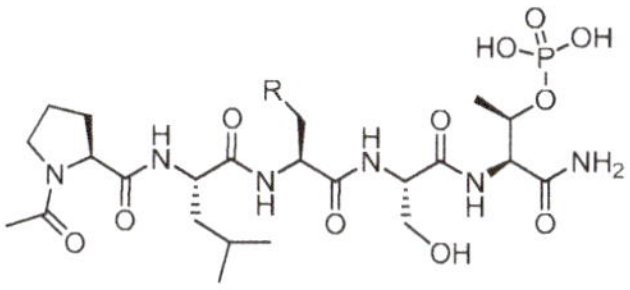

General Structure

Peptide	R	IC_{50} (nM)		
		PLK1 PBD	PLK2 PBD	PLK3 PBD
1 [i]	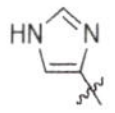	650 ± 39	ND [iv]	ND
17		1000 ± 140	ND	ND
13	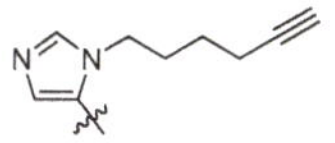	1100 ± 45	ND	ND
2a [ii]	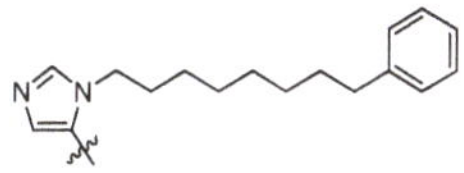	15 ± 0.94	220 ± 15	1100 ± 230
2b [iii]	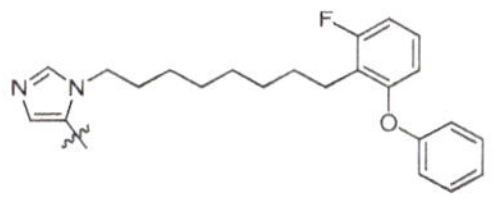	15 ± 0.33	180 ± 14	450 ± 87
3a	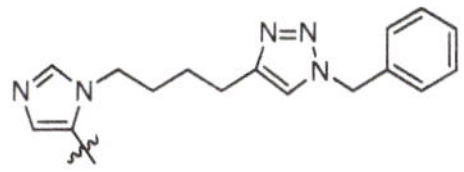	110 ± 6.6	ND	ND
3b	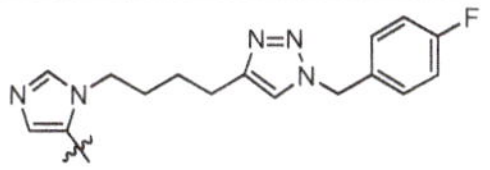	100 ± 19	ND	ND
3c	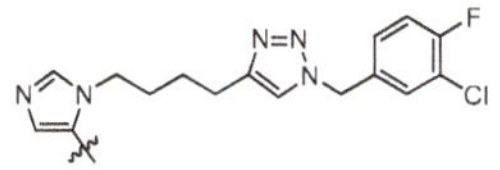	130 ± 9.8	ND	ND
3d	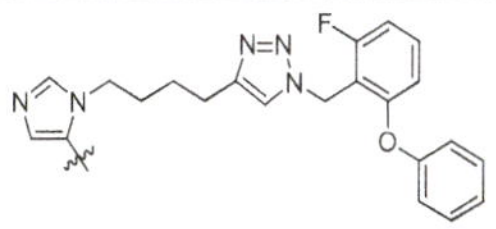	25 ± 1.6	5900 ± 420	9900 ± 2200
4b	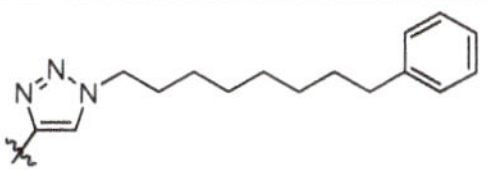	17 ± 0.17	690 ± 20	3400 ± 130

[i] See reference [14]; [ii] See reference [15]; [iii] See references [25,26]; [iv] Not determined.

Peptides **3a–3d** represent a series of analogs having 1,4-substituted triazoles tethered from the His $N(\pi)$-position by $-(CH_2)_4-$ chains. Similar to **2a** and **2b**, this results in a total chain extension of 8-units between the His $N(\pi)$-nitrogen and the terminal aryl group. We had previously shown that this is an optimal length by examining a series of sequentially lengthened tethers [15]. Introducing a 4-fluoro substituent (**3b**, IC_{50} = 100 nM, Table 1) or 3-chloro-4-fluoro substituents (**3c**, IC_{50} = 130 nM, Table 1) were intended to potentially enhance interactions with the hydrophobic cryptic pocket. However, these did not significantly alter affinity relative to **3a**. The reasons for this are not clear. Although peptide **3a** was designed to mimic peptide **2a**, it shows an approximate 8-fold relative loss of Plk1 PBD-binding affinity (**3a**, IC_{50} = 110 nM, Table 1). In contrast to the marked loss of affinity incurred by introducing the triazole ring to **2a**, the triazole-containing mimetic of **2b** showed good retention of Plk1 PBD-binding (**3d**, IC_{50} = 25 nM). While peptides **3a–3c** contain a single tethered phenyl ring, peptide **3d** has a bis-aryl system. The greater extension afforded by this latter arrangement may permit better retention of binding interactions with the cryptic pocket than is afforded by peptides have a single phenyl ring. Importantly, **3d** showed extremely high selectivity for Plk1 relative to Plk2 (IC_{50} = 5900 nM) and Plk3 (IC_{50} = 9900 nM) (Table 1).

In contrast to peptides **3a–3d**, where triazole rings were inserted into His-$N(\pi)$-tethered chains to potentially induce conformational constraint proximal to the cryptic binding pocket, peptide **4b** represents a triazole mimetic of the His imidazole ring. In our previous efforts to access the cryptic pocket using a variety of amino acid derivatives at the pT-2 position, the highest affinities were obtained using His residues, with alkylation at the His-$N(\pi)$ position (**2a**, Figure 1) being significantly preferred to alkylation at the isomeric His-$N(\tau)$ position (**4a**, Figure 1) [24]. In spite of the fact that the 1,4-triazole substitution pattern of **4b** does not appear to optimally replicate the geometry of the His-$N(\pi)$-1,2-imidazole pattern shown by **2a**, its Plk1 binding affinity (IC_{50} = 17 nM) equals that of **2a** (Table 1). The Plk1 PBD selectivity of **4b** is slightly better than **2a** against the Plk2 and Plk3 PBDs (690 nM and 3400 nM, respectively).

It is known that auto-inhibitory interdomain interactions between the KD and PBD can result in decreased potencies in assays that employ full-length Plk1 relative to assays that use isolated PBD preparations, which lack a KD component [23]. The selectivity data shown in Table 1 were obtained using fluorescence polarization assays with isolated PBDs. In contrast, Table 2 shows binding data from an ELISA assay employing full-length Plk1 (Figure S2 in Supplementary Material). Peptides possessing His-$N(\pi)$-tethered chains showed an approximate order-of-magnitude potency reduction in the full-length assay relative to the isolated PBD assay (27-fold and 19-fold reductions for **2a** and **2b**, respectively). However, triazole-containing peptides experienced significantly greater losses of inhibitory potency (160-fold for **4b** and 480-fold for **3d**). The larger differences may indicate a reduced ability of these peptides to effectively relieve auto-inhibition or to engage the PBD cryptic pocket in the full-length construct.

Although there are no crystals structure of full-length Plk1, which might clarify the mechanisms of autoinhibition, a co-crystal structure of Map205-stabilized isolated Plk1 KD and PBD has been solved (PDB accession code: 4J7B) [46]. In this structure the KD is situated on the face of the PBD opposite the phosphopeptide-binding site. In such an orientation, the KD displaces downward an extended loop of the PBD (residues 490–510) from where it is typically observed in isolated PBD crystal structures with bound phosphopeptides. This conformational change prevents the loop from participating in an extensive network of water-mediated hydrogen bonds with the peptide phosphate group. This may be related to the ability of the KD to inhibit ligand binding to the PBD in full-length Plk1. It is unclear from this how access to the cryptic pocket would be adversely impacted in full-length Plk1 or why the triazole-containing peptides would be more sensitive to these effects. However, it is intriguing that this loop originates from the αB helix (residues 470–489), which forms an important component of the cryptic binding pocket.

Table 2. PBD-binding affinities of peptides against full-length Plk1 using an ELISA assay.

Peptide	IC_{50} (nM)
2a [i]	400 ± 32 (27×) [iii]
2b [ii]	290 ± 6.7 (19×)
3d	12000 ± 2100 (480×)
4b	2700 ± 190 (159×)

[i] See reference [15]; [ii] See references [25,26]; [iii] Fold-change relative to isolated PBD value.

3. Experimental Section

3.1. *Synthesis*

3.1.1. General Procedures

As previously reported [26], proton (^{1}H) and carbon (^{13}C) NMR spectra were recorded on a Varian 400 MHz spectrometer or a Varian 500 MHz spectrometer (Varian, Palo Alto, CA, USA) and are reported in ppm relative to tetramethylsilane (TMS) and referenced to the solvent in which the spectra were collected. Solvent was removed by rotary evaporation under reduced pressure and anhydrous solvents were obtained commercially and used without further drying. Purification by silica gel chromatography was performed using Combiflash instruments (Telenyde ISCO, Lincoln, NE, USA) with EtOAc-hexanes or CH_2Cl_2-MeOH solvent systems. Preparative high pressure liquid chromatography (HPLC) was conducted using a Waters Prep LC4000 system (Waters, Milford, MA, USA) having photodiode array detection and C18 columns (catalogue No. 00G4436-P0-AX, 250 mm × 21.2 mm 10 μm particle size, 110 Å pore, Phenomenex, Torrance, CA, USA) at a flow rate of 10 mL/min. Binary solvent systems consisting of A = 0.1% aqueous TFA and B = 0.1% TFA in acetonitrile were employed with gradients as indicated. Products were obtained as amorphous solids following lyophilization. Electrospray ionization-mass spectra (ESI-MS) were acquired with an Agilent LC/MSD system (Agilent, Santa Clara, CA, USA) equipped with a multimode ion source. High resolution mass spectrometric (HRMS, ThermoFisher Scientific, Grand Island, NY, USA) were acquired by LC/MS-ESI with a LTQ-Orbitrap-XL at 30 K resolution.

3.1.2. Synthesis of 2-Fluoro-6-phenoxybenzaldehyde (**6**)

According to the literatures [25,47], to a solution of 2,6-difluorobenzaldehyde (**5**) (11 mL, 102 mmol) and phenol (9.6 g, 102 mmol) in dimethylacetamide (DMA) (50 mL) was added potassium carbonate (14 g, 102 mmol) and the mixture was heated and refluxed (165 °C, 2 h). The mixture was cooled to room temperature, diluted with H_2O (100 mL), extracted with CH_2Cl_2 and the combined organic extract was dried (Na_2SO_4) and concentrated. The resulting residue was purified by silica gel chromatography to afford product **6** as a colorless oil (14.1 g, 64% yield). ^{1}H-NMR (400 MHz, $CDCl_3$) δ 10.52 (s, 1H), 7.47–7.40 (m, 3H), 7.23 (t, *J* = 7.4 Hz, 1H), 7.09 (dd, *J* = 8.6, 1.2 Hz, 2H), 6.89–6.85 (m, 1H), 6.66 (d, *J* = 8.5 Hz, 1H). ^{13}C-NMR (101 MHz, $CDCl_3$) δ 186.79 (1C, d, *J* = 2.3 Hz), 162.90 (1C, d, *J* = 263.4 Hz), 160.50 (1C, d, *J* = 5.2 Hz), 155.63, 135.73 (1C, d, *J* = 11.6 Hz), 130.19 (2C), 124.90, 119.85 (2C), 116.03 (1C, d, *J* = 9.5 Hz), 113.48 (1C, d, *J* = 3.7 Hz), 110.81 (d, *J* = 21.2 Hz). ESI-MS *m*/*z*: 239.0 [M + Na^+].

3.1.3. Synthesis of (2-Fluoro-6-phenoxyphenyl)methanol (**7**)

To a solution of 2-fluoro-6-phenoxybenzaldehyde (**6**) (5.9 g, 27 mmol) in MeOH (100 mL) was added sodium borohydride (1.0 g, 27 mmol) portion-wise at 0 °C and the mixture was stirred (0 °C, 30 min), then concentrated. The resulting residue was partitioned between EtOAc and brine, dried (Na_2SO_4), concentrated and purified by silica gel chromatography to afford product **7** as a colorless oil (5.7 g, 96% yield). ^{1}H-NMR (500 MHz, $CDCl_3$) δ 7.40–7.37 (m, 2H), 7.23–7.16 (m, 2H), 7.06–7.04 (m, 2H), 6.86 (t, *J* = 8.9 Hz, 1H), 6.66 (d, *J* = 8.3 Hz, 1H), 4.85 (s, 2H).^{13}C-NMR (126 MHz, $CDCl_3$) δ

161.70 (1C, d, *J* = 247.3 Hz), 156.95 (1C, d, *J* = 7.4 Hz), 156.62, 129.98 (2C), 129.57 (1C, d, *J* = 10.5 Hz), 124.02, 119.41 (1C, d, *J* = 18.0 Hz), 119.04 (2C), 113.77 (1C, d, *J* = 3.3 Hz), 110.48 (1C, d, *J* = 22.6 Hz), 54.02 (1C, d, *J* = 5.1 Hz).

3.1.4. Synthesis of 2-(Bromomethyl)-1-fluoro-3-phenoxybenzene (**8d**)

According to the literature [38], triphenylphosphine (10 g, 39 mmol) was added to a solution of (2-fluoro-6-phenoxyphenyl)-methanol (**7**) (5.7 g, 26 mmol) in acetonitrile (70 mL) and the suspension was cooled to 0 °C and carbon tetrabromide (13 g, 39 mmol) was added. The suspension turned to a clear brown solution and then to a white suspension after 2 min. The reaction suspension was stirred (room temperature, 30 min), then diluted with EtOAc and the organic phase was concentrated and purified by silica gel chromatography to provide product **8d** as a colorless oil (7.4 g, 99% yield). ^{1}H-NMR (500 MHz, $CDCl_3$) δ 7.43–7.40 (m, 2H), 7.23–7.19 (m, 2H), 7.12–7.09 (m, 2H), 6.86 (t, *J* = 9.2 Hz, 1H), 6.63 (d, *J* = 8.4 Hz, 1H), 4.70 (d, *J* = 1.3 Hz, 2H). ^{13}C-NMR (126 MHz, $CDCl_3$) δ 161.56 (1C, d, *J* = 250.5 Hz), 156.91 (1C, d, *J* = 6.4 Hz), 156.34, 130.16 (1C, d, *J* = 10.5 Hz), 129.98 (2C), 124.30, 119.61 (2C), 117.10 (1C, d, *J* = 17.2 Hz), 113.42 (1C, d, *J* = 3.2 Hz), 110.11 (1C, d, *J* = 21.6 Hz), 20.10 (1C, d, *J* = 5.4 Hz).

3.1.5. General Procedure A for the Synthesis of Azides **9a–9d** and **16**

To a solution of bromides **8a–8d** or commercially available (8-bromooctyl)benzene (7.0 mmol) in acetone (10 mL) and H_2O (2.0 mL) was added sodium azide (1.8 g, 28 mmol) and the mixture was stirred (55 °C, 15 h). The reaction was quenched by the addition of H_2O, extracted with Et_2O and the combined organic phase was washed with brine, dried (Na_2SO_4), concentrated and purified by silica gel chromatography to provide the target azides **9a–9d,** and **16**.

3.1.6. Synthesis of (Azidomethyl)benzene (**9a**)

According to the literature [48], treatment of (bromomethyl)benzene (**8a**) [48] as outlined in general procedure A provided title compound **9a** as a colorless oil (57% yield). ESI-MS *m*/*z*: 106.1 ($MH^+ - N_2$).

3.1.7. Synthesis of 1-(Azidomethyl)-4-fluorobenzene (**9b**)

Treatment of 1-(bromomethyl)-4-fluorobenzene (**8b**) as outlined in general procedure A provided the title compound **9b** as a colorless oil (82% yield). ^{1}H-NMR (500 MHz, $CDCl_3$) δ 7.32 (dd, *J* = 8.4, 5.4 Hz, 2H), 7.10 (t, *J* = 8.6 Hz, 2H), 4.34 (s, 2H). ESI-MS *m*/*z*: 124.1 ($MH^+ - N_2$).

3.1.8. Synthesis of 4-(Azidomethyl)-2-chloro-1-fluorobenzene (**9c**)

Treatment of 4-(bromomethyl)-2-chloro-1-fluorobenzene (**8c**) as outlined in general procedure A provided the title compound **9c** as a colorless oil (49% yield). ^{1}H-NMR (500 MHz, $CDCl_3$) δ 7.40 (dd, *J* = 6.9, 2.1 Hz, 1H), 7.22 (ddd, *J* = 7.0, 4.7, 2.1 Hz, 1H), 7.18 (t, *J* = 8.5 Hz, 1H), 4.34 (s, 2H). ^{13}C-NMR (126 MHz, $CDCl_3$) δ157.94 (d, *J* = 249.9 Hz), 132.53 (d, *J* = 4.0 Hz), 130.37, 127.85 (d, *J* = 7.3 Hz), 121.46 (d, *J* = 18.0 Hz), 116.96 (d, *J* = 21.4 Hz), 53.54. ESI-MS *m*/*z*: 158.1 ($MH^+ - N_2$)

3.1.9. Synthesis of 2-(Azidomethyl)-1-fluoro-3-phenoxybenzene (**9d**)

Treatment of 2-(bromomethyl)-1-fluoro-3-phenoxybenzene (**8d**) as outlined in general procedure A provided the title compound **9d** as a colorless oil (58% yield). ^{1}H-NMR (400 MHz, $CDCl_3$) δ 7.79 (t, *J* = 7.9 Hz, 2H), 7.67–7.63 (m, 1H), 7.61–7.57 (m, 1H), 7.47–7.45 (m, 2H), 7.28 (t, *J* = 8.6 Hz, 1H), 7.05 (d, *J* = 8.4 Hz, 1H), 4.91 (s, 2H). ^{13}C-NMR (101 MHz, $CDCl_3$) δ 162.04 (d, *J* = 248.7 Hz), 157.26 (d, *J* = 7.0 Hz), 156.14, 130.29 (d, *J* = 10.5 Hz), 130.00 (2C), 124.30, 119.47 (2C), 114.17 (d, *J* = 18.2 Hz), 113.12 (d, *J* = 3.3 Hz), 110.09 (d, *J* = 22.2 Hz), 42.55 (d, *J* = 4.0 Hz). ESI-MS *m*/*z*: 216.1 ($MH^+ - N_2$).

3.1.10. Synthesis of (8-Azidooctyl)benzene (**16**)

Treatment of commercially available (8-bromooctyl)benzene as outlined in general procedure A provided the title compound **16** as a colorless oil (68% yield). ^{1}H-NMR (400 MHz, $CDCl_3$) δ 7.32–7.28 (m, 2H), 7.22–7.18 (m, 3H), 3.28 (t, J = 7.0 Hz, 2H), 2.64 (t, J = 7.7 Hz, 2H), 1.66–1.58 (m, 4H), 1.41–1.33 (m, 8H). ^{13}C-NMR (101 MHz, $CDCl_3$) δ 142.82, 128.39 (2C), 128.23 (2C), 125.59, 51.49, 35.96, 31.45, 29.34, 29.19, 29.08, 28.84, 26.71. ESI-MS *m*/*z*: 204.2 ($MH^+ - N_2$).

3.1.11. Synthesis of N^{α}-(((9*H*-Fluoren-9-yl)methoxy)carbonyl)-N^{π}-(hex-5-yn-1-yl)-L-histidine (**11**)

As previously reported [39], to a solution of trifluoromethanesulfonic anhydride (2.8 mL, 2.8 mmol) in CH_2Cl_2 (5.0 mL) was added a solution of hex-5-yn-1-ol (0.31 mL, 2.8 mmol) and *N*-ethyl-*N*-isopropylpropan-2-amine (0.49 mL, 2.8 mmol, 1.0 M in CH_2Cl_2) in CH_2Cl_2 (10 mL) dropwise under argon at −78 °C and the mixture was stirred at −78 °C (20 min). To this was added a solution of (*S*)-2,4-dimethoxybenzyl 2-((((9*H*-fluoren-9-yl)methoxy)carbonyl)amino)-3-(1-trityl-1*H*-imidazol-4-yl)propanoate (**10**) [24] (2.0 g, 2.5 mmol) in CH_2Cl_2 (5.0 mL) at −78 °C and the mixture was allowed to come to room temperature and stirred (overnight). The solvent was removed by evaporation and a solution of TFA:TIS (10:1, 10 mL) was added and the mixture was stirred at room temperature (2 h). The reaction mixture was concentrated and the resulting residue was purified by silica gel chromatography to provide the title compound **11** as a colorless sticky oil (0.53 g, 46% yield). ESI-MS *m*/*z*: 458.2 (MH^+).

3.2. *Peptide Synthesis*

3.2.1. General Solid-Phase Peptide Synthesis (SPPS)

As previously reported [26], the protected amino acids used were Fmoc-L-Thr(PO(OBzl)OH)-OH, Fmoc-L-Ser(O^{t}Bu)-OH, Fmoc-L-Leu-OH, and Fmoc-L-Pro-OH (purchased from Novabiochem, MilliporeSigma, Burlington, MA, USA). Peptides were synthesized on a NovaSyn® TGR resin (Novabiochem Cat#. 855009) using standard Fmoc SPPS protocols in *N*-methyl-2-pyrrolidone (NMP). Coupling reagents used were 1-[bis(dimethylamino)methylene]-1*H*-1,2,3-triazolo[4,5-b]pyridinium 3-oxid hexafluorophosphate (HATU) (5.0 equivalents) and *N*,*N*-diisopropylethylamine (DIPEA) (10 equivalents). Non-coded amino acid residues were coupled using 2.5 equivalents amino acids. Deprotection was performed using 20% piperidine in DMF (15 min, twice). Amino-terminal acetylation was performed using 1-acetylimidazole. Finished resins were washed with NMP, MeOH, CH_2Cl_2, and Et_2O, dried under vacuum and cleaved by treatment with a solution of TFA:H_2O:TIS (95:2.5:2.5) (5 h). The resin was removed by filtration, and the filtrate was concentrated under vacuum and the resulting residue was dissolved in 50% aqueous acetonitrile (5 mL) and purified by reverse-phase HPLC as outline above in General Synthetic Procedures.

3.2.2. Synthesis of Peptides **3a–3d** and **4b** Using On-resin Copper-catalyzed Alkyne-azide Cycloaddition Reaction (CuAAC)

By sequential coupling, Fmoc-Thr(PO(OBzl)OH)-OH, Fmoc-Ser(O^{t}Bu)-OH, alkynyl-labelled *N(π)*-alkylated Fmoc-His-OH (**11**) or Fmoc-L-propargylglycine (**14**), Fmoc-Leu-OH, and Fmoc-Pro-OH were loaded onto NovaSyn® TGR resin using the general SPPS protocols outlined above. The pre-loaded resin (**12** or **15**, 0.02 mmol) was mixed with a solution of azides (**9a–9d** or **16**) (0.14 mmol), copper(I) iodide (0.26 mmol), DIEA (0.34 mmol) and L-ascorbic acid (0.14 mmol) in BuOH:DMF:pyridine (5:3:2, 1.5 mL) and the mixture was stirred (17 h). The resin was washed with NMP, MeOH, CH_2Cl_2, and Et_2O, dried under vacuum and then cleaved by treatment with a solution of TFA:H_2O:TIS (95:2.5:2.5) (5 h). The resin was removed by filtration and the filtrate was concentrated under vacuum and the resulting residue was subjected to preparative HPLC purification.

3.2.3. Synthesis of Peptide **4b** Using On-resin Ruthenium-catalyzed Alkyne-azide Cycloaddition Reaction (RuAAC)

According to literature [36,49], pre-loaded alkyne-labeled NovaSyn® TGR resin **15** (0.049 mmol) was mixed with Cp*RuCl(PPh_3)$_2$ [pentamethylcyclopentadienylbis(triphenylphosphine) ruthenium (II) chloride] (0.049 mmol) in DMF (1.0 mL) at room temperature (1 h). A solution of (8-azidooctyl)benzene (**16**) (56 mg, 0.24 mmol) in DMF (1.0 mL) was added and the mixture was stirred at room temperature (24 h). The resulting dark brown resin was washed with NMP, MeOH, CH_2Cl_2, and Et_2O, dried under vacuum and cleaved by treatment with a solution of TFA:H_2O:TIS (95:2.5:2.5) (5 h). The resin was removed by filtration and the filtrate was concentrated under vacuum and the resulting residue was purified by preparative HPLC.

3.2.4. Peptide Data

Peptide **3a**. Linear gradient of 0% B to 80% B over 30 min, retention time = 16.0 min. ESI-MS *m/z*: 888.4 (MH^+). HRMS calcd $C_{39}H_{59}N_{11}O_{11}P(MH^+)$, 888.4128; found, 888.4139.

Peptide **3b**. Linear gradient of 0% B to 80% B over 30 min, retention time = 16.4 min. ESI-MS *m/z*: 906.4 (MH^+). HRMS calcd $C_{39}H_{58}FN_{11}O_{11}P$ (MH^+), 906.4033; found, 906.4045.

Peptide **3c**. Linear gradient of 0% B to 80% B over 30 min, retention time = 17.0 min. ESI-MS *m/z*: 940.3 (MH^+). HRMS calcd $C_{39}H_{57}ClFN_{11}O_{11}P$ (MH^+), 940.3644; found, 940.3650.

Peptide **3d**. Linear gradient of 0% B to 80% B over 30 min, retention time = 17.8 min. ESI-MS *m/z*: 998.2 (MH^+). HRMS calcd $C_{45}H_{62}FN_{11}O_{12}P(MH^+)$, 998.4296; found, 998.4311.

Peptide **4b**. Linear gradient of 0% B to 80% B over 30 min, retention time = 22.6 min. ESI-MS *m/z*: 864.4 (MH^+). HRMS calcd $C_{39}H_{63}N_9O_{11}P$ (MH^+): 864.4379; found, 864.4365.

Peptide **13**. Linear gradient of 0% B to 80% B over 30 min, retention time = 14.8 min. ESI-MS *m/z*: 755.3 (MH^+). HRMS calcd $C_{32}H_{52}N_8O_{11}P$ (MH^+): 755.3488; found, 755.3497.

Peptide **17**. Linear gradient of 0% B to 80% B over 30 min, retention time = 15.0 min. ESI-MS *m/z*: 633.2 (MH^+). HRMS calcd $C_{25}H_{42}N_6O_{11}P$ (MH^+), 633.2644; found, 633.2625.

3.3. Determination of Binding Selectivity against the PBDs of Plks 1–3 Using Fluorescence Polarization

3.3.1. Expression and Purification of Isolated PBDs of Plks 1–3 for Fluorescence Polarization Assays

As previously reported [25,26,50], a plasmid encoding myc-tagged Plk1 PBD was purchased from Addgene (Plasmid #41162, Watertown, MA, USA) [51]. Plasmids encoding the myc-tagged PBDs of Plk2 and Plk3 were generous gifts from Prof. Erich Nigg (Univ. of Basel, Basel, Switzerland) [51]. ~20 M HEK (human embryonic kidney)-293T cells (2 × 15 cm plates) were transfected with each plasmid using TurboFect reagent. Following 24 h expression, cells were harvested, lysed in buffer [phosphate buffered saline (PBS, pH 7.4) containing 0.5% NP-40 and protease/phosphatase inhibitor cocktail] using freeze/thaw cycles (3×) and centrifuged at 12,500× *g* for 10 min at 4 °C. The supernatant containing expressed protein was diluted into 8 mL of PBS (pH 7.4) containing protease/phosphatase inhibitor cocktail. This protein solution was added to a 1 mL bed of myc-agarose resin (Thermo Scientific, Waltham, MA, USA) and allowed to bind for 2 h at 4 °C with gentle rotation. The lysate was eluted and the resin was washed 4× with 4-(2-hydroxyethyl)-1-piperazineethanesulfonic acid (HEPES) buffered saline (HBS) containing 0.05% Tween-20, 1 mM dithiothreitol (DTT) and 1 mM ethylenediaminetetraacetic acid (EDTA). The bound PBD protein was then eluted with a 1 mg/mL solution of myc peptide (EQKLISEEDL) in HBS + 1 mM DTT and 1 mM EDTA. The purified PBD protein was dialyzed 5× with HBS + 1 mM DTT and 1 mM EDTA using a 10 kDa molecular weight cut-off (MWCO) filter (Sigma-Aldrich, St. Louis, MO, USA) fixed angle rotor at 7500× *g*, 4 °C, 10 min). The concentration of the final protein solution was determined by absorbance at 280 nm and purity was determined by SDS-PAGE (sodium dodecyl sulfate-polyacrylamide gel electrophoresis) with Coomassie staining.

3.3.2. Evaluation of Binding Affinities against the Isolated PBDs of Plk1, Plk2 and Plk3 Using Fluorescence Polarization Assays

As previously reported [25,26,50], isolated PBD protein was diluted to a 2× working dilution in assay buffer (HEPES-buffered saline with 0.05% Tween-20, 1 mM DTT, and 1 mM EDTA). The following final protein concentrations used were: 80 nM for Plk1 PBD; 80 nM for Plk2 PBD and 130 nM for Plk3 PBD. These concentrations represent the approximate K_d values determined for the respective fluorescence polarization probe sequences. Inhibitors were serially diluted to generate 4× working dilutions in assay buffer containing 4% DMSO. 20 μL of 2× PBD solution was added to each well of a 384-well plate (0% binding controls received 20 μL of assay buffer). 10 μL of the 4× inhibitor solution (or DMSO blank) was added to corresponding wells and allowed to pre-incubate at RT for 30 min with shaking. The following sequences were utilized as fluorescent probes: 5CF-GPMQSpTPLNG-NH_2 for Plk1 PBD; 5CF-GPMQTSpTPKNG-NH_2 for Plk2 PBD and 5CF-PLATSpTPKNG-NH_2 for Plk3 PBD [10]. Fluorescent probes were diluted to 40 nM (4×) in assay buffer and then 10 μL was added to each well. The plate was allowed to equilibrate at room temperature for (30 min) with shaking. The FP was read using a BioTek Synergy 2 plate reader (BioTek, Winooski, VT, USA) with 485/20 excitation and 528/20 emission. The FP values were obtained in triplicate and normalized to 100% (no inhibitor) and 0% binding (no protein) controls. Normalized values were plotted versus concentration and analyzed using non-linear regression in GraphPad Prism 8 (GraphPad Software, San Diego, CA, USA) [log(inhibitor) vs. response-variable slope (four parameter) model]. IC_{50} values are presented in Table 1 and represent average ± standard error of the mean (SEM).

3.4. Evaluation of Binding Affinities against Full-length Plk1 Using ELISA Assays

3.4.1. Lysate Production for ELISA-based Inhibition Assay against Full Length Plk1

Assays were conducted as previously reported [25,26,50]. To summarize, a plasmid encoding myc-tagged full-length Plk1 (Addgene, Plasmid #41160) [52] was transiently transfected into HEK (human embryonic kidney)-293T cells using the TurboFect reagent (Thermo Scientific, Waltham, MA, USA) according to manufacturer's instructions. Following 48 h expression, cells were harvested, lysed in buffer (PBS, pH 7.4 with 0.5% NP-40 and protease/phosphatase inhibitor cocktail) using freeze/thaw cycles (3×) and centrifuged at 10,000× *g* for 10 min at 4 °C. The supernatant was removed to provide a crude cytosolic lysate containing overexpressed, myc-tagged Plk1 (total protein concentration determined by bicinchoninic acid (BCA) assay).

3.4.2. Determination of Inhibitory Potency in an ELISA Assay Using Full-Length Plk1

As previously reported [25,26,50] a biotinylated phosphopeptide (sequence: Biotin-Ahx-PMQS(pT)PLN-NH_2) was diluted to 1 μM (from a 2 mM DMSO stock solution) in PBS (pH 7.4) and loaded onto the wells of a 96-well Neutravidin-coated plate (Pierce Biotechnology, ThermoFisher Scientific, Waltham, MA, USA) at 100 μL per well for 1 h (background control contained no biotinylated peptide). The wells were washed once with 150 μL PBST (PBS, pH 7.4 + 0.05% Tween-20), and then 100 μL of 1% BSA in PBS (pH 7.4) (blocking buffer) was added for 1 h. A cytosolic lysate-containing transiently expressed myc-tagged Plk1 protein was diluted to 300 μg/mL in PBS (pH 7.4) containing protease/phosphatase inhibitors (Pierce Biotechnology), mixed with competitive inhibitor (from a 10× stock in ~4% DMSO/PBS), and allowed to pre-incubate for 1 h (100 μL per well in a 96-well plate, 30 μg total protein). The blocked ELISA plate was washed 2× with PBST (PBS, pH 7.4 + 0.05% Tween-20) (150 μL) and the pre-incubated lysates were added to the plate and incubated (1 h). The wells were washed 4× with PBST (150 μL) and then treated with anti-myc primary antibody (1:1500 dilution in PBS, mouse monoclonal, Pierce Biotechnology) for 1 h. The wells were then washed 4×

with PBST (150 μL), and incubated with rabbit anti-mouse horseradish peroxidase (HRP) conjugate [1:3000 dilution in 1% (%*w*/*v*) BSA in PBS, Pierce Biotechnology] for 1 h. The wells were then washed 5× with PBST (150 μL) and incubated with Turbo TMB (3,3′,5,5′-tetramethyl benzidine substrate)-ELISA solution (Pierce Biotechnology) until the desired absorbance was reached (5–10 min). The reaction was quenched by the addition of 2 N aqueous H_2SO_4 and the absorbance was measured at 450 nm using a BioTek Synergy 2 96-well plate reader. Absorbance was plotted versus concentration (logM) and fit to a non-linear regression analysis using GraphPad Prism 8 software [model: log(inhibitor) vs. response-variable slope (four parameters)]. The calculated IC_{50} values presented in Table 2 are from multiple independent experiments and were normalized and averaged to provide values ± SEM.

4. Conclusions

Presented herein are the design of the triazole-containing conformationally constrained peptides **3a**–**3d** and the His mimic-containing peptide **4b** as well as their facile preparation using on-resin azide-alkyne cycloaddition reactions. The resulting peptides were evaluated in FP binding assays using isolated PBDs of Plk1, Plk2 and Plk3 and in ELISA assays against full-length Plk1. Certain of these new ligands retain the high Plk1 PBD-binding affinity of the parent peptide **2a**, while having enhanced selectivity for the PBD of Plk1 relative to the PBDs of Plk2 and Plk3. It is interesting that peptides **4b** and **3d** show significantly greater than anticipated reduced affinities in full-length Plk1 ELISA assays relative to values obtained with the isolated PBD (160-fold for **4b** and 480-fold for **3d**). The larger differences may indicate a reduced ability of these triazole-containing peptides to effectively relieve auto-inhibition arising from interdomain interactions between the KD and PBD or to engage the PBD cryptic pocket in the full-length construct. These observations are noteworthy, in that they potentially indicate structural interactions of the KD and PBD in full-length Plk1 that are not anticipated by the previous co-crystal structure of isolated KD and PBD in the presence of Map205.

Supplementary Materials: Supplementary material associated with this article is available online. Figures S1 and S2 reporting FP binding data against the isolated PBDs of Plk1, Plk2 and Plk3 and ELISA binding assays against full-length Plk1.

Author Contributions: X.Z.Z. designed and synthesized the peptides. K.T. and D.H. performed the biological evaluation. X.Z.Z., K.T., D.H. and T.R.B.Jr. interpreted the data and wrote the paper. All authors have approved the final manuscript.

Funding: This work was supported by the Intramural Research Program of the NIH, Center for Cancer Research, National Cancer Institute, National Institutes of Health. This work was supported in part by a JSPS Research Fellowship for Japanese Biomedical and Behavioral Researchers at NIH.

Acknowledgments: We thank Joseph Barchi (Chemical Biology Laboratory, NCI, NIH) for helpful discussion concerning NMR and James A. Kelley and Christopher C. Lai (Chemical Biology Laboratory, NCI, NIH) for HRMS data.

Conflicts of Interest: The authors declare no conflict of interest.

References

1. Zitouni, S.; Nabais, C.; Jana, S.C.; Guerrero, A.; Bettencourt-Dias, M. Polo-like kinases: Structural variations lead to multiple functions. *Nat. Rev. Mol. Cell Biol.* **2014**, *15*, 433–452. [CrossRef] [PubMed]
2. Park, J.-E.; Erikson, R.L.; Lee, K.S. Feed-forward mechanism of converting biochemical cooperativity to mitotic processes at the kinetochore plate. *Proc. Natl. Acad. Sci. USA* **2011**, *108*, 8200–8205. [CrossRef] [PubMed]
3. Lowery, D.M.; Lim, D.; Yaffe, M.B. Structure and function of polo-like kinases. *Oncogene* **2005**, *24*, 248–259. [CrossRef] [PubMed]
4. Strebhardt, K.; Ullrich, A. Targeting polo-like kinase 1 for cancer therapy. *Nat. Rev. Cancer* **2006**, *6*, 321–330. [CrossRef]
5. Park, J.-E.; Soung, N.-K.; Johmura, Y.; Kang, Y.H.; Liao, C.; Lee, K.H.; Park, C.H.; Nicklaus, M.C.; Lee, K.S. Polo-box domain: A versatile mediator of polo-like kinase function. *Cell. Mol. Life Sci.* **2010**, *67*, 1957–1970. [CrossRef]

6. Strebhardt, K. Multifaceted polo-like kinases: Drug targets and antitargets for cancer therapy. *Nat. Rev. Drug Discov.* **2010**, *9*, 643–660. [CrossRef]
7. Lee, K.S.; Burke, T.R., Jr.; Park, J.-E.; Bang, J.K.; Lee, E. Recent advances and new strategies in targeting Plk1 for anticancer therapy. *Trends Pharmacol. Sci.* **2015**, *36*, 858–877. [CrossRef]
8. Archambault, V.; Lepine, G.; Kachaner, D. Understanding the polo kinase machine. *Oncogene* **2015**, *34*, 4799–4807. [CrossRef]
9. Jang, Y.-J.; Lin, C.-Y.; Ma, S.; Erikson, R.L. Functional studies on the role of the C-terminal domain of mammalian polo-like kinase. *Proc. Nat. Acad. Sci. USA* **2002**, *99*, 1984–1989. [CrossRef]
10. Reindl, W.; Yuan, J.; Kraemer, A.; Strebhardt, K.; Berg, T. Inhibition of polo-like kinase 1 by blocking polo-box domain-dependent protein-protein interactions. *Chem. Biol.* **2008**, *15*, 459–466. [CrossRef]
11. Reindl, W.; Graeber, M.; Strebhardt, K.; Berg, T. Development of high-throughput assays based on fluorescence polarization for inhibitors of the polo-box domains of polo-like kinases 2 and 3. *Anal. Biochem.* **2009**, *395*, 189–194. [CrossRef]
12. Gjertsen, B.T.; Schoffski, P. Discovery and development of the polo-like kinase inhibitor volasertib in cancer therapy. *Leukemia* **2015**, *29*, 11–19. [CrossRef]
13. Berg, A.; Berg, T. Inhibitors of the polo-box domain of polo-like kinase 1. *ChemBioChem* **2016**, *17*, 650–656. [CrossRef]
14. Yun, S.-M.; Moulaei, T.; Lim, D.; Bang, J.K.; Park, J.-E.; Shenoy, S.R.; Liu, F.; Kang, Y.H.; Liao, C.; Soung, N.-K.; et al. Structural and functional analyses of minimal phosphopeptides targeting the polo-box domain of polo-like kinase 1. *Nat. Struct. Mol. Biol.* **2009**, *16*, 876–882. [CrossRef]
15. Liu, F.; Park, J.-E.; Qian, W.-J.; Lim, D.; Graber, M.; Berg, T.; Yaffe, M.B.; Lee, K.S.; Burke, T.R., Jr. Serendipitous alkylation of a Plk1 ligand uncovers a new binding channel. *Nat. Chem. Biol.* **2011**, *7*, 595–601. [CrossRef]
16. Liu, F.; Park, J.-E.; Qian, W.-J.; Lim, D.; Scharow, A.; Berg, T.; Yaffe, M.B.; Lee, K.S.; Burke, T.R., Jr. Identification of high affinity polo-like kinase 1 (Plk1) polo-box domain binding peptides using oxime-based diversification. *ACS Chem. Biol.* **2012**, *7*, 805–810. [CrossRef]
17. Liu, F.; Park, J.-E.; Qian, W.-J.; Lim, D.; Scharow, A.; Berg, T.; Yaffe, M.B.; Lee, K.S.; Burke, T.R., Jr. Peptoid-peptide hybrid ligands targeting the polo box domain of polo-like kinase 1. *ChemBioChem* **2012**, *13*, 1291–1296. [CrossRef]
18. Qian, W.-J.; Park, J.-E.; Grant, R.; Lai, C.C.; Kelley, J.A.; Yaffe, M.B.; Lee, K.S.; Burke, T.R., Jr. Neighbor-directed histidine N(τ)–alkylation: A route to imidazolium-containing phosphopeptide macrocycles. *Pept. Sci.* **2015**, *104*, 663–673. [CrossRef]
19. Hymel, D.; Grant, R.A.; Tsuji, K.; Yaffe, M.B.; Burke, T.R., Jr. Histidine N(τ)-cyclized macrocycles as a new genre of polo-like kinase 1 polo-box domain-binding inhibitors. *Bioorg. Med. Chem. Lett.* **2018**, *28*, 3202–3205. [CrossRef]
20. Sledz, P.; Stubbs, C.J.; Lang, S.; Yang, Y.-Q.; McKenzie, G.J.; Venkitaraman, A.R.; Hyvoenen, M.; Abell, C. From crystal packing to molecular recognition: Prediction and discovery of a binding site on the surface of polo-like kinase 1. *Angew. Chem. Int. Ed. Engl.* **2011**, *50*, 4003–4006. [CrossRef]
21. Tan, Y.S.; Śledź, P.; Lang, S.; Stubbs, C.J.; Spring, D.R.; Abell, C.; Best, R.B. Using ligand-mapping simulations to design a ligand selectively trgeting a cryptic surface pocket of polo-like kinase 1. *Angew. Chem. Int. Ed. Engl.* **2012**, *51*, 10078–10081. [CrossRef]
22. Śledź, P.; Lang, S.; Stubbs, C.J.; Abell, C. High-throughput interrogation of ligand binding mode using a fluorescence-based assay. *Angew. Chem. Int. Ed. Engl.* **2012**, *51*, 7680–7683. [CrossRef]
23. Elia, A.E.; Rellos, P.; Haire, L.F.; Chao, J.W.; Ivins, F.J.; Hoepker, K.; Mohammad, D.; Cantley, L.C.; Smerdon, S.J.; Yaffe, M.B. The molecular basis for phosphodependent substrate targeting and regulation of Plks by the polo-box domain. *Cell* **2003**, *115*, 83–95. [CrossRef]
24. Qian, W.-J.; Park, J.-E.; Lee, K.S.; Burke, T.R., Jr. Non-proteinogenic amino acids in the pThr-2 position of a pentamer peptide that confer high binding affinity for the polo box domain (PBD) of polo-like kinase 1 (Plk1). *Bioorg. Med. Chem. Lett.* **2012**, *22*, 7306–7308. [CrossRef]
25. Zhao, X.Z.; Hymel, D.; Burke, T.R., Jr. Application of oxime-diversification to optimize ligand interactions within a cryptic pocket of the polo-like kinase 1 polo-box domain. *Bioorg. Med. Chem. Lett.* **2016**, *26*, 5009–5012. [CrossRef]
26. Zhao, X.Z.; Hymel, D.; Burke, T.R., Jr. Enhancing polo-like kinase 1 selectivity of polo-box domain-binding peptides. *Bioorg. Med. Chem.* **2017**, *25*, 5041–5049. [CrossRef]

27. Angell, Y.L.; Burgess, K. Peptidomimetics via copper-catalyzed azide-alkyne cycloadditions. *Chem. Soc. Rev.* **2007**, *36*, 1674–1689. [CrossRef]
28. Yoo, B.; Shin, S.B.Y.; Huang, M.L.; Kirshenbaum, K. Peptoid macrocycles: Making the rounds with peptidomimetic oligomers. *Chem. Eur. J.* **2010**, *16*, 5528–5537. [CrossRef]
29. Kappe, C.O.; Van der Eycken, E. Click chemistry under non-classical reaction conditions. *Chem. Soc. Rev.* **2010**, *39*, 1280–1290. [CrossRef]
30. Pedersen, D.S.; Abell, A. 1,2,3-Triazoles in peptidomimetic chemistry. *Eur. J. Org. Chem.* **2011**, *13*, 2399–2411. [CrossRef]
31. Ahmad Fuaad, A.A.; Azmi, F.; Skwarczynski, M.; Toth, I. Peptide conjugation via CuAAC 'click' chemistry. *Molecules* **2013**, *18*, 13148–13174. [CrossRef]
32. Das, R.; Majumdar, N.; Lahiri, A. A review on 1,3-dipolar cycloaddition reactions in bioconjugation and it's importance in pharmaceutical chemistry. *Int. J. Res. Pharm. Chem.* **2014**, *4*, 467–472. [CrossRef]
33. Fehlhammer, W.P.; Beck, W. Azide chemistry—An inorganic perspective, part II [3+2]-cycloaddition reactions of metal azides and related systems. *Z. Anorg. Allg. Chem.* **2015**, *641*, 1599–1678. [CrossRef]
34. Johansson, J.R.; Beke-Somfai, T.; Said Stålsmeden, A.; Kann, N. Ruthenium-catalyzed azide alkyne cycloaddition reaction: Scope, mechanism, and applications. *Chem. Rev.* **2016**, *116*, 14726–14768. [CrossRef] [PubMed]
35. Barlow, T.M.A.; Tourwé, D.; Ballet, S. Cyclisation to form small, medium and large rings by use of catalysed and uncatalysed azide–alkyne cycloadditions (AACs). *Eur. J. Org. Chem.* **2017**, *32*, 4678–4694. [CrossRef]
36. Buysse, K.; Farard, J.; Nikolaou, A.; Vanderheyden, P.; Vauquelin, G.; Sejer Pedersen, D.; Tourwé, D.; Ballet, S. Amino triazolo diazepines (Ata) as constrained histidine mimics. *Org. Lett.* **2011**, *13*, 6468–6471. [CrossRef]
37. Chen, Y.; Li, Z.; Liu, Y.; Lin, T.; Sun, H.; Yang, D.; Jiang, C. Identification of novel and selective non-peptide inhibitors targeting the polo-box domain of polo-like kinase 1. *Bioorg. Chem.* **2018**, *81*, 278–288. [CrossRef]
38. Appel, R. Tertiary phosphane/tetrachloromethane, a versatile reagent for chlorination, dehydration, and phosphorus-nitrogen linkage. *Angew. Chem. Int. Ed. Engl.* **1975**, *14*, 801–811. [CrossRef]
39. Qian, W.; Liu, F.; Burke, T.R., Jr. Investigation of unanticipated alkylation at the N(pi) position of a histidyl residue under Mitsunobu conditions and synthesis of orthogonally protected histidine analogues. *J. Org. Chem.* **2011**, *76*, 8885–8890. [CrossRef]
40. Tornoe, C.W.; Christensen, C.; Meldal, M. Peptidotriazoles on solid phase: [1,2,3]-triazoles by regiospecific copper(I)-catalyzed 1,3-dipolar cycloadditions of terminal alkynes to azides. *J. Org. Chem.* **2002**, *67*, 3057–3064. [CrossRef]
41. Rostovtsev, V.V.; Green, L.G.; Fokin, V.V.; Sharpless, K.B. A stepwise Huisgen cycloaddition process: Copper(I)-catalyzed regioselective "ligation" of azides and terminal alkynes. *Angew. Chem. Int. Ed. Engl.* **2002**, *41*, 2596–2599. [CrossRef]
42. Tron, G.C.; Pirali, T.; Billington, R.A.; Canonico, P.L.; Sorba, G.; Genazzani, A.A. Click chemistry reactions in medicinal chemistry: Applications of the 1,3-dipolar cycloaddition between azides and alkynes. *Med. Res. Rev.* **2008**, *28*, 278–308. [CrossRef]
43. Zhang, L.; Chen, X.; Xue, P.; Sun, H.H.Y.; Williams, I.D.; Sharpless, K.B.; Fokin, V.V.; Jia, G. Ruthenium-catalyzed cycloaddition of alkynes and organic azides. *J. Am. Chem. Soc.* **2005**, *127*, 15998–15999. [CrossRef]
44. Rasmussen, L.K.; Boren, B.C.; Fokin, V.V. Ruthenium-catalyzed cycloaddition of aryl azides and alkynes. *Org. Lett.* **2007**, *9*, 5337–5339. [CrossRef]
45. Creary, X.; Anderson, A.; Brophy, C.; Crowell, F.; Funk, Z. Method for assigning structure of 1,2,3-triazoles. *J. Org. Chem.* **2012**, *77*, 8756–8761. [CrossRef]
46. Xu, J.; Shen, C.; Wang, T.; Quan, J. Structural basis for the inhibition of polo-like kinase 1. *Nat. Struct. Mol. Biol.* **2013**, *20*, 1047–1053. [CrossRef]
47. Fish, P.V.; Ryckmans, T.; Stobie, A.; Wakenhut, F. [4-(Phenoxy)pyridin-3-yl]methylamines: A new class of selective noradrenaline reuptake inhibitors. *Bioorg. Med. Chem. Lett.* **2008**, *18*, 1795–1798. [CrossRef]
48. Siebertz, K.D.; Hackenberger, C.P.R. Chemoselective triazole-phosphonamidate conjugates suitable for photorelease. *Chem. Commun.* **2018**, *54*, 763–766. [CrossRef]
49. Boren, B.C.; Narayan, S.; Rasmussen, L.K.; Zhang, L.; Zhao, H.; Lin, Z.; Jia, G.; Fokin, V.V. Ruthenium-catalyzed azide–alkyne cycloaddition: Scope and mechanism. *J. Am. Chem. Soc.* **2008**, *130*, 8923–8930. [CrossRef]

50. Hymel, D.; Burke, T.R., Jr. Phosphatase-stable phosphoamino acid mimetics that enhance binding affinities with the polo-box domain of polo-like kinase 1. *ChemMedChem* **2017**, *12*, 202–206. [CrossRef]
51. Hanisch, A.; Wehner, A.; Nigg, E.A.; Sillje, H.H.W. Different Plk1 functions show distinct dependencies on polo-Box domain-mediated targeting. *Mol. Biol. Cell* **2006**, *17*, 448–459. [CrossRef]
52. Golsteyn, R.M.; Schultz, S.J.; Bartek, J.; Ziemiecki, A.; Ried, T.; Nigg, E.A. Cell cycle analysis and chromosomal localization of human Plk1, a putative homologue of the mitotic kinases Drosophila polo and Saccharomyces cerevisiae Cdc5. *J. Cell Sci.* **1994**, *107*, 1509–1517.

Sample Availability: Samples of select peptides may be available from the authors in limited quantities.

molecules

MDPI

Article

A Stapled Peptide Mimic of the Pseudosubstrate Inhibitor PKI Inhibits Protein Kinase A

Jascha T. Manschwetus [1,†], George N. Bendzunas [2,†], Ameya J. Limaye [2], Matthias J. Knape [1,‡], Friedrich W. Herberg [1,*] and Eileen J. Kennedy [2,*]

1 Department of Biochemistry, Institute for Biology, University of Kassel, Heinrich-Plett-Str. 40, 34132 Kassel, Germany; j.manschwetus@uni-kassel.de (J.T.M.); maknape@googlemail.com (M.J.K.)

2 Department of Pharmaceutical and Biomedical Sciences, College of Pharmacy, University of Georgia, 240 W. Green St, Athens, GA 30602, USA; georgenb@uga.edu (G.N.B.); ameya.limaye@uga.edu (A.J.L.)

* Correspondence: herberg@uni-kassel.de (F.W.H.); ekennedy@uga.edu (E.J.K.); Tel.: +49-561-804-4511 (F.W.H.); +1-706-542-6497 (E.J.K.)

† These Authors contributed equally to this work.

‡ Current address: Boehringer Ingelheim Pharma GmbH & Co. KG, Analytical Developments Biologicals, Birkendorfer Strasse 65, 88397 Biberach an der Riss, Germany.

Academic Editors: Henry Mosberg, Tomi Sawyer and Carrie Haskell-Luevano
Received: 30 March 2019; Accepted: 19 April 2019; Published: 20 April 2019

check for updates

Abstract: Kinases regulate multiple and diverse signaling pathways and misregulation is implicated in a multitude of diseases. Although significant efforts have been put forth to develop kinase-specific inhibitors, specificity remains a challenge. As an alternative to catalytic inhibition, allosteric inhibitors can target areas on the surface of an enzyme, thereby providing additional target diversity. Using cAMP-dependent protein kinase A (PKA) as a model system, we sought to develop a hydrocarbon-stapled peptide targeting the pseudosubstrate domain of the kinase. A library of peptides was designed from a Protein Kinase Inhibitor (PKI), a naturally encoded protein that serves as a pseudosubstrate inhibitor for PKA. The binding properties of these peptide analogs were characterized by fluorescence polarization and surface plasmon resonance, and two compounds were identified with K_D values in the 500–600 pM range. In kinase activity assays, both compounds demonstrated inhibition with 25–35 nM IC_{50} values. They were also found to permeate cells and localize within the cytoplasm and inhibited PKA activity within the cellular environment. To the best of our knowledge, these stapled peptide inhibitors represent some of the highest affinity binders reported to date for hydrocarbon stapled peptides.

Keywords: PKA; stapled peptide; PKI; pseudosubstrate; kinase inhibitor; IP20

1. Introduction

Protein kinases play pivotal roles as key modulators of cellular signaling events and are involved in numerous and diverse processes, including hormone response signaling, gene transcription, cell differentiation and apoptosis [1]. More than 500 eukaryotic protein kinases are encoded by the human genome and thus tight regulation of enzymatic activity and substrate interactions is essential for proper kinase function [2]. Aberrant signaling by this important enzyme class is linked to a broad spectrum of health issues such as cancer, diabetes and neurodegenerative diseases [3]. Due to the wide-ranging implications by kinases in signaling and biology, significant efforts have been put forth to develop selective kinase inhibitors that can be applied as either research tools or therapeutic inhibitors [4]. The majority of kinase inhibitors target the ATP binding site as it forms a deep pocket that is amenable for small molecule targeting [3]. Since the ATP pocket resides within the kinase domain and is therefore conserved across the kinase superfamily [5], specificity has remained a challenge. Alternatively, allosteric inhibitors may overcome the challenge of specificity by targeting more evolutionarily divergent surfaces or pockets for a kinase of interest.

As a model system, we focused on one of the best understood kinases, cAMP-dependent protein kinase (PKA). The PKA tetrameric holoenzyme complex consists of a regulatory subunit dimer and two monomeric catalytic subunits [6]. The catalytically inactive holoenzyme is activated by increased levels of the second messenger cAMP upon extracellular or intracellular stimuli, triggering the R subunits to undergo a conformational change that can then result in release of the catalytic subunits (PKA-C) [7]. PKA-C phosphorylates a vast variety of intracellular substrates that regulate a myriad of cellular processes via phosphorylation of the consensus sequence Arg-Arg-X-Ser/Thr-y, where X represents a small residue and y represents a large hydrophobic residue [8].

Nearly 50 years ago, a naturally encoded protein was discovered that could inhibit the catalytic activity of PKA, termed Protein Kinase Inhibitor (PKI) [9]. It was later discovered that only a short fragment of PKI was required for inhibition [10–13]. This 20-residue fragment derived from the N-terminal residues 5–24 of PKI, termed IP20, was found to be highly specific for PKA and could inhibit activity with K_D values in the single nanomolar range by binding the catalytic subunit of PKA as a pseudosubstrate, thereby preventing substrate engagement with the kinase (Figure 1a). IP20 includes a cluster of basic arginine residues as well as a hydrophobic portion in the pseudosubstrate sequence (Arg^{15}-Thr-Gly-Arg-Arg-Asn-Ala-Ile^{22}, where Ala substitutes for the phosphorylatable Ser/Thr). The charged residues, in particular the P-3 Arg, are a requisite for high-affinity binding to PKA-C [10,13,14] in addition to Mg^{2+} and ATP [14]. Although this 20-residue peptide, IP20 ($PKI^{5–24}$), has been used for many years as an investigative tool in biochemical assays, the peptide itself is not membrane permeable and requires modifications such as myristoylation to promote cell permeation [15,16]. However, a major drawback of this reagent is that the hydrophobic nature of the myristoylation moiety can intrinsically promote membrane interactions/embedding, thereby leading to potential mislocalization of the peptide and limiting its interactions with PKA-C at various intracellular locations.

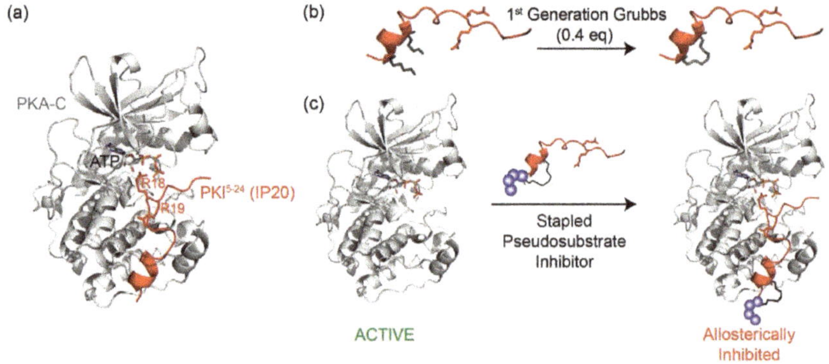

Figure 1. Design of a stapled pseudosubstrate inhibitor for the catalytic subunit of Protein Kinase A (PKA-C): (**a**) Crystal structure of PKA-C (gray, PDB ID: 1ATP) bound to a Protein Kinase Inhibitor ($PKI^{5–24}$) (IP20, red). The side chains of Arg 18 and 19 are shown and are critical for pseudosubstrate inhibition; (**b**) Peptide stapling was performed on-resin with ring-closing metathesis chemistry using the 1st Generation Grubbs catalyst to introduce a staple in the N-terminal alpha-helix; and (**c**) An analog of IP20 is designed by incorporating a hydrocarbon staple into the N-terminus of the PKI-derived peptide to serve as a non-catalytic, allosteric inhibitor for PKA-C. Structures were rendered using PyMol.

Due to its high target specificity and affinity for PKA-C, we explored whether the PKA pseudosubstrate peptide IP20 could be modified through hydrocarbon peptide stapling to improve cell permeability in the absence of lipidation (Figure 1b,c). Several analogs were designed and characterized for their affinity to PKA-C. While the stapled analogs of IP20 were found to have worsened affinities for PKA-C, we found that elongation of the sequence and reposition of the staple restored affinities to mid-picomolar range as measured by both fluorescence polarization (FP) and Surface Plasmon Resonance (SPR), representing one of the highest affinity binders reported to date for hydrocarbon stapled peptides. These peptides were further shown to inhibit the catalytic activity of PKA-C in vitro and could permeate cells and inhibit PKA phosphorylation within the cellular environment. Thus, the constrained peptides developed in this study represent a novel, non-lipidated, cell permeable tool for allosteric inhibition of PKA.

2. Results and Discussion

In order to determine whether a constrained peptide could be developed to mimic the pseudosubstrate inhibitory properties of PKI, analogs of the 20-mer peptide IP20 were first designed (compounds **1–4**, Table 1). Based on the crystal structure of IP20 with PKA-C, the peptide largely interacts with the catalytic subunit in an elongated fashion that lacks an ordered secondary structure [17]. However, a single alpha-helical turn is present in the N-terminus of the peptide structure (PKI residues 5–13) and thus provided a potential point for incorporation of the hydrocarbon staple. Based on this, an olefinic amino acid ((*S*)-*N*-Fmoc-2-(4′-pentenyl) alanine) was introduced into positions four and eight of the 20 amino acid peptide sequence so as to constrain a portion of the peptide while trying to minimize any structural impact on the C-terminal portion of the sequence. Peptides were synthesized using standard Fmoc solid phase chemistry. The olefinic amino acids were cyclized on solid support using ring closing metathesis (RCM) chemistry with 0.4 equivalents of 1st Generation Grubbs catalyst for two 1-h treatments in 1,2-dichloroethane (DCE) (Figure 1b). Cyclization yields ranged from 87–98% for each of the peptide products. Additionally, the N-terminus was modified to contain either a hydrophobic linker (β-alanine, βA, compound **2**) or hydrophilic linker (PEG_3, compound 4). Non-stapled peptides bearing the same N-terminal modifications were also synthesized as controls (compounds 1 and 3). Peptides products were confirmed by ESI-MS and purified by RP-HPLC over a Zorbax SB-C18 column prior to use. Overall yields ranged from 1–2%.

Table 1. IP20 Analogs developed as potential pseudosubstrate inhibitors for the catalytic subunit of Protein Kinase A (PKA-C) and summary of measured binding affinities (K_D, [nM]) of peptides towards the human PKA catalytic isoforms Cα and Cβ1 as measured by fluorescence polarization (FP). Mean values of three independent measurements are given.

Compound	Sequence [1]	Cα	Cβ1
PKI^{5-24}	TTYADFIASGRTGRRNAIHD	n.d. [2]	
1	βA-TTYADFIASGRTGRRNAIHD	0.7 ± 0.1	
2	βA-TTY*DFI*SGRTGRRNAIHD	5.2 ± 0.3	n.d. [2]
3	PEG_3-TTYADFIASGRTGRRNAIHD	0.8 ± 0.1	
4	PEG_3-TTY*DFI*SGRTGRRNAIHD	5.4 ± 0.9	
PKI^{1-24}	TDVETTYADFIASGRTGRRNAIHD	n.d. [2]	
5	βA-TDVETTYADFIASGRTGRRNAIHD	0.4 ± 0.1	0.4 ± 0.1
6	βA-TDV*TTY*DFIASGRTGRRNAIHD	0.6 ± 0.1	0.8 ± 0.3
7	PEG_3-TDVETTYADFIASGRTGRRNAIHD	0.5 ± 0.1	0.5 ± 0.1
8	PEG_3-TDV*TTY*DFIASGRTGRRNAIHD	0.7 ± 0.2	0.9 ± 0.3

[1] Stars represent positions where 2-(4′-pentenyl) alanine was inserted into the sequence. [2] n.d.–not determined.

In order to determine whether the constrained peptides retained their binding affinity towards PKA-C, FP studies were performed (Figures 2a and S5). N-terminally fluorescein-labeled peptides were incubated with a concentration range of recombinant human PKA-Cα. The non-stapled controls (compounds **1** and **3**) had measured K_D values ranging from 0.7–0.8 nM which is comparable to the previously reported K_D value of 1 nM by IP20 for PKA-Cα [18]. Unfortunately, the stapled versions of IP20 (compounds **2** and **4**) appeared to detrimentally affect binding for PKA-Cα with K_D values ranging around 5–5.5 nM (Table 1). A one-way ANOVA (Tukey test) showed that the approximately 7-fold decrease in affinity was significant.

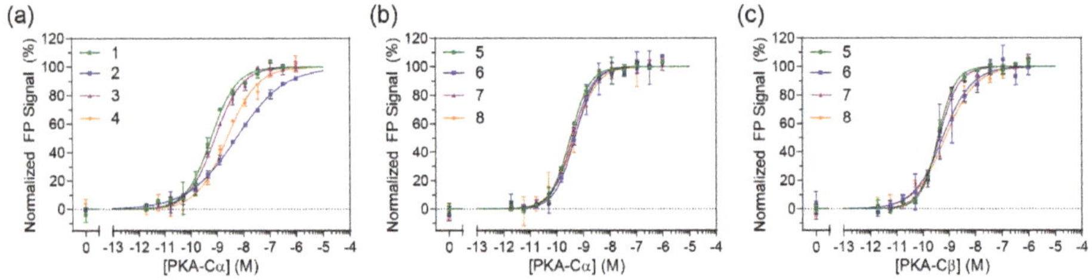

Figure 2. Direct binding measurements of fluorescein-labeled peptides by fluorescence polarization (FP): (**a**) Binding measurements of $PKI^{5\text{-}24}$ analogs to PKA-Cα demonstrate that stapling the 20-residue peptide negatively impacts binding; (**b**) Binding measurements of PKI^{1-24} analogs to PKA-Cα show no negative effect when stapling the 24-residue peptide; and (**c**) Binding measurements of PKI^{1-24} analogs to PKA-Cβ1 reveal that the stapled 24-mer analogs also retain high affinity for the Cβ1 isoform.

Based on these findings, we sought to explore whether the parent IP20 peptide could be modified in such a way that the staple wouldn't detrimentally affect its binding towards PKA-C. It was previously shown that extending IP20 by four residues (PKI^{1-24}) had inhibitory properties on PKA-C that were on par with IP20 [12], however, this would provide additional space to shift the staple closer to the N-terminus. Using PKI^{1-24} as a parent sequence, a subsequent set of stapled analogs was synthesized as before with either a βA or PEG_3 linker on the N-terminus (compounds 6 and 8). Non-stapled analogous controls were also synthesized (compounds **5** and **7**). FP measurements were subsequently performed on FAM-labeled peptides with PKA-Cα (Figure 2b). Under these conditions, no notable differences could be detected between the stapled and unstapled versions, indicating that the introduction of a staple to this longer sequence did not impede binding to PKA-C. Further, as compared to the PKI^{5-24} analogs, binding affinities were notably improved with K_D values ranging from 600–700 pM. To determine whether these stapled compounds could detect other PKA-C isoforms, they were also tested for binding to PKA-Cβ1 (Figure 2c and Table 1). Under these conditions, there was no significant loss in affinities as compared to their non-stapled counterparts, and all peptides retained K_D values in the mid-high picomolar range.

Since **6** and **8** were found to have sub-nanomolar affinities for PKA-C, we wanted to kinetically characterize this interaction using SPR. For this, an N-terminally GST-tagged PKA-C (GST-PKA-Cα) was captured on a CM5 chip surface via immobilized α-GST antibodies. The test compounds **6** and **8** were injected as an analyte over a concentration ranging from 0.05 to 28 nM. Association and dissociation rate constants were determined using a 1:1 Langmuir binding model. Both compounds **6** and **8** were found to have K_D values in the 500–600 pM range (Figure 3). As compared to the unstapled parent control peptide (PKI^{1-24}), both stapled analogs appear to have improved affinities for PKA-Cα. Notably, while the stapled and parent compounds were found to have similar association rates, it appears that the non-stapled peptide has significantly faster dissociation rates as identified using one-way ANOVA analysis (Dunnet test), resulting in an overall reduction in K_D (Tables 2 and S1).

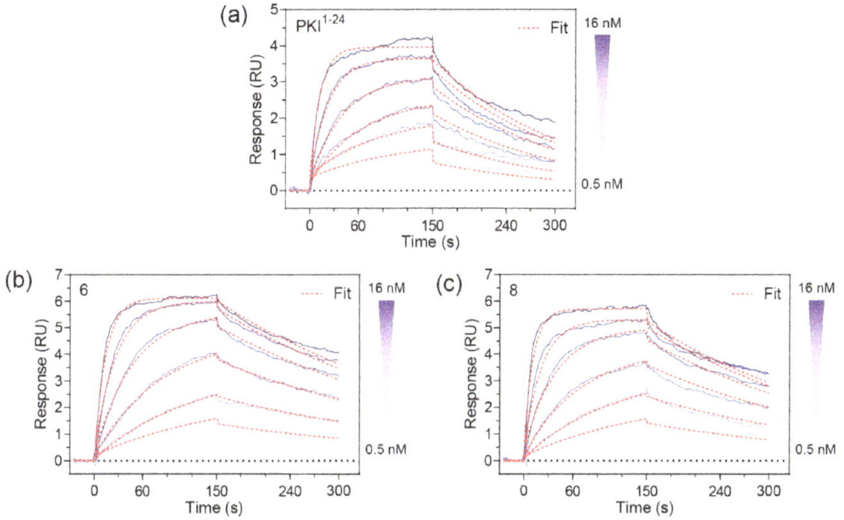

Figure 3. Binding interaction studies by Surface Plasmon Resonance (SPR): (**a**) Binding measurements of the non-modified PKI$^{1-24}$ control; (**b**) Binding measurements of Compound **6**; and (**c**) Binding measurements of Compound **8**. Compounds **6** and **8** demonstrated K_D values of 500 and 600 pM, respectively and demonstrate slightly slower dissociation rates as compared to the non-modified PKI$^{1-24}$ control.

Table 2. Summary of SPR analysis. Values were obtained from at least three independent measurements and are given with SD.

Compound	k_a (×10^6 M^{-1} s^{-1})	k_d (×10^{-3} s^{-1})	K_D (nM)
PKI$^{1-24}$	6.3 ± 1.7	7.2 ± 1.0	1.2 ± 0.2
6	8.0 ± 2.2	3.4 ± 0.4	0.5 ± 0.2
8	6.2 ± 1.4	3.5 ± 0.3	0.6 ± 0.2

Although constrained peptides **6** and **8** demonstrated high affinities for their target, PKA-C, it was unclear whether they could effectively inhibit the catalytic activity of their target kinase. In order to assess whether these constrained peptides could still serve as pseudosubstrate inhibitors, microfluidic electrophoretic mobility shift assays (MMSA) were used to analyze kinase function by monitoring phosphorylation of a substrate peptide (Kemptide, LRRASLG) using recombinant PKA-Cα (Figures 4 and S7). Peptides **6** and **8**, along with the non-constrained peptide control (PKI$^{1-24}$) were applied in serial dilutions ranging from 17 pM to 9 μM to determine half-maximal inhibitory concentrations (IC_{50} values). While the non-modified control was found to have an IC_{50} value of 17 nM, the stapled versions **6** and **8** had values ranging from 25–35 nM (Tables 3 and S2). Overall, it appears that the stapled peptides are comparable to the non-modified parent peptide under substrate saturation conditions and still have considerable potency for kinase inhibition in the lower nanomolar range.

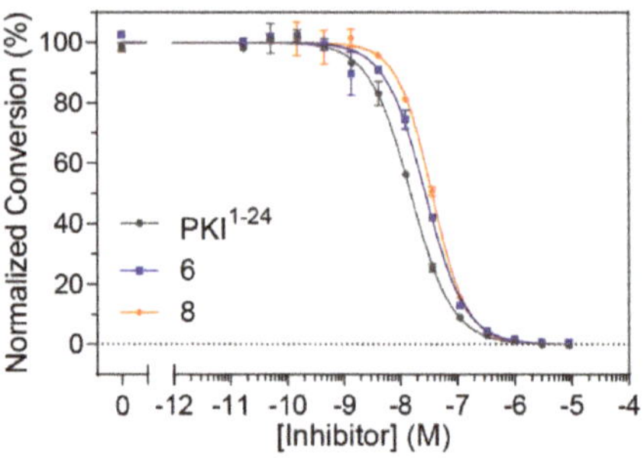

Figure 4. Kinase activity assays using microfluidic electrophoretic mobility shift assays (MMSA): Phosphorylation of a fluorescently-labeled substrate peptide by PKA-Cα was monitored over a concentration range of inhibitor peptides **6** and **8** as well as PKI^{1-24}. Both **6** and **8** were found to have IC_{50} values that compare to the non-modified parent control, PKI^{1-24}, thereby indicating that the introduction of a staple does not impair its inhibitory activity on PKA-Cα.

Table 3. Summary of microfluidic electrophoretic mobility shift assays (MMSA) analysis. Values were obtained from at least three independent measurements and are reported with SD.

Compound	IC_{50} (nM)
PKI^{1-24}	17.0 ± 3.4
6	24.8 ± 3.1
8	34.9 ± 5.2

Following in vitro characterization of these peptides, we next wanted to determine whether the staple would provide additional benefits for cell-based assays including improved cell permeation and *in cellulo* inhibition. Cell permeation experiments were performed using HEK293 cells. Cells were grown on chamber slides in complete media and 5 μM of each respective peptide analog of PKI^{1-24} was added to the media. Following an 8 h incubation, cells were imaged to monitor for intracellular localization (Figures 5a, S8 and S9). While the stapled versions **6** and **8** were found to readily permeate cells, their non-stapled counterparts (**5** and **7**) were not notably detected in cells.

Based on the cell uptake experiments, coupled with the observation that **8** appeared to have greater solubility in aqueous cell-based assays, we chose to further characterize **8** in a cell-based inhibition assay (Figure 5b). Following an 18 h incubation period in serum-free media to downregulate intrinsic PKA activity, HEK293 cells were pre-treated with compound **8** at different concentrations for 6 h. At this 24 h time point, cells were stimulated with forskolin, an adenylyl cyclase activator, to stimulate PKA activity for 30 min prior to lysis. The ATP-competitive catalytic inhibitor H89 (50 μM) was used as a negative control. PKA activity was monitored as a function of substrate phosphorylation using a phospho-Ser/Thr-PKA substrate antibody and tubulin was detected as a loading control. In the absence of stimulation, PKA substrate phosphorylation is downregulated to a basal level that is comparable to forskolin-stimulated cells that are co-treated with H89. Constrained peptide **8** was found to inhibit PKA substrate phosphorylation in a dose-dependent manner with a notable decrease in phosphorylated substrates at the 5 and 10 μM dosing range. Taken together, it appears that compound **8** can act as a cell permeable pseudosubstrate inhibitor of PKA-C.

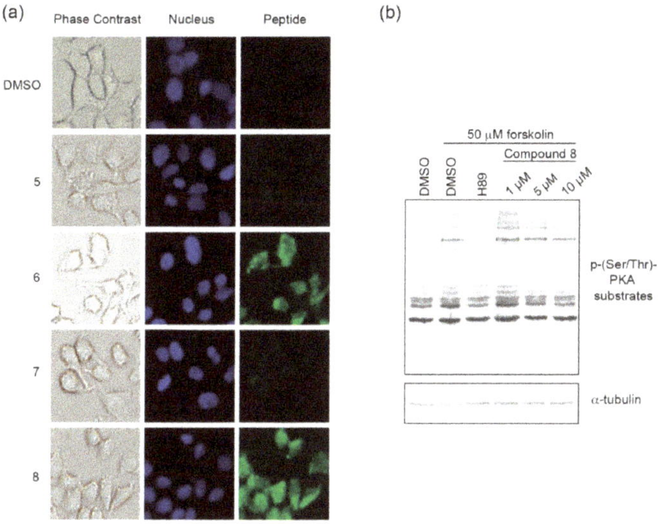

Figure 5. Cell-based uptake and inhibition: (**a**) Cell permeation is detected for stapled compounds **6** and **8** but not their unstapled counterparts after an 8 h incubation period; and (**b**) Cell-based inhibition by monitoring PKA activity in cells. In the presence of **8**, PKA substrate phosphorylation is inhibited in a dose-dependent manner.

Since protein kinases are key regulators of diverse signaling pathways and diseases, they are attractive targets for manipulation both in basic research as well as therapeutic intervention. Significant efforts have been put forth to develop inhibitors/modulators of kinase activity, however the majority of these compounds target the highly conserved ATP pocket and numerous shortcomings have been noted including lack of specificity and therefore cross-reactivity, poor inhibitory potency, and clinical usage often results in rapid development of resistance [5].

As a research tool, the ATP-competitive small molecule inhibitor H89 has been widely used as a PKA-C inhibitor due to its ability to readily permeate cells and its K_i of 48 nM [19]. However, H89 was found to not only inhibit PKA-C but was also shown to inhibit other kinases with even greater potency than PKA [20]. After short peptides derived from PKI were found to inhibit PKA-C with high specificity [12], they became valuable research tools for in vitro studies. A shortcoming of these peptides is that they are not intrinsically cell permeable, however a derivative was later developed that contained the addition of a myristoyl group (myr-PKI$^{14-22}$) [16]. The addition of the myristoyl moiety to PKI-derived peptides may significantly alter its interactions within a cellular environment, and thus alternative analogs lacking this moiety would expand the repertoire of reagents available for studying PKA-C in cells. Furthermore, several other kinases also contain a pseudosubstrate domain analogous to PKA-C including PKC and PKG [16,21] and thus this domain may serve more broadly as a viable target for selective, allosteric kinase inhibition. An alternative strategy has been employed by generating bi-substrate inhibitors of PKA where an ATP-competitive small molecule is conjugated to a peptidic moiety [22]. While some adenosine-oligoarginine conjugates (ARCs) were found to have high potency with K_D values as low as 3 pM and IC_{50} values in the low nanomolar range due to avidity effects [23], ease of synthesis of these compounds and cell permeation remains a challenge.

In contrast to ATP-competitive inhibitors, kinase-targeting peptide inhibitors often mimic protein-protein interaction sites [24–26]. Peptide-based inhibitors unite the benefits of both small-molecules and proteins, potentially resulting in high specificity, high potency, membrane permeability, conformational restriction and metabolic stability [27]. The compounds developed in this study offer many advantages for PKA targeting including ease of synthesis and its ability to permeate cells without the need for other modifications. Moreover, these peptides have an extremely high affinity for their target. The SPR data fit very well with a 1:1 model of Langmuir binding and the association rates detected for **6** and **8** approach the limitations of the Biacore instrumentation. The stapled peptide affinities are surprisingly comparable to the full-length PKI protein which has an affinity of approximately 0.5 nM as measured by SPR (Figure S6 and [28]). The stapled peptides developed in this work can be applied as unique tools for various investigations such as competitive displacement studies with substrates and pseudosubstrates. Additionally, one could envision taking advantage of its high affinity by further functionalizing it into various forms including a proteolysis-targeting chimera (PROTAC) or bi-substrate inhibitors.

3. Materials and Methods

3.1. General Information

Standard N-a-Fmoc amino acids and rink amide MBHA resin LL were purchased from Novabiochem (Millipore Sigma, Burlington, MA, USA). (*S*)-*N*-Fmoc-2-(4′-pentenyl) alanine (Fmoc-S_5) and 1st Generation Grubbs catalyst (Bis(tricyclohexylphosphine)benzylidene ruthenium(IV) chloride) were purchased from Sigma. 2-(6-Chloro-1-*H*-benzotrizole-1-yl)-1,1,3,3-tetramethylaminium hexafluorophosphate (HCTU) and Fmoc-11-amino-3,6,9-trioxaundecanoic acid (Fmoc-PEG_3) were purchased from ChemPep (Wellington, FL, USA). Unless noted, all other reagents and solvents were purchased from Fisher Scientific (Hampton, NH, USA), Carl Roth (Karsruhe, Germany), Sigma Aldrich (St. Louis, MO, USA), AppliChem (Darmstadt, Germany). and Merck (Darmstadt, Germany). HPLC-grade acetonitrile, trifluoroacetic acid and methanol were used for peptide purification by HPLC and MS analysis.

3.2. Cell Culture

HEK293 cells were cultured in Dulbecco's Modified Eagle Medium (DMEM) with glucose and L-glutamine (Lonza, Alpharetta, GA, USA), 10% fetal bovine serum (Thermo Scientific, Waltham, MA, USA), and penicillin/streptomycin (VWR Life Science, Radnor, PA, USA).

3.3. Peptide Synthesis

Synthesis was performed on MBHA resin LL using standard solid phase synthesis. Deprotection steps were performed using 25% (*v*/*v*) piperidine in 1-methyl-2-pyrrolidinone (NMP) for 25 min with gentle agitation. Coupling reactions with standard amino acids were performed using 10 eq amino acid, 9.9 eq HCTU and 20 eq *N*,*N*-diisopropylethylamine (DIEA) at room temperature for at least 45 min. Couplings with Fmoc-S_5 and Fmoc-PEG_3 were performed using 4 eq at room temperature for at least 60 min. Ring-closing metathesis of the olefinic amino acids ((*S*)-*N*-Fmoc-2-(4′-pentenyl) alanine) was performed on-resin in 1,2-dichloroethane (DCE) with 0.4 eq of 1st Generation Grubbs catalyst for two 1 h treatments. For N-terminal 5(6)-caroboxyfluorescein (FAM) labeling, 2 eq FAM were added along with 1.8 eq HCTU and 4.6 eq DIEA in DMF overnight with gentle agitation. For N-terminal biotin labeling, 10 eq of D-Biotin (Anaspec) was added along with 9.9 eq HCTU and 20 eq DIEA in a 1:1 mixture of DMF and DMSO overnight. Resin cleavage was performed in 95% (*v*/*v*) trifluoroacetic acid (TFA), 2.5% (*v*/*v*) triisopropylsilane and 2.5% (*v*/*v*) water for 4–5 h at room temperature, followed by precipitation in methyl-*tert*-butyl ether at 4 °C.

Peptides were characterized by ESI-MS (Agilent 6120 Single Quadrupole, Santa Clara, CA, USA) after HPLC separation over a Zorbax analytical SB-C18 column (Agilent 1200). Peptides were separated by reversed phase HPLC over a 10–100% gradient of water:acetonitrile with 0.1% TFA using a linear gradient and flow rate of 0.5 mL/min. Purification was performed using the same conditions except over a semi-preparatory column with a flow rate of 4 ml/min. FAM-labeled peptides were quantified based on absorbance at 495 nm in 10 mM Tris pH 8 (Bio-Tek Synergy 2) using an extinction coefficient of e = 68,000 $M^{-1}cm^{-1}$ as previously described [29]. Biotin-labeled peptides were quantified by measuring decreased absorbance of the 2-hydroxyazobenzen-4′-carboxylic acid (HABA)-avidin complex at 500 nm. Spectra for compounds **5–8** are shown in Figures S1–S4.

Peptide masses for each FAM-labeled product are as follows: 1 = 2649.9 (expected mass = 2650.8); 2 = 2758.2 (expected mass = 2759.0); 3 = 2769.6 (expected mass = 2768.9); 4 = 2876.4 (expected mass = 2877.1); 5 = 3094.8 (expected mass = 3095.3); 6 = 3145.2 (expected mass = 3145.3); 7= 3212.8 (expected mass = 3213.4); and 8 = 3262.4 (expected mass = 3263.5).

Peptide masses for each biotin-labeled product are as follows: 2 = 2625.9 (expected mass = 2627.0); 3 = 2635.8 (expected mass = 2636.9); 4 = 2744.4 (expected mass = 2745.1); 5 = 2962.2 (expected mass = 2963.2); 6 = 3012.6 (expected mass = 3013.4); 7 = 3080.4 (expected mass = 3081.4); and 8 = 3130.8 (expected mass = 3131.5).

Peptide mass for the unlabeled version of compound 5 unlabeled = 2665.2 (expected mass= 2665.8). Peptide mass for the PKI^{5-24} FF negative control (βA-TTY*DFI*SGRTGFFNAIHD): 2740.2 (expected mass = 2740.9).

3.4. Protein Expression and Preparation

Human wildtype PKA catalytic subunit, isoform α1 (PKA-Cα in pET30a), was expressed in *E. coli* T7 Express lysY/I^q cells, while both isoform β1 (PKA-Cβ in pET30a) and N-terminally GST-tagged murine isoform α1 (GST-PKA-Cα in pGEX-KG) were expressed in *E. coli* BL21-CodonPlus(DE3)-RIL cells for 16 h at RT after induction with 0.4 M IPTG. All PKA-C isoforms were purified using IP20-resin affinity chromatography as previously described [30]. All isoforms were stored in elution buffer (50 mM Tris-HCl pH 7.4, 200 mM L-arginine, 1 mM EDTA, 50 mM NaCl). Prior to further use, the buffer was exchanged to buffer A (20 mM MOPS pH 7, 150 mM NaCl, 2 mM β-mercaptoethanol) for both PKA-Cα and PKA-Cβ1. Full-length PKI was expressed and purified as previously described [31].

3.5. Fluorescence Polarization (FP)

Direct binding studies of peptides to PKA-C were performed using FP as previously described by Saldanha, et al. [32] and adapted by Bendzunas, et al. [33]. Each FAM-labeled peptide was plated to have a final concentration of 0.5 nM after the addition of protein in 384-well microtiter plates (BRAND GmbH + Co KG, BRANDplates, pureGrade, black). Three-fold dilution series of PKA-Cα or PKA-Cβ1, respectively, were mixed in the peptide wells in a 1:1 ratio to have at least 12 final concentrations ranging from 1 μM to 0.2 pM. The assay was performed in FP buffer (20 mM MOPS pH 7, 150 mM NaCl, 0.005 % CHAPS, 1 mM ATP, 10 mM $MgCl_2$) at room temperature. Focus height (7.6 mm) and gain (35 mPol) adjustments were performed on reaction mixtures without PKA-C. The following settings were utilized on a CLARIOstar (BMG LABTECH) plate reader in a top optic format: excitation/emission/dichroic filters: 482–16 nm/530–40 nm/LP 504; 50 flashes per well; settling time: 0.1 s. GraphPad Prism 6.01 (GraphPad Software, San Diego, CA, USA) was used to perform non-linear regression (sigmoidal dose response) on FP signals which were plotted against log-scale protein concentrations to determine equilibrium dissociation constants (K_D). At least two protein preparations were used for three independent duplicate measurements.

3.6. Surface Plasmon Resonance Spectroscopy (SPR)

GST-PKA-Cα was captured by polyclonal α-GST antibodies (Carl Roth) which were covalently immobilized on a Series S Sensor Chip CM5 (Biacore, GE Healthcare) surface using standard NHS/EDC chemistry with a Biacore T200 instrument (Biacore, GE Healthcare) to approximately 3000–13,000 response units (RU) as previously described [28]. Required dilutions of the analytes were injected to the flow cells containing GST-PKA-Cα before proceeding to a buffer or regeneration run, respectively. All measurements were simultaneously performed on reference flow-cells with α-GST Ab only and next to blank runs without analytes to be subtracted as non-specific binding. Unless otherwise noted, all analyses and coupling/capture steps were performed in HBS-P+ running buffer (10 mM HEPES, pH 7.4, 150 mM NaCl, 0.05 % Surfactant P20). Measurements were analyzed and fitted using the Biacore

T200 Evaluation Software 3.0 (GE Healthcare). Data sets were exported to and further processed in GraphPad Prism 6.01 (GraphPad Software).

For biochemical and biophysical assays, peptide concentrations were reapproved using calibration-free concentration analysis (CFCA). Diffusion coefficients of peptides at 20 °C were calculated using the online Biacore tool termed Diffusion Coefficient Calculator [34] The molecular weight of each peptide was entered and all compounds were assumed to be in elongated shape (frictional ratio 2.5). The sample compartment temperature was set to 15 °C while the analysis was performed at 20 °C. Two variable dilutions were prepared and adjusted for each peptide in HBS-P+ buffer containing 1 mM ATP and 10 mM $MgCl_2$. First, GST-PKA-Cα was captured to saturation with a flow rate of 30 µL/min resulting in capture levels of 750 RU to 2700 RU (high density). The adjusted peptide dilutions (ranging from as low as 1:150,000 to as high as 1:3,500,000) were subsequently injected for 45 s with flow rates of 5 µL/min and 100 µL/min, respectively, for each dilution. Between every peptide injection, PKA subunits were successfully regenerated by injecting elution buffer (described above) for 210 s with a flow rate of 30 µL/min.

To monitor association and dissociation of the biotin-labeled PKI^{1-24} analogs, interaction studies were adapted from [35]. Briefly, GST-PKA-Cα was injected to obtain capture levels of approximately 130–220 RU (low density) in each cycle. Two-fold peptide dilution series ranging from 50 pM to 28 nM were subsequently injected for 150 s (association) before initiating the dissociation phase by injecting buffer without analyte for another 150 s. Finally, regeneration of the immobilized α-GST antibodies was achieved by injecting 10 mM glycine (pH 1.9) for 30–60 s. All measurements were performed at 25 °C in HBS-P+ buffer containing 1 mM ATP and 10 mM $MgCl_2$ at a flow rate of 30 µL/min. The equilibrium dissociation constant (K_D) was subsequently calculated by dividing the dissociation rate constant (k_d) from the association rate constant (k_a) which were obtained by applying a 1:1 binding model (global fit, Langmuir conditions). Kinetic interaction analyses were performed in 3–5 independent repetitions with at least three protein preparations.

3.7. Microfluidic Electrophoretic Mobility Shift Assay (MMSA)

Kinase activity was determined by monitoring phosphorylation of the fluorescently-labeled substrate Kemptide (FITC-LRRASLG) in an MMSA to determine the amount of compound needed for half-maximal inhibition (IC_{50}) as previously described [36]. Off-chip reaction mixtures were prepared in 384-well plates (Corning, low volume, nonbinding surface) containing 10 mM HEPES pH 7.4, 150 mM NaCl, 0.1 mg/ml BSA, 1 mM DTT, 0.1 % L-31, 1 mM ATP, 10 mM $MgCl_2$, 250 µM Kemptide (GeneCust), 10 µM FITC-Kemptide (GL Biochem Ltd.) as well as 0.5 nM PKA-Cα or Cβ. Biotin-labeled peptides were tested over a 3-fold dilution series ranging from 17 pM to 9 µM. To remain maximum reaction velocity, Kemptide was applied at saturating concentrations of 260 µM [37]. After 45 min (PKA-Cα or 20 min (PKA-Cβ) of incubation in the dark at RT, samples were drawn into a four-sipper mode ProfilerPro Chip (Perkin Elmer) using a LabChip DeskTop Profiler (Caliper Life Sciences). While applying an upstream voltage of −1800 V and a downstream voltage of −150 V, substrate and product underwent electrophoretic separation in LabChip ProfilerPro Separation Buffer (PerkinElmer, Waltham, MA, USA) with a screening pressure of −1.7 PSI. Duplicate measurements were independently repeated 3–4 times with at least two separate protein preparations. Substrate conversion was plotted against log-scale inhibitor concentrations and fitted with nonlinear regression (sigmoidal dose-response curves) to determine IC_{50} values using GraphPad Prism 6.01 (GraphPad Software).

3.8. Cell Permeation Assays

HEK293 cells per well were seeded at 100,000 cells/well on 8-well chamber slides (BD Biosciences). Cells were grown overnight in DMEM medium with 10% fetal bovine serum. Next, 5 µM 5(6)-carboxyfluorescein-labeled peptides were added to the medium and incubated at 37 °C for 8 h before fixation in 2% paraformaldehyde. Slides were imaged using an Olympus IX71 microscope. Uptake experiments were repeated at least three times.

3.9. Cell-Based PKA Activity Assay

HEK293 cells were grown on 12-well culture plates (BD Biosciences). Cells were serum-starved for 24 h in serum-free DMEM with penicillin/streptomycin, glucose and L-glutamine. Peptides were added to cells at either 1, 5, or 10 μM concentrations for 6 h, followed by stimulation with 50 μM forskolin for 30 min. As a negative control, cells were treated with H89 (50 μM) for 30 min prior to forskolin stimulation. Cells were lysed in Laemmli sample buffer and analyzed by western blotting. Anti-phospho serine/threonine PKA substrate (1:1000, Cell Signaling Technology) or anti-tubulin (1:2000, DSHB) primary antibodies were used, followed by anti-rabbit IRDye 800CW (1:25,000) or anti-mouse IRDye 680LT secondary antibodies (1:30,000) (LI-COR Biosciences). Blots were imaged using an Odyssey Fc imaging system. Three independent replicates were performed.

Supplementary Materials: The following are available online, Figure S1–S9; Table S1–S2.

Author Contributions: Author contributions are as follows: conceptualization, E.J.K. and F.W.H.; methodology, G.N.B., J.T.M. and M.J.K.; software, G.N.B. and J.T.M.; validation, G.N.B. and J.T.M.; formal analysis, G.N.B., J.T.M., E.J.K. and F.W.H.; investigation, G.N.B., J.T.M., M.J.K. and A.J.L.; resources, G.N.B., J.T.M. and A.J.L.; data curation, G.N.B., J.T.M. and A.J.L.; writing—original draft preparation, J.T.M., G.N.B., E.J.K. and F.W.H; writing—review and editing, G.N.B., J.T.M., A.J.L., M.J.K., E.J.K. and F.W.H; supervision, E.J.K. and F.W.H.; project administration, E.J.K. and F.W.H.; funding acquisition, E.J.K. and F.W.H.

Funding: This research was funded by National Institutes of Health, grant numbers CA154600 and CA188439 to E.J.K.; the Department of Defense, grant number W81XWH-17-1-0290 to E.J.K.; the Deutsche Forschungsgemeinschaft, grant number He1818/10 and the funding line Future (PhosMOrg) to F.W.H.; and the Otto-Braun Fund Predoctoral Fellowship for J.T.M.

Acknowledgments: The authors would like to thank Leah Helton and Daniela Bertinetti for helpful discussions.

Conflicts of Interest: The authors declare no conflict of interest.

References

1. Manning, G.; Whyte, D.B.; Martinez, R.; Hunter, T.; Sudarsanam, S. The protein kinase complement of the human genome. *Science* **2002**, *298*, 1912–1934. [CrossRef]
2. Brognard, J.; Hunter, T. Protein kinase signaling networks in cancer. *Curr. Opin. Genet. Dev.* **2011**, *21*, 4–11. [CrossRef] [PubMed]
3. Ferguson, F.M.; Gray, N.S. Kinase inhibitors: The road ahead. *Nat. Rev. Drug Discov.* **2018**, *17*, 353–377. [CrossRef] [PubMed]
4. Muller, S.; Chaikuad, A.; Gray, N.S.; Knapp, S. The ins and outs of selective kinase inhibitor development. *Nat. Chem. Biol.* **2015**, *11*, 818–821. [CrossRef]
5. Zhang, J.; Yang, P.L.; Gray, N.S. Targeting cancer with small molecule kinase inhibitors. *Nat. Rev. Cancer* **2009**, *9*, 28–39. [CrossRef] [PubMed]
6. Taylor, S.S.; Zhang, P.; Steichen, J.M.; Keshwani, M.M.; Kornev, A.P. PKA: Lessons learned after twenty years. *Biochim. Biophys. Acta* **2013**, *1834*, 1271–1278. [CrossRef] [PubMed]
7. Taylor, S.S.; Ilouz, R.; Zhang, P.; Kornev, A.P. Assembly of allosteric macromolecular switches: Lessons from PKA. *Nat. Rev. Mol. Cell Biol.* **2012**, *13*, 646–658. [CrossRef] [PubMed]
8. Kemp, B.E.; Pearson, R.B. Protein kinase recognition sequence motifs. *Trends Biochem. Sci.* **1990**, *15*, 342–346. [CrossRef]
9. Walsh, D.A.; Ashby, C.D.; Gonzalez, C.; Calkins, D.; Fischer, E.H. Krebs EG: Purification and characterization of a protein inhibitor of adenosine 3′,5′-monophosphate-dependent protein kinases. *J. Biol. Chem.* **1971**, *246*, 1977–1985.
10. Scott, J.D.; Fischer, E.H.; Demaille, J.G.; Krebs, E.G. Identification of an inhibitory region of the heat-stable protein inhibitor of the cAMP-dependent protein kinase. *Proc. Natl. Acad. Sci. USA* **1985**, *82*, 4379–4383. [CrossRef]
11. Scott, J.D.; Fischer, E.H.; Takio, K.; Demaille, J.G.; Krebs, E.G. Amino acid sequence of the heat-stable inhibitor of the cAMP-dependent protein kinase from rabbit skeletal muscle. *Proc. Natl. Acad. Sci. USA* **1985**, *82*, 5732–5736. [CrossRef] [PubMed]

12. Scott, J.D.; Glaccum, M.B.; Fischer, E.H.; Krebs, E.G. Primary-structure requirements for inhibition by the heat-stable inhibitor of the cAMP-dependent protein kinase. *Proc. Natl. Acad. Sci. USA* **1986**, *83*, 1613–1616. [CrossRef] [PubMed]
13. Cheng, H.C.; van Patten, S.M.; Smith, A.J.; Walsh, D.A. An active twenty-amino-acid-residue peptide derived from the inhibitor protein of the cyclic AMP-dependent protein kinase. *Biochem. J.* **1985**, *231*, 655–661. [CrossRef] [PubMed]
14. Whitehouse, S.; Walsh, D.A. Mg X ATP2-dependent interaction of the inhibitor protein of the cAMP-dependent protein kinase with the catalytic subunit. *J. Biol. Chem.* **1983**, *258*, 3682–3692.
15. Glass, D.B.; Cheng, H.C.; Mende-Mueller, L.; Reed, J.; Walsh, D.A. Primary structural determinants essential for potent inhibition of cAMP-dependent protein kinase by inhibitory peptides corresponding to the active portion of the heat-stable inhibitor protein. *J. Biol. Chem.* **1989**, *264*, 8802–8810.
16. Eichholtz, T.; de Bont, D.B.; de Widt, J.; Liskamp, R.M.; Ploegh, H.L. A myristoylated pseudosubstrate peptide, a novel protein kinase C inhibitor. *J. Biol. Chem.* **1993**, *268*, 1982–1986.
17. Knighton, D.R.; Zheng, J.H.; Ten Eyck, L.F.; Ashford, V.A.; Xuong, N.H.; Taylor, S.S.; Sowadski, J.M. Crystal structure of the catalytic subunit of cyclic adenosine monophosphate-dependent protein kinase. *Science* **1991**, *253*, 407–414. [CrossRef]
18. Knape, M.J.; Ballez, M.; Burghardt, N.C.; Zimmermann, B.; Bertinetti, D.; Kornev, A.P.; Herberg, F.W. Divalent metal ions control activity and inhibition of protein kinases. *Metallomics* **2017**, *9*, 1576–1584. [CrossRef]
19. Lochner, A.; Moolman, J.A. The many faces of H89: A review. *Cardiovasc Drug Rev.* **2006**, *24*, 261–274. [CrossRef] [PubMed]
20. Davies, S.P.; Reddy, H.; Caivano, M.; Cohen, P. Specificity and mechanism of action of some commonly used protein kinase inhibitors. *Biochem. J.* **2000**, *351*, 95–105. [CrossRef]
21. Mitchell, R.D.; Glass, D.B.; Wong, C.W.; Angelos, K.L.; Walsh, D.A. Heat-stable inhibitor protein derived peptide substrate analogs: Phosphorylation by cAMP-dependent and cGMP-dependent protein kinases. *Biochemistry* **1995**, *34*, 528–534. [CrossRef] [PubMed]
22. Viht, K.; Schweinsberg, S.; Lust, M.; Vaasa, A.; Raidaru, G.; Lavogina, D.; Uri, A.; Herberg, F.W. Surface-plasmon-resonance-based biosensor with immobilized bisubstrate analog inhibitor for the determination of affinities of ATP- and protein-competitive ligands of cAMP-dependent protein kinase. *Anal. Biochem.* **2007**, *362*, 268–277. [CrossRef]
23. Ivan, T.; Enkvist, E.; Viira, B.; Manoharan, G.B.; Raidaru, G.; Pflug, A.; Alam, K.A.; Zaccolo, M.; Engh, R.A.; Uri, A. Bifunctional Ligands for Inhibition of Tight-Binding Protein-Protein Interactions. *Bioconjug. Chem.* **2016**, *27*, 1900–1910. [CrossRef] [PubMed]
24. Hanold, L.E.; Fulton, M.D.; Kennedy, E.J. Targeting kinase signaling pathways with constrained peptide scaffolds. *Pharmacol. Ther.* **2017**, *173*, 159–170. [CrossRef] [PubMed]
25. Fulton, M.D.; Hanold, L.E.; Ruan, Z.; Patel, S.; Beedle, A.M.; Kannan, N.; Kennedy, E.J. Conformationally constrained peptides target the allosteric kinase dimer interface and inhibit EGFR activation. *Bioorg. Med. Chem.* **2018**, *26*, 1167–1173. [CrossRef] [PubMed]
26. Flaherty, B.R.; Ho, T.G.; Schmidt, S.H.; Herberg, F.W.; Peterson, D.S.; Kennedy, E.J. Targeted Inhibition of Plasmodium falciparum Calcium-Dependent Protein Kinase 1 with a Constrained J Domain-Derived Disruptor Peptide. *ACS Infect. Dis.* **2019**. [CrossRef]
27. Hill, T.A.; Shepherd, N.E.; Diness, F.; Fairlie, D.P. Constraining cyclic peptides to mimic protein structure motifs. *Angew. Chem. Int. Ed. Engl.* **2014**, *53*, 13020–13041. [CrossRef]
28. Zimmermann, B.; Schweinsberg, S.; Drewianka, S.; Herberg, F.W. Effect of metal ions on high-affinity binding of pseudosubstrate inhibitors to PKA. *Biochem. J.* **2008**, *413*, 93–101. [CrossRef]
29. Hanold, L.E.; Oruganty, K.; Ton, N.T.; Beedle, A.M.; Kannan, N.; Kennedy, E.J. Inhibiting EGFR dimerization using triazolyl-bridged dimerization arm mimics. *PLoS ONE* **2015**, *10*, e0118796. [CrossRef]
30. Olsen, S.R.; Uhler, M.D. Affinity purification of the C alpha and C beta isoforms of the catalytic subunit of cAMP-dependent protein kinase. *J. Biol. Chem.* **1989**, *264*, 18662–18666. [PubMed]
31. Thomas, J.; Van Patten, S.M.; Howard, P.; Day, K.H.; Mitchell, R.D.; Sosnick, T.; Trewhella, J.; Walsh, D.A.; Maurer, R.A. Expression in Escherichia coli and characterization of the heat-stable inhibitor of the cAMP-dependent protein kinase. *J. Biol. Chem.* **1991**, *266*, 10906–10911. [PubMed]

32. Saldanha, S.A.; Kaler, G.; Cottam, H.B.; Abagyan, R.; Taylor, S.S. Assay principle for modulators of protein-protein interactions and its application to non-ATP-competitive ligands targeting protein kinase A. *Anal. Chem.* **2006**, *78*, 8265–8272. [CrossRef] [PubMed]
33. Bendzunas, N.G.; Dorfler, S.; Autenrieth, K.; Bertinetti, D.; Machal, E.M.F.; Kennedy, E.J.; Herberg, F.W. Investigating PKA-RII specificity using analogs of the PKA:AKAP peptide inhibitor STAD-2. *Bioorg. Med. Chem.* **2018**. [CrossRef] [PubMed]
34. Diffusion Coefficient Calculator/Converter. Available online: https://www.biacore.com/lifesciences/Application_Support/laboratory-guidelines/Diffusion_Coefficient_Calculator/index.html?section=lifesciences&realsection=lifesciences (accessed on 19 April 2019).
35. Knape, M.J.; Ahuja, L.G.; Bertinetti, D.; Burghardt, N.C.; Zimmermann, B.; Taylor, S.S.; Herberg, F.W. Divalent Metal Ions Mg(2)(+) and Ca(2)(+) Have Distinct Effects on Protein Kinase A Activity and Regulation. *ACS Chem. Biol.* **2015**, *10*, 2303–2315. [CrossRef]
36. Huang, G.Y.; Kim, J.J.; Reger, A.S.; Lorenz, R.; Moon, E.W.; Zhao, C.; Casteel, D.E.; Bertinetti, D.; Vanschouwen, B.; Selvaratnam, R.; et al. Structural basis for cyclic-nucleotide selectivity and cGMP-selective activation of PKG I. *Structure* **2014**, *22*, 116–124. [CrossRef]
37. Zimmermann, B.; Chiorini, J.A.; Ma, Y.; Kotin, R.M.; Herberg, F.W. PrKX Is a Novel Catalytic Subunit of the cAMP-dependent Protein Kinase Regulated by the Regulatory Subunit Type I. *J. Biol. Chem.* **1999**, *274*, 5370–5378. [CrossRef] [PubMed]

Sample Availability: Samples of the compounds are available from the authors.

molecules

MDPI

Article

Small AntiMicrobial Peptide with In Vivo Activity Against Sepsis

Héloise Boullet [1], Fayçal Bentot [1], Arnaud Hequet [2], Carine Ganem-Elbaz [2], Chérine Bechara [1], Emeline Pacreau [3], Pierre Launay [3], Sandrine Sagan [1], Claude Jolivalt [2], Claire Lacombe [1,4], Roba Moumné [1] and Philippe Karoyan [1,5,6,*]

1. Sorbonne Université, École Normale Supérieure, PSL University, CNRS, Laboratoire des Biomolécules, LBM, 75005 Paris, France; hel.boullet@gmail.com (H.B.); faycal.bentot@gmail.com (F.B.); cherine.bechara@umontpellier.fr (C.B.); sandrine.sagan@sorbonne-universite.fr (S.S.); claire.lacombe.s@gmail.com (C.L.); roba.moumne@sorbonne-universite.fr (R.M.)
2. Laboratoire Charles Friedel, UMR7223, École Nationale Supérieure de Chimie de Paris, 11 rue Pierre et Marie Curie, 75005 Paris, France; arhequet@gmail.com (A.H.); carine.ganem-elbaz@curie.fr (C.G.-E.); claude.jolivalt@sorbonne-universite.fr (C.J.)
3. Inserm U1149, Labex Inflammex, Bichat Medical School, 75005 Paris, France; emeline.pacreau@inserm.fr (E.P.); pierre.launay@inserm.fr (P.L.)
4. Faculté des Sciences et Technologie, Univ Paris Est-Créteil Val de Marne, 94000 Créteil, France
5. Kayvisa, AG, Industriestrasse, 44, 6300 Zug, Switzerland
6. Kaybiotix, GmbH, Zugerstrasse 32, 6340 Baar, Switzerland

* Correspondence: philippe.karoyan@sorbonne-universite.fr; Tel.: +33-44274469

Academic Editors: Henry Mosberg, Tomi Sawyer and Carrie Haskell-Luevano
Received: 30 March 2019; Accepted: 17 April 2019; Published: 1 May 2019

check for updates

Abstract: Antimicrobial peptides (AMPs) are considered as potential therapeutic sources of future antibiotics because of their broad-spectrum activities and alternative mechanisms of action compared to conventional antibiotics. Although AMPs present considerable advantages over conventional antibiotics, their clinical and commercial development still have some limitations, because of their potential toxicity, susceptibility to proteases, and high cost of production. To overcome these drawbacks, the use of peptides mimics is anticipated to avoid the proteolysis, while the identification of minimalist peptide sequences retaining antimicrobial activities could bring a solution for the cost issue. We describe here new polycationic β-amino acids combining these two properties, that we used to design small dipeptides that appeared to be active against Gram-positive and Gram-negative bacteria, selective against prokaryotic versus mammalian cells, and highly stable in human plasma. Moreover, the in vivo data activity obtained in septic mice reveals that the bacterial killing effect allows the control of the infection and increases the survival rate of cecal ligature and puncture (CLP)-treated mice.

Keywords: polycationic β-amino acids; small antimicrobial peptides; sepsis

1. Introduction

If the discovery of antibiotics is one of the major medical breakthroughs of the last century, bacterial resistance has consecutively emerged as a main medical problem [1]. Indeed, the number of infections caused by bacterial strains resistant to conventional antibiotics is rising and despite the success of genomics in identifying new essential bacterial genes, there is a lack of sustainable leads in antibacterial drug discovery to address these increasing multidrug-resistant (MDR) microorganisms [2]. The search for novel antibiotics with original mechanism of action is of particular interest. In this context, Antimicrobial Peptides (AMPs) are considered as an inspirational source for future antibiotics [3,4]. Indeed, although their mechanism of action is still a matter of basic research, it is generally admitted that most of them act directly on the bacterial membrane (membranolytic) and thus likely escape the mechanisms of bacterial resistance [5]. Although AMPs present considerable advantages as new generation antibiotics, their development as therapeutics is still limited by peptide drawbacks, such as their potential toxicity, susceptibility to proteases, and high manufacturing costs. To overcome these limitations, different strategies have been investigated: The use of unnatural amino acids is anticipated to enhance their proteolytic stability [6], while the identification of small antimicrobial peptides (SAMP) [7] with sequence length ranging from 2 to 10 amino acids is suggested as an interesting solution for the cost issue. Small non peptidic scaffolds that mimic their mechanism of action have also been recently reported [8,9].

AMPs are usually amphipathic sequences and contain several basic residues, i.e., lysine and arginine, as well as a hydrophobic core, which are critical for their activity. The lysine and arginine side-chains are positively charged at physiological pH and direct these amphiphilic peptides to the anionic surface of bacterial cell membranes, allowing the interaction of hydrophobic residues with the hydrocarbon core of the lipid bilayer. In the aim of identifying minimalist sequence that act like AMP, the use of building blocks bearing multi-cationic groups at physiological pH could be an interesting strategy. Aussedat et al. have previously reported a small achiral tetravalent template, the "α-bis-arginine", which contains twice the side chain of arginine, and thus increases the charge density of the peptide sequence [10]. Although a promising tool, the steric hindrance of the α-bis-arginine quaternary center adjacent to the amine and acid functions rendered its peptidic coupling difficult in SPPS or LPPS (Solid and Liquid Phase Peptide Syntheses). The use of additional non-bulky spacers such as glycine or β-alanine residues was necessary to incorporate this α-amino acid into peptides. Consequently, even if the number of charged residues could be reduced through the use of this multi-charged amino acid, the overall size of the peptide cannot be shortened. We report here new residues that combine the advantage of the α-bis-arginine but can be easily oligomerized leading to small peptides with potential therapeutic applications: the $\beta^{2,2}$- and $\beta^{3,3}$-*homo*-bis-arginine derivatives, homologated respectively on the carboxylate or on the amino side (Figure 1). We postulated that the additional methylene group of β-amino acids (in green in Figure 1) would limit the steric hindrance around the quaternary center (in red in Figure 1) and facilitate their incorporation into peptides. Oligomers of β-amino acids represent one of the most studied class of foldamers. Since the pioneer work of Seebach et al. [11], only few studies dealing with $\beta^{2,2}$- or $\beta^{3,3}$-amino acids have been reported in the literature [12–14]. Noticeably, while the use of lipophilic $\beta^{2,2}$-amino acids has proven valuable for the design of both antibacterial [15] and anticancer peptides [16,17], geminally disubstituted residues with basic side-chains have not been reported so far.

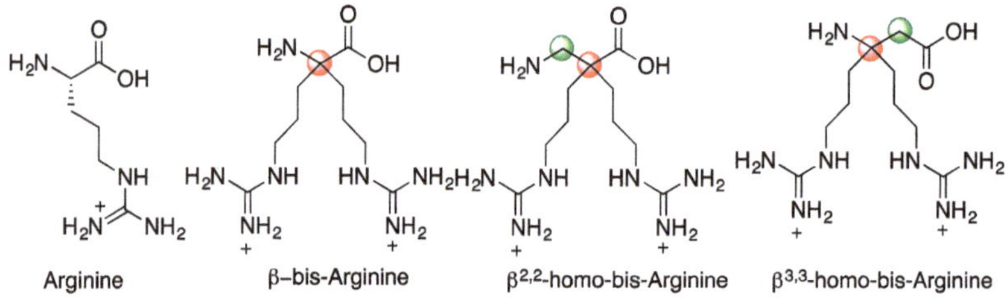

Figure 1. Bis-disubstituted-arginine analogues.

We report here the syntheses of $\beta^{2,2}$- and $\beta^{3,3}$-bis-*homo*-ornithine/arginine, and their use to design small cationic peptides. These peptides were evaluated as antimicrobial agents against Gram-positive and Gram-negative bacteria, and their cytotoxicity against eukaryotic cells as well as their stability in human serum were assessed. This work led to the selection of a dipeptide as a lead for in vivo studies for the treatment of sepsis in mice. Remarkably, the in vivo results revealed that the bacterial killing effect of this cationic dipeptide allows the control of the infection and sustains the immune response in the remediation of sepsis.

2. Results

2.1. Amino Acids Syntheses

The $\beta^{2,2}$- (**1** and **2**) and $\beta^{3,3}$-bis-*homo*-ornithine derivatives (**3**) required for the synthesis of the cationic dipeptides were prepared suitably protected for dipeptide syntheses (Figure 2).

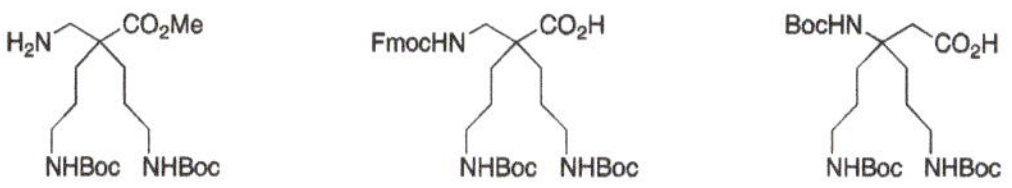

1 2 3

Figure 2. $\beta^{2,2}$- and $\beta^{3,3}$-bis-*homo*-ornithine derivatives suitably protected for peptide syntheses.

The $\beta^{2,2}$-*homo*-bis-ornithine methyl ester **1** and the Fmoc-protected $\beta^{2,2}$-*homo*-bis-ornithine **2** were both obtained from methyl cyanoacetate, respectively, in three and four steps (Scheme 1).

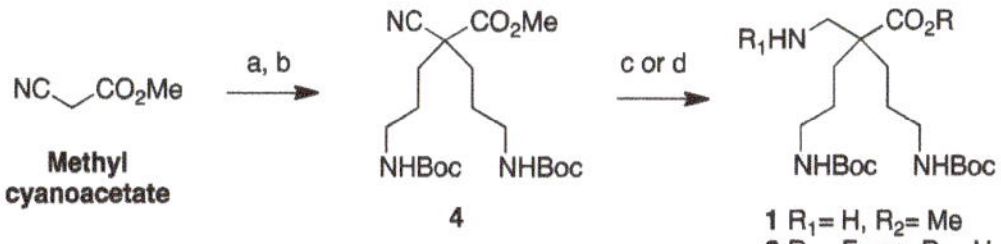

Scheme 1. $\beta^{2,2}$-*homo*-bis-ornithine derivatives 1 and 2 syntheses. (**a**) CH_2=CHCN, $LiClO_4$, NEt_3 (93%); (**b**) H_2, PtO_2, Boc_2O, MeOH (21%); (**c**) H_2, Ni Raney, MeOH (**1**, 98%); (**d**) 1/H_2, Ni Raney, NaOH (2 M), THF/EtOH 2/FmocOSu, K_2CO_3, H_2O, dioxane (**2**, 72%).

The double Michael addition on acrylonitrile [18] followed by selective reduction of the nitrile groups in γ-position over PtO_2 and simultaneous Boc-protection of the resulting amines gave the key intermediate **4** with moderate yields (21%). Improvement of this yield could be realized using a large excess of Raney Nickel (50% Yields) but was not relevant for safety reason and large-scale synthesis. Reduction of the α-nitrile by Raney nickel catalyzed hydrogenation in methanol led to the amine-free, acid-protected $\beta^{2,2}$-*homo*-bis-ornithine derivative **1** that could be directly used in peptide coupling on the amine side. The *N*-protected, acid-free counterpart **2** was obtained when the reduction of **4** was performed in the presence of sodium hydroxide, followed by a Fmoc-protection. Boc-protected $\beta^{3,3}$-*homo*-bis-ornithine derivative **3** was obtained starting from *tert*-butyl benzyl malonate (Scheme 2).

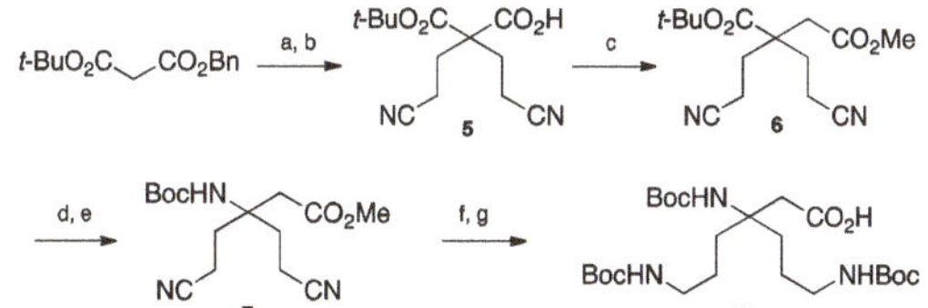

Scheme 2. $\beta^{3,3}$-*homo*-bis-ornithine derivatives 3 synthesis. (**a**) CH_2=CHCN $LiClO_4$, NEt_3 (88%); (**b**) $NH_4^+HCO_2^-$, Pd/C, MeOH (83%); (**c**) 1/1-chloro-*N*,*N*,2-trimethyl-1-propenylamine, DCM 2/TMSCHN_2, DIEA, CH3CN 3/Ag_2O, DMF/MeOH, reflux (21%); (**d**) TFA/TIS/DCM (86%); (**e**) 1/$ClCO_2Et$, NEt_3, acetone, 0 °C 2/NaN_3, H_2O 3/toluene, *tert*-BuOH, reflux (35%); (**f**) 1/PtO_2, H_2, $CHCl_3$/MeOH 2/K_2CO_3, Boc_2O, H_2O/THF (62%); (**g**) LiOH, CH_3CN/H_2O (98%).

The double Michael addition on acrylonitrile followed by selective benzyl ester hydrogenolysis using ammonium formate on palladium charcoal gave compound **5**. Arndt–Eistert homologation catalyzed by silver oxide led to compound **6** with 21% yields over the three steps. After deprotection of the *t*-Bu ester, the acid group was converted to Boc-protected amine via a Curtius rearrangement. Reduction of the nitrile groups in γ-position was then achieved by platinum oxide catalyzed hydrogenation. Finally, protection of the amino groups as Boc-carbamate and saponification of the methyl ester gave access to compound **3** readily usable for peptide coupling on the acid side.

2.2. Peptides Design and Syntheses

With these compounds in hand, we have designed antimicrobial dipeptides inspired by the work of Svendsen and co-workers, who defined the minimal set of functional motifs required to develop short AMPs as two cationic charges and two bulky hydrophobic aromatic units [19,20]. Based on this minimalist pharmacophore model, they indeed developed promising antibacterial tripeptides composed of a central 2,5,7-tri-tertbutyltryptophan (Tbt) flanked by two arginine residues. These peptides have anti-infectious properties and have reached phase-II clinical studies [21–23]. Several other groups have then reported the successful implementation of this pharmacophore model [24–26]. Starting from the peptide reported by Svendsen et al., the two arginine residues were replaced by one dicationic amino acid, leading to dipeptides **8–13** containing a tryptophan derivative (Trp or Tbt) and a dicationic $\beta^{2,2}$- or $\beta^{3,3}$-amino acid: Trp-$\beta^{2,2}$-*h*-bis-Orn-OMe (**8**), Tbt-$\beta^{2,2}$-*h*-bis-Orn-OMe (**9**), Gdm-Trp-$\beta^{2,2}$-*h*-bis-Arg-OMe (**10**), Tbt-$\beta^{2,2}$-*h*-bis-Arg-OMe (**11**), Gdm-Tbt-$\beta^{2,2}$-*h*-bis-Arg-OMe (**12**), and $\beta^{3,3}$-*h*-bis-Arg-Tbt-OMe (**13**) (Figure 3). In order to investigate the effect of the positive charge segregation on the antimicrobial activity of the compound [27], we also synthesized peptide **14** (Gdm-$\beta^{2,2}$-*h*-bis-Arg-Tbt-OMe), in which the sequence of dipeptide **11** is reversed.

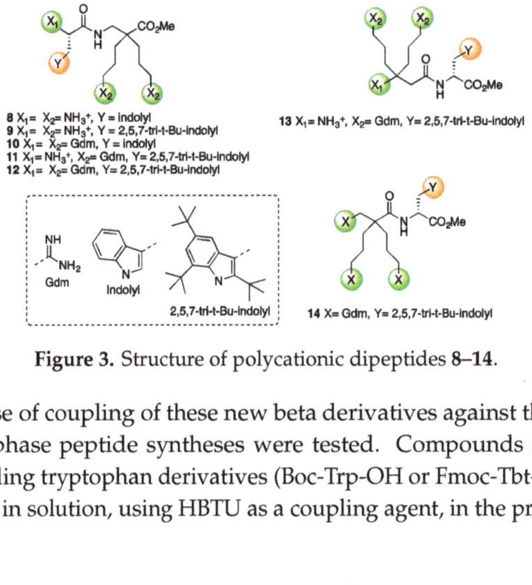

Figure 3. Structure of polycationic dipeptides **8–14**.

To evaluate the ease of coupling of these new beta derivatives against their alpha counterparts, both liquid and solid phase peptide syntheses were tested. Compounds **8–12** were prepared by coupling the corresponding tryptophan derivatives (Boc-Trp-OH or Fmoc-Tbt-OH) with the $\beta^{2,2}$-*h*-bis-ornithine methyl ester **1** in solution, using HBTU as a coupling agent, in the presence of DIEA, in DMF (Scheme 3).

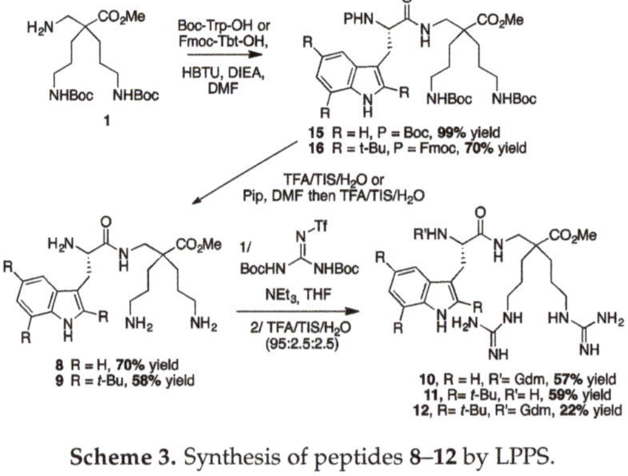

Scheme 3. Synthesis of peptides **8–12** by LPPS.

The fully protected dipeptides **15** and **16** were obtained from Boc-Trp-OH and Fmoc-Tbt-OH, in respectively 99% and 70% yields. Noticeably, the α-bis-ornithine derivative coupling failed in the same conditions. Deprotection of the amines gave access to the corresponding $\beta^{2,2}$-*h*-bis-Ornitine derivatives **8** and **9**. Introduction of the guanidinium group (Gdm) on these two compounds followed by Boc-deprotection using a TFA cocktail led to the $\beta^{2,2}$-*h*-bis-Arg derivatives. While a unique tri-guanylated compound was obtained for the tryptophan containing dipeptide **10**, two products were isolated for the Tbt-derived compound in respectively 59% and 22% yields: One with the guanidinium groups on the side chains of the amino acids (**11**) only, and one with an additional guanidinium group on the β-amine (**12**).

The synthesis of peptides **13** and **14** was achieved by SPPS, starting from a HMBA resin-bound Tbt (Scheme 4).

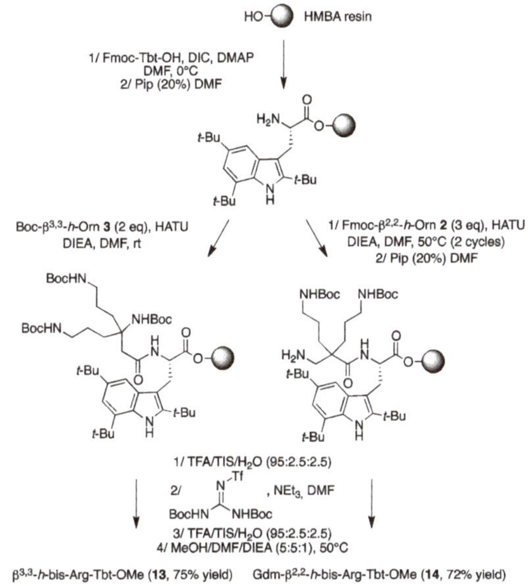

Scheme 4. Synthesis of peptides **13** and **14** by SPPS.

In both cases coupling of Fmoc-$\beta^{2,2}$-*h*-bis-Orn-OH **2** and Boc-$\beta^{3,3}$-*h*-bis-Orn-OH **3** was achieved through HATU activation, in the presence of DIEA, in DMF. However, because of the steric hindrance of its carboxyl group, heating at 50 °C as well as a second coupling round were necessary to ensure the complete conversion of **2**. As anticipated, the improved reactivity of the carboxyl group of this residue with its $\beta^{3,3}$-counterpart confirms that an additional methylene near the quaternary center is an effective strategy to facilitate the incorporation of the bis-ornithine derivative into a peptide sequence. After piperidine-mediated Fmoc-deprotection and/or removal of the acid labile protective groups by treatment with a trifluoroacetic acid (TFA)-triisopropylsilane (TIS)-H_2O cocktail, introduction of the guanidine moiety was performed using an excess of 1,3-di-Boc-2-(trifluoromethylsulfonyl)guanidine in DMF, in the presence of triethylamine, followed by removal of the Boc-protective groups. Cleavage of peptides **13** and **14** from the resin was achieved by treatment with methanol in the presence of DIEA and DMF giving direct access to the methyl ester protected dipeptide. Compound **14** was obtained as a tri-guanylated derivative. On the contrary, as expected, the steric hindrance of the quaternary β-amino group of compound **13** prevents any reaction on the backbone amine. In addition, NMR analysis confirmed that peptide **13** was only guanylated on the amine side-chains. Several studies have reported that the N-terminal capping of cationic peptides with a fatty acid moiety enhances their antimicrobial activity [28,29]. Thus, in order to further improve the potency of **11**, an additional hydrophobic group was incorporated, first on the N-terminal end of the sequence. (Figure 4, peptides **17–19**).

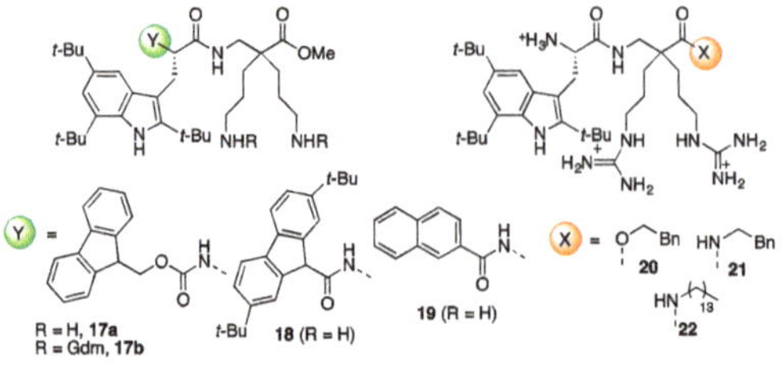

Figure 4. Pharmacomodulation of antimicrobial peptide.

We also evaluated whether such a capping effect could be also observed in this series of peptides. The biological activities of Fmoc-protected derivatives Fmoc-Tbt-$\beta^{2,2}$-*h*-bis-Orn-OMe **17a** and Fmoc-Tbt-$\beta^{2,2}$-*h*-bis-Arg-OMe **17b** were synthesized in addition to the ones of the two compounds **18** and **19** capped through a more robust amide bond at their N-terminal end. All peptides were purified to >95% homogeneity by preparative RP-HPLC and the mass of each purified peptide was checked by MALDI MS (see Supporting Information).

Finally, in order to study the influence Trp- and Tbt derivatives, we compared the retention time in RP-HPLC of selected peptides (Figure 5).

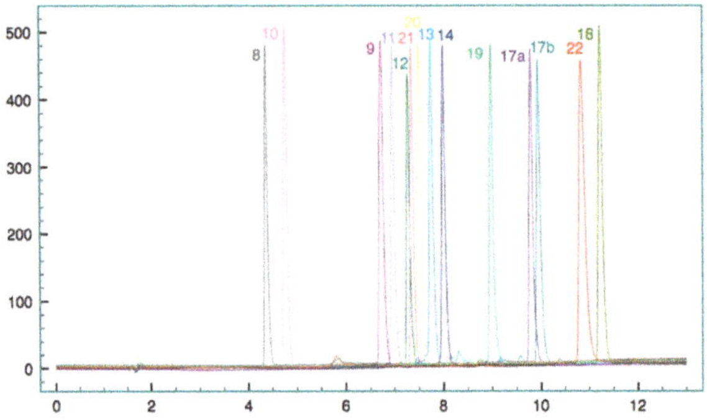

Figure 5. Superimposition of the analytical HPLC of peptides **8** to **22** on a C18 column, using as eluting gradient H_2O containing 0.1% TFA with 5% to 100% with MeCN containing 0.1% TFA.

2.3. *Biological Activities*

2.3.1. Antimicrobial, Hemolytic, and Cytotoxic Activities and Serum Stability

The antibacterial activities of the peptides were then investigated in the conditions reported by Svendsen, by determining the Minimal Inhibitory Concentration (MIC, µg/mL) on six strains of bacteria; three Gram-positive, *Staphylococcus aureus* ATCC25923, *Enterococcus faecalis* ATCC29212, and the methicillin resistant *Staphylococcus aureus* SA-1199B, and three Gram-negative, *Escherichia coli* ATCC25922, *Pseudomonas aeruginosa* ATCC27853, and *Acinetobacter baumannii* ATCC19606 [14] (Table 1). The tri-peptide Arg-Tbt-Arg-NH_2 reported by Svendsen (called here peptide A), and the dipeptide Tbt-Arg-OMe (called here peptide B), were used as positive controls of our experimental conditions.

The hemolytic and cytotoxic activities against human cells of all active peptides were assessed (Table 1, Figures 6 and 7 and Supporting Information).

Table 1. Biological activity, hemolytic activities, and cytotoxicity.

	MIC in µg/mL (µM)						% Hemolysis		% Cytotoxicity[a]	
	S. aureus ATCC25923	*S. aureus* 1199B	*E. faecalis* ATCC29212	*E. coli* ATCC25922	*P. aeruginosa* ATCC27853	*A. baumannii* ATCC19606	10 µM	50 µM	10 µM	50 µM
A	8 (12)	16 (23)	32 (47)	>64 (>93)	32 (47)	>64 (>93)	ND	ND	ND	ND
B	8 (15)	16 (30)	16 (30)	>64 (>120)	>64 (>120)	>64 (>120)	ND	ND	ND	ND
8	>64 (>16)	>64 (16)	>64 (>16)	>64 (>16)	>64 (>16)	>64 (>16)	ND	ND	ND	ND
9	8 (14)	>64 (112)	>64 (112)	>64 (112)	>64 (112)	>64 (112)	ND	ND	ND	ND
10	64 (120)	>64 (120)	>64 (120)	>64 (120)	>64 (120)	>64 (120)	ND	ND	ND	ND
11	2 (3)	16 (24)	16 (24)	8 (12)	4 (6)	64 (97)	<1	20	<1	<1
12	2 (3)	8 (12)	8 (12)	2 (3)	2 (3)	64 (92)	<1	30	<1	<1
13	2 (3)	2 (3)	4 (6)	8 (12)	8 (12)	>64 (97)	<1	10	<1	<1
14	8 (12)	8 (12)	8 (12)	32 (46)	>64 (92)	64 (92)	<1	20	<1	<1
17a	4 (5)	2 (2.5)	2 (2.5)	>64 (80)	>64 (80)	4 (5)	80	ND	45	85
17b	4 (4)	2 (2)	2 (2)	>64 (73)	>64 (73)	4 (4)	70	ND	10	80
18	8 (9)	8 (9)	8 (9)	>64 (73)	>64 (73)	64 (73)	20	ND	50	80
19	2 (3)	2 (3)	2 (3)	8 (11)	16 (22)	32 (44)	25	ND	55	80
20	1 (1.5)	2 (3)	2 (3)	2 (3)	8 (11)	8 (11)	2	30	<1	55
21	2 (3)	4 (6)	8 (11)	8 (11)	>64 (88)	8 (11)	5	30	<1	<1
22	32 (48)	>64 (96)	>64 (96)	>64 (96)	>64 (96)	>64 (96)	ND	ND	ND	ND

Minimal inhibitory concentrations (MIC in µg/mL) were measured against three Gram-positive (*S. aureus* ATCC25923, *S. aureus* 1199B, and *E. faecalis* ATCC29212) and three Gram-negative strains (*E. coli* ATCC25922, *P. aeruginosa* ATCC27853, and *A. baumannii* ATCC19606). Hemolytic activity against juvenile rat cells (Figure 6) and cytotoxicity against human SHSY5 cells (Figure 7) were measured after incubation of the peptides at 10 and/or 50 µM, respectively for one and three hours. ND: not determined.

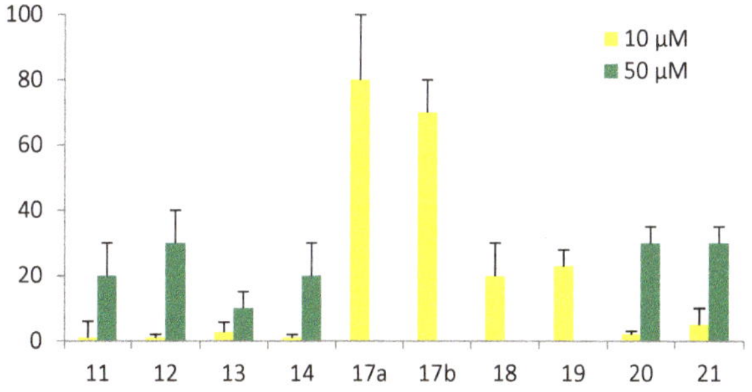

Figure 6. Percentage of hemolysis (see Supporting Information). The given results correspond to a percentage calculated as follows: %age = absorbance obtained with the peptide - absorbance obtained with the negative control (=buffer alone)/absorbance obtained with the positive control (=triton). * The haemolytic activities of peptides **17a**, **17b**, **18**, and **19** were not measured at 50 µM because of their poor solubility at such concentration.

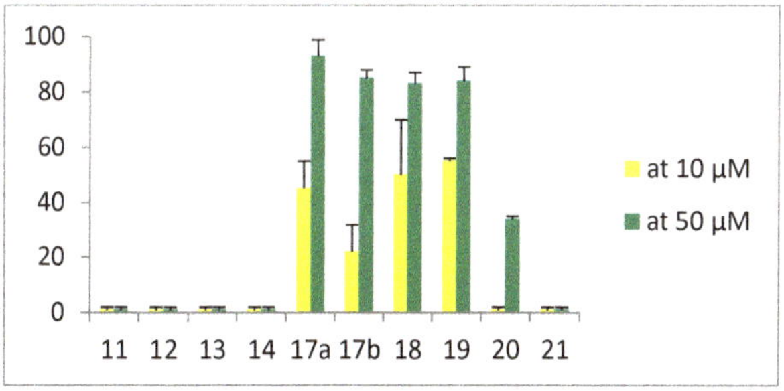

Figure 7. Percentage of cell death (see Supporting Information).

2.3.2. Interaction with Membrane Model

Although the mechanism of action of AMPs is still an active field of research, it is generally admitted that a common primary mode of action involves the disruption of cellular membrane. In order to get some insights into the mechanism of action, biophysical studies were conducted with membrane model. We used the intrinsic fluorescent properties of the tryptophan residue, as initial analysis of the bactericidal mechanism [30]. Depending on its environment in peptides, the wavelength of the fluorescence light emitted by the aromatic tryptophan residues varies. In a polar environment (water), λmax is circa 357 nm, whereas in a non-polar one, λmax shifts to shorter wavelengths (blue-shift). Moreover, the emission intensity increases when the tryptophan residue enters into a hydrophobic environment [31]. We therefore recorded the fluorescence of the most active peptide **11** and compared it to the inactive one **10** (Figure 8).

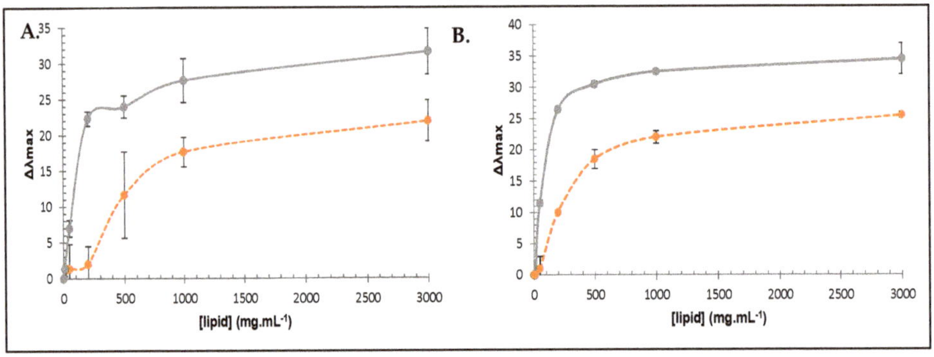

Figure 8. Lipid-induced changes in tryptophan fluorescence of peptide **11** (full line) and **10** (dashed line). Blue-shift for tryptophan in the wavelength of maximal emission in the presence of large unilamellar vesicles (LUVs) produced from *S. aureus* ATCC25923′ phospholipids (**A**) and from *E. coli* K12 (**B**) (see Supporting Information).

2.3.3. In Vivo Experiment Studies

In vivo experiment studies were conducted on septic mice. Sepsis is a life-threatening condition described as a syndrome of infection complicated by acute organ dysfunction. It is still a leading cause of death in intensive care units despite early antibiotic strategies to control bacterial infection [32]. Therefore, the rapidity and efficacy of antibacterial strategies are highly connected to the outcome of this acute disease and patient survival. After acute cecal ligature and puncture (CLP), peptide **11** or PBS (negative control) were injected to mice and survival was observed (Figure 9).

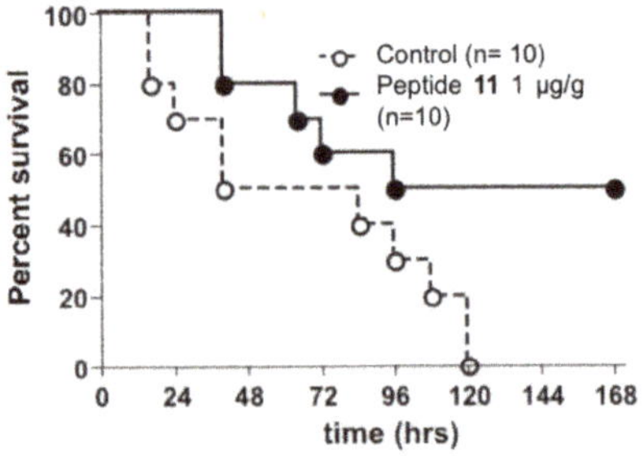

Figure 9. Survival after acute cecal ligature and puncture (CLP) in PBS-injected mice (open circle; n = 10) and peptide 11-injected mice (closed circle; n = 10). Kaplan–Meier curves and log-rank test were used to analyze the mortality rate; P = 0.0299.

3. Discussion

We have designed small AMPs based on new polycationic β-amino acids, $\beta^{2,2}$- and $\beta^{3,3}$-*homo*-bis-ornithine derivatives. These moieties mimic the cationic side chains of two lysine residues or two arginine residues and thus allow shortening the cationic AMP size. Their combination with the supertryptophan residue (2,5,7-tri-tertbutyltryptophane) reported by Svendsen and co-workers allows obtaining highly active antimicrobial dipeptides. They exhibit activity in the range of 2 to 16 µg/mL (Table 1), values that are promising for compounds to enter into clinical trials. Among the different peptides tested, several $\beta^{2,2}$- and $\beta^{3,3}$-*bis* cationic derivatives (peptides **11–14**) were potent killing agents against the different strains, with MIC values comparable to or lower than that of the positive controls, and no significant difference was observed between the compound derived from the $\beta^{2,2}$- (**11**) and $\beta^{3,3}$-*h*-bis-Arg (**13**). Noticeably, the $\beta^{2,2}$-amino acid derivatives are easier to synthesize.

Some structure activity relationships can be drawn from these results. First, the importance of the guanidinium groups for the antimicrobial activity is highlighted, since peptide **9**, containing the $\beta^{2,2}$-*h*-bis-Orn, shows little antimicrobial activity against all strains (except *S. aureus*) compared to the $\beta^{2,2}$-*h*-bis-Arg analog **11**. This net difference in the antimicrobial activity of arginine- and lysine-containing compounds agrees with the literature and is believed to result from the stronger ability of the guanidinium group to form bidentate hydrogen bonds with the phosphate moiety of phospholipid polar heads, in addition to electrostatic interactions [33]. Oppositely, the absence of difference in the antimicrobial activity of peptides **11** and **12** indicates that the additional guanidinium group on the β-amine has little influence, suggesting that the cationic group on the N-terminal end is not involved in the pharmacophore of the peptide.

Another important point is the positive influence of the *t*-Bu group on the tryptophan moiety, similar to the peptide reported by Svendsen et al. Indeed, in comparison to **11** or **12**, peptide **10** presents no activity on the tested strains. This lack of activity can be related to the lower lipophilicity of tryptophan compared to the Tbt derivatives **11** and **12**, confirmed by its lower retention time in RP-HPLC (Figure 5) together with its lower capacity to interact with membrane. Indeed, the larger size of Tbt compared to Trp (around 2.5-fold) could allow a deeper penetration of this hydrophobic residue into the phospholipid bilayer and an effective disruption of the membrane that is not allowed by the smaller indole moiety. In order to evaluate this hypothesis, we recorded the fluorescence of the active peptide **11**, and compared it to the inactive peptide **10**. The tryptophan fluorescence spectra of both peptides in aqueous buffer had a maximum emission at 355 nm. Addition of increasing concentration of large unilamellar vesicles (LUVs), prepared from phospholipids directly extracted from *S. epidermidis*, showed large blue-shift (near 35 nm) in the emission maxima of peptide **11**, characteristic of the embedding of Trp side chain into the hydrophobic medium of the negatively charged phospholipid (Figure 2). For peptide **10**, the blue-shift was 10 nm smaller with apparent binding constant K_L (lipid concentration that induced 50% of maximal blue-shift) about 3 times lower for peptide **11** (90 ± 2 mg·mL^{-1} s and 100 ± 1.5 mg·mL^{-1}, respectively with *S. aureus* LUVs and *E. coli* LUVs) than for peptide **10** (280 ± 1.5 mg·mL^{-1} and 500 ± 6 mg·mL^{-1} with *S. aureus* LUVs and *E. coli* LUVs). These preliminary biophysical studies on the interaction of **11** with model membrane suggested that this compound indeed could act as an antimicrobial peptide, by destabilizing the bacterial membrane. We are aware that deeper investigations might be performed in order to assess the mechanism by which this membrane permeabilization occurs.

Interestingly, the sequence of the dipeptides seemed to have an influence on the bacterial activity. Indeed, even though the reverse peptide **14** had a similar activity against Gram-positive bacteria as the one of peptide **12**, its potency against some of the Gram-negative strains was significantly lower. This decreased activity was accompanied by a higher hydrophobicity according to its longer retention time on reversed-phase HPLC (Figure 5). We anticipate that since the chemical composition of these peptides is similar, these different behaviors are likely related to a different spatial arrangement of the cationic and hydrophobic side-chains, giving a different amphiphilicity to peptide **14** vs. **12**. Indeed, AMPs usually adopt facially amphiphilic conformations in which cationic hydrophilic and hydrophobic side chains segregate onto opposite regions of the molecular surface. The importance of this overall topology and not the precise sequence, secondary structure, or chirality of the peptides has been highlighted as key features for their cell-killing activity [34]. Seminal works from Seebach [11] and more recently from Balaram [13,35] suggest that achiral $\beta^{2,2}$-amino acids are β-turn inducers. In order to get some insight into the solution structure of these peptides, ^{1}H NMR studies were conducted in D_2O. Assignment of the proton signals was achieved by combination of COSY, TOCSY, and NOESY measurements. The data reveal that for peptides **9**, **11**, and **12**, one of the two β-protons CH_2NH of the $\beta^{2,2}$-*h*bis-Arg is significantly down-field shifted (2.4, 1.8 ppm, and 2.8 ppm respectively for **9**, **11**, and **12**) compared to the other (3.5 ppm), which is not the case for peptide **14**. Moreover, the presence of the *t*Bu group on the indole moiety has an important effect on the chemical shift of this proton since for peptides **8** and **10**, the chemical shift of this proton is 3.1–3.2 ppm. Altogether, these data suggest a close proximity between the β-protons CH_2NH of the $\beta^{2,2}$-*h*bis-Arg and the indole moiety in peptides **9**, **11**, and **12**, most likely because of cation-π interactions. Regardless of its nature, this specific conformation might favor the interaction of the peptide with the bacterial membrane and bring an explanation for the different biological behaviors of the two isomers **12** and **14** towards Gram-negative bacteria.

Regarding hemolysis (Figure 6), significant hemolytic effect was observed only at concentrations much higher than the antibacterial MIC values for the four most active peptides **11–14**, indicating a good selectivity of the compounds for bacterial cells over mammalian cells. Moreover, no cytotoxicity was observed for the 4 peptides **11–14** on human SHSYS5 cells. Finally, while introduction of fluorenyl or naphtyl group led to improved antibacterial activity for peptides **17–19**, this enhancement was, however, accompanied by a decreased selectivity on bacteria, and a significant increase in hemolysis and cytotoxicity on human cells (Table 1). We then evaluated the influence of an additional hydrophobic group on the C-terminal end (peptides **20–22**). While replacement of methyl ester with benzyl ester (**20**) or benzamide (**21**) gave peptides with enhanced efficiency, the incorporation of an alkyl chain (**22**) completely abolished the antimicrobial activity, probably reflecting an inappropriate balance between hydrophobicity and charge in this peptide.

Altogether, we selected peptide **11** as the best candidate for further analysis of its potential as therapeutic agent, thanks to its lack of haemolytic and cytolytic activity on mammalian cells and the easier synthesis of $\beta^{2,2}$-*h*-bis-Orn-OH compared to $\beta^{3,3}$-*h*-bis-Orn-OH. Since the incorporation of β-amino acids into peptides is known to improve their metabolic stability, the serum stability of this compound was first evaluated in human plasma (See Figure 10), where it appeared to be completely stable over 24 h, as expected for β-amino acids containing peptides sequences compared to a positive control peptide (4NGG) that was fully degraded in 20 mn (See 4. Materials and Methods).

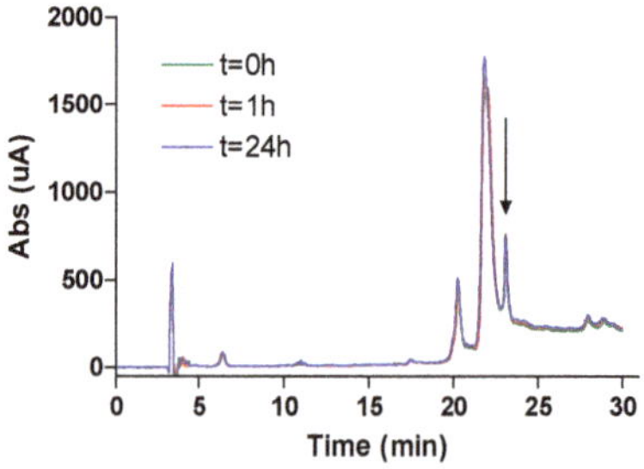

Figure 10. Serum stability of compound **11** evaluated in human plasma (See Supporting Information).

The potency of peptide **11** was finally assessed in vivo in septic mice. In order to analyze its potential, mice were subjected to the acute model of sepsis "high grad sepsis" in which less than 50% of the mice survived to the procedure (See SI). In our technical conditions, 100% of the CLP-induced control mice succumbed during the five days following the induction of sepsis (Figure 9). However, the mice treated with one peritoneal injection of the peptide at 1 µg/g show a significant increase of the survival rate. Indeed, 50% of the mice treated with peptide **11** survived the acute peritonitis. The results revealed that the injection of peptide **11** induced an increase in the survival rate of CLP-treated mice.

Finally, this study validates these polycationic residues as new tools for the design of short bioactive antimicrobial cationic peptides. These new unnatural arginine analogs might be useful tools for other applications for which cationic residues are a key player, such as cell-penetrating peptides or RNA ligands.

4. Materials and Methods

4.1. General Considerations

All reactions were carried out under argon atmosphere with dry commercial or freshly distilled solvents under anhydrous conditions unless otherwise stated. All reagents were purchased from commercial suppliers and used without further purification. Flash chromatography was performed using silica gel Merck 60 (0.040–0.063 μm, Molsheim, France). Analytical thin-layer chromatography (TLC) was performed using silica gel Merck 60 on alumina, visualized by UV fluorescence at 254 nm, and revealed with ninhydrin (0.3% in *n*-butanol/AcOH) or phosphomolybdic acid (solution in EtOH).

4.2. Solid Phase Peptide Synthesis

All reactions were carried out in Polypropylene Torviq syringes (sizes 5, 10, 20, or 50 mL) equipped with a porous polypropylene disc at the bottom and closed with an appropriate cap. HMBA resin (4-(Hydroxymethyl)benzoyl-aminoethyl) polystyrene (200–400 mesh, 0.8–1.2 mmol/g) was purchased from Iris Biotech (Marktredwitz, Germany). The loading of the Fmoc amino acid coupled resin was determined using a Cary3 *Uv/v*IS spectrometer (Agilent, Santa-Clara, CA, USA). *O*-(Benzotriazol-1-yl)-*N,N,N′,N′*-tetramethyluronium hexafluorophosphate (HBTU) and 2-(1H-9-azabenzotriazole-1-yl)-1,1,3,3-tetramethyluronium hexafluorophosphate (HATU) were purchased from Iris Biotech. Solvents were purchased from VWR in HPLC grade and used without further purification. Purifications were performed by reverse-phase HPLC either on a Waters preparative HPLC system connected to a Breeze software (Fisher Scientific, Illkirch, France), using a *Waters XBridge* column (RP C18, 19 × 50 mm, 5 μm, 135 Å) at a flow rate of 14 mL/min or a Dionex semi-preparative HPLC-system connected to a Chromeleon software (Fisher Scientific, Illkirch, France), using a C18 semi-preparative column from AIT at a flow rate of 5 mL/min; and using as eluent A, H_2O containing 0.1% of TFA, and as eluent B, CH_3CN containing 0.1% of TFA. UV detection was done at 220 nm and 280 nm. Purification gradients were chosen to get a ramp of approximately 1% solution B per minute in the interest area. Peptide fractions from purification were analyzed by analytical HPLC, pooled according to their purity, partly concentrated under vacuum, and freeze-dried on an Alpha 2/4 freeze dryer from Bioblock Scientific (Fisher Bioblock Scientific, Rungis, France) to get the expected peptide as a powder.

4.3. Product Characterisation

NMR spectra were recorded on Bruker ARX 250 (Bruker, France SAS, Wissembourg, France) or Brucker Avance III 300 spectrometers (Bruker, France SAS, Wissembourg, France) unless otherwise noted. Proton chemical shifts values (δ) are reported in parts per million (ppm) downfield from tetramethylsilane (TMS) unless noted otherwise. Coupling constants (*J*) are reported in Hertz (Hz). Carbon chemical shifts values (δ) are reported in parts permillion (ppm) with reference to internal solvent $CDCl_3$ (77.00 ppm) or CD_3OD (49.00 ppm). Multiplicities are abbreviated as follows: Singlet (s), doublet (d), triplet (t), quartet (q), multiplet (m), and broad singlet (bs). Signal assignments were made using COSY and HSQC experiments, and for peptides NOESY (250 ms mixing time), TOCSY (80 ms mixing time), and DQF-COSY spectra. High-resolution mass spectra (HRMS) were obtained on a Finnigan MAT 95 instrument and are given as experimental (found) and theoretical (calcd). Analytical RP-HPLC were performed on either a Waters system connected to a Breeze software or a Dionex system connected to a Chromeleon software. Waters system consisted of a binary pump (Waters 1525) and a dual wavelength Uv/visible Absorbance detector (Waters 2487, Saint-Quentin-en-Yveline, France). Dionex system consisted in an analytical automated LC system (Ultimate 3000) equipped with an auto sampler, a pump block composed of two ternary gradient pumps, and a dual wavelength detector. The analyses were performed on C18 analytical columns (from AIT (Paris, France) or Higgins (San Diego, CA, USA)) using as eluent A, H_2O containing 0.1% of TFA and as eluent B, CH_3CN containing 0.1% of TFA, at a flow rate of 1 mL/min. UV detection was done at 220 and 280 nm. Peptides were characterized by MALDI-TOF MS (DE-Pro, PerSeptive Biosystems, Framingham, MA, USA) in positive ion reflector mode using the matrix α-cyano-4-hydroxy-cinnamic acid (CHCA). Peptide molecular weights were determined for the free amine and not for the TFA salts.

4.3.1. Synthesis of H-$\beta^{2,2}$ *h*bis-Orn(Boc)$_2$OMe 1 and Fmoc $\beta^{2,2}$ *h*bis-Orn(Boc)$_2$OH 2 (Scheme 5)

Methyl 2,4-dicyano-2-(2-cyanoethyl)butanoate **23**: Methyl 2-cyanoacetate (10 g, 100 mmol) was mixed with acrylonitrile (11.7 g, 220 mmol) in a three-necked round bottom flask equipped with a condenser and an addition funnel. Triethylamine (6.8 mL, 50 mmol) was added dropwise at 0 °C through the addition funnel. The reaction was stirred continuously and allowed to react overnight at rt. After confirming completion of the reaction by TLC, AcOEt was added. The organic layer was washed with 5% citric acid solution and brine, dried over $MgSO_4$, filtered, and evaporated. The product precipitated overnight. The solid was washed with AcOEt and obtained as a pale yellow powder (19.27 g, 93% yield); $\mathbf{R_f}$ (Cy/AcOEt, 1:1) = 0.47; ^{1}H NMR (250 MHz, $CDCl_3$) δ 3.87 (s, 3H, CO_2CH_3), 2.37–2.62 (m, 4H, $CH_2\beta$), 2.31 (ddd, *J* = 15.5 Hz, 8.6 Hz, 6.8 Hz, 2H, $CH_2\gamma$), 2.14 (ddd, *J* = 14.2 Hz, 8.6 Hz, 6.1 Hz, 2H, $CH_2\gamma$); ^{13}C NMR (75 MHz, $CDCl_3$): δ 166.6 (C, C=O), 117.2 (2C, C≡Nγ), 116.1 (C, C≡N α), 54.30 (CH_3, CO_2CH_3), 47.6 (C, Cα), 32.1 (2CH_2, $CH_2\beta$), 13.6 (2CH_2, $CH_2\gamma$); MS-ESI+: calcd for $C_{10}H_{11}N_3O_2$ 205.09, calcd for $C_{10}H_{11}N_3O_2Na$ 228.08, found 228.07 $[M + Na]^+$.

Methyl 2-cyano-4-(Boc)amine-2-(3-(Boc)amine propyl)pentanoate **4**: Compound **23** (10 g, 49 mmol) was dissolved in methanol (25 mL). Boc_2O (23.5 g, 108 mmol) and PtO_2 (2.2 g, 9.8 mmol) were added and the reaction mixture was stirred at rt for 3 days under 5 bars of H_2 pressure. The reaction mixture was filtered through a celite pad and evaporated to dryness. The crude compound was purified by flash chromatography (Cy/AcOEt 100:0 → 70:30) to afford yellowish oil (5 g, 21% yield); $\mathbf{R_f}$ (Cy/AcOEt, 1:1) = 0.56; ^{1}H NMR (300 MHz, $CDCl_3$): δ (ppm) 4.69 (bs, 2H, *NH*), 3.76 (s, 3H, CO_2CH_3), 3.08–3.20 (m, 4H, $CH_2\delta$), 1.44–2 (m, 8H, $CH_2\beta\alpha\nu\delta CH_2\gamma$), 1.37–1.50 (m, 18H, $C(CH_3)_3$).; ^{13}C NMR (62.5 MHz, $CDCl_3$) δ 169.1 (C, C=O ester), 155.8 (2C, C=O carbamate), 118.7 (C, C≡N), 79.3 (2C, $C(CH_3)_3$), 53.3 (CH_3, CO_2CH_3), 49.1 (C, Cα), 39.7 (2CH_2, $CH_2\delta$), 34.4 (2CH_2, $CH_2\beta$), 28.2 (6CH_3, $C(CH_3)_3$), 26.1 (2CH_2, $CH_2\gamma$).; MS-ESI+: calcd for $C_{20}H_{35}N_3O_6$ 413.25, calcd for $C_{20}H_{35}N_3O_6Na$ 436.24, found 436.24 $[M + Na]^+$.

*H-$\beta^{2,2}$ h*bis-*Orn(Boc)$_2$OMe* **1**: Compound **4** (2.35 g, 4.9 mmol) was dissolved in methanol (100 mL). Raney nickel was added, and the mixture was stirred under 5 bars of H_2 pressure at rt for 3 days. The reaction mixture was filtered through a celite pad and evaporated to dryness. The product was used in peptide synthesis without further purification. (2.0 g, 98% yield); $\mathbf{R_f}$ (Cy/AcOEt, 1:1) = 0.56; ^{1}H NMR (300 MHz, MeOD) δ 3.68 (s, 3H, CO_2CH_3), 3.01 (t, *J* = 6.7 Hz, 4H, $CH_2\delta$), 2.77 (s, 2H, $CH_2\beta\varepsilon$), 1.55–1.60 (m, 4H, $CH_2\beta$), 1.32–1.43 (m, 22H, $CH_2\gamma$ and $C(CH_3)_3$); ^{13}C NMR (75 MHz, MeOD) δ 177.9 (C, C=O ester), 158.6 (2C, C=O carbamate), 79.9 (2C, $C(CH_3)_3$), 52.4 (CH_3, CO_2CH_3), 51.5 (C, Cα), 45.9 (CH_2, $CH_2\beta\varepsilon$), 41.6 (2CH_2, $CH_2\delta$), 31.2 (2CH_2, $CH_2\beta$), 28.8 (6CH_3, $C(CH_3)_3$), 25.4 (2CH_2, $CH_2\gamma$); HRMS-ESI+: calcd for $C_{20}H_{39}N_3O_6$ 417.2839, found 418.2915 $[M + H]^+$.

*Fmoc $\beta^{2,2}$ h*bis-*Orn(Boc)$_2$OH* **2**: Compound **4** (2.3 g, 5.6 mmol) was dissolved in methanol (125 mL). An aqueous solution of sodium hydroxide (2 M) (12.5 mL, 25 mmol) and Raney nickel were added. The mixture was stirred under 5 bars of H_2 pressure at rt for 7 days. The reaction mixture was filtered through a celite pad and evaporated to dryness. The crude compound was dissolved in a 1:1 mixture of THF and water (150 mL). FmocOSu (2.3 g, 6.8 mmol) and K_2CO_3 (1.7 g, 12.2 mmol) were added.

The solution was allowed to react at rt overnight. After confirming the completion of the reaction by TLC, THF was evaporated. The resulting aqueous solution was acidified to pH = 2 by dropwise addition of 1M hydrochloric acid at 0 °C. The product was extracted with AcOEt, dried over $MgSO_4$, filtered, and concentrated *in vacuo*. The crude compound was purified by flash chromatography (Cy/AcOEt/AcOH 100:0:1 → 75:25:1) to afford a white powder (2.5 g, 72% yield); $\mathbf{R_f}$ (Cy/AcOEt/AcOH, 7:3:0.1) = 0.27; ^{1}H NMR (250 MHz, $CDCl_3$) δ 7.75 (d, *J* = 7.2 Hz, 2H, *CH* Ar), 7.58 (d, *J* = 7.2 Hz, 2H, *CH* Ar), 7.19–7.39 (m, 4H, *CH* Ar), 5.54 (bs, 1H, *NH* Fmoc), 4.95 (bs, 2H, *NH Boc*), 4.40 (d, *J* = 6.5 Hz, 2H, CH_2 Fmoc), 4.20 (t, *J* = 6.5 Hz, 1H, *CH* Fmoc), 3.38–3.41 (m, 2H, $CH_2\beta\varepsilon$), 3.07 (m, 4H, $CH_2\delta$), 1.20–1.67 (m, 26H, $CH_2\beta$, $CH_2\gamma$ and $C(CH_3)_3$); ^{13}C NMR (62.5 MHz, $CDCl_3$) δ 176.5 (C, C=O acid), 157.20, 156.4 (3C, C=O carbamate), 143.9, 141.3 (4C, *C* Ar), 129.1, 128.2, 127.7, 127.1, 125.3, 125.1, 120.0 (8CH, CH Ar), 79.3 (2C, *C*$(CH_3)_3$), 67.0 (CH_2, CH_2 Fmoc), 49.8 (CH_2, $CH_2\beta\varepsilon$), 47.2 (CH, CH Fmoc), 40.7 ($2CH_2$, $CH_2\delta$), 40.6 (C, Cα), 30.6 ($2CH_2$, $CH_2\beta$), 28.4 ($6CH_3$, $C(CH_3)_3$), 24.3 ($2CH_2$, $CH_2\gamma$); HRMS-ESI+: calcd for $C_{34}H_{47}N_3O_8$ 625.3255, calcd for $C_{34}H_{47}N_3O_8Na$ 648,3153, found 648.3261 $[M + Na]^+$.

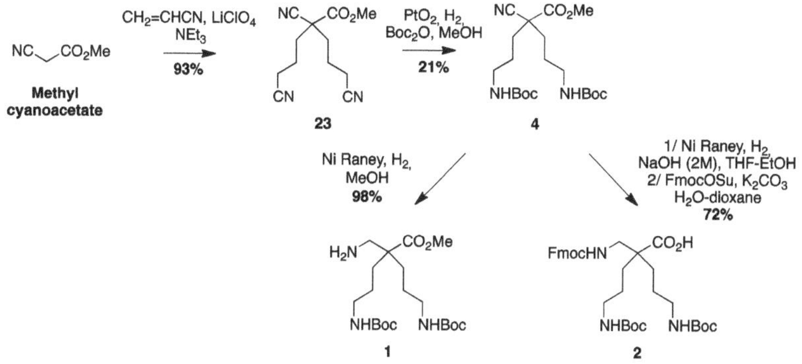

Scheme 5. Synthesis of H-$\beta^{2,2}$ h bis-Orn$(Boc)_2$OMe 1 and Fmoc $\beta^{2,2}$ h bis-Orn$(Boc)_2$OH.

4.3.2. Synthesis of Boc-$\beta^{3,3}$ *h*bis-Orn$(Boc)_2$OH **3** (Scheme 6)

*1-Benzyl 3-*tert*-butyl 2,2-bis(2-cyanoethyl)malonate* **24**: Benzyl *tert*-butylmalonate (25 g, 96.4 mmol) was mixed with acrylonitrile (14 mL, 210 mmol). Triethylamine (5.3 mL, 40 mmol) was added dropwise, followed by lithium perchlorate (5.4 g, 50 mmol). The reaction was stirred continuously and allowed to react overnight. After confirming completion of the reaction by TLC, AcOEt was added to the reaction mixture. The organic layer was washed with 5% citric acid solution and brine, dried over $MgSO_4$, filtered, and evaporated. The crude compound was purified by flash chromatography (Cy/AcOEt, 100:0 to 8:2) to afford a yellow oil (30.2 g, 88% yield); $\mathbf{R_f}$ (Cy/AcOEt, 8:2) = 0.37; ^{1}H NMR (250 MHz, $CDCl_3$) δ 7.37 (m, 5H, *CH* Ar), 5.20 (s, 2H, CH_2Ph), 2.17–2.43 (m, 8H, $CH_2\beta\alpha\nu\delta CH_2\gamma$), 1.35 (s, 9H, $C(CH_3)_3$); ^{13}C NMR (62.5 MHz, $CDCl_3$) δ 169.2, 167.9 (2C, C=O), 134.5 (C, *C* Ar), 128.9, 128.8, 128.5, 127, 126.2 (5CH, CH Ar), 118.5 (2C, C≡N), 84 (C, *C*$(CH_3)_3$), 67.9 (CH_2, CH_2Ph), 56.2 (C, Cα), 29.5 ($2CH_2$, $CH_2\beta$), 27.6 ($3CH_3$, $C(CH_3)_3$), 13 ($2CH_2$, $CH_2\gamma$); HRMS-ESI+: calcd for $C_{20}H_{24}N_2O_4$ 356.1736, calcd for $C_{20}H_{24}N_2O_4Na$ 379,1634, found 379.1628 $[M + Na]^+$.

2-(Tert-butoxycarbonyl)-4-cyano-2-(2-cyanoethyl)butanoic acid **5**: Compound **24** (18 g, 51 mmol) was dissolved in MeOH (500 mL). Ammonium formate (16.7 g, 265 mmol) and Pd/C (5.1 g, 100 mg/mmol) were added and the reaction mixture was stirred for 3 h. Afterward, the reaction mixture was filtered through a celite pad to remove the Pd/C before evaporation to dryness. The product was diluted with dichloromethane. The organic layer was washed with 10% citric acid solution and brine, dried over $MgSO_4$, filtered, and evaporated to afford an oil. The product was used in the following step without further purification. (11.34 g, 83% yield); $\mathbf{R_f}$ (Cy/AcOEt/AcOH, 8:2:0.1) = 0.1; ^{1}H NMR (250 MHz, $CDCl_3$) δ 2.41–2.54 (m, 4H, $CH_2\beta$), 2.20 (t, *J* = 7.5 Hz, 4H, $CH_2\gamma$), 1.51 (s, 9H, $C(CH_3)_3$); ^{13}C NMR

(62.5 MHz, $CDCl_3$) δ 173.1 (C, C=O acid), 168.3 (C, C=O ester), 118.5 (2C, C≡N), 84.8 (C, $C(CH_3)_3$), 56.2 (C, Cα), 30.0 (2CH_2, CH_2β), 27.8 (3CH_3, $C(CH_3)_3$), 13.1 (2CH_2, CH_2γ); HRMS-ESI+: calcd for $C_{13}H_{18}N_2O_4$ 266.1267, calcd for $C_{13}H_{18}N_2O_4Na$ 289,1165, found 289.1159 $[M + Na]^+$.

1-Tert-butyl 4-methyl 2,2-bis(2-cyanoethyl)succinate **6**: Compound **5** (9.0 g, 34 mmol) was dissolved in DCM under Argon. 1-Chloro-*N*,*N*-2-trimethylpropenylamine (9.0 mL, 68 mmol) was added. The solution was stirred for 2 h then concentrated *in vacuo*. The residue was dissolved in dry acetonitrile (170 mL) and cooled to 0 °C. DIEA (11.9 mL, 68 mmol) and a 2M solution of trimethylsilyldiazomethane in Et_2O (34 mL, 68 mmol) was added. The reaction mixture was stirred at 0 °C for 16 h. The organic solvents were evaporated *in vacuo*. The residue was dissolved in AcOEt and washed with 10% citric acid, saturated $NaHCO_3$ and brine. Finally, the organic layer was dried over $MgSO_4$, filtered, and evaporated to dryness. The crude compound was dissolved in DMF (180 mL) and MeOH (90 mL) then Ag_2O (39.4 g, 170 mmol) was added. The reaction mixture was refluxed for 10 min. After evaporation of MeOH, diethyl ether and a saturated solution of NH_4Cl were added slowly and the mixture was filtered through a celite pad. The organic layer was separated and washed with a saturated solution of NH_4Cl, dried over $MgSO_4$, filtered, and evaporated. The crude compound was purified by flash chromatography (Cy/AcOEt, 100:0 to 60:40) to afford a yellow oil (2.1 g, 21% yield); $\mathbf{R_f}$ (Cy/AcOEt, 1:1) = 0.6; ^{1}H NMR (300 MHz, $CDCl_3$) δ 3.71 (s, 3H, CO_2CH_3), 2.61 (s, 2H, CH_2α), 2.27–2.37 (m, 4H, CH_2γ), 1.91–2.07 (m, 4H, CH_2δ), 1.48 (s, 9H, $C(CH_3)_3$); ^{13}C NMR (75 MHz, $CDCl_3$) δ 171.4, 170.1 (2C, C=O), 118.8 (2C, C≡N), 82.5 (C, $C(CH_3)_3$), 51.6 (CH_3, CO_2CH_3), 46.6 (CH_2, CH_2α), 37.4 (C, Cβ), 30.6 (2CH_2, CH_2γ), 27.5 (3CH_3, $C(CH_3)_3$), 12.3 (2CH_2, CH_2δ); HRMS-ESI+: calcd for $C_{15}H_{22}N_2O_4$ 294.1580, calcd for $C_{15}H_{22}N_2O_4Na$ 317,1478, found 317.4718 $[M + Na]^+$.

2,2-Bis(2-cyanoethyl)-4-methoxy-4-oxobutanoic acid **25**: Compound **6** (1.3 g, 4.4 mmol) was dissolved in DCM (40 mL). Triisopropylsilane (900 μL, 4.4 mmol) and TFA (40 mL) were added. The reaction mixture was stirred for 1 hour before evaporation to dryness. The crude compound was purified by flash chromatography (Cy/AcOEt/AcOH, 100:0:1 to 50:50:1) to afford a colorless oil (900 mg, 86% yield); $\mathbf{R_f}$ (Cy/AcOEt/AcOH, 5:5:0.1) = 0.34; ^{1}H NMR (300 MHz, $CDCl_3$) δ 3.66 (s, 3H, CO_2CH_3), 2.65 (s, 2H, CH_2α), 2.30–2.49 (m, 4H, CH_2γ), 1.98–2.16 (m, 4H, CH_2δ); ^{13}C NMR (75 MHz, $CDCl_3$) δ 177.9 (C, C=O acid), 170.5 (C, C=O ester), 118.7 (2C, C≡N), 52.4 (CH_3, CO_2CH_3), 46.3 (C, C β), 37.0 (CH_2, CH_2α), 30.8 (2CH_2, CH_2γ), 12.8 (2CH_2, CH_2δ); HRMS-ESI+: calcd for $C_{11}H_{14}N_2O_4$ 238.0954, calcd for $C_{11}H_{14}N_2O_4Na$ 261,0852, found 261.0845 $[M + Na]^+$.

Methyl 3-((tert-butoxycarbonyl)amino)-5-cyano-3-(2-cyanoethyl)pentanoate **7**: Compound **25** (450 mg, 1.9 mmol) was dissolved in dry acetone (15 mL) and cooled to 0° C. NEt_3 (300 μL, 2.3 mmol) and $ClCO_2Et$ (200 μL, 2.1 mmol) were added. The reaction mixture was stirred for 1.5 h. A solution of NaN_3 (309 mg, 4.75 mmol) in H_2O (8.5 mL) was added and the mixture was stirred at 0 °C for 2 additional hours. Acetone was evaporated and the compound was extracted with toluene. The organic layer was dried over $MgSO_4$ and filtered. The volume was reduced by evaporation to 20 mL. *tert*-BuOH (15 mL) was added and the reaction was refluxed for 16 h. The solvent was evaporated and the crude compound purified by flash chromatography (Cy/AcOEt, 100:0 to 7:3) to afford a white powder (200 mg, 35% yield); $\mathbf{R_f}$ (Cy/AcOEt, 1:1) = 0.44; ^{1}H NMR (300 MHz, $CDCl_3$) δ 5.17 (bs, 1H, *N*HBoc), 3.71 (s, 3H, CO_2CH_3), 2.60 (s, 2H, CH_2α), 2.22–2.45 (m, 6H, CH_2γ and $CH_2δ_1$), 1.99–2.12 (m, 2H, $CH_2δ_2$), 1.40 (s, 9H, $C(CH_3)_3$); ^{13}C NMR (75 MHz, $CDCl_3$) δ 170.4 (C, C=O ester), 154.3 (C, C=O carbamate), 119.2 (2C, C≡N), 80.5 and 80.4 (2C, $C(CH_3)_3$), 55.3 (C, Cβ), 52.4 (CH_3, CO_2CH_3), 39.5 (CH_2, CH_2α), 31.8 (2CH_2, CH_2γ), 28.3 (3CH_3, $C(CH_3)_3$), 12.0 (2CH_2, CH_2δ); HRMS-ESI+: calcd for $C_{15}H_{23}N_3O_4$ 309.1689, calcd for $C_{15}H_{23}N_3O_4Na$ 332,1587, found 332.1581 $[M + Na]^+$.

Methyl-3,6-bis((tert-butoxycarbonyl)amino)-3-(3-((tert-butoxycarbonyl)amino)propyl) hexanoate **26**: Compound **7** (145 mg, 0.47 mmol) was dissolved in a 9:1 mixture of methanol and chloroform. PtO_2 (16 mg, 0.07 mmol) was added and the reaction mixture was stirred under 5 bars of H_2 pressure at rt for 3 days. The reaction mixture was filtered through a celite pad and evaporated to dryness. The crude product was dissolved in a 1:1 mixture of THF/H_2O and Boc_2O was added. After stirring overnight, THF was evaporated and the product was extracted with DCM. The organic layer was washed with brine, dried over $MgSO_4$, filtered, and evaporated *in vacuo*. The crude compound was purified by flash chromatography (Cy/AcOEt, 7:3) to afford a colorless oil (150 mg, 62% yield); $\mathbf{R_f}$ (Cy/AcOEt, 1:1) = 0.68; ^{1}H NMR (300 MHz, $CDCl_3$) δ 4.85 (bs, 1H, *NH* Boc), 4.72 (bs, 2H, *NH* Boc), 3.64 (s, 3H, CO_2CH_3), 3.02–3.11 (m, 4H, $CH_2ε$), 2.61 (s, 2H, $CH_2α$), 1.56–1.77 (m, 4H, $CH_2γ$), 1.34–1.48 (m, 31H, $CH_2δ$ and $C(CH_3)_3$); ^{13}C NMR (75 MHz, $CDCl_3$) δ 171.7 (C, C=O ester), 156.0 (2C, C=O carbamate), 154.5 (C, C=O carbamate), 79.1 (3C, $C(CH_3)_3$), 56.1 (C, Cβ), 51.6 (CH_3, CO_2CH_3), 40.5 ($2CH_2$, $CH_2ε$), 40.3 (CH_2, $CH_2α$), 33.3 ($2CH_2$, $CH_2β$), 28.4 ($9CH_3$, $C(CH_3)_3$), 23.8 ($2CH_2$, $CH_2γ$); HRMS-ESI+: calcd for $C_{25}H_{47}N_3O_8$ 517.3363, calcd for $C_{25}H_{47}N_3O_8Na$ 540,3261, found 540.3255 $[M + Na]^+$.

*Boc-$β^{3,3}$ h*bis-*Orn(Boc)$_2$OH* **3**: *Compound* **26** (0.130 g, 0.25 mmol) was dissolved in a 1:1 mixture of THF/H_2O. LiOH (12 mg, 0.5 mmol) was added and the reaction mixture was stirred at rt for 5 days. THF was evaporated and the resulting aqueous solution was acidified to pH = 2 by dropwise addition of 1 M hydrochloric acid at 0 °C. The product was extracted with DCM and the organic layer was washed with brine, dried over $MgSO_4$, filtered, and evaporated to afford a white powder (120 mg, 98% yield). The product was used in following step without any further purification; $\mathbf{R_f}$ (Cy/AcOEt, 1:1) = 0.20; ^{1}H NMR (300 MHz, MeOD) δ 3.01 (t, *J* = 6.6 Hz, 4H, $CH_2ε$), 2.62 (s, 2H, $CH_2α$), 1.73 (m, 4H, $CH_2γ$), 1.42 (m, 31H, $CH_2δ$ and $C(CH_3)_3$); ^{13}C NMR (75 MHz, MeOD) δ 158.6 (3C, C=O carbamate), 80.0 (3C, $C(CH_3)_3$), 57.2 (C, Cβ), 41.7 ($3CH_2$, $CH_2α$ and $CH_2ε$), 34.3 ($2CH_2$, $CH_2γ$), 29.0 ($9CH_3$, $C(CH_3)_3$), 25.0 ($2CH_2$, $CH_2δ$); HRMS-ESI+: calcd for $C_{24}H_{45}N_3O_8$ 503.3207, calcd for $C_{24}H_{45}N_3O_8Na$ 526,3105, found 526.3099 $[M + Na]^+$; IR (ATR) υ (cm^{-1}): 3346.9 (-OH acid), 2962.3, 2975.8, 2872.9, 2495.0, 1686.5 (C=O acid), 1514.6, 1479.5, 1453.5, 1392.0, 1365.3, 1273.7, 1248.7, 1162.3, 1092.6, 985.2, 866.5, 778.8.

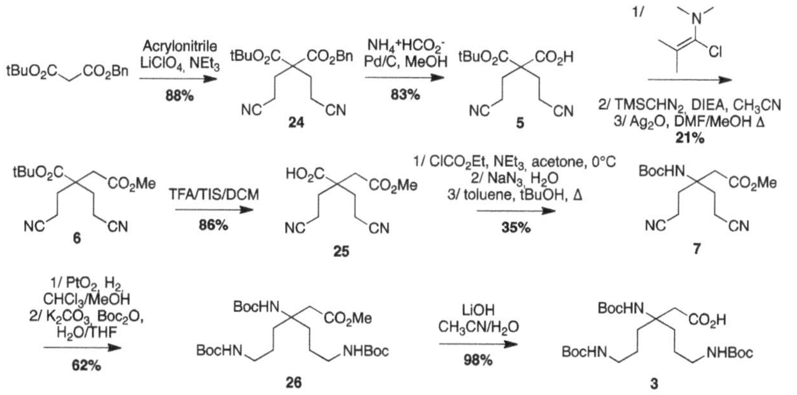

Scheme 6. Synthesis of Boc-$β^{3,3}$ *h*bis-Orn(Boc)$_2$OH **3**.

4.3.3. Synthesis of Fmoc-Tbt-OH (Scheme 7)

(S)-2-((((9H-Fluoren-9-yl)methoxy)carbonyl)amino)-3-(2,4,6-tri-tert-butyl-1H-indol-3-yl) propanoic Acid: A mixture of H-Trp-OH (3 g, 14.6 mmol) and *tert*-BuOH (31 mL, 323 mmol) in TFA (90 mL) was stirred at rt for 20 days. The resulting dark solution was evaporated to dryness to give a black oil, and water (50 mL) was added. To the resulting suspension was added $KHCO_3$ until pH = 8–9. THF (50 mL) and FmocOSu (5.4 g, 16.0 mmol) were added and the mixture was stirred for 16 h. THF was evaporated and the solution was acidified to pH = 2. The compound was extracted with AcOEt, dried over $MgSO_4$, filtered, and concentrated *in vacuo*. The crude compound was purified by flash chromatography (Cy/AcOEt/AcOH 100:0:1 to 50:50:1) to afford a white powder (6 g, 70% yield); $\mathbf{R_f}$ (Cy/AcOEt/AcOH, 5:5:0.1) = 0.66; ^{1}H NMR (300 MHz, $CDCl_3$) δ 7.12–8.08 (m, 10H, *CH* Ar), 4.65–4.88 (m, 1H, *CH* Fmoc), 4.22–4.43 (m, 2H, CH_2 Fmoc), 4.17 (t, *J* = 6.8 Hz, 1H, *CH*α), 3.56-3.74 (m, 1H, $CH_2β_1$), 3.42 (dd, *J* =

14.8 Hz, 9.1 Hz, 1H, $CH_2\beta_2$), 1.57 (s, 18H, $C(CH_3)_3$), 1.45 (s, 9H, $C(CH_3)_3$); ^{13}C NMR (75 MHz, $CDCl_3$) δ 177.7 (C, C=O acid), 156.1 (C, C=O carbamate), 143.8, 143.7, 142.9, 142.7, 141.2, 132.0, 130.2, 129.8 (9C, C Ar), 127.6, 127.0, 125.2, 125.1, 119.8, 116.9, 111.6 (10C, CH Ar), 103.9 (C, C Ar), 67.2 (CH_2, CH_2 Fmoc), 55.3 (CH, CHα), 47.0 (CH, CH Fmoc), 34.8 (2C, $C(CH_3)_3$), 33.1 (C, $C(CH_3)_3$), 32.0, 30.9, 30.6 ($9CH_3$, $C(CH_3)_3$), 27.6 (CH_2, $CH_2\beta$); HRMS-ESI+: calcd for $C_{38}H_{46}N_2O_4$ 594.3458, calcd for $C_{38}H_{46}N_2O_4Na$ 617.3356, found 617.3350 $[M + Na]^+$.

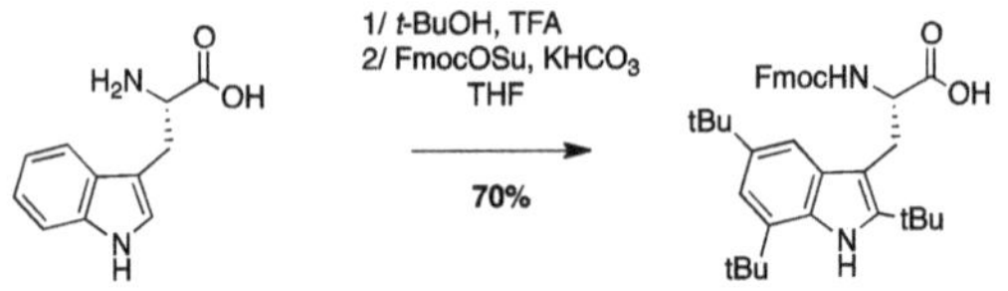

Scheme 7. Synthesis of Fmoc-Tbt-OH.

4.3.4. Synthesis of Peptide A: Arg-Tbt-Arg-NH_2

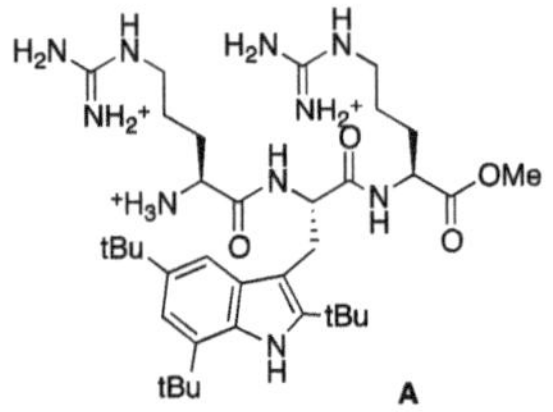

Fmoc Rink Amide resin loaded at 0.43 mmol/g (162 mg, 0.07 mmol) was washed with DMF and allowed to swell in DMF for 15 min. Fmoc deprotection was achieved through treatment of the resin with a solution of 20% piperidine (*v:v*) in DMF (5 min, 3 times), followed by washing with NMP. Fmoc-Arg(Pbf)-OH (4 eq, 0.28 mmol, 182 mg) was dissolved in dry NMP and HATU (3.6 eq, 0.25 mmol, 95 mg) and DIEA (10 eq, 0.7 mmol, 130 μL) were added. The resulting solution was added to the resin and the mixture was stirred for 2 h then filtrated and washed with NMP. Removal of the Fmoc protecting group was achieved by treatment of the resin with 20% (*v:v*) piperidine in DMF (3 times for 5 min). The resin was washed with NMP. Fmoc-Tbt-OH (4 eq, 0.28 mmol, 166 mg) was dissolved in NMP (1.5 mL). HATU (3.6 eq, 0.25 mmol, 95 mg) and DIEA (10 eq, 0.7 mmol, 130 μL) were added. The solution was added to the resin and the coupling reaction was allowed to proceed for 1.5 h at room temperature. The solution was removed by filtration and the resin was washed with DMF. After removal of the Fmoc protective group (20% piperidine in DMF, 5 min, 3 times) and washing of the resin with NMP, a solution of Fmoc-Arg(Pbf)-OH (4 eq, 0.28 mmol, 182 mg), HATU (3.6 eq, 0.25 mmol, 95 mg), and DIEA (10 eq, 0.7 mmol, 130 μL) in NMP (2 mL) was added and the reaction mixture was stirred for 2 h then filtrated and washed with NMP. Simultaneous final deprotection and cleavage from the resin was achieved by treating the resin with a TFA/TIS/H_2O cocktail (95:2.5:2.5, 3 mL) for 4 h. The crude peptide was precipitated through addition of cold diethyl ether. Purification by preparative RP-HPLC using a gradient of 15% to 90% MeCN in 30 min gives after lyophilisation peptide A as a white powder with a purity of >95%. MALDI-TOF: calcd for $C_{36}H_{62}N_{10}O_3$ 683, found 684.4 $[M + H]^+$, 706.4 $[M + Na]^+$, 722.4 $[M + K]^+$; HPLC (Water/ACN (0.1% TFA); 15% to 100% ACN in 30 min): tr = 10.19 min.

4.3.5. Synthesis of Peptide B, Tbt-Arg-OMe B (Scheme 8)

Boc-Tbt-OH (50 mg, 0.11 mmol) was dissolved in DMF. HBTU (42 mg, 0.11 mmol) and DIEA (40 μL, 0.22 mmol) were added and the mixture was stirred for 5 min before addition of H-Apγ(Pbf)OMe (52 mg, 0.11 mmol). The reaction mixture was stirred at room temperature for 5 h, then diluted with Et_2O and washed with an aqueous saturated solution of NH_4Cl. The organic layer was dried over $MgSO_4$, filtered, and evaporated to dryness. The crude compound was purified by flash chromatography (Cy/AcOEt, 100:0 to 50:50) to afford the pure protected dipeptide as a white powder (80 mg, 80% yield). Treatment of this compound with a cocktail of TFA/TIS/H_2O (95:2.5:2.5) for 4 h, followed by evaporation to dryness lead to peptide **B**, which was purified by preparative RP-HPLC using a gradient of 30% to 50% MeCN in 30 min. After lyophilisation, peptide **B** was obtained as white powder with purity >98%; ^1H NMR (300 MHz, MeOD) δ 7.24 (s, 1H, *CH* indole), 7.11 (s, 1H, *CH* indole), 4.25 (t, *J* = 6, 1H, *CH*α Arg), 4.08 (t, *J* = 8.1, 1H, *CH*α Tbt), 3.42 (d, *J* = 8.1, 1H, *CH*$_2$β Tbt), 3.39 (s, 3H, COO*CH*$_3$), 3.09–3.15 (m, 2H, *CH*$_2$δ Arg), 1.70–1.74 (m, 1H, *CH*$_2$γ$_1$ Arg), 1.44–1.57 (m, 3H, *CH*$_2$γ$_2$ and *CH*$_2$β Arg), 1.54 (s, 9H, C(*CH*$_3$)$_3$), 1.50 (s, 9H, C(*CH*$_3$)$_3$), 1.37 (s, 9H, C(*CH*$_3$)$_3$); MALDI-TOF: calcd for $C_{30}H_{50}N_6O_3$ 542.4, found 543.2 $[M + H]^+$, 565.2 $[M + Na]^+$; HPLC (Water/ACN (0.1% TFA); 5% to 100% ACN in 30 min: tr = 15.15 min.

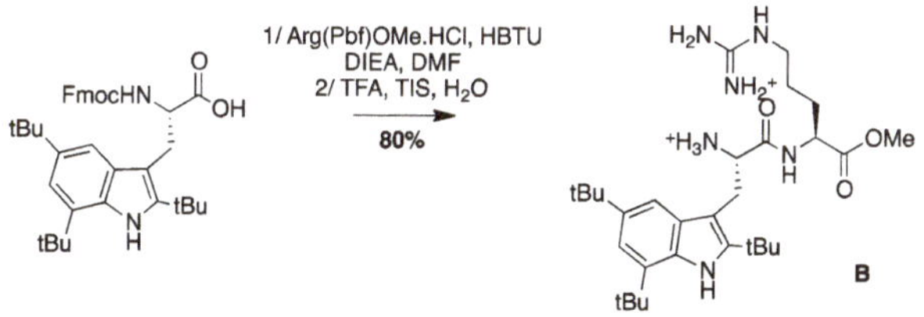

Scheme 8. Synthesis of Peptide B, Tbt-Arg-OMe B.

4.3.6. Synthesis of Peptides **8–12** by LPPS (Scheme 9)

Synthesis of Trp-$\beta^{2,2}$ *h*bis-Orn-OMe **8** and Gdm-Trp-$\beta^{2,2}$ *h*bis-Arg-OMe **10**

*Boc Trp-$\beta^{2,2}$ h*bis-*Orn(Boc)$_2$-OMe* **15:** Boc-Tbt-OH (60 mg, 0.2 mmol) was dissolved in DMF (6 mL). HBTU (76 mg, 0.2 mmol) and DIEA (80 µL, 0.4 mmol) were added and the mixture was stirred for 5 min before addition of H-$\beta^{2,2}$ *h*bis-Orn(Boc)$_2$OMe **1** (84 mg, 0.2 mmol). The reaction mixture was stirred at room temperature overnight, then diluted with Et_2O and washed with an aqueous saturated solution of NH_4Cl. The organic layer was dried over $MgSO_4$, filtered, and evaporated to dryness. The crude compound was purified by flash chromatography (Cy/AcOEt, 70:30) to afford **15** as a white powder (140 mg, 99% yield). ^1H NMR (300 MHz, MeOD) δ 7.71 (d, *J* = 7.8, 1H, *CH* Ar), 7.38 (d, *J* = 7.2, 1H, *CH* Ar), 7.19 (td, *J* = 7.2, 1.1, 1H, *CH* Ar), 7.13 (td, *J* = 7.8, 1.1, 1H, *CH* Ar), 7.06 (d, *J* = 2.1, 1H, *CH* Ar), 5.91 (br, 1H, N*H* Boc), 5.36 (br, 1H, N*H* Boc), 4.78 (br, 1H, *CH*α Trp), 4.72 (br, 1H, *CH*$_2$β$_1$ Trp), 4.52 (br, 1H, *CH*$_2$β$_2$ Trp), 3.66 (s, 3H, CO$_2$*CH*$_3$), 3.30–3.35 (m, 2H, *CH*$_2$βε$_1$β^{2,2}*h*bis-Orn), 3.09–3.23 (m, 2H, *CH*$_2$βε$_2$β^{2,2}*h*bis-Orn), 2.95–3.04 (m, 4H, *CH*$_2$δβ^{2,2}*h*bis-Orn), 1.52 (s, 27H, C(*CH*$_3$) $_3$), 1.42–1.15 (m, 8H, *CH*$_2$βανδ*CH*$_2$γβ^{2,2}*h*bis-Orn).

Trp-$\beta^{2,2}$ h bis-Orn-OMe **8:** Compound **15** (70 mg, 0.1 mmol) was dissolved in DCM (~0.4 M) and an equivalent volume of TFA/TIS/H_2O (95:2.5:2.5). The mixture was stirred at rt for 1 h then evaporated to dryness. The crude product was purified by preparative RP-HPLC using a gradient of 10% to 50% MeCN in 30 min. After lyophilisation compound **8** was obtained as white powder with purity >95% (30 mg, 70% yield); ^1H NMR (500 MHz, D_2O) δ 7.68 (d, *J* = 8, 1H, *CH* Ar), 7.55 (d, *J* = 12.8, 1H, *CH* Ar), 7.33 (s, 1H, *CH* Ar), 7.30 (t, *J* = 8, 1H, *CH* Ar), 7.22 (t, *J* = 7.5, 1H, *CH* Ar), 4.42 (dd, *J* = 9.5, 6, 1H, *CH*α Trp), 3.66 (s, 3H, CO$_2$*CH*$_3$), 3.51 (d, *J* = 14.5, 1H, *CH*$_2$βε$_1$ β^{2,2} *h* bis-Arg), 3.41 (dd, *J* = 14.2, 6, 1H, *CH*$_2$β$_1$ Trp), 3.35 (dd, *J* = 14.2, 9.5, 1H, *CH*$_2$β$_2$ Trp), 3.15 (d, *J* = 14.5, 1H, *CH*$_2$βε$_2$ β^{2,2} *h*bis-Arg), 2.81 (t, *J* = 7.8, 1H, *CH*$_2$δ$_1$ β^{2,2} *h* bis-Arg), 2.71 (t, *J* = 7.8, 1H, *CH*$_2$δ$_2$ β^{2,2} *h* bis-Arg), 1.49–1.53 (m, 1H, *CH*$_2$γ$_1$ β^{2,2} *h* bis-Arg), 1.35–1.39 (m, 3H, *CH*$_2$γ$_{1'}$ and *CH*$_2$γ$_2$ β^{2,2} *h* bis-Arg), 1.24 (td, *J* = 13.2, 3.7, 1H, *CH*$_2$β$_1$ β^{2,2} *h* bis-Arg), 1.05–1.12 (m, 2H, *CH*$_2$β$_{1'}$ and *CH*$_2$β$_2$β^{2,2} *h*bis-Arg), 0.88–0.95 (m, 1H, *CH*$_2$β$_{2'}$β^{2,2} *h*bis-Arg); MALDI-TOF: calcd for $C_{21}H_{33}N_5O_3$ 403.3, calcd for $C_{21}H_{33}N_5O_3Na$ 426.3, found 404.5 $[M + H]^+$, 426.5 $[M + Na]^+$, 442.5 $[M + K]^+$; HPLC (Water/ACN (0.1% TFA); 5% to 100% ACN in 30 min): tr = 7.18 min (Figure 11).

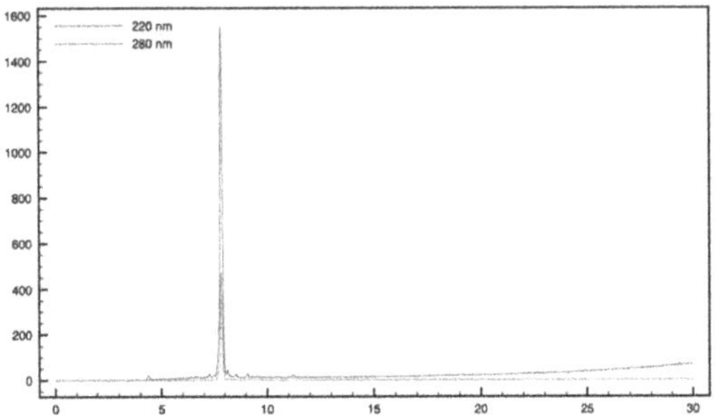

Figure 11. HPLC profile of *Trp-β*^{2,} *h bis-Orn-OMe* **8**.

Gdm-Trp-β^{2,2} *h*bis-*Arg-OMe* **10:** Compound **15** (70 mg, 0.1 mmol) was dissolved in DCM (~0.4 M) and an equivalent volume of TFA/TIS/H_2O (95:2.5:2.5). The mixture was stirred at rt for 1.5 h then evaporated to dryness. The crude compound was dissolved in 6 mL of THF 1,3-Di-Boc-2-(trifluoromethylsulfonyl)guanidine (137 mg, 0.35 mmol) and NEt_3 (60 μL, 0.4 mmol) were added and the reaction mixture was stirred at rt overnight. After evaporation of THF, a solution of TFA/TIS/H_2O (95:2.5:2.5) was added and the mixture was stirred at rt for 2 h. The crude product was purified by preparative RP-HPLC using a gradient of 10% to 50% MeCN in 30 min. After lyophilisation, compound **10** was obtained as white powder with purity >98% (31 mg, 57% yield); ^{1}H NMR (300 MHz, D_2O) δ 7.69 (d, *J* = 7.5, 1H, *CH* Ar), 7.36 (d, *J* = 8.1, 1H, *CH* Ar), 7.31 (s, 1H, *CH* Ar), 7.26 (td, *J* = 7.5, 0.9, 1H, *CH* Ar), 7.22 (td, *J* = 7.2, 0.9, 1H, *CH* Ar), 4.62 (t, *J* = 7.5, 1H, *CH*α Trp), 3.69 (s, 3H, CO_2CH_3), 3.47 (d, *J* = 14.1, 1H, $CH_2β ε_1$ $β^{2,2}$ *h*bis-Arg), 3.35 (d, *J* = 7.5, 2H, $CH_2β$ Trp), 3.21 (d, *J* = 14.4, 1H, $CH_2β ε_2$ $β^{2,2}$ *h*bis-Arg), 3.05 (t, *J* = 6.6, 1H, $CH_2δ_1$ $β^{2,2}$ *h* bis-Arg), 2.98 (dd, *J* = 11.7, 6.6, 1H, $CH_2δ_2$ $β^{2,2}$ *h* bis-Arg), 1.29–1.43 (m, 4H, $CH_2γ$ $β^{2,2}$ *h*bis-Arg), 1.09-1.28 (m, 4H, $CH_2β$ $β^{2,2}$ *h*bis-Arg); MALDI-TOF: calcd for $C_{32}H_{57}N_5O_3$ 529.3, calcd for $C_{32}H_{57}N_5O_3Na$ 552.3, found 530.6 $[M + H]^+$, 552.6 $[M + Na]^+$, 513.6 $[M + H - NH_3]^+$; HPLC (Water/ACN (0.1% TFA); 5% to 100% ACN in 30 min): tr = 9.62 min (Figure 12).

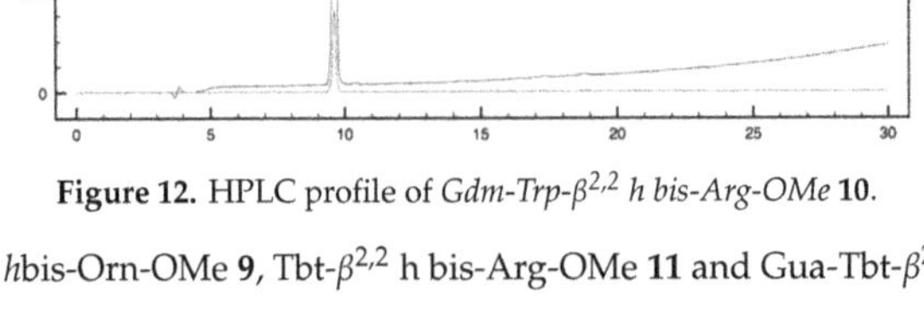

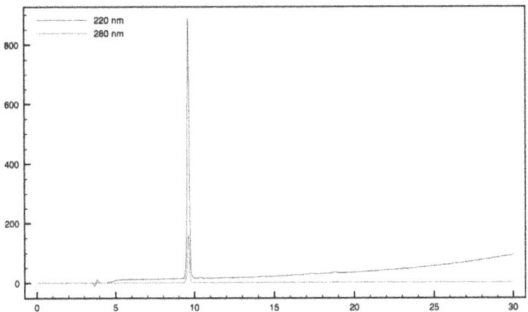

Figure 12. HPLC profile of *Gdm-Trp-β*^{2,2} *h bis-Arg-OMe* **10**.

Synthesis of Tbt-*β*^{2,2} *h*bis-Orn-OMe **9**, Tbt-*β*^{2,2} h bis-Arg-OMe **11** and Gua-Tbt-*β*^{2,2} h bis-Arg-OMe **12**

Fmoc-Tbt-β^{2,2} *h*bis-*Orn(Boc)*$_2$*OMe* **16:** Fmoc-Tbt-OH (400 mg, 0.64 mmol) was dissolved in DMF (24 mL). HBTU (244 mg, 0.64 mmol) and DIEA (240 μL, 1.28 mmol) were added and the mixture was stirred for 3 h before addition of H-$β^{2,2}$ *h* bis-Orn(Boc)$_2$OMe **1** (268 mg, 0.64 mmol). The reaction mixture was stirred at room temperature overnight, then diluted with Et_2O and washed with an aqueous saturated solution of NH_4Cl. The organic layer was dried over $MgSO_4$, filtered, and evaporated to dryness. The crude compound was purified by flash chromatography (Cy/AcOEt, 100:0 to 70:30) to afford the pure protected dipeptide as a white powder (450 mg, 70% yield). ^{1}H NMR (300 MHz, MeOD) δ 8.22 (s,

1H, NH indole), 7.75 (d, J = 7.2, 1H, CH Ar Fmoc), 7.55 (d, J = 7.2, 1H, CH Ar Fmoc), 7.41 (s, 1H, CH Ar indole), 7.35 (t, J = 7.2, 1H, CH Ar Fmoc), 7.24 (dt, J = 11.7 and 7.2, 1H, CH Ar Fmoc), 7.12 (s, 1H, CH indole), 4.27–4.33 (m, 3H, CHα Tbt and CH_2 Fmoc), 4.12 (t, J = 6.9, 1H, CH Fmoc), 3.55 (s, 3H, CO_2CH_3), 3.43 (dd, J = 14.1 9.3, 1H, $CH_2\beta_1$ Tbt), 3.39 (d, J = 14.1, 1H, $CH_2\beta\varepsilon_1$ $\beta^{2,2}$ h bis-Orn), 3.23 (dd, J = 14.4, 6.3, 1H, $CH_2\beta_2$ Tbt), 2.9 (m, 4H, $CH_2\delta$ $\beta^{2,2}$ h bis-Orn), 2.79 (d, J = 14.1, 1H, $CH_2\beta\varepsilon_2$ $\beta^{2,2}$ hbis-Orn), 1.52 (s, 9H, $C(CH_3)_3$ indole), 1.47 (s, 9H, $C(CH_3)_3$ indole), 1.36–1.44 (m, 35H, $C(CH_3)_3$ indole, $C(CH_3)_3$ Boc, $CH_2\beta$ $\beta^{2,2}$ hbis-Orn and $CH_2\gamma$ $\beta^{2,2}$ hbis-Orn); ^{13}C NMR (75 MHz, MeOD) δ 177.1 (C, C=O amide), 174.9 (C, C=O ester), 158.4 (C=O Boc), 157.9 (C=O Fmoc), 145.2, 145.1, 143.6, 142.9, 142.5, 133.1, 131.8, 131.3 (8C, C Ar), 128.7, 128.2, 126.2, 120.9 (4CH, CH Ar Fmoc), 117.3, 113.4 (2CH, CH Ar indole), 106.2 (C, C Ar), 79.8 (C, $C(CH_3)_3$ Boc), 68.1 (CH_2, CH_2 Fmoc), 58.5 (CH, CHα Tbt), 52.3 (CH_3, CO_2CH_3), 50.7 (C, Cα $\beta^{2,2}$ hbis-Orn), 48.3 (CH, CH Fmoc), 42.9 (CH_2, $CH_2\beta\varepsilon$ $\beta^{2,2}$ hbis-Orn), 41.6 (CH_2, $CH_2\delta$ $\beta^{2,2}$ hbis-Orn), 35.7, 35.5 and 34.3 (3C, $C(CH_3)_3$ indole), 32.7 (CH_3, $C(CH_3)_3$ indole), 32.4 and 32.1 (CH_2, $CH_2\gamma$ $\beta^{2,2}$ h bis-Orn), 31.3 (CH_3, $C(CH_3)_3$ indole), 30.9 (CH_3, $C(CH_3)_3$ indole), 29 (CH_2, $CH_2\beta$ Tbt), 28.8 ($6CH_3$, $C(CH_3)_3$ Boc), 25.5 and 25.3 (CH_2, $CH_2\beta$ $\beta^{2,2}$ h bis-Orn).

H-Tbt-$\beta^{2,2}$ h bis-OrnOMe **9:** Compound **16** (60 mg, 0.06 mmol) was dissolved in a 20% solution of piperidine in DCM and allowed to react for 1 h before evaporation to dryness. A solution of TFA/TIS/H_2O (95:2.5:2.5) was added and the mixture was stirred at rt for 1 h. The crude product was purified by preparative RP-HPLC using a gradient of 30% to 50% MeCN in 30 min. After lyophilisation **9** was obtained as white powder with a purity of 98% (20 mg, 58% yield); ^1H NMR (300 MHz, D_2O) δ 8.54 (s, 1H, NH indole), 7.26 (s, 1H, CH Ar), 7.22 (s, 1H, CH Ar), 4.03 (dd, J = 9.3, 6, 1H, CHα Tbt), 3.50 (s, 3H, CO_2CH_3), 3.37 (d, J = 14.2, 1H, $CH_2\beta\varepsilon_1$ $\beta^{2,2}$ h bis-Orn), 3.34 (d, J = 14.1, 2H, $CH_2\beta$ Tbt), 2.80 (m, 4H, $CH_2\delta$ $\beta^{2,2}$ h bis-Orn), 2.33 (d, J = 14.2, 1H, $CH_2\beta\varepsilon_2$ $\beta^{2,2}$ h bis-Orn), 1.31–1.44 (m, 35H, $CH_2\beta$ $\beta^{2,2}$ h bis-Orn, $CH_2\gamma$ $\beta^{2,2}$ h bis-Orn and $C(CH_3)_3$); MALDI-TOF: calcd for $C_{32}H_{57}N_5O_3$ 571.5, found 572.6 $[M + H]^+$; HPLC (Water/ACN (0.1% TFA); 30% to 50% ACN in 30 min): tr = 12.73 min (Figure 13).

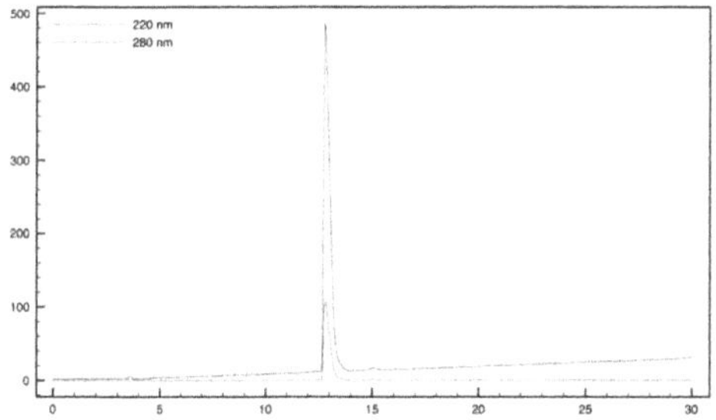

Figure 13. HPLC profile of *H-Tbt-$\beta^{2,2}$ h bis-OrnOMe* **9**.

H-Tbt-$\beta^{2,2}$ h bis-Arg-OMe 11 and Gua-Tbt-$\beta^{2,2}$ h bis-Arg-OMe **12:** Compound **9** (10 mg, 0.013 mmol) was dissolved in 1 mL of THF. 1,3-Di-Boc-2-(trifluoromethylsulfonyl) guanidine (30 mg, 0.08 mmol) and DIEA (27 μL, 0.156 mmol) were added and the reaction mixture was stirred at rt for 2 h. After evaporation of THF, a solution of TFA/TIS/H_2O (95:2.5:2.5) was added and the mixture was stirred at rt for 2 h. The crude product was evaporated *in vacuo* and purified by preparative RP-HPLC using a gradient of 30% to 50% MeCN in 30 min. Two pics were collected separately at 14 and 18 min corresponding, respectively, to compounds **11** and **12**. After lyophilisation, the two compounds **11** (5 mg, 59% yield) and **12** (2 mg, 22% yield) were obtained as white powders with purity >99%.

H-Tbt-$\beta^{2,2}$ h bis-Arg-OMe **11**: ^1H NMR (500 MHz, D_2O) δ 7.29 (s, 1H, CH indole), 7.27 (s, 1H, CH indole), 4.14 (dd, J = 11.2, 5.5, 1H, CHα Tbt), 3.61 (dd, J = 14.5, 5, 1H, $CH_2\beta_1$ Tbt), 3.57 (s, 3H, CO_2CH_3), 3.44 (dd, J = 13.5, 12, 2H, $CH_2\beta_2$ Tbt), 3.21 (d, J = 14.5, 1H, $CH_2\beta\varepsilon_1$ $\beta^{2,2}$ h bis-Arg), 3.04 (m, J = 4H, $CH_2\delta$ $\beta^{2,2}$ h bis-Arg), 1.83 (d, J = 14.5, 1H, $CH_2\beta\varepsilon_2$ $\beta^{2,2}$ h bis-Arg), 1.55 (s, 9H, $C(CH_3)_3$), 1.49 (s, 9H, $C(CH_3)_3$), 1.39 (s, 9H, $C(CH_3)_3$), 1.1-1.34 (m, 8H, $CH_2\beta$ $\beta^{2,2}$ h bis-Arg and $CH_2\gamma$ $\beta^{2,2}$ h bis-Arg); MALDI-TOF:

calcd for $C_{35}H_{61}N_5O_3$ 655.5, calcd for $C_{35}H_{61}N_5O_3Na$ 678.5, found 656.4 $[M + H]^+$, 678.4 $[M + Na]^+$, 694.4 $[M + K]^+$, 639.4 $[M + H - NH_3]^+$; HPLC (Water/ACN (0.1% TFA); 30% to 50% ACN in 30 min: tr = 16.11 min (Figure 14).

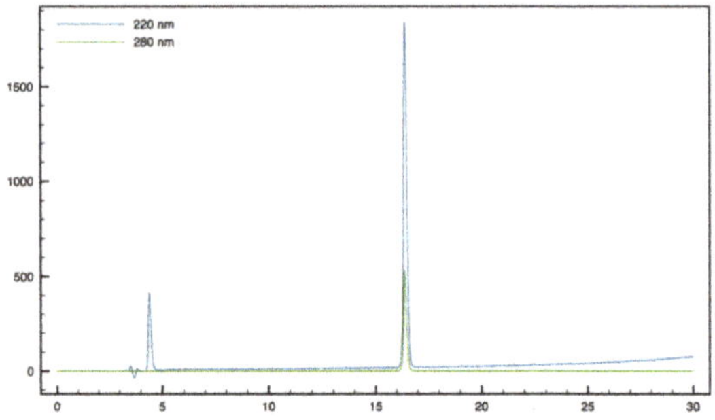

Figure 14. HPLC profile of *H-Tbt-$\beta^{2,2}$ h bis-Arg-OMe* **11**.

Gua-Tbt-$\beta^{2,2}$ h bis-Arg-OMe **12**: ^{1}H NMR (300 MHz, MeOD) δ 8.35 (s, 1H, *N*H indole), 7.31 (d, *J* = 1.5, 1H, *C*H Ar), 7.14 (d, *J* = 1.5, 1H, *C*H Ar), 4.39 (t, *J* = 7.2, 1H, *C*Hα Tbt), 3.65 (s, 3H, CO_2CH_3), 3.52 (d, *J* = 14.2, 1H, $CH_2\beta\varepsilon_1$ $\beta^{2,2}$ *h* bis-Arg), 3.47 (dd, *J* = 11.1, 7.2, 2H, $CH_2\beta$ Tbt), 3.01–3.13 (m, 4H, $CH_2\delta$ $\beta^{2,2}$ *h* bis-Arg), 2.82 (d, *J* = 14.2, 1H, $CH_2\beta\varepsilon_2$ $\beta^{2,2}$ *h* bis-Arg), 1.26–1.64 (m, 35H, $CH_2\beta$ $\beta^{2,2}$ *h* bis-Arg, $CH_2\gamma$ $\beta^{2,2}$ *h* bis-Arg and $C(CH_3)_3$); MALDI-TOF: calcd for $C_{36}H_{63}N_{11}O_3$ 697.5, calcd for $C_{36}H_{63}N_{11}O_3Na$ 720.5, found 698.4 $[M + H]^+$, 720.4 $[M + Na]^+$, 736.3 $[M + K]^+$, 681.3 $[M + H - NH_3]^+$; HPLC (Water/ACN (0.1% TFA); 30% to 70% ACN in 30 min): tr = 14.08 min (Figure 15).

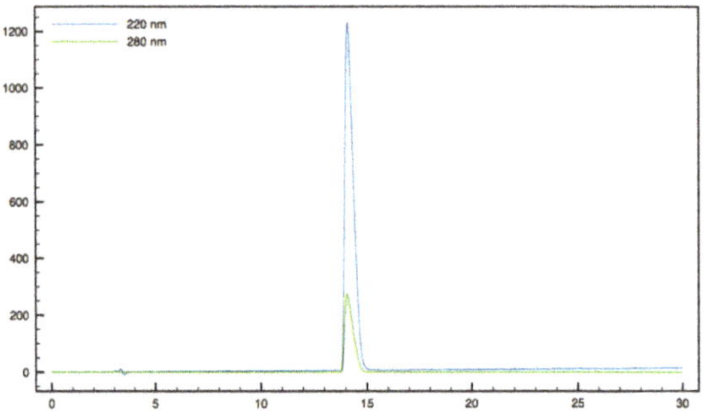

Figure 15. HPLC profile of *Gua-Tbt-$\beta^{2,2}$ h bis-Arg-OMe* **12**.

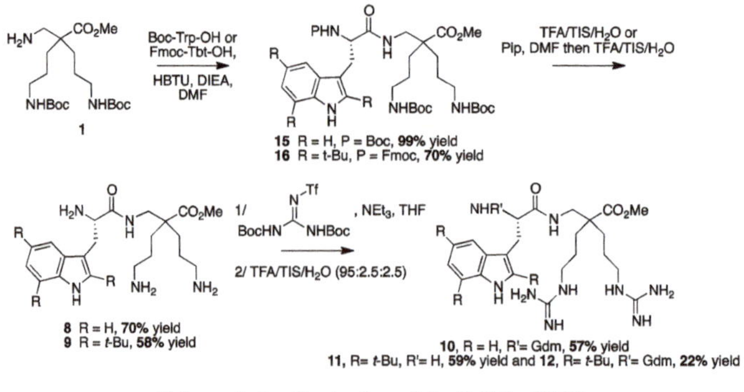

Scheme 9. Synthesis of peptides 8–12 by LPPS.

4.3.7. Synthesis of Peptides 13 and 14 by SPPS (Scheme 10)

H-β^{3,3}-h-bis-Arg-Tbt-OMe **13**: HMBA-AM resin (108 mg, 0.1 mmol) was washed five times with DMF, DCM, and DMF, then allowed to swell in DMF for 30 min. Fmoc-Tbt-OH (4 eq, 0.4 mmol, 238 mg) was dissolved in dry DCM. The solution was cooled to 0 °C, DIC (4 eq, 0.4 mmol, 60 µL) was added. The reaction was stirred for 1.5 h and the solvent was then removed *in vacuo*. The resulting anhydride was dissolved in DMF and added to the resin. A solution of DMAP (0.1 eq, 0.04 mmol, 5 mg) in DMF was added and the resin was shaken for 1 h before washing with DMF, DCM, and DMF (resin loading = 0.84 mmol/g). Removal of the Fmoc protecting group was achieved by treatment of the resin with 20% (*v*:*v*) piperidine in DMF 3 times for 5 min. The resin was washed five times with DMF. Boc-β^{3,3} *h* bis-Orn(Boc)$_2$OH **3** (2 eq, 0.18 mmol, 90 mg) was dissolved in DMF (1.2 mL). HATU (1.8 eq, 0.17 mmol, 65 mg) and DIEA (2 eq, 0.18 mmol, 23 µL) were added. The solution was added to the resin (0.09 mmol, 108 mg) and the coupling reaction was allowed to proceed for 2 h at room temperature. The solution was removed by filtration and the resin was washed with DMF five times. Reaction completion was monitored by Kaiser test. Boc removal was performed by treating the resin with a TFA/TIS/H_2O cocktail (95:2.5:2.5) for 5 h. The free amines were then reacted with 1,3-Di-Boc-2-(trifluoromethylsulfonyl)guanidine (10 eq, 1.8 mmol, 700 mg) and NEt_3 (10 eq, 1.8 mmol, 240 µL) in DMF overnight. The resin was filtrated and the Boc groups were removed with a TFA/TIS/H_2O cocktail (95:2.5:2.5) at rt for 3 h. After filtration, peptide **14** was cleaved from the resin using a mixture of MeOH/DMF/DIEA (5:5:1) for 16 h at 50 °C. The solution was filtrated, and solvents were evaporated. The crude product was purified by preparative RP-HPLC using a gradient of 30% to 70% MeCN in 30 min. After lyophilisation peptide **13** was obtained as a white powder with a purity of >95% (47 mg, 75% yield); ^{1}H NMR (500 MHz, D_2O) δ 7.37 (d, *J* = 1.7, 1H, *CH* Ar indole), 7.28 (d, *J* = 1.7, 1H, *CH* Ar indole), 4.69 (t, *J* = 7.5, 1H, *CH*α Tbt), 3.48–3.53 (m, 1H, *CH*$_2$β$_1$ Tbt), 3.68 (dd, *J* = 10.5, 1, 1H, *CH*$_2$β$_2$ Tbt), 3.25 (t, *J* = 6.5, 1H, *CH*$_2$ε$_1$ β^{2,2} *h* bis-Arg), 3.17 (t, *J* = 6.5, 1H *CH*$_2$ε$_2$ β^{2,2} *h* bis-Arg), 2.69 (d, *J* = 16, 1H, *CH*$_2$α$_1$ β^{2,2} *h* bis-Arg), 2.55 (d, *J* = 16, 1H, *CH*$_2$α$_2$ β^{2,2} *h* bis-Arg), 1.70–1.75 (m, 4H, *CH*$_2$γ β^{2,2} *h* bis-Arg), 1.64-1.68 (m, 2H, *CH*$_2$δ$_1$ β^{2,2} *h* bis-Arg), 1.55–1.61 (m, 2H, *CH*$_2$δ$_2$ β^{2,2} *h* bis-Arg), 1.42 (s, 9H, C(*CH*$_3$)$_3$), 1.40 (s, 9H, C(*CH*$_3$)$_3$), 1.29 (s, 9H, C(*CH*$_3$)$_3$); MALDI-TOF: calcd for $C_{35}H_{61}N_9O_2$ 655.5, calcd for $C_{35}H_{61}N_9O_2Na$ 678.5, found 656.5 [M + H]$^+$, 678.5 [M + Na]$^+$, 694.5 [M + K]$^+$; HPLC (Water/ACN (0.1% TFA); 5% to 100% ACN in 30 min): tr = 19.29 min (Figure 16).

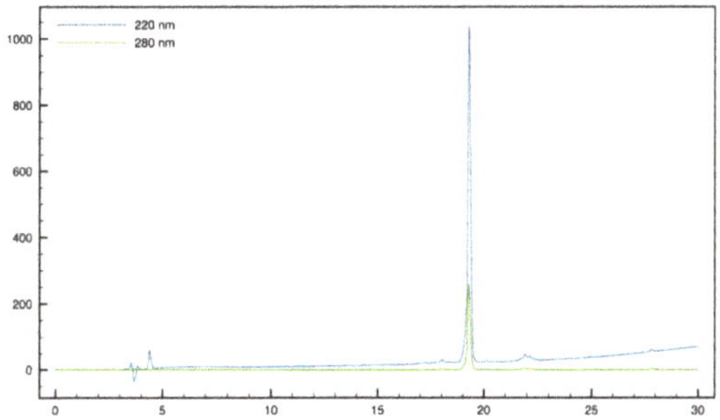

Figure 16. HPLC profile of *H-β^{3,3}*-h-*bis-Arg-Tbt-OMe* **13**.

Gdm-β^{2,2}-h-bis-Arg-Tbt-OMe **14:** HMBA-AM resin (185 mg, 0.2 mmol) was washed five times with DMF, DCM. and DMF, then allowed to swell in DMF for 30 min. Fmoc-Tbt-OH (4 eq, 0.4 mmol, 238 mg) was dissolved in dry DCM. The solution was cooled to 0 °C, and DIC (4 eq, 0.4 mmol, 60 µL) was added. The reaction was stirred for 30 min and the solvent was then removed *in vacuo*. The resulting anhydride was dissolved in DMF and added to the resin. A solution of DMAP (0.1 eq, 0.04 mmol, 5 mg) in DMF was added and the resin was shaken for 1 h before washing with DMF, DCM, and DMF (resin loading = 0.4 mmol/g). Removal of the Fmoc protecting group was achieved by treatment of the resin with 20% (*v:v*) piperidine in DMF 3 times for 5 min. The resin was washed five times with DMF. Fmoc-$\beta^{2,2}$ *h* bis-Orn(Boc)$_2$OH **2** (3 eq, 0.22 mmol, 141 mg) was dissolved in DMF (1.5 mL). HATU (1.8 eq, 0.21 mmol, 80 mg) and DIEA (4 eq, 0.88 mmol, 150 μL) were added. The solution was added to the resin (0.07 mmol, 185 mg) and the reaction was allowed to proceed at 50 °C for 16 h. The solution was removed by filtration and the resin was washed with DMF five times. The reaction being incomplete as revealed by a Kaiser test, the same coupling procedure was repeated a second time. The resin was then treated with a 20% solution of piperidine in DMF for 5 min 3 times. Boc removal was performed by treatment with a TFA/TIS/H_2O cocktail (95:2.5:2.5) for 1 h. The free amines were then reacted with 1,3-Di-Boc-2-(trifluoromethylsulfonyl)guanidine (5 eq, 0.35 mmol, 137 mg) and NEt_3 (10 eq, 0.7 mmol, 90 μL) in DMF overnight. The resin was filtrated and the Boc groups were removed with a TFA/TIS/H_2O cocktail (95:2.5:2.5) at rt for 3 h. After filtration, peptide **14** was cleaved from the resin using a mixture of MeOH/DMF/DIEA (5:5:1) for 16 h at 50 °C. The solution was filtrated, and solvents were evaporated. The crude product was purified by preparative RP-HPLC using a gradient of 40% to 90% MeCN in 30 min. After lyophilisation, peptide **14** was obtained as white powder with a purity of >95% (34 mg, 72% yield); ^{1}H NMR (300 MHz, D_2O) δ 7.36 (s, 1H, *CH* indole), 7.19 (s, 1H, *CH* indole), 4.7 (m, 1H, *CH*α Tbt), 3.61 (s, 3H, CO_2CH_3), 3.53 (dd, *J* = 15.3, 6.6, 1H, $CH_2\beta_1$ Tbt), 3.31–3.36 (m, 2H, $CH_2\beta_2$ Tbt and $CH_2\beta\varepsilon_1$ $\beta^{2,2}$ *h* bis-Arg), 2.88 (t, *J* = 7, 1H, $CH_2\delta_1$ $\beta^{2,2}$ *h* bis-Arg), 2.85 (t, *J* = 7, 1H, $CH_2\delta_2$ $\beta^{2,2}$ *h* bis-Arg), 2.83 (d, *J* = 14.5, 1H, $CH_2\beta\varepsilon_2$ $\beta^{2,2}$ *h* bis-Arg), 1.42 (s, 9H, $C(CH_3)_3$), 1.39 (s, 9H, $C(CH_3)_3$), 1.27 (s, 9H, $C(CH_3)_3$), 1.14–1.33 (m, 8H, $CH_2\beta$ and $CH_2\gamma$ $\beta^{2,2}$ *h* bis-Arg); MALDI-TOF: calcd for $C_{36}H_{63}N_{11}O_3$ 697.5, calcd for $C_{36}H_{63}N_{11}O_3Na$ 720.5, found 698.5 $[M + H]^+$, 720.4 $[M + Na]^+$, 736.4 $[M + K]^+$; HPLC (Water/ACN (0.1% TFA); 30% to 70% ACN in 30 min): tr = 16.5 min (Figure 17).

4.3.8. Synthesis of Fmoc-Tbt-$\beta^{2,2}$-*h*-bis-Orn-OMe **17a** and Fmoc-Tbt-$\beta^{2,2}$-*h*-bis-Arg-OMe **17b** (Scheme 11)

Fmoc-Tbt-$\beta^{2,2}$-h-bis-Orn-OMe **17a**: Compound **16** (42 mg, 0.042 mmol) was treated with a mixture of TFA/TIS/H_2O (95:2.5:2.5, V = 1mL) at rt for 3 h and then evaporated to dryness. The crude product was purified by preparative RP-HPLC using a gradient of 50% to 100% MeCN in 30 min. After lyophilisation compound **17a** was obtained as white powder with purity >99% (27 mg, 95% yield); ^{1}H NMR (300 MHz, CD_3OD) δ 7.80 (d, *J* = 7.5 Hz, 2H, *CH* Fmoc), 7.60 (t, *J* = 8.8 Hz, 2H, *CH* Fmoc), 7.37–7.42 (m, 5H, *CH* indole and *CH* Fmoc), 7.13 (d, *J* = 1.4 Hz, 1H, *CH* indole), 4.44 (dt, *J* = 9.8 Hz, 7.7 Hz, 1H, *CH* Fmoc), 4.17–4.24 (m, 3H, CH_2 Fmoc and *CH*α Tbt), 3.59 (d, *J* = 14.2 Hz, 1H, $CH_2\beta\varepsilon_1$ $\beta^{2,2}$ *h* bis-Arg), 3.41 (dd, *J* = 14.6 Hz, 9 Hz, 1H, $CH_2\beta_1$ Tbt), 3.26 (dd, *J* = 14.2 Hz, 5.8 Hz, 1H, $CH_2\beta_2$ Tbt), 2.88 (d, *J* = 14.2 Hz, 1H, $CH_2\beta\varepsilon_2$ $\beta^{2,2}$ *h* bis-Arg), 2.79–2.82 (m, 4H, $CH_2\delta$ $\beta^{2,2}$ *h* bis-Arg), 1.22–1.69 (m, 35H, $C(CH_3)_3$, $CH_2\beta$ $\beta^{2,2}$ *h* bis-Arg and $CH_2\gamma$ $\beta^{2,2}$ *h* bis-Arg); **MALDI-TOF**: calcd for $C_{48}H_{67}N_5O_5$ 793.5, found 794.5 $[M + H]^+$, 816.4 $[M + Na]^+$, 832.4 $[M + K]^+$; **HPLC** (Water/ACN (0.1% TFA); 50% to 100% ACN in 10 min: tr = 6.29 min (Figure 18).

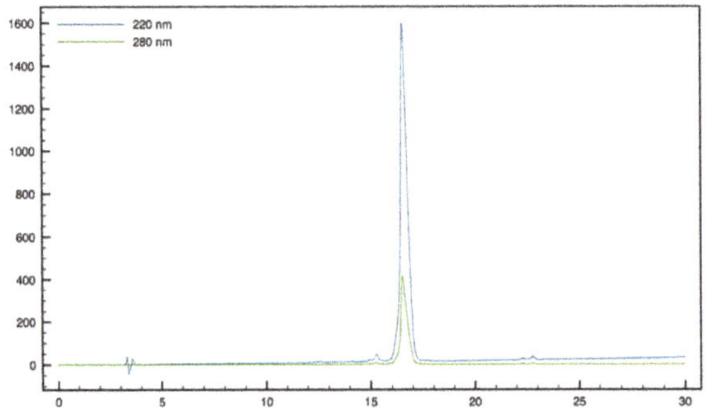

Figure 17. HPLC profile of *Gdm-$\beta^{2,2}$*-h-*bis-Arg-Tbt-OMe* **14**.

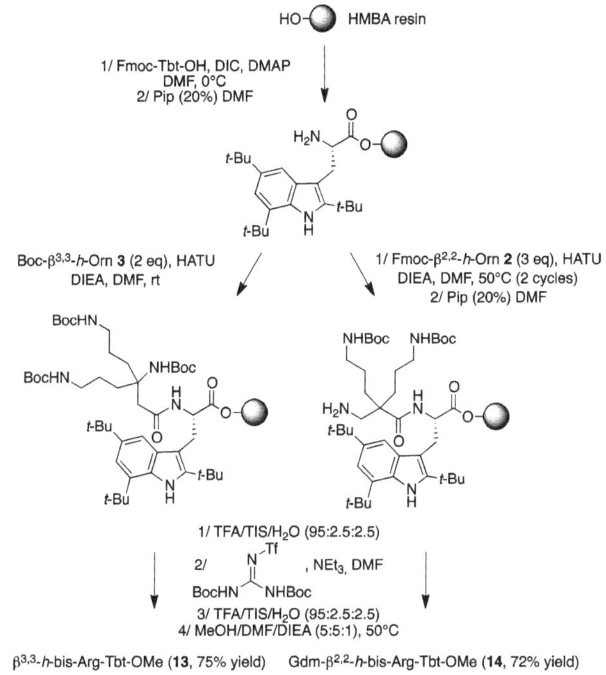

Scheme 10. Synthesis of peptides 13 and 14 by SPPS.

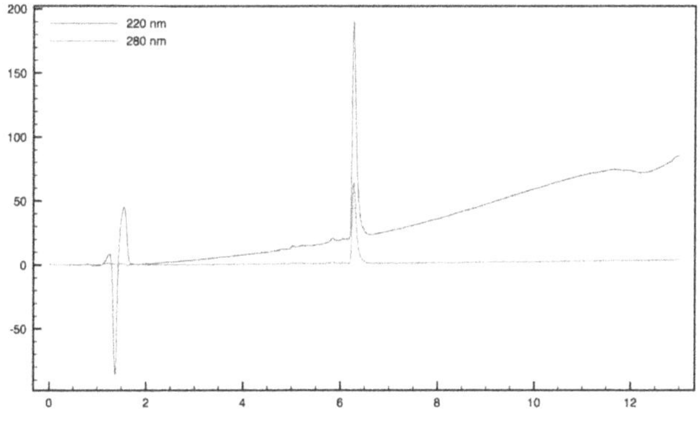

Figure 18. HPLC profile of *Fmoc-Tbt-$\beta^{2,2}$*-h-*bis-Orn-OMe* **17a**.

Synthesis of Fmoc-Tbt-$\beta^{2,2}$-*h*-bis-Arg-OMe **17b**

Compound **17a** (50 mg, 0.05 mmol) was dissolved 1 mL of THF. 1,3-Di-Boc-2-(trifluoromethylsulfonyl)guanidine (51 mg, 0.13 mmol) and NEt_3 (35 μL, 0.26 mmol) were added and the reaction mixture was stirred at rt for 24 h. After evaporation of THF, a solution of TFA/TIS/H_2O (95:2.5:2.5, 2 mL) was added and the mixture was stirred at rt for 45 min. The crude product was evaporated *in vacuo* and purified by preparative RP-HPLC using a gradient of 30% to 100% MeCN in 30 min. After lyophilisation compound **17b** was obtained as white powders with purity >99% (25 mg, 57% yield); ^{1}H NMR (300 MHz, CD_3OD) δ 7.80 (d, *J* = 7.5 Hz, 2H, *CH* arom Fmoc), 7.60 (d, *J* = 7.5 Hz, 2H, *CH* arom Fmoc), 7.39 (t, *J* = 7.5 Hz, 2H, *CH* arom Fmoc), 7.33 (s, *1*H, *CH* arom indole), 7.27 (t, *J* = 7.5 Hz, 2H, *CH* arom Fmoc), 7.13 (s, 1H, *CH* indole), 4.27–4.38 (m, 2H, *CH*$_2$ Fmoc), 4.18–4.22 (m, 2H, *CH* Fmoc and *CH*α Tbt), 3.56 (d, *J* = 11.8 Hz, 1H, *CH*$_2$βε$_1$ β^{2,2} *h* bis-Arg), 3.40 (dd, *J* = 14.6 Hz, 9.1 Hz,

1H, $CH_2\beta_1$ Tbt), 3.25 (dd, *J* = 14.6 Hz, 5.5 Hz, 1H, $CH_2\beta_2$ Tbt), 3–3.07 (m, 4H, $CH_2\delta$ $\beta^{2,2}$ *h* bis-Arg), 2.72 (d, *J* = 14.3 Hz, 2H, $CH_2\beta\varepsilon_2$ $\beta^{2,2}$ *h* bis-Arg), 1.34–1.53 (m, 35H, $C(CH_3)_3$, $CH_2\beta$ $\beta^{2,2}$ *h* bis-Arg and $CH_2\gamma$ $\beta^{2,2}$ *h* bis-Arg); MALDI-TOF: calcd for $C_{50}H_{71}N_9O_5$ 877.6, found 878.4 $[M + H]^+$, 916.4 $[M + K]^+$; HPLC (Water/ACN (0.1% TFA); 5% to 100% ACN in 30 min: tr = 24.59 min (Figure 19).

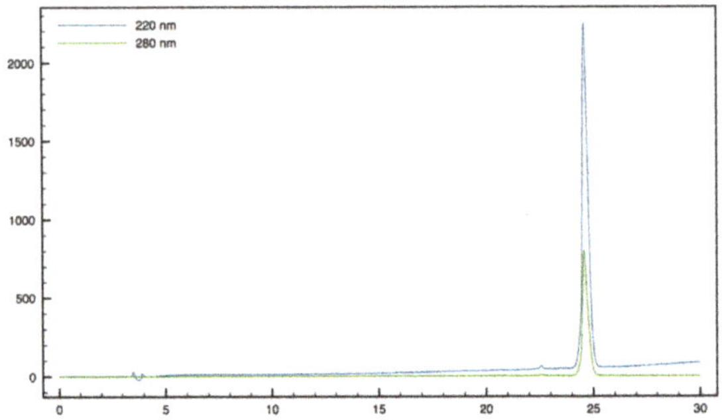

Figure 19. HPLC profile of Fmoc-Tbt-$\beta^{2,2}$-*h*-bis-Arg-OMe **17b**.

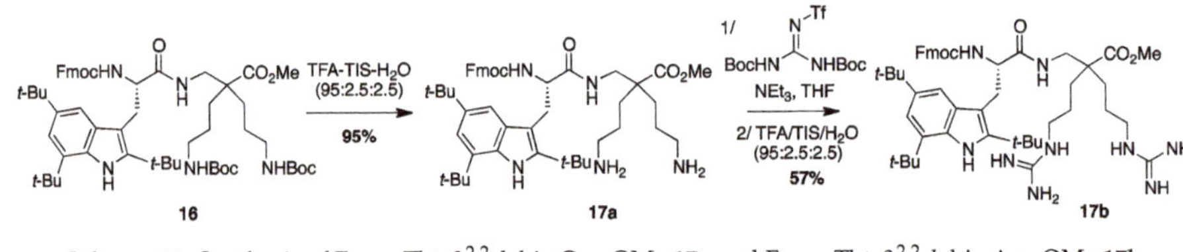

Scheme 11. Synthesis of Fmoc-Tbt-$\beta^{2,2}$-*h*-bis-Orn-OMe **17a** and Fmoc-Tbt-$\beta^{2,2}$-*h*-bis-Arg-OMe **17b**.

4.3.9. Synthesis of Fluo-Tbt-$\beta^{2,2}$ h bis-Orn-OMe 18 (Scheme 12)

Compound **16** (43 mg, 0.043 mmol) was dissolved in THF (1 mL) and treated with DBU (0.2 μL, 0.0013 mmol) and octanethiol (75 μL, 0.43 mmol) at rt for 10 min and then evaporated to dryness. The crude compound was purified by flash chromatography (DCM/MeOH/NEt_3, 100:0:0 to 80:20:1) affording a white powder (17 mg, 99% yield). The product was dissolved in 2 mL of THF. 2,7-di-*tert*-butylfluorène-9-carboxylic acid (17 mg, 0.05 mmol), HBTU (16 mg, 0.043 mmol), and DIEA (75 μL, 0.43 mmol) were added and the reaction mixture was stirred at rt overnight. After evaporation of THF, a solution of TFA/TIS/H_2O (95:2.5:2.5, 2 mL) was added and the mixture was stirred at rt for 45 min and then evaporated. The crude product was purified by preparative RP-HPLC using a gradient of 50% to 100% MeCN in 30 min. After lyophilisation compound **18** was obtained as white powder with purity >99% (24 mg, 65% yield); ^1H NMR (300 MHz, CD_3OD) δ 7.79 (s, *CH* arom fluorenyl), 7.71 (d, *J* = 8 Hz, 2H, *CH* arom fluorenyl), 7.59 (s, *CH* arom fluorenyl), 7.49 (d, *J* = 8 Hz, 2H, *CH* arom fluorenyl), 7.36 (s, 1H, *CH* indole), 7.14 (s, 1H, *CH* indole), 4.38 (dd, *J* = 10 Hz, 4 Hz, 1H, *CH*α Tbt), 3.65 (d, *J* = 14 Hz, 1H, $CH_2\beta\varepsilon_1$ $\beta^{2,2}$ *h* bis-Arg), 3.56 (dd, *J* = 14.8 Hz, 10.5 Hz, 1H, $CH_2\beta_1$ Tbt), 3.39 (dd, *J* = 14.8 Hz, 4 Hz, 1H, $CH_2\beta_2$ Tbt), 2.65 (d, *J* = 14.3 Hz, 2H, $CH_2\beta\varepsilon_2$ $\beta^{2,2}$ *h* bis-Arg), 2.52–2.66 (m, 2H, $CH_2\delta_1$ $\beta^{2,2}$ *h* bis-Arg), 2.38–2.45 (m, 2H, $CH_2\delta$ $\beta^{2,2}$ *h* bis-Arg), 1.30–1.53 (m, 35H, $C(CH_3)_3$, $CH_2\beta$ $\beta^{2,2}$ *h* bis-Arg and $CH_2\gamma$ $\beta^{2,2}$ *h* bis-Arg); MALDI-TOF: calcd for $C_{55}H_{81}N_5O_4$ 875.6, found 876.6 $[M + H]^+$, 898.6 $[M + Na]^+$, 914.6 $[M + K]^+$; HPLC (Water/ACN (0.1% TFA); 45% to 100% ACN in 30 min: tr = 21.9 min (Figure 20).

4.3.10. Synthesis of Np-Tbt-$\beta^{2,2}$ h bis-Orn-OMe 19 (Scheme 13)

Compound **16** (50 mg, 0.05 mmol) was dissolved in THF (1 mL) and treated with DBU (0.3 μL, 0.002 mmol) and octanethiol (90 μL, 0.5 mmol) at rt for 10 min and then evaporated to dryness. The crude compound was purified by flash chromatography (DCM/MeOH/NEt_3, 100:0:0 to 80:20:1) affording a white powder (34 mg, 87% yield). This compound was dissolved in 4 mL of THF. 2-Naphtoyl chloride (9.5 mg, 0.05 mmol) and NEt_3 (14 µL, 0.1 mmol) were added and the reaction mixture was stirred at rt overnight. After evaporation of THF, a solution of TFA/TIS/H_2O (95:2.5:2.5, 2 mL) was added and the mixture was stirred at rt for 30 min and then evaporated. The crude product was purified by preparative RP-HPLC using a gradient of 30% to 100% MeCN in 30 min. After lyophilisation compound **19** was obtained as white powder with 96% purity (22 mg, 60% yield); ^{1}H NMR (300 MHz, CD_3OD) δ 8.06 (s, 1H, *CH* Np), 7.91 (d, *J* = 8.4 Hz, 2H, *CH* Np), 7.86 (d, *J* = 7.8 Hz, 1H, *CH* Np), 7.75 (d, *J* = 8.4 Hz, 1H, *CH* Np), 7.60 (t, *J* = 6.4 Hz, 1H, *CH* Np), 7.56 (t, *J* = 6.4 Hz, 1H, *CH* Np), 7.41 (s, 1H, *CH* indole), 7.18 (s, 1H, *CH* indole), 4.57 (t, *J* = 7.5 Hz, 1H, CHα Tbt), 3.69 (d, *J* = 14.2, 2H, $CH_2\beta\varepsilon_1$ $\beta^{2,2}$ *h* bis-Arg), 3.63 (dd, *J* = 14.7 Hz, 8.3 Hz, 1H, $CH_2\beta_1$ Tbt), 3.48 (dd, *J* = 14.7 Hz, 6.6 Hz, 1H, $CH_2\beta_2$ Tbt), 2.99 (d, *J* = 14.2, 2H, $CH_2\beta\varepsilon_1$ $\beta^{2,2}$ *h* bis-Arg), 2.78–2.88 (m, 4H, $CH_2\delta$ $\beta^{2,2}$ *h* bis-Arg), 1.18–1.37 (m, 35H, $C(CH_3)_3$, $CH_2\beta$ $\beta^{2,2}$ *h* bis-Arg and $CH_2\gamma$ $\beta^{2,2}$ *h* bis-Arg); MALDI-TOF: calcd for $C_{44}H_{65}N_5O_5$ 725.5, found 726.4 $[M + H]^+$, 748.4 $[M + K]^+$, 764.4 $[M + K]^+$; HPLC (Water/ACN (0.1% TFA); 5% to 100% ACN in 30 min: tr = 21.9 min (Figure 21).

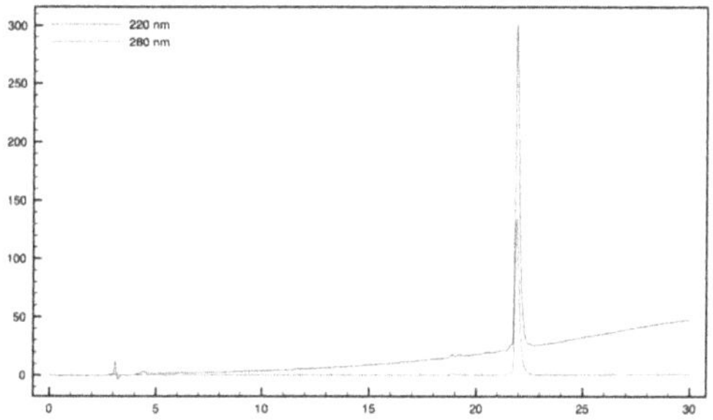

Figure 20. HPLC profile of Fluo-Tbt-$\beta^{2,2}$ h bis-Orn-OMe **18**.

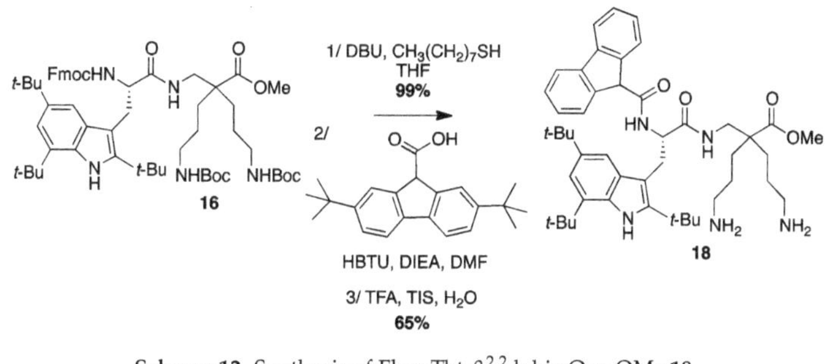

Scheme 12. Synthesis of Fluo-Tbt-$\beta^{2,2}$ h bis-Orn-OMe **18**.

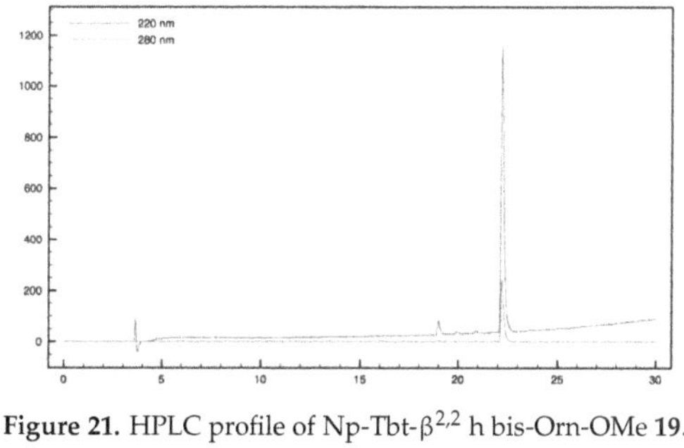

Figure 21. HPLC profile of Np-Tbt-$\beta^{2,2}$ h bis-Orn-OMe **19**.

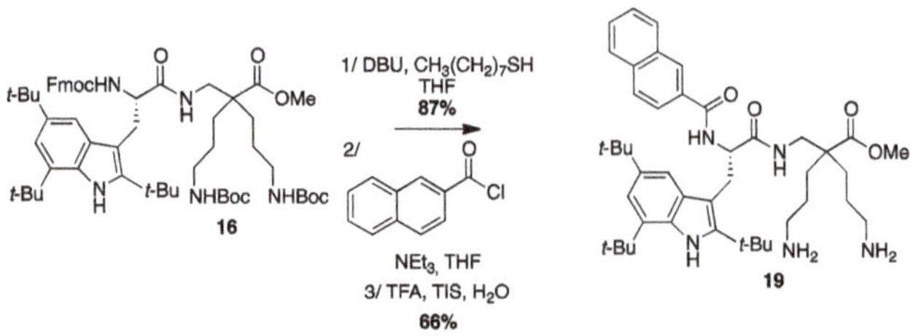

Scheme 13. Synthesis of Np-Tbt-$\beta^{2,2}$ h bis-Orn-OMe **19**.

4.3.11. Synthesis of Tbt-$\beta^{2,2}$ h bis-Arg-OBn **20** (Scheme 14)

$\beta^{2,2}$-h-bis-Orn(Boc)$_2$OBn **27**: Fmoc $\beta^{2,2}$-*h*-bis-Orn(Boc)$_2$OH **2** (300 mg, 0.48 mmol) was dissolved in MeCN (1.7 mL). After addition of Cs_2CO_3 (188 mg, 0.58 mmol) and benzyl bromide (63 µL, 0.53 mmol), the reaction mixture was heated at 60 °C under microwave (150W) for 10 min. The solution was filtered and evaporated to dryness. The crude compound was dissolved in AcOEt and washed with an aqueous solution of $NaHCO_3$ 5% followed by a solution of citric acid 5%, then dried over $MgSO_4$, filtered, and concentrated *in vacuo*. The crude compound was purified by flash chromatography (DCM/MeOH/NEt_3 100:0:0.1 to 95:5:0.1) to afford a white powder (80 mg, 28% yield); ^{1}H NMR (300 MHz, CD_3OD) δ 7.34–7.43 (m, 5H, *CH* Ar), 5.17 (s, 2H, CH_2Ph), 3.01 (t, *J* = 6.8 Hz, 4H, $CH_2\delta$), 2.84 (s, 2H, $CH_2\beta\varepsilon$), 1.62 (dd, *J* = 9.3 Hz, 5.3 Hz, 4H, $CH_2\beta$), 1.43 (s, 18H, $C(CH_3)_3$), 1.24–1.41 (m, 4H, $CH_2\gamma$); ^{13}C NMR (75 MHz, CD_3OD) δ 176.9 (C, C=O ester), 158.5 (2C, C=O carbamate), 137.5 (C, C Ar), 129.6, 129.4, 129.3 (3CH, CH Ar), 79.9 (2C, $C(CH_3)_3$), 67.5 (CH_2, CH_2Ph), 51.3 (CH_2, $CH_2\beta\varepsilon$), 45.5 (C, Cα), 41.5 (2CH_2, $CH_2\delta$), 31.1 (2CH_2, $CH_2\beta$), 28.8 (6CH_3, $C(CH_3)_3$), 25.3 (2CH_2, $CH_2\gamma$); HRMS-ESI+: calcd for $C_{26}H_{43}N_3O_6$ 493.3152, found 494.3225 $[M + H]^+$.

Fmoc-Tbt-$\beta^{2,2}$-h-bis-Orn(Boc)$_2$OBn **28:** Fmoc-Tbt-OH (83 mg, 0.14 mmol) was dissolved in DMF (6 mL). HBTU (53 mg, 0.14 mmol) and DIEA (24 µL, 0.14 mmol) were added and the mixture was stirred for 5 min before addition of H-$\beta^{2,2}$-*h*-bis-Orn(Boc)$_2$OBn **28** (70 mg, 0.14 mmol). The reaction mixture was stirred at room temperature overnight, then diluted with Et_2O and washed with an aqueous saturated solution of NH_4Cl. The organic layer was dried over $MgSO_4$, filtered, and evaporated to dryness. The crude compound was purified by flash chromatography (Cy/AcOEt, 100:0 to 70:30) to afford the pure protected dipeptide as a white powder (67 mg, 45% yield). ^{1}H NMR (300 MHz, MeOD) δ 7.91 (s, 1H, *NH* indole), 7.66 (d, *J* = 7.5, 1H, *CH* Ar Fmoc), 7.45 (d, *J* = 7.2, 1H, *CH* Ar Fmoc), 7.37 (s, 1H, *CH* Ar indole), 7.3 (t, *J* = 7.5, 1H, *CH* Ar Fmoc), 7.18 (dt, *J* = 14.7 and 6.9, 1H, *CH* Ar Fmoc), 7.09 (s, 1H, *CH* indole), 5.89 (bs, 2H, *NH* Boc), 5.71 (bs, 1H, *NH* Fmoc), 4.87 (s, 2H, CH_2Ph), 4.20–4.34 (m, 3H, *CH*α Tbt and CH_2 Fmoc), 4.09 (t, *J* = 7.2, 1H, *CH* Fmoc), 3.37 (d, *J* = 14.1, 1H, $CH_2\beta\varepsilon_1$ $\beta^{2,2}$ *h* bis-Orn), 3.31 (d, *J* = 7.5 Hz, 2H, $CH_2\beta$ Tbt), 2.86 (m, 4H, $CH_2\delta$ $\beta^{2,2}$ *h* bis-Orn), 2.55 (d, *J* = 14.1, 1H, $CH_2\beta\varepsilon_2$ $\beta^{2,2}$ *h* bis-Orn), 1.52 (s, 9H, $C(CH_3)_3$ indole), 1.47 (s, 9H, $C(CH_3)_3$ indole), 1.36–1.44 (m, 35H, $C(CH_3)_3$ indole, $C(CH_3)_3$ Boc, $CH_2\beta$ $\beta^{2,2}$ *h* bis-Orn and $CH_2\gamma$ $\beta^{2,2}$ *h* bis-Orn).

H-Tbt-$\beta^{2,2}$ h bis-Arg-OBn **20:** Compound **28** (68 mg, 0.064 mmol) was dissolved in DCM (~0.4 M) and an equivalent volume of TFA. The mixture was stirred at rt for 1.5 h then evaporated to dryness. The crude compound was dissolved in 4 mL of THF.

1,3-Di-Boc-2-(trifluoromethylsulfonyl)guanidine (50 mg, 0.128 mmol) and NEt_3 (500 µL, 3.2 mmol) were added and the reaction mixture was stirred at rt for 16 h. After evaporation of THF, the crude mixture was dissolved in a 20% solution of piperidine in DCM and allowed to react for 2 h before evaporation to dryness. A solution of TFA/TIS (95:5) was added and the mixture was stirred at rt for 1.5 h. After evaporation, the crude product was purified by preparative RP-HPLC using a gradient of 20% to 90% MeCN in 30 min. After lyophilisation compound **20** was obtained as white powder with purity >99% (10 mg, 22% yield); ^{1}H NMR (300 MHz, CD_3OD) δ 8.36 (s, 1H, *NH* indole), 7.20–7.32 (m, 5H, *CH* Ph), 7.28 (s, 1H, *CH* indole), 7.15 (s, 1H, *CH* indole), 5.03 (d, *J* = 12 Hz, 1H, CH_2 Ph), 5.01 (d, *J* =

12 Hz, 1H, CH_2 Ph), 4.03 (t, *J* = 6.1 Hz, 1H, CHα Tbt), 3.60 (d, *J* = 14.2, 1H, $CH_2\beta\varepsilon_1$ $\beta^{2,2}$ *h* bis-Arg), 3.42 (d, *J* = 6.6 Hz, 2H, $CH_2\beta$ Tbt), 2.97–3 (m, 4H, $CH_2\delta$ $\beta^{2,2}$ *h* bis-Arg), 2.33 (d, *J* = 1.24 Hz, 1H, $CH_2\beta\varepsilon_2$ $\beta^{2,2}$ *h* bis-Arg), 1.20–1.59 (m, 35H, $C(CH_3)_3$, $CH_2\beta$ $\beta^{2,2}$ *h* bis-Arg and $CH_2\gamma$ $\beta^{2,2}$ *h* bis-Arg); MALDI-TOF: calcd for $C_{48}H_{67}N_5O_5$ 731.5, found 732.4 $[M + H]^+$, 770.3 $[M + K]^+$, 716.3 $[M + H - NH_3]^+$; HPLC (Water/ACN (0.1% TFA); 40% to 90% ACN in 10 min: tr = 7.51 min (Figure 22).

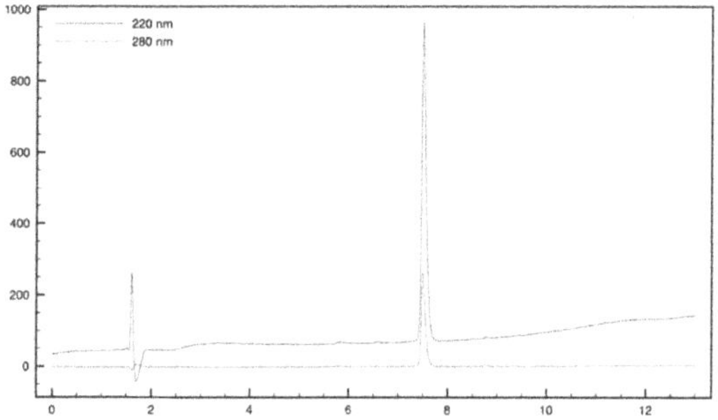

Figure 22. HPLC profile of *H-Tbt-$\beta^{2,2}$ h bis-Arg-OBn* **20**.

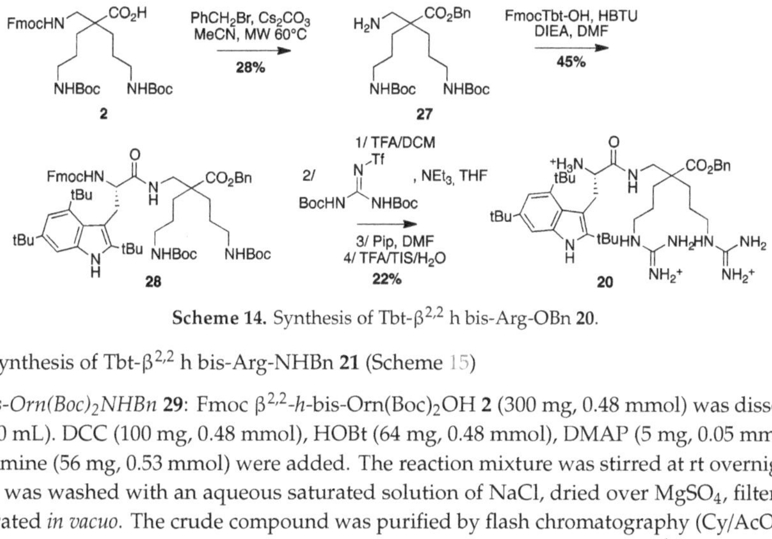

Scheme 14. Synthesis of Tbt-$\beta^{2,2}$ h bis-Arg-OBn **20**.

4.3.12. Synthesis of Tbt-$\beta^{2,2}$ h bis-Arg-NHBn **21** (Scheme 15)

$\beta^{2,2}$-h-bis-Orn(Boc)$_2$NHBn **29**: Fmoc $\beta^{2,2}$-*h*-bis-Orn(Boc)$_2$OH **2** (300 mg, 0.48 mmol) was dissolved in DCM (20 mL). DCC (100 mg, 0.48 mmol), HOBt (64 mg, 0.48 mmol), DMAP (5 mg, 0.05 mmol), and benzyl amine (56 mg, 0.53 mmol) were added. The reaction mixture was stirred at rt overnight. The solution was washed with an aqueous saturated solution of NaCl, dried over $MgSO_4$, filtered, and concentrated *in vacuo*. The crude compound was purified by flash chromatography (Cy/AcOEt 100:0 to 50:50) to afford a colorless oil (251 mg, 73% yield); $\mathbf{R_f}$ (Cy/AcOEt, 7:3) = 0.5; ^1H NMR (300 MHz, $CDCl_3$) δ 7.76 (d, *J* = 7.5 Hz, 2H, *CH* Ar), 7.58 (d, *J* = 7.5 Hz, 2H, *CH* Ar), 7.40 (t, *J* = 7.5 Hz, 2H, *CH* Ar), 7.25–7.33 (m, 7H, *CH* Ar), 6.48 (bs, 1H, *NH* amide), 5.47 (bs, 1H, *NH* Fmoc), 4.78 (bs, 2H, *NH* Boc), 4.36–4.42 (m, 4H, CH_2Ph, CH_2 Fmoc), 4.15–4.20 (m, 1H, *CH* Fmoc), 3.36–3.38 (m, 2H, $CH_2\beta\varepsilon$), 2.98–3.04 (m, 4H, $CH_2\delta$), 1.31–1.69 (m, 26H, $CH_2\beta$, $C(CH_3)_3$, $CH_2\gamma$); ^{13}C NMR (75 MHz, CD_3OD) δ 175.3 (C, C=O amide), 157.3 (C, C=O carbamate), 156.3 (C, C=O carbamate), 143.9, 141.4, 138.3 (3C, *C* Ar), 128.8, 127.8, 127.6, 127.1, 125.1, 120.1 (6CH, *C*H Ar), 79.2 (C, $C(CH_3)_3$), 66.9 (CH_2, CH_2 Fmoc), 49.8 (C, *C*α), 47.3 (CH, *C*H Fmoc), 44.6 (CH_2, $CH_2\beta\varepsilon$), 43.8 (CH_2, CH_2Ph), 40.7 (CH_2, $CH_2\delta$), 30.8 (CH_2, $CH_2\beta$), 29.0 (CH_3, $C(CH_3)_3$), 24.2 (CH_2, $CH_2\gamma$); Fmoc $\beta^{2,2}$-*h*-bis-Orn(Boc)$_2$NHBn (251 mg, 0.35 mmol) was dissolved in THF (6 mL). Octanethiol (600 μL, 3.5 mmol) and DBU (1.5 μL, 0.01 mmol) were added. The reaction mixture was stirred for 15 min then concentrated *in vacuo*. The crude compound was purified by flash chromatography (DCM/MeOH/NEt_3 100:0:0 to 80:20:0.1) to afford **29** as a colorless oil (150 mg, 87% yield); ^1H NMR (300 MHz, $CDCl_3$) δ 8.94 (bs, 2H, NH_2), 7.15–7.24 (m, 5H, *CH* Ar), 4.75 (bs, 2H, *NH* Boc), 4.33–4.35 (m, 2H, CH_2Ph), 2.98–3.11 (m, 4H, $CH_2\delta$), 2.80 (s, 2H, $CH_2\beta\varepsilon$), 1.01–1.73

(m, 26H, $CH_2\beta$, $C(CH_3)_3$, $CH_2\gamma$); ^{13}C NMR (75 MHz, CD_3OD) δ 176.3 (C, C=O amide), 156.1 (C, C=O carbamate), 139 (C, *C* Ar), 128.5, 127.3, 127 (3CH, *C*H Ar), 78.9 (C, *C*(CH_3)$_3$), 47.3 (C, Cα), 45.3 (CH_2, $CH_2\beta\varepsilon$), 42.9 (CH_2, CH_2Ph), 40.8 (CH_2, $CH_2\delta$), 31.6 (CH_2, $CH_2\beta$), 28.4 (CH_3, $C(CH_3)_3$), 22.4 (CH_2, $CH_2\gamma$); HRMS-ESI+: calcd for $C_{26}H_{44}N_4O_5$ 492.3312, found 515.3199 $[M + Na]^+$.

Fmoc-Tbt-$\beta^{2,2}$ *h bis-Orn(Boc)*$_2$*NHBn* **30**: Fmoc-Tbt-OH (90 mg, 0.15 mmol) was dissolved in DMF (6 mL). HBTU (57 mg, 0.15 mmol) and DIEA (30 μL, 0.15 mmol) were added and the mixture was stirred for 5 min before addition of H-$\beta^{2,2}$ *h* bis-Orn(Boc)$_2$NHBn **29** (75 mg, 0.15 mmol). The reaction mixture was stirred at room temperature overnight, then diluted with Et_2O and washed with an aqueous saturated solution of NH_4Cl. The organic layer was dried over $MgSO_4$, filtered, and evaporated to dryness. The crude compound was purified by flash chromatography (Cy/AcOEt, 100:0 to 60:40) to afford the pure protected dipeptide **30** as a white powder (64 mg, 40% yield). ^{1}H NMR (300 MHz, MeOD) δ 7.91 (s, 1H, *NH* indole), 7.65 (d, *J* = 7.5, 2H, *CH* Ar Fmoc), 7.40 (d, *J* = 7.4, 2H, *CH* Ar Fmoc), 7.35 (s, 1H, *CH* Ar indole), 7.28 (t, *J* = 7.4, 2H, *CH* Ar Fmoc), 7.03–7.20 (m, 8H, *CH* Ar Fmoc, *CH* indole, *CH* benzyl), 6.35 and 6.19 (2 bs, 1H, *NH* Amide), 5.61 (bs, 1H, *NH* Fmoc), 4.69 and 4.76 (2bs, 2H, *NH* Boc), 4.15–4.27 (m, 5H, *CH*α Tbt, CH_2 Fmoc, CH_2Ph), 4.08 (t, *J* = 76.8, 1H, *CH* Fmoc), 3.24–3.39 (m, 3H, $CH_2\beta_1$ Tbt, $CH_2\beta\varepsilon$ $\beta^{2,2}$ *h* bis-Orn), 2.84–2.94 (m, 4H, $CH_2\delta$ $\beta^{2,2}$ *h* bis-Orn), 2.67–2.74 (m, 1H, $CH_2\beta_2$ Tbt), 1.30–1.34 (m, 53H, $C(CH_3)_3$ indole, $C(CH_3)_3$ Boc, $CH_2\beta$ $\beta^{2,2}$ *h* bis-Orn and $CH_2\gamma$ $\beta^{2,2}$ *h* bis-Orn) ^{13}C NMR (75 MHz, CD_3OD) δ 175.1 and 172.4 (C, C=O amide), 156.2 (C, C=O carbamate), 143.9, 143.6, 142.8, 142.6, 141.3, 141.2, 138.3, 132.1, 130.2, 129.8 (10C, *C* Ar), 128.7, 127.7, 127.4, 127.1, 125.3, 125.2, 120, 116.8, 112.1 (9CH, CH Ar), 104.5 (C, *C* indolyl), 79.1 (C, *C*(CH_3)$_3$), 67.2 (CH_2, CH_2 Fmoc), 56.7 (CH, CHα Tβτ), 49.2 (C, *C*α $\beta^{2,2}$ *h* bis-Orn), 47.1 (CH, CH Fμοχ), 43.6 (CH_2, CH_2Ph), 42.9 (CH_2, $CH_2\beta$ Tbt), 40.7 (2CH_2, $CH_2\delta$ $\beta^{2,2}$ *h* bis-Orn), 34.9, 34.7, 33.1 (3CH_2, $CH_2\beta$ ανδ $CH_2\beta'$ $\beta^{2,2}$ *h* bis-Orn), 32.2, 30.9, 30.8, 30.7 (4CH_3, $C(CH_3)_3$), 24.2, 24.3 (2CH_2, $CH_2\gamma$).

H-Tbt-$\beta^{2,2}$ *h bis-Arg-NHBn* **21:** Compound **30** (64 mg, 0.06 mmol) was dissolved in DCM (~0.4 M) and an equivalent volume of TFA containing 5% of TIS. The mixture was stirred at rt for 2 h then evaporated to dryness. The crude compound was dissolved in 4 mL of THF. 1,3-Di-Boc-2-(trifluoromethylsulfonyl)guanidine (117 mg, 0.3 mmol) and NEt_3 (80 μL, 0.6 mmol) were added and the reaction mixture was stirred at rt for 48 h. After evaporation of THF, the crude mixture was dissolved in a 20% solution of piperidine in DCM and allowed to react for 2 h before evaporation to dryness. A solution of TFA/TIS (95:5) in DCM was added and the mixture was stirred at rt for 1.5 h. After evaporation, the crude product was purified by preparative RP-HPLC using a gradient of 40% to 100% MeCN in 30 min. After lyophilisation, compound **21** was obtained as white powder with purity >99% (20 mg, 45% yield); ^{1}H NMR (300 MHz, CD_3OD) δ 7.32 (s, 1H, *CH* indole), 7.25–7.32 (m, 5H, *CH* arom), 7.17 (s, 1H, *CH* indole), 4.28 (s, 2H, CH_2Ph), 4.06 (dd, *J* = 9.4 Hz, 6.1 Hz, 1H, CHα Tbt), 3.44–3.56 (m, 3H, $CH_2\beta\varepsilon_1$ $\beta^{2,2}$ *h* bis-Arg and $CH_2\beta$ Tbt), 3.11–3.17 (m, 4H, $CH_2\delta$ $\beta^{2,2}$ *h* bis-Arg), 2.39 (d, *J* = 14 Hz, 1H, $CH_2\beta\varepsilon_2$ $\beta^{2,2}$ *h* bis-Arg), 1.22–1.54 (m, 35H, $C(CH_3)_3$, $CH_2\beta$ $\beta^{2,2}$ *h* bis-Arg and $CH_2\gamma$ $\beta^{2,2}$ *h* bis-Arg); MALDI-TOF: calcd for $C_{41}H_{66}N_{10}O_2$ 730.5, found 731.6 $[M + H]^+$; HPLC (Water/ACN (0.1% TFA); 40% to 100% ACN in 30 min: tr = 13.57 min (Figure 23).

4.3.13. Synthesis of Tbt-$\beta^{2,2}$ h bis-Arg-NH(CH_2)$_{13}$$CH_3$ 22 (Scheme 16)

$\beta^{2,2}$*-h-bis-Orn(Boc)*$_2$*NH(CH*$_2$*)*$_{13}$*CH*$_3$ **31**: Fmoc $\beta^{2,2}$ *h* bis-Orn(Boc)$_2$OH **2** (300 mg, 0.48 mmol) was dissolved in DCM (25 mL). DCC (109 mg, 0.53 mmol), HOBt (72 mg, 0.53 mmol), DMAP (5 mg, 0.05 mmol), and tetradecyl amine (113 mg, 0.53 mmol) were added. The reaction mixture was stirred at for 4 h. The solution was washed with brine, dried over $MgSO_4$, filtered, and concentrated *in vacuo*. The crude compound was purified by flash chromatography (Cy/AcOEt 100:0 to 50:50) to afford a colorless oil (390 mg, 99% yield); $\mathbf{R_f}$ (Cy/AcOEt, 1:1) = 0.76; ^{1}H NMR (300 MHz, $CDCl_3$) δ 7.67 (d, *J* = 7.3 Hz, 2H, *CH* Ar), 7.51 (d, *J* = 7.3 Hz, 2H, *CH* Ar), 7.31 (t, *J* = 7.3 Hz, 2H, *CH* Ar), 7.22 (t, *J* = 7.3 Hz, 2H, *CH* Ar), 6.05 (bs, 1H, *NH* amide), 5.65 and 5.47 (2bs, 1H, *NH* Fmoc), 4.80 (bs, 2H, *NH* Boc), 4.30 (d, *J* = 6.2 Hz, 2H, CH_2 Fmoc), 4.11 (t, *J* = 6.9 Hz, 1H, *CH* Fmoc), 3.28 (d, *J* = 6.1 Hz,

1H, $CH_2\beta\varepsilon$ $\beta^{2,2}$ *h* bis-Orn), 3.13 (m, 2H, $CH_2C_{13}H_{27}$), 3 (m, 4H, $CH_2\delta$ $\beta^{2,2}$ *h* bis-Orn), 1.41 (m, 4H, $CH_2\gamma$ $\beta^{2,2}$ *h* bis-Orn), 1.17-1.35 (m, 46H, $C(CH_3)_3$ Boc, $(CH_2)_{12}CH_3$ and $CH_2\beta$ $\beta^{2,2}$ *h* bis-Orn), 0.8 (t, 3H, $(CH_2)_{12}CH_3$); ^{13}C NMR (75 MHz, CD_3OD) δ 175.2 (C, C=O amide), 157.3 and 156.3 (2C, C=O carbamate), 143.9 and 141.3 (C, *C* arom Fmoc), 127.7, 127.1, 125.1, 120 (5CH, *C*H arom Fmoc), 79.1 (C, $C(CH_3)_3$), 66.9 (CH_2, CH_2 Fmoc), 49.6 (C, *C*α $\beta^{2,2}$ *h* bis-Orn), 47.2 (C, CH Fmoc), 44.6 (CH_2, $CH_2\beta\varepsilon$ $\beta^{2,2}$ *h* bis-Orn), 40.7 (CH_2, $CH_2C_{13}H_{27}$), 39.8 (CH_2, $CH_2\delta$ $\beta^{2,2}$ *h* bis-Orn), 33.9 (CH_2, $CH_2C_{12}H_{25}$), 31.9 (CH_2, $CH_2\beta$ $\beta^{2,2}$ *h* bis-Orn), 30.8 (CH_2, $CH_2C_{11}H_{23}$), 29.72, 29.68, 29.62, 29.59, 29.39, 29.33 (CH_2, $CH_2C_7H_{17}$), 28.4 (CH_3, $C(CH_3)_3$), 27.1, 27.0, 24.2 (CH_2, $(CH_2)_3CH_3$), 22.7 (CH_2, $CH_2\gamma$ $\beta^{2,2}$ *h* bis-Orn), 14.2 (CH_3, $(CH_2)_{13}CH_3$); HRMS-ESI+: calcd for $C_{48}H_{76}N_4O_7$ 820.5714, found 843.5606 $[M + Na]^+$. The obtained Fmoc $\beta^{2,2}$-*h*-bis-Orn$(Boc)_{22}NH(CH_2)_{13}CH_3$ (130 mg, 0.12 mmol) was dissolved in THF (2 mL). Octanethiol (210 μL, 1.2 mmol) and DBU (0.5 μL, 0.0036 mmol) were added. The reaction mixture was stirred for 20 min then concentrated *in vacuo*. The crude compound was purified by flash chromatography (DCM/MeOH/NEt_3 100:0:0.1 to 80:20:0.1) to afford a colorless oil (58 mg, 81% yield); ^1H NMR (300 MHz, CD_3OD) δ 3.21 (t, *J* = 7.2 Hz, 2H, $CH_2C_{12}H_{27}$), 33.04 (t, *J* = 6.9 Hz, 4H, $CH_2\delta$ $\beta^{2,2}$ *h* bis-Orn), δ 2.78 (s, 2H, $CH_2\beta'$ $\beta^{2,2}$ *h* bis-Orn), 1.32-1.58 (m, 48H, $C(CH_3)_3$ Boc, $CH_2(CH_2)_{11}CH_3$, $CH_2\beta$ $\beta^{2,2}$ *h* bis-Orn and $CH_2\gamma$ $\beta^{2,2}$ *h* bis-Orn), 0.93 (t, 3H, *J* = 6.6 Hz, $(CH_2)_{13}CH_3$); ^{13}C NMR (75 MHz, CD_3OD) δ 178.2 (C, C=O amide), 159.4 (C, C=O carbamate), 79.8 (C, $C(CH_3)_3$), 50.2 (C, Cα), 45.8 (CH_2, $CH_2\beta'$), 41.7 (CH_2, $CH_2\delta$), 40.4 (CH_2, $CH_2(CH_2)_{12}CH_3$), 33.1, 31.6, 30.8, 30.5 ($4CH_2$), 28.8, ($6CH_3$, $C(CH_3)_3$), 28.2, 25.3, 23.7 (CH_2), 14.5 (CH_3, CH_2CH_3); HRMS-ESI+: calcd for $C_{33}H_{66}N_4O_5$ 598.5033, found 599.5112 $[M + H]^+$.

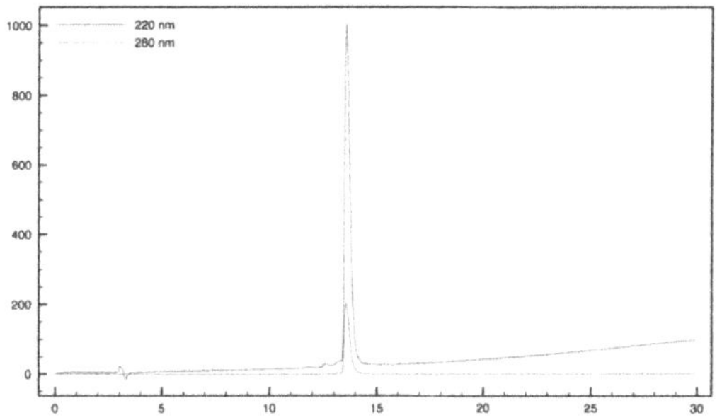

Figure 23. HPLC profile of *H-Tbt-β*^{2,2} *h bis-Arg-NHBn* **21**.

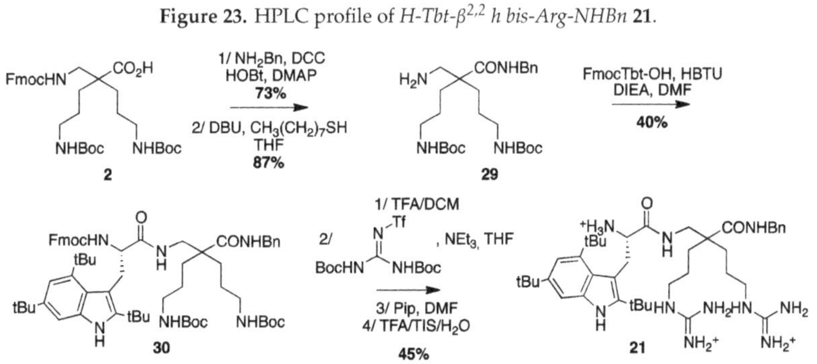

Scheme 15. Synthesis of Tbt-$\beta^{2,2}$ h bis-Arg-NHBn **21**.

Fmoc-Tbt-β^{2,2}*-h-bis-Orn(Boc)*$_2$*NH(CH*$_2$*)*$_{13}$*CH*$_3$ **32**: Fmoc-Tbt-OH (54 mg, 0.09 mmol) was dissolved in DMF (5 mL). HBTU (34 mg, 0.09 mmol) and DIEA (20 μL, 0.09 mmol) were added and the mixture was stirred for 5 min before addition of $\beta^{2,2}$-*h*-bis-Orn$(Boc)_2NH(CH_2)_{13}CH_3$ 31 (55 mg, 0.09 mmol). The reaction mixture was stirred at room temperature for 4 h, then diluted with Et_2O and washed with an aqueous saturated solution of NH_4Cl. The organic layer was dried over $MgSO_4$, filtered, and evaporated to dryness. The crude compound was purified by flash chromatography (Cy/AcOEt, 100:0 to 50:50) to afford the pure protected dipeptide as a white powder (70 mg, 66% yield). ^{1}H NMR (300 MHz, $CDCl_3$) δ 7.99 (s, 1H, *NH* indole), 7.23 (d, *J* = 7.5, 2H, *CH* Ar Fmoc), 7.50 (d, *J* = 7.2, 2H, *CH* Ar Fmoc), 7.43 (s, 1H, *CH* Ar indole), 7.38 (t, *J* = 7.5, 2H, *CH* Ar Fmoc), 7.24 (t, *J* = 7.5, 2H, *CH* Ar Fmoc), 7.17 (s, 1H, *CH* indole), 6.23 (bs, 1H, *NH* amide), 5.92 and 5.66 (2bs, 1H, *NH* Fmoc), 4.78 and 4.86 (2bs, 2H, *NH* Boc), 4.25–4.37 (m, 3H, *CH*α Tbt and CH_2 Fmoc), 4.13–4.17 (m, 1H, *CH* Fmoc), 3.33–3.44 (m, 3H, CH_2βε $\beta^{2,2}$ *h* bis-Orn and $CH_2\beta_1$ Tbt), 3.02 (m, 6H, CH_2δ $\beta^{2,2}$ *h* bis-Orn and $CH_2(CH_2)_{12}CH_3$), 2.75–2.80 (m, 1H, $CH_2\beta_2$ Tβτ), 1.30–1.47 (m, 77H, $3C(CH_3)_3$ indole, $CH_2(CH_2)_{12}CH_3$, $2C(CH_3)_3$ Boc, $2CH_2\beta$ $\beta^{2,2}$ *h* bis-Orn and $2CH_2\gamma\beta^{2,2}$*h* bis-Orn), 0.86 (t, *J* = 6.9, 3H, $(CH_2)_{13}CH_3$) ^{13}C NMR (75 MHz, $CDCl_3$) δ 174.8 and 172.3 (C, C=O amide), 156.1 and 156.2 (C, C=O carbamate), 143.9, 143.6, 142.8, 142.6, 141.3, 141.2, 132.1, 130.2, 129.8 (9C, *C* Ar), 127.7, 127.1, 125.3, 125.2, 120, 116.8, 112.1 (7CH, CH Ar), 104.5 (C, *C* indolyl), 79.1 (C, *C*($CH_3)_3$), 67.2 (CH_2, CH_2 Fmoc), 56.7 (CH, CHα Tβτ), 49.2 (C, Cα $\beta^{2,2}$ *h* bis-Orn), 47.1 (CH, CH Fμοχ), 43 (CH_2, $CH_2\beta$ Tbt), 40.7 (CH_2, $CH_2C_{13}H_{29}$, 39.7 ($2CH_2$, $CH_2\delta$ $\beta^{2,2}$ *h* bis-Orn), 34.9 (CH_2, $CH_2C_{12}H_{27}$), 34.8 (CH_2, $CH_2C_{11}H_{25}$), 33.1 (CH_2, $CH_2C_{10}H_{23}$), 32.1 (CH_3, $C(CH_3)_3$), 32 (CH_2, $CH_2C_9H_{21}$), 30.6 and 30.9 ($2CH_3$, $C(CH_3)_3$), 29.8, 29.7, 29.6, 29.5, 29.4, 29.3 ($7CH_2$, $(CH_2)_8CH_3$), 28.5 ($2CH_3$, $C(CH_3)_3$ Boc), 27 and 26.9 ($2CH_2$, $CH_2\beta$ $\beta^{2,2}$ *h* bis-Orn), 24.2 (CH_2, $CH_2\beta\varepsilon$ $\beta^{2,2}$ *h* bis-Orn), 22.7 ($2CH_2$, $CH_2\gamma$), 14.2 (CH_3, $(CH_2)_{13}CH_3$).

H-Tbt-$\beta^{2,2}$*h bis-Arg-NH(CH*$_2$*)*$_{13}$*CH*$_3$ **22:** Compound **32** (52 mg, 0.045 mmol) was dissolved in DCM (3 mL) and a mixture of TFA/TIS/H_2O (3 mL/150 μL/150 μL) as added. The solution was stirred at rt for 4 h then evaporated to dryness. The crude compound was dissolved in 4 mL of THF. 1,3-Di-Boc-2-(trifluoromethylsulfonyl)guanidine (53 mg, 0.135 mmol) and NEt_3 (40 μL, 0.27 mmol) were added and the reaction mixture was stirred at rt overnight. After evaporation of THF, the crude mixture was dissolved in a 20% solution of piperidine in DCM and allowed to react for 2 h before evaporation to dryness. A solution of TFA/TIS/H_2O (95:2.5:2.5) in DCM was added and the mixture was stirred at rt for 3 h. After evaporation, the crude product was purified by preparative RP-HPLC using a gradient of 40% to 90% MeCN in 30 min. After lyophilisation, compound **22** was obtained as white powder with purity >99% (12 mg, 40%); ^{1}H NMR (300 MHz, CD_3OD) δ 8.33 (s, 1H, *NH* indole), 7.60 (t, *J* = 5.6 Hz, 1H, NH amide), 7.30 (d, *J* = 1.5 Hz, 1H, *CH* indole), 7.15 (d, *J* = 1.5 Hz, 1H, *CH* indole), 4.06 (dd, *J* = 10.1 Hz, 5.6 Hz, CHα Tbt), 3.34–3.55 (m, 3H, $CH_2\beta\varepsilon_1$ $\beta^{2,2}$ *h* bis-Arg and $CH_2\beta$ Tbt), 3.11-3.17 (m, 2H, $CH_2C_{13}H_{29}$), 3.01–3.09 (m, 4H, $CH_2\delta$ $\beta^{2,2}$ *h* bis-Arg), 2.37 (d, *J* = 14.1 Hz, 1H, $CH_2\beta\varepsilon_2$ $\beta^{2,2}$ *h* bis-Arg), 1.68–1.84 (m, 2H, $CH_2C_{12}H_{27}$), 1.16–1.62 (m, 57H, $3C(CH_3)_3$, $(CH_2)_{11}CH_3$, $CH_2\beta$ $\beta^{2,2}$ *h* bis-Arg and $CH_2\gamma$ $\beta^{2,2}$ *h* bis-Arg), 0.90 (t, *J* = 6.7, 3H, $(CH_2)_{13}CH_3$); MALDI-TOF: calcd for $C_{48}H_{88}N_{10}O_2$ 836.7, found 837.6 $[M + H]^+$, 859.6 $[M + Na]^+$; HPLC (Water/ACN (0.1% TFA); 50% to 100% ACN in 10 min: tr = 8.09 min (Figure 24).

4.4. Antimicrobial Assays

4.4.1. Bacterial Strains and Media

Three Gram-negative strains (*Escherichia coli* ATCC25922, *Acinetobacter baumannii* ATCC19606, and *Pseudomonas aeruginosa* ATCC29853) and three Gram-positive strains (*Staphylococcus aureus* ATCC25923, *Staphylococcus aureus* SA-1199B, and *Enterrococcus faecalis* ATCC29212) were used in this study. *Staphylococcus aureus* SA-1199B is resistant to fluoroquinolones due notably to the overexpression of the membrane-associated NorA efflux pump [36].

All these strains were grown in Mueller–Hinton Broth media (MH, BioRad 69444, Mitry Mory, France) overnight at 37 °C without shaking, before being diluted in 1% Bacto Peptone water (Conda 1616.00, batch n°30927). Counting was realized on MH agar plates (MH, BioRad 64884, Mitry Mory, France). Colony forming unit (CFU) counting, used to check the bacterial density at T0 in the antibacterial activity test, was carried out by counting colonies present in 2 × 10 μL of serial log dilutions of bacteria inoculum spotted on MH agar plates. Plates were examined for growth after one night at 37 °C.

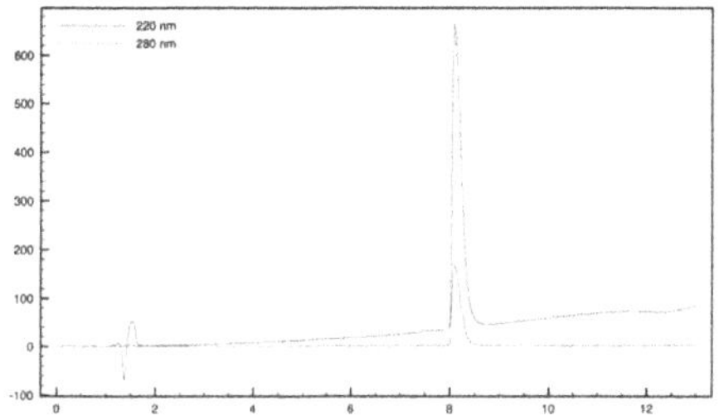

Figure 24. H-Tbt-$\beta^{2,2}$ h bis-Arg-$NH(CH_2)_{13}CH_3$ **22**.

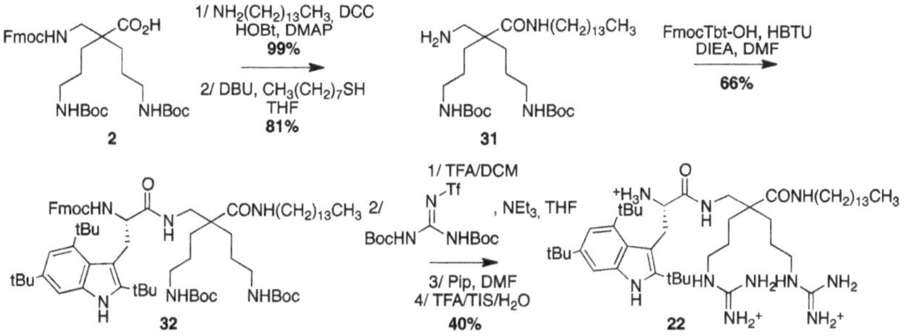

Scheme 16. Synthesis of Tbt-$\beta^{2,2}$ h bis-Arg-$NH(CH_2)_{13}CH_3$ **22**.

4.4.2. Antibacterial Activity

The antibacterial activity was evaluated in 1% Bacto Peptone. First, the peptides (solubilized in H_2O or in DMSO according to their own solubility), were dispensed in a 96-wells microplate by 2-fold serial dilutions in 1% Bacto Peptone water using a handling robot (Biomek 2000, Beckman, Fullerton, CA, USA). The final volume in each well was 100 µL. Then, 100 µL of an overnight grown bacterial culture diluted in 1% Bacto Peptone water was added in order to reach a bacterial concentration comprised between 10^5 and 10^6 CFU/mL. The final range of peptide concentrations were 64, 32, 16, 8, 4, 2, 1, 0.5, 0.25, 0.125, and 0.06 µg/mL, and the highest final concentration of DMSO or H_2O was less than 1.3% in all experiments. Growth at 37 °C without shaking was assayed using a microplate reader (DTX880, Beckman) by monitoring the absorption at 620 nm, at 0, 1, 4, 7, and 24 h. A solution of 2.6% DMSO was used as negative control, and peptide **A** was used as positive control. For each experiment, MICs of reference antibiotics were also measured and compared to the reported one in order to validate the assay. The minimal inhibitory concentrations (MIC) of the different peptides were defined as the lowest concentration of compound that completely inhibits cell growth during 24 h incubation. All peptides were tested at least twice in parallel.

4.5. Hemolytic Activities

Red blood cells (RBCs) were isolated from rat blood and re-suspended in PBS (4% *v*/*v*). RBC suspensions (100 µL) were introduced into a 96-microwell plate and either 1 µL (final concentration of 10 µM) or 5 µL (final concentration of 50 µM)* of peptides solutions in PBS (1 mM) were added to the wells. PBS was used as negative control while a solution of 1% triton ×100 in PBS was used as positive control. The plate was incubated for 1 h at 37 °C. After the incubation, the plate was centrifuged at 1500 rpm for 5 min. The absorbance of the supernatant 550 nm was measured and percentage of hemolysis was determined as (A − APBS)/(Atriton − A0) × 100, where A is the absorbance of the tested well, APBS the absorbance of the negative control, and Atriton the absorbance of the positive control.

4.6. Cytotoxicity on Human SH-SYS5 Cells

The cytotoxicity of the compounds was evaluated on SH-SYS5 neuroblastoma adherent cells (Figure 7). The SH-SYS5 cells were seeded (40,000 cells per well) in 96-well microplates the day before, then incubated at 37 °C, with 0, 1, 10, 50, or 100 μM compounds in RPMI for 2 h. The cell-counting kit solution was used as indicated by the supplier (Dojindo Laboratories). Absorbance at 450 nm (and reference at 620 nm) is directly related to the number of living cells. Experiments were done in triplicates and repeated two-times independently. Results are normalized to the control cells, in the absence of any compound.

4.7. In Vivo Experiments

Mice were bred and maintained at the mouse facilities of the Bichat Medical School campus. All experiments were performed in accordance with the French Council of Animal Care guidelines and national ethical guidelines of INSERM Animal Care Committee (Animal Use Protocol number 75-1596).

4.8. Cecal Ligation and Puncture (CLP)

Bl6 mice (only male 12 weeks old) were anesthetized and the cecum exposed by a 1 cm midline incision on the abdomen. The distal half of the cecum was ligated with a 5-0 silk suture and punctured with a 21-gauge needle. The cecum was replaced, and 1 ml of sterile saline injected into the peritoneal cavity. The incision was closed using surgical sutures. Mice were monitored every 8 h for the first 3 days and then every 12 h until death or day 7, when they were euthanized. For the peptide **11** treatment, 1 ug/g of mice (on average 20 g) was injected (intraperitoneal injection) during the surgical suture at the end of the CLP procedure.

4.9. Peptide Hydrophobicity

Analytical HPLC on C18 column (Higgins RS 1046 D183, 100*4.6 mm) using as eluent a 5% to 100% gradient of MeCN containing 0.1% TFA in water containing 0.1% TFA, in 30 min, and UV detection was done at 220 and 280 nm.

4.10. Stability of Peptide in Human Serum

To a mixture of 250 μL of human serum and 750 μL of RPMI 1640 were added 20 μL of the peptide solution at 10 mg/mL. The mixture was incubated at 37 °C. Aliquots of 100 μL were removed from the medium at different time, mixed with 100 μL of ethanol and 5 μL of 1M NaOH, and incubated at 4 °C for at least 15 min to precipitate all the serum proteins. After centrifugation at 12,000 rpm for 2 min, 50 μL of the supernatant were injected in HPLC with a a linear gradient from 5% to 50% ACN [0.1% (*v*/*v*) TFA in acetonitrile] in aqueous 0.1% (*v*/*v*) TFA. The relative concentrations of the remaining soluble peptides were analyzed by the integration of the absorbance at 220 nm as a function of retention time.

To ensure the serum activity, the peptide 4NGG [37] is used as positive control (Figure 25):

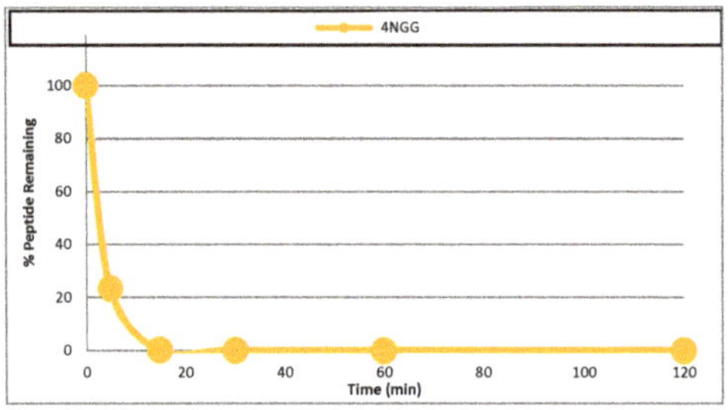

Figure 25. Serum activity evaluated with the 4NGG peptide degraded in 15 min.

5. Patents

The patent application WO2014191392 A1 (PCT/EP2014/060917) included results from this paper. The authors declare that no other competing interest exist.

Supplementary Materials: The following are available online. ^{1}H and ^{13}C NMR Spectra of all compounds.

Author Contributions: H.B. performed amino acids, peptides syntheses and metabolic stability assay under the supervision of R.M. and P.K. A.H., C.G.-E. performed the antimicrobial assays under the supervision of C.J. C.B. and H.B. performed the cytotoxicity assays under the supervision of S.S. E.P. performed the in vivo assays under the supervision of P.L. F.B. and C.L. performed the study of Interaction with membrane model. P.K. and R.M. wrote the manuscript with the assistance of the others authors. P.K. designed the AMPs and led the project. All authors have given approval to the final version of the manuscript.

Funding: H.B. was recipient of a MERS fellowship from the french Ministère de l'Enseignement Supérieure et de la Recherche. P.K. is grateful to SATT-Lutech and DGRTT (Sorbonne-Université) for financial and logistic supports in patent filing.

Conflicts of Interest: The authors declare no conflict of interest.

References

1. Jones, D. The antibacterial lead discovery challenge. *Nat. Rev. Drug Discov.* **2010**, *9*, 751–752.
2. Bax, B.D.; Chan, P.F.; Eggleston, D.S.; Fosberry, A.; Gentry, D.R.; Gorrec, F.; Giordano, I.; Hann, M.M.; Hennessy, A.; Hibbs, M.; et al. Type IIA topoisomerase inhibition by a new class of antibacterial agents. *Nature* **2010**, *466*, 935–940. [CrossRef] [PubMed]
3. Fjell, C.D.; Hiss, J.A.; Hancock, R.E.W.; Schneider, G. Designing antimicrobial peptides: Form follows function. *Nat. Rev. Drug Discov.* **2011**, *1*, 37–51.
4. Uggerhøj, L.E.; Poulsen, T.J.; Munk, J.K.; Fredborg, M.; Sondergaard, T.E.; Frimodt-Moller, N.; Hansen, P.R.; Wimmer, R. Rational design of alpha-helical antimicrobial peptides: Do's and don'ts. *ChemBioChem* **2015**, *16*, 242–253. [CrossRef] [PubMed]
5. Shai, Y. Mode of action of membrane active antimicrobial peptides. *Biopolymers* **2002**, *66*, 236–248. [CrossRef] [PubMed]
6. Tew, G.N.; Scott, R.W.; Klein, M.L.; DeGrado, W.F. De Novo Design of Antimicrobial Polymers, Foldamers, and Small Molecules: From Discovery to Practical Applications. *Acc. Chem. Res.* **2010**, *43*, 30–39. [CrossRef]
7. Ramesh, S.; Govender, T.; Kruger, H.G.; de la Torre, B.G.; Albericio, F. Short AntiMicrobial Peptides (SAMPs) as a class of extraordinary promising therapeutic agents. *J. Pept. Sci.* **2016**, *22*, 438–451. [CrossRef]
8. Teng, P.; Nimmagadda, A.; Su, M.; Hong, Y.; Shen, N.; Li, C.; Tsai, L.-Y.; Cao, J.; Li, Q.; Cai, J. Novel bis-cyclic guanidines as potent membrane-active antibacterial agents with therapeutic potential. *Chem Commun.* **2017**, *53*, 11948–11951. [CrossRef]
9. Niu, Y.; Wang, M.; Yafei Cao, Y.; Nimmagadda, A.; Hu, J.; Wu, Y.; Cai, J.; Ye, X.-S. Rational Design of Dimeric Lysine N-Alkylamide as Potent and Broad Spectrum Antibacterial Agents. *J. Med. Chem.* **2018**, *61*, 2865–2874. [CrossRef]
10. Aussedat, B.; Dupont, E.; Sagan, S.; Joliot, A.; Lavielle, S.; Chassaing, G.; Burlina, F. Modifications in the chemical structure of Trojan carriers: Impact on cargo delivery. *Chem. Commun.* **2008**, 1398–1400. [CrossRef]
11. Seebach, D.; Abele, S.; Sifferlen, T.; Hänggi, M.; Gruner, S.; Seiler, P. Disubstituted $\beta^{2,2}$ and $\beta^{3,3}$ amino Acids. A Turn Motif for β-peptides. *Helv. Chim. Acta* **1998**, *81*, 2218–2243. [CrossRef]
12. Yu, J.-S.; Noda, H.; Shibasaki, M. Quaternary $\beta^{2,2}$-Amino Acids: Catalytic Asymmetric Synthesis and Incorporation into Peptides by Fmoc-Based Solid-Phase Peptide Synthesis. *Angew. Chem. Int. Ed.* **2018**, *57*, 818–822. [CrossRef] [PubMed]
13. Basuroy, K.; Rajagopal, A.; Raghothama, S.; Shamala, N.; Balaram, P. β-Turn analogues in model αβ-hybrid peptides: Structural characterization of peptides containing β(2,2)Ac6c and β(3,3)Ac6c residues. *Chem. Asian J.* **2012**, *7*, 1671–1678. [CrossRef] [PubMed]
14. García-González, I.; Mata, L.; Corzana, F.; Jiménez-Osés, G.; Avenoza, A.; Busto, J.H.; Peregrina, J.M. Synthesis and conformational analysis of hybrid α/β-dipeptides incorporating S-glycosyl-β(2,2)-amino acids. *Chemistry* **2015**, *21*, 1156–1168. [CrossRef]

15. Hansen, T.; Ausbacher, D.; Flaten, G.E.; Havelkova, M.; Strøm, M.B. Synthesis of cationic antimicrobial β(2,2)-amino acid derivatives with potential for oral administration. *J. Med. Chem.* **2012**, *54*, 858–868. [CrossRef]
16. Tørfoss, V.; Ausbacher, D.; de A. Cavalcanti-Jacobsen, C.; Hansen, T.; Brandsdal, B.-O.; Havelkova, M.; Strøm, M.B. Synthesis of anticancer heptapeptides containing a unique lipophilic β(2,2)-amino acid building block. *J. Pept. Sci.* **2012**, *18*, 170–176. [CrossRef]
17. Hansen, T.; Ausbacher, D.; Zachariassen, Z.G.; Anderssen, T.; Havelkova, M.; Strøm, M.B. Anticancer activity of small amphipathic $\beta^{2,2}$-amino acid derivatives. *Eur. J. Med. Chem.* **2012**, *58*, 22–29. [CrossRef] [PubMed]
18. Saidi, M.R.; Azizi, N.; Akbari, E.; Ebrahimi, F. LiCO4/Et3N: Highly efficient and active catalyst for selective Michael addition of active methylene compounds under solvent-free condition. *J. Mol. Catal. A Chem.* **2008**, *292*, 44–48. [CrossRef]
19. Strøm, M.B.; Rekdal, Ø.; Svendsen, J.S. Antimicrobial activity of short arginine- and tryptophan-rich peptides. *J. Pept. Sci.* **2002**, *8*, 431–437. [CrossRef] [PubMed]
20. Strøm, M.B.; Haug, B.E.; Skar, M.L.; Stensen, W.; Stiberg, T.; Svendsen, J.S. The pharmacophore of short cationic antibacterial peptides. *J. Med. Chem.* **2003**, *46*, 1567–1570. [CrossRef] [PubMed]
21. Haug, B.E.; Stensen, W.; Stiberg, T.; Svendsen, J.S. Bulky nonproteinogenic amino acids permit the design of very small and effective cationic antibacterial peptides. *J. Med. Chem.* **2004**, *47*, 4159–4162. [CrossRef] [PubMed]
22. Haug, B.E.; Stensen, W.; Kalaaji, M.; Rekdal, Ø.; Svendsen, J.S. Synthetic antimicrobial peptidomimetics with therapeutic potential. *J. Med. Chem.* **2008**, *51*, 4306–4314. [CrossRef] [PubMed]
23. Isaksson, J.; Brandsdal, B.O.; Engqvist, M.; Flaten, G.E.; Svendsen, J.S.M.; Stensen, W. A synthetic antimicrobial peptidomimetic (LTX 109): Stereochemical impact on membrane disruption. *J. Med. Chem.* **2011**, *54*, 5786–5795. [CrossRef] [PubMed]
24. Sharma, R.K.; Reddy, R.P.; Tegge, W.; Jain, R. Discovery of Trp-His and His-Arg analogues as new structural classes of short antimicrobial peptides. *J. Med. Chem.* **2009**, *52*, 7421–7431. [CrossRef] [PubMed]
25. Hansen, T.; Alst, T.; Havelkova, M.; Strøm, M.B. Antimicrobial activity of small beta-peptidomimetics based on the pharmacophore model of short cationic antimicrobial peptides. *J. Med. Chem.* **2010**, *53*, 595–606. [CrossRef] [PubMed]
26. Bremner, J.B.; Keller, P.A.; Pyne, S.G.; Boyle, T.P.; Brkic, Z.; David, D.M.; Garas, A.; Morgan, J.; Robertson, M.; Somphol, K.; et al. Binaphthyl-based dicationic peptoids with therapeutic potential. *Angew. Chem. Int. Ed.* **2010**, *49*, 537–540. [CrossRef] [PubMed]
27. Rekdal, Ø.; Haug, B.E.; Kalaaji, M.; Hunter, H.N.; Lindin, I.; Israelsson, I.; Solstad, T.; Yang, N.; Brandl, M.; Mantzilas, D.; Vogel, H.J. Relative spatial positions of tryptophan and cationic residues in helical membrane-active peptides determine their cytotoxicity. *J. Biol. Chem.* **2012**, *287*, 233–244. [CrossRef] [PubMed]
28. Thennarasu, S.; Lee, D.-K.; Tan, A.; Prasad Kari, U.; Ramamoorthy, A. Antimicrobial activity and membrane selective interactions of a synthetic lipopeptide MSI-843. *Biochim. Biophys. Acta* **2005**, *1711*, 49–58. [CrossRef] [PubMed]
29. Das, S.; Ben Haj Salah, K.; Wenger, E.; Martinez, J.; Kotarba, J.; Andreu, V.; Ruiz, N.; Savini, F.; Stella, L.; Didierjean, C.; et al. Enhancing the Antimicrobial Activity of Alamethicin F50/5 by Incorporating N-terminal Hydrophobic Triazole Substituents. *Chemistry* **2017**, *23*, 17964–17972. [CrossRef] [PubMed]
30. Ladokhin, A.S.; Jayasinghe, S.; White, S.H. How to measure and analyze tryptophan fluorescence in membranes properly, and why bother? *Anal. Biochem.* **2000**, *285*, 235–245. [CrossRef] [PubMed]
31. Killian, J.A.; Keller, R.C.A.; Struyve, M.; De Kroon, A.; Tommassen, J.; De Kruijff, B. Tryptophan fluorescence study on the interaction of the signal peptide of the Escherichia coli outer membrane protein PhoE with model membranes. *Biochemistry* **1990**, *29*, 8131–8137. [CrossRef] [PubMed]
32. Pinheiro da Silva, F.; Aloulou, M.; Skurnik, D.; Benhamou, M.; Andremont, A.; Velasco, I.T.; Chiamolera, M.; Verbeek, J.S.; Launay, P.; Monteiro, R.C. CD16 promotes Escherichia coli sepsis through an FcR gamma inhibitory pathway that prevents phagocytosis and facilitates inflammation. *Nat. Med.* **2007**, *13*, 1368–1374. [CrossRef] [PubMed]
33. Svenson, J.; Karstad, R.; Flaten, G.E.; Brandsdal, B.-O.; Brandl, M.; Svendsen, J.S. Altered activity and physicochemical properties of short cationic antimicrobial peptides by incorporation of arginine analogues. *Mol. Pharm.* **2009**, *6*, 996–1005. [CrossRef] [PubMed]

34. Bisello, A.; Sala, S.; Tonello, A.; Signor, G.; Melotto, E.; Mammi, S.; Peggion, E. Conformation and interactions of all-D-, retro-all-D- and retro-bombolitin III analogues in aqueous solution and in the presence of detergent micelles. *Int. J. Biol. Macromol.* **1995**, *17*, 273–282. [CrossRef]
35. Basuroy, K.; Karuppiah, V.; Shamala, N.; Balaram, P. The Structural Characterization of Folded Peptides Containing the Conformationally Constrained β-Amino Acid Residue $\beta^{2,2}Ac_6c$. *Helv. Chim.* **2012**, *95*, 2589–2603. [CrossRef]
36. Sabatini, S.; Gosetto, F.; Manfroni, G.; Tabarrini, O.; Kaatz, G.W.; Patel, D.; Cecchetti, V. Evolution from a natural flavones nucleus to obtain 2-(4-Propoxyphenyl)quinoline derivatives as potent inhibitors of the S. aureus NorA efflux pump. *J. Med. Chem.* **2011**, *54*, 5722–5736. [CrossRef] [PubMed]
37. Denèfle, T.; Boullet, H.; Herbi, L.; Newton, C.; Martinez-Torres, A.C.; Guez, A.; Pramil, E.; Quiney, C.; Pourcelot, M.; Levasseur, M.D.; et al. Thrombospondin-1 Mimetic Agonist Peptides Induce Selective Death in Tumor Cells: Design, Synthesis, and Structure-Activity Relationship Studies. *J. Med. Chem.* **2016**, *59*, 8412–8421. [CrossRef] [PubMed]

Sample Availability: Sample of the compound **11** is available from the authors.

molecules

MDPI

Article

Triazolopeptides Inhibiting the Interaction between Neuropilin-1 and Vascular Endothelial Growth Factor-165

Bartlomiej Fedorczyk [1,*], Piotr F. J. Lipiński [2], Anna K. Puszko [1], Dagmara Tymecka [1], Beata Wilenska [1], Wioleta Dudka [3], Gerard Y. Perret [4], Rafal Wieczorek [1] and Aleksandra Misicka [1,2,*]

1 Faculty of Chemistry, University of Warsaw, Pasteura 1, 02-093 Warsaw, Poland; apuszko@chem.uw.edu.pl (A.K.P.); dulok@chem.uw.edu.pl (D.T.); bwilenska@chem.uw.edu.pl (B.W.); wieczorek@chem.uw.edu.pl (R.W.)

2 Department of Neuropeptides, Mossakowski Medical Research Centre, Polish Academy of Sciences, Pawinskiego 5, 02-106 Warsaw, Poland; plipinski@imdik.pan.pl

3 Laboratory of Cytometry, Nencki Institute of Experimental Biology, Polish Academy of Sciences, Pasteura 3, 02-093 Warsaw, Poland; wioletadudka@gmail.com

4 Université Paris 13, Sorbonne Paris Cité, INSERM U1125, 74 rue Marcel Cachin, 93017 Bobigny, France; perretgerard@sfr.fr

* Correspondence: bfedorczyk@chem.uw.edu.pl (B.F.); misicka@chem.uw.edu.pl (A.M.)

Academic Editor: Henry Mosberg
Received: 29 March 2019; Accepted: 4 May 2019; Published: 6 May 2019

check for updates

Abstract: Inhibiting the interaction of neuropilin-1 (NRP-1) with vascular endothelial growth factor (VEGF) has become an interesting mechanism for potential anticancer therapies. In our previous works, we have obtained several submicromolar inhibitors of this interaction, including branched pentapeptides of general structure Lys(Har)-Xxx-Xxx-Arg. With the intent to improve the proteolytic stability of our inhibitors, we turned our attention to 1,4-disubstituted 1,2,3-triazoles as peptide bond isosteres. In the present contribution, we report the synthesis of 23 novel triazolopeptides along with their inhibitory activity. The compounds were synthesized using typical peptide chemistry methods, but with a conversion of amine into azide completely on solid support. The inhibitory activity of the synthesized derivatives spans from 9.2% to 58.1% at 10 μM concentration (the best compound Lys(Har)-GlyΨ[Trl]GlyΨ[Trl]Arg, **3**, IC_{50} = 8.39 μM). Synthesized peptidotriazoles were tested for stability in human plasma and showed remarkable resistance toward proteolysis, with half-life times far exceeding 48 h. In vitro cell survival test resulted in no significant impact on bone marrow derived murine cells 32D viability. By means of molecular dynamics, we were able to propose a binding mode for compound **3** and discuss the observed structure–activity relationships.

Keywords: peptidomimetics; $VEGF_{165}$; neuropilin-1; molecular dynamics; structure–activity relationship

1. Introduction

Neuropilin-1 (NRP-1), vascular endothelial growth factor receptor type-2 (VEGFR-2) and vascular endothelial growth factor 165 ($VEGF_{165}$) form a complex (VEGFR-2/NRP-1/$VEGF_{165}$), which modulates the process of angiogenesis [1]. The interaction of $VEGF_{165}$ with NRP-1 significantly increases $VEGF_{165}$/VEGFR-2 binding strength [2,3] and, as a result, it increases the proangiogenic signal exerted by this complex. NRP-1 is not only expressed by endothelial cells of blood vessels, but also by several immune system cell types such as plasmacytoid dendritic cells [4] or regulatory T cells (Tregs) [5]. The protein is thus involved in the regulation of immune response [6].

Aside from the part that NRP-1 plays in physiological processes, it plays many roles in cancer. The protein is expressed by numerous types of cancer cells [7] and its overexpression was found to be related to tumor malignancy and poor prognosis [8,9]. It is believed that this phenomenon is caused by an autocrine pathway through the $VEGF_{165}$/NRP-1 axis, which favors cancer cells' migration, proliferation, and growth [10], and also increases their survivability [11]. Additionally, Tregs tend to express large amounts of NRP-1 on their surface. Thanks to this, they migrate toward the source of the chemoattractant, tumor originated $VEGF_{165}$, and are recruited into the tumor microenvironment, causing cancer-associated immunosuppression [12].

The involvement of $VEGF_{165}$/NRP-1 interaction in cancer pathology makes its inhibition an interesting approach for finding novel anticancer therapies [13–15]. Several groups (including ours) proposed a number of different $VEGF_{165}$/NRP-1 inhibitors. These include small molecules [16–21], $VEGF_{165}$ derived peptides [22,23], or cyclic peptides [24–26]. Another set of the inhibitors proposed so far consists of the peptide A7R (ATWLPPR) [27] and derivatives inspired by this sequence [28–30]. A7R exhibits a relatively good inhibition in in vitro tests with an IC_{50} of 5.86 μM [24]. Further, the compound has been proven to be active in vivo in nude mice xenografted with drug-resistant MDA-MB-231 human breast cancer cells [31].

In our previous works, we aimed at modifying the A7R sequence in order to improve the activity and stability of the inhibitors. In their course, we have obtained branched pentapeptides of the general structure Lys(Har)-Xaa-Xaa-Arg [29]. The results of their in vitro testing and that of the other derivatives of ours [31–33] led us to the conclusion that N-terminus branching is beneficial for inhibitory activity of the $VEGF_{165}$/NRP-1 interaction.

Regarding stability, we tested the degradation pathway under proteolytic conditions of the strongest inhibitors Lys(Har)-Dab/Dap-Pro-Arg (IC_{50} = 0.2 μM) and Lys(Har)-Pro-Ala/Dab-Arg (IC_{50} = 0.2/0.3 μM, respectively) [29]. There, we observed that first enzymatic cleavage occurred in the middle part of the molecule, leading to splitting of the molecule into halves possessing no inhibitory activity. For this reason, we decided to prepare derivatives with a non-classical peptide bond bioisostere at the sites prone to proteolysis (in the middle part of the molecule). Our attention was turned to the 1,4-disubstituted 1,2,3-triazole ring. Incorporation of triazoles into a peptide chain is a popular approach for the preparation of mimetics [33,34] owing to its efficient and easy preparation step through 1,3-dipolar cycloaddition catalyzed with copper ions, a click reaction [35,36].

In the present contribution, we report the synthesis and in vitro inhibitory activity of 23 triazolopeptide analogues. Further, the rationalization for the observed structure–activity trends is provided based on molecular dynamics simulations. For the best hits, we have also investigated their proteolytic resistance in human plasma as well as viability against normal cell lines.

2. Results and Discussion

Previous works have shown that strong inhibition of the NRP-1/$VEGF_{165}$ interaction is obtained when the structure contains a C-terminal arginine ("anchor") and a certain positively charged residue at the N-terminus ("arm"), spaced by two residues in the middle part ("linker") [28–30,32]. Modifying this "linker" part by introducing triazole rings (in a glycyl-1,2,3-triazole unit—Figure 1) as peptide bond mimetics changes the flexibility of the backbone. Furthermore, it increases the geometrical distance between the "arm" and the "anchor" (Figure 2). The replacement of a peptide bond for a triazole ring elongates the distance between neighboring Cα atoms by about 10 nm.

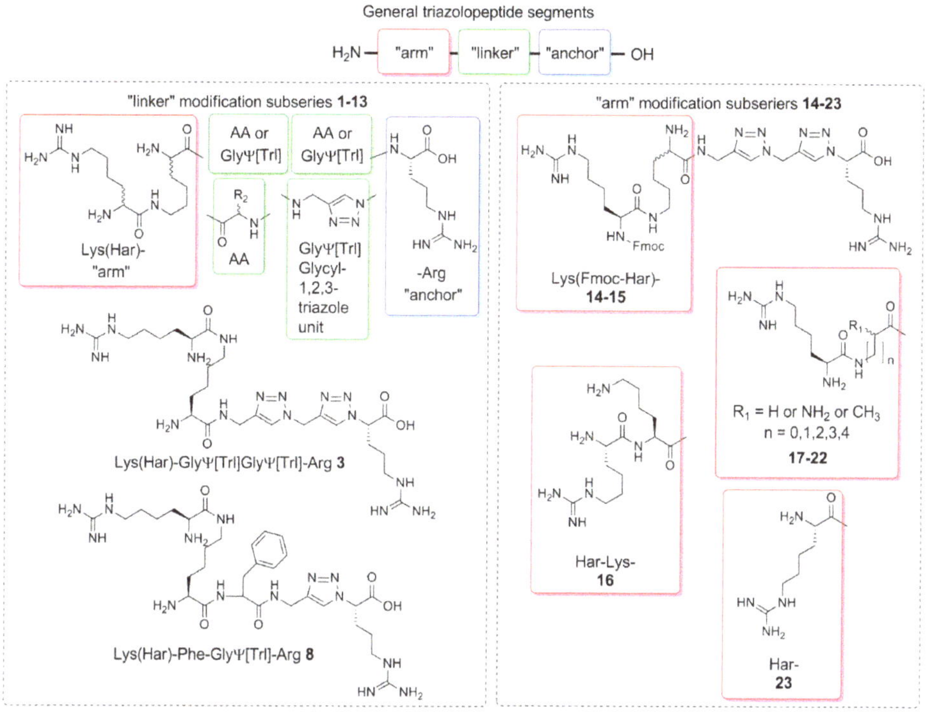

Figure 1. The general description of used notation and two exemplary structures **3** and **8**. Between the N-terminal Har and C-terminal Arg, there are two or three amino acids/glycyl-1,2,3-triazole units in various configurations, where AA stands for canonical amino acid residue and GlyΨ[Trl] is a glycyl-1,2,3-triazole unit mimicking glycine (triazole ring substitution instead of peptide bond). All analogues were divided into two subseries with modification in the "linker" site of the molecule and at the "arm" site.

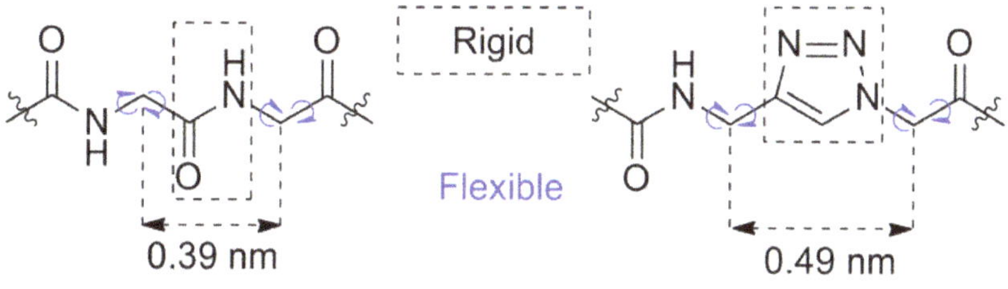

Figure 2. General comparison of trans peptide bond and 1,4-disubstituted 1,2,3-triazole ring as trans peptide bond non-classical bioisostere, adapted from the work of [37]. Every such triazole ring modification leads to backbone elongation and different conformational latitude.

Both changes (flexibility and length) can be expected to influence the activity. Therefore, we set out for rational investigation of structure–activity relationships within the triazolopeptide inhibitors. The research focused on two lines of variation. First, we modified the "linker" ("linker" subseries) with the aim to establish the best configuration of triazole rings in the backbone. Then, the "arm" was subjected to variation ("arm" subseries). On the basis of best hits from "linker" subseries, we wanted to see if changes related to backbone elongation can be compensated by modification of the "arm" (Figure 1). The scheme of the modifications is given in Figure 1. The full list of compounds with their sequences is presented in Table 1.

Table 1. Systematic characterization of synthesized triazolopeptides **1–23**.

No.	Sequence	RT [min.]	General Formula	Calc. MS [*m*/*z*]	Meas. MS [*m*/*z*]
		"linker" subseries			
1	Lys(Har)-GlyΨ[Trl]Arg	11.98 [1]	C22H43N13O4	554.3634 [4]	554.3640 [4]
2	D-Lys(Har)-GlyΨ[Trl]Arg	11.96 [1]	C22H43N13O4	554.3634 [4]	554.3656 [4]
3	Lys(Har)-GlyΨ[Trl]GlyΨ[Trl]Arg	13.22 [1]	C25H46N16O4	635.3961 [4]	635.3979 [4]
4	D-Lys(Har)-GlyΨ[Trl]GlyΨ[Trl]Arg	13.30 [1]	C25H46N16O4	635.3961 [4]	635.3980 [4]
5	D-Lys(D-Har)-GlyΨ[Trl]GlyΨ[Trl]Arg	13.33 [1]	C25H46N16O4	635.3961 [4]	635.3982 [4]
6	Lys(Har)-Pro-GlyΨ[Trl]Arg	14.65 [1]	C27H50N14O5	651.4161 [4]	651.4187 [4]
7	D-Lys(Har)-Pro-GlyΨ[Trl]Arg	14.65 [1]	C27H50N14O5	651.4161 [4]	651.4190 [4]
8	Lys(Har)-Phe-GlyΨ[Trl]Arg	14.89 [2]	C31H52N14O5	701.4318 [4]	701.4339 [4]
9	D-Lys(Har)-Phe-GlyΨ[Trl]Arg	15.04 [2]	C31H52N14O5	701.4318 [4]	701.4338 [4]
10	Lys(Har)-GlyΨ[Trl]Ala-Arg	13.17 [1]	C25H48N14O5	625.4005 [4]	625.3994 [4]
11	Lys(Har)-GlyΨ[Trl]Gly-Arg	12.19 [1]	C24H46N14O5	611.3848 [4]	611.3878 [4]
12	Har-Pro-GlyΨ[Trl]Arg	13.78 [1]	C21H38N12O4	523.3212 [4]	523.3221 [4]
13	Har-GlyΨ[Trl]GlyΨ[Trl]GlyΨ[Trl]Arg	14.52 [1]	C22H37N17O3	588.3338 [4]	588.3362 [4]
		"arm" subseries			
14	Lys(Fmoc-Har)-GlyΨ[Trl]GlyΨ[Trl]Arg	16.50 [3]	C40H56N16O6	429.2357 [5]	429.2371 [5]
15	D-Lys(Fmoc-Har)-GlyΨ[Trl]GlyΨ[Trl]Arg	16.53 [3]	C40H56N16O6	429.2357 [5]	429.2373 [5]
16	Har-Lys-GlyΨ[Trl]GlyΨ[Trl]Arg	13.05 [1]	C25H46N16O4	635.3961 [4]	635.3991 [4]
17	Dab(Har)-GlyΨ[Trl]GlyΨ[Trl]Arg	12.46 [1]	C23H42N16O4	607.3648 [4]	607.3675 [4]
18	Dap(Har)-GlyΨ[Trl]GlyΨ[Trl]Arg	11.92 [1]	C22H40N16O4	593.3491 [4]	593.3517 [4]
19	Har-6Ahx-GlyΨ[Trl]GlyΨ[Trl]]Arg	16.83 [1]	C25H45N15O4	620.3852 [4]	620.3878 [4]
20	Har-5Ava-GlyΨ[Trl]GlyΨ[Trl]Arg	15.23 [1]	C24H43N15O4	606.3695 [4]	606.3721 [4]
21	Har-Ala-GlyΨ[Trl]GlyΨ[Trl]]Arg	13.46 [1]	C22H39N15O4	578.3382 [4]	578.3406 [4]
22	Har-Gly-GlyΨ[Trl]GlyΨ[Trl]Arg	13.06 [1]	C21H37N15O4	564.3226 [4]	564.3244 [4]
23	Har-GlyΨ[Trl]GlyΨ[Trl]Arg	13.06 [1]	C19H34N14O3	507.3020 [4]	507.3011 [4]

[1] linear increase of phase B from 1% to 21% in 20 min; [2] linear increase of phase B from 10% to 40% in 20 min; [3] linear increase of phase B from 20% to 40% in 20 min; [4] pseudomolecular ion $[M + H]^+$; [5] pseudomolecular ion $[M + 2H]^{2+}$.

2.1. *Synthesis of Triazolopeptides on Solid Support*

The designed triazolopeptides were prepared on solid support, using standard polystyrene Wang resin preloaded with Fmoc-Arg(Pbf). Fmoc group deprotection (20% piperidine in DMF) and amino acid coupling (DIC/OxymaPure/Fmoc-AA) steps were proceeded in the standard manner. What is less usual, we incorporated 1,4-disubstituted 1,2,3-triazole moiety in the peptide backbone, completely on solid support. For this purpose, a modification of a standard solid phase peptide synthesis was carried out. The general synthesis scheme of triazole rings is shown in Figure 3.

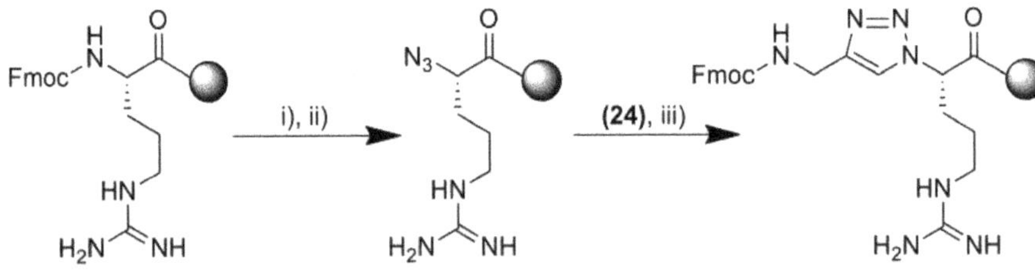

Figure 3. The general scheme of triazole rings synthesis on solid support. Reagents and conditions: (i) 20% piperidine in DMF; (ii) trifluoromethanesulfonyl azide in DCM, MeOH and K_2CO_3, $CuSO_4$ in H_2O (2:1:1 *v*/*v*/*v*), and Fmoc-propargylamine **24**; (iii) THF and $CuSO_4$, sodium ascorbate in H_2O (2:1 *v*/*v*).

2.1.1. Conversion of Primary Amine Group into Azide on Solid Support

First, we transformed primary amine group of peptidyl-resin into N-terminal azide. To achieve this, we used the Wong diazotransfer reaction [38], carried out according to protocol from the literature [39], but adjusted to proceed directly on the solid support. Peptidyl-resin was treated with mixture of trifluoromethanesulfonyl azide (c.a. 2 eq.) in DCM, MeOH, and H_2O with dissolved potassium carbonate (1 eq.) and copper(II) sulfate pentahydrate (0.067 eq.). Solvents volume ratio was 2:1:1 (DCM/MeOH/H_2O). The reaction was left overnight with constant shaking, not stirring. Completion of the reaction was monitored by Kaiser test (negative result after one repetition).

2.1.2. Click Reaction on Solid Support

The peptidyl-resin with N-terminal azide group was treated with a mixture of Fmoc-propargylamine (**24**) (2 eq.) dissolved in THF and copper(II) sulfate pentahydrate (0.2 eq) reduced by sodium ascorbate (0.67 eq.), both dissolved in H_2O. The solvent volume ratio was 2:1 (THF:H_2O). The reaction was left for at least 10 h under an argon atmosphere. Completion of the reaction was determined by modified Kaiser test with azide reduction beforehand according to the procedure described in the literature [40] (negative result after one repetition).

2.1.3. Homoarginine (Har) Synthesis on Solid Support

Har residue was obtained through guanylation reaction of ε-amino group of Boc-Lys(Fmoc) after Fmoc deprotection. For this purpose, we used 3,5-dimethylpyrazole-1-carboxamidine nitrate (10 eq.) and DIPEA (to pH c.a. 10–11), following a procedure described in the literature [41].

2.1.4. Final Cleavage from Solid Support and Triazolopeptides Isolation

The complete sequence was cleaved from solid support with the mixture of TFA/TIS/H_2O with a volume ratio of 95:2.5:2.5. The reaction was carried out for at least three hours. Then, the resin was filtrated and washed with neat TFA three times. Solvents were connected and evaporated. To the residual oil, a cold diethyl ether was added in c.a. 15 times volume to precipitate triazolopeptides. Further, the crude product was filtered off, analyzed, purified on RP-HPLC with C-12 resin, and characterized with mass spectrometry. Analytical data for the compounds **1–23** are given in Table 1.

2.2. *Inhibition of NRP-1/VEGF-A*

The inhibitory activity of obtained triazolopeptides **1–23** toward binding of $VEGF_{165}$ to NRP-1 was measured with the enzyme-linked immunosorbent assay (ELISA). This protocol was described earlier in the literature [42] and was broadly used by our group [24,26,28–30,32]. $VEGF_{165}$ was used in biotinylated form (bt-$VEGF_{165}$).

The inhibitory activity listed in Table 2 (at 10 μM, denoted further as *inh*) of the obtained derivatives spans from 9.2% (**12**) to 58.1% (**3**). None of the compounds described here are better than reference A7R (IC_{50} = 5.86) [24] or than the best of the branched pentapeptides that we have reported before (IC_{50} ~ 0.2 μM) [29]. Thus, at least within the structural space explored herein, triazole mimetics of the peptide bond are not very favourable for the activity on their own.

Table 2. Inhibitory activity of the synthesized triazolopeptides.

No	Sequence	Inhibition of bt-VEGF165 Binding to NRP-1 [10 μM] [1]	IC_{50} [μM]
A7R	Ala-Thr-Trp-Lys-Pro-Pro-Arg	61.0 ± 0.4 [3]	5.86 [3]
KPPR	Lys-Pro-Pro-Arg	64.5	4.60 [4]
	Lys(Har)-Dap/Dab-Pro-Arg	96.8/98.5	0.2/0.2 [4]
	"linker" subseries		
1	Lys(Har)-GlyΨ[Trl]Arg	28.1 ± 1.2	-
2	D-Lys(Har)-GlyΨ[Trl]Arg	33.1 ± 1.9	-
3	Lys(Har)-GlyΨ[Trl]GlyΨ[Trl]Arg	58.1 ± 2.1	8.39 [2]
4	D-Lys(Har)-GlyΨ[Trl]GlyΨ[Trl]Arg	52.6 ± 1.3	10.22 [2]
5	D-Lys(D-Har)-GlyΨ[Trl]GlyΨ[Trl]Arg	48.5 ± 2.9	9.11 [2]
6	Lys(Har)-Pro-GlyΨ[Trl]Arg	18.3 ± 0.9	-
7	D-Lys(Har)-Pro-GlyΨ[Trl]Arg	38.4 ± 1.5	-
8	Lys(Har)-Phe-GlyΨ[Trl]Arg	30.9 ± 2.1	-
9	D-Lys(Har)-Phe-GlyΨ[Trl]Arg	37.9 ± 1.1	-
10	Lys(Har)-GlyΨ[Trl]Ala-Arg	43.2 ± 1.5	-
11	Lys(Har)-GlyΨ[Trl]Gly-Arg	30.6 ± 1.1	-
12	Har-Pro-GlyΨ[Trl]Arg	9.2 ± 0.8	-
13	Har-GlyΨ[Trl]GlyΨ[Trl]GlyΨ[Trl]Arg	34.8 ± 1.5	-
	"arm" subseries		
14	Lys(Fmoc-Har)-GlyΨ[Trl]GlyΨ[Trl]Arg	57.7 ± 1.8	-
15	D-Lys(Fmoc-Har)-GlyΨ[Trl]GlyΨ[Trl]Arg	43.7 ± 0.5	-
16	Har-Lys-GlyΨ[Trl]GlyΨ[Trl]Arg	36.5 ± 1.4	-
17	Dab(Har)-GlyΨ[Trl]GlyΨ[Trl]Arg	41.3 ± 0.5	-
18	Dap(Har)-GlyΨ[Trl]GlyΨ[Trl]Arg	25.3 ± 3.5	-
19	Har-6Ahx-GlyΨ[Trl]GlyΨ[Trl]Arg	30.5 ± 0.6	-
20	Har-5Ava-GlyΨ[Trl]GlyΨ[Trl]Arg	29.7 ± 1.8	-
21	Har-Ala-GlyΨ[Trl]GlyΨ[Trl]Arg	27.8 ± 2.1	-
22	Har-Gly-GlyΨ[Trl]GlyΨ[Trl]Arg	35.7 ± 1.6	-
23	Har-GlyΨ[Trl]GlyΨ[Trl]Arg	20.0 ± 2.1	-

[1] Percentage value for inhibition of vascular endothelial growth factor 165 ($VEGF_{165}$) binding to neuropilin-1 (NRP-1) (P) was calculated according to the equation P = 100% − [(S − NS)·100%/(P − NS)], where S is signal intensity measured, N is signal measured in negative control, and P is the maximum binding signal obtained with (bt)-VEGF-A165 without triazolopeptide **1**–**23**. The values represent mean ± S.D of at least two independent experiences performed in triplicate; [2] **3** $\log IC_{50} = -5.076 \pm 0.06$, $R^2 = 0.9859$; **4** $\log IC_{50} = -4.991 \pm 0.05$, $R^2 = 0.9921$; **5** $\log IC_{50} = -5.040 \pm 0.1417$, $R^2 = 0.9358$; [3] values taken from the work of [24]; [4] values taken from the work of [29].

The obtained derivatives were grouped into two lines of structural variation ("linker" and "arm" subseries). The first one was aimed at deciphering the optimal triazole-containing spacer for H-Lys(Har)-linker-Arg-OH structure ("linker" series). Among the studied bridges, -GlyΨ[Trl]Arg-; -Pro-GlyΨ[Trl]-; -Phe-GlyΨ[Trl]-; -GlyΨ[Trl]Ala-; -GlyΨ[Trl]Gly-; -GlyΨ[Trl]GlyΨ[Trl]-; -GlyΨ[Trl]GlyΨ[Trl]GlyΨ[Trl]-; and the one containing two triazole units, -GlyΨ[Trl]GlyΨ[Trl]-, seem to provide the best spacing. This bridge is present in the strongest derivative presented here, H-Lys(hArg)-GlyΨ[Trl]GlyΨ[Trl]Arg-OH (cmpd **3**, *inh* = 58.1%, IC_{50} = 8.39). The isomer of this compound with D-Lys at the first position exhibits a slightly lower inhibition **4** (*inh* = 52.6%, IC_{50} = 10.22). If there is a simultaneous exchange for D-Har at the branched side-chain **5**, (*inh* = 48.5%, IC_{50} = 9.11), the inhibition is in between. As to the remaining bridges of the "linker" series, shorter derivatives **1** and **2** (containing -GlyΨ[Trl]Arg) are significantly worse inhibitors (~30% of inhibition). Elongating this spacer by a natural AA, either before or after the triazole-AA, usually improves the inhibition, but not to a large extent and not in each case (**6**–**11**).

Having identified -GlyΨ[Trl]GlyΨ[Trl]- as the optimal spacer, we conceived the design of several analogues of structure **3**, in which the N-terminal residue is varied ("arm" subseries). Here, it turned out that free amine at the Har residue is not of crucial importance. When it is masked by Fmoc (**14**, *inh* = 57.7%), there is no drop in inhibitory activity compared with compound **3**. Some decrease upon Fmoc-masking of this amine, however, is observed in the derivative pair with D-Lys at the first position (**15**, *inh* = 43.7%).

The shortening of the first position's side chain is adverse to activity (**17**, *inh* = 41.3%; **18**, *inh* = 25.3%). Additionally, it is to be noted that 6Ahx, which replaces Lys in this derivative, differs from the latter by the lack of an α-NH_2 group. In fact, the lack of the N-terminal amine group seems to be deteriorating to activity as the derivative with 6-aminohexanoic acid (**19**, *inh* = 30.5%) and 5-aminopentanoic acid (**20**, *inh* = 29.7%) are significantly worse than the parent.

Derivatives in which Har is attached to the backbone (via Cα and not via the side-chain) are significantly worse than the parent **3** (cmpds **12**, **16**, **21**, **22**, **23**, inhibitory activity in the range of 9.2% to 36.5%), indicating that Har residue must be attached at the side chain of the lysine.

Correlation Analysis

The discussed observations are also quantitatively captured by correlation analysis. Herein, we correlated activity against variables describing the presence/absence of particular structural features and other structural characteristics. The former were accounted for by descriptors of binary type (with values, 1—presence and 0—absence). Other types of variables included topological distance between important structural features. The descriptor matrix used for the analysis is provided in Supporting Materials (Table SM-COR-1).

According to the correlation analysis, a single structural factor able to explain as much as 54% (Model 1, coefficient of determination, R^2 = 0.54, Figure 4) of the observed variance is the topological distance between guanidine groups at the N- and C-termini of the ligands ($dis_{N\text{-}C}$). Thus, within our set of compounds, the larger the separation of the guanidines, the higher the observed inhibitory activity. Including more explanatory variables obviously improves the model (listing SM-COR-1); however, owing to a rather small number of points analyzed, this improvement cannot be stated to be statistically robust. Nevertheless, as the variables included are structurally well-understood, the models provide at least approximate explanation of the tendencies.

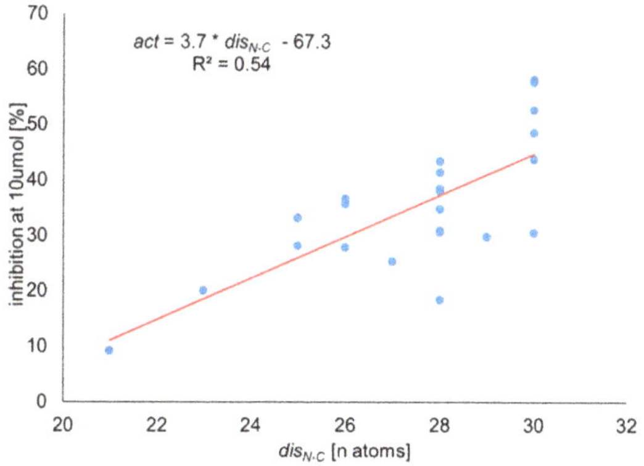

Figure 4. Correlation of inhibitory activity at 10 μM with the topological distance between guanidine groups at the N- and C-termini of the ligands (Model 1).

The best tradeoff between quality of fit and number of variables is obtained when three variables are used (Model 2, Figure 5): (a) (normalized) topological distance between guanidine groups at the N- and C-termini of the ligands ($dis_{N\text{-}C,\,norm}$); (b) triazole unit instead of the second amide/peptide bond (C to N direction) ($2Trl_{C\text{-}N}$); (c) free amine present by the second amide/peptide bond (going from the

N-terminus or from the residue attached to the N-terminal side chain) (am_{2N}). The model equation reads as follows:

$$inh = 8.6\ (\pm\ 5.0) + 20.9\ (\pm\ 8.6) * dis_{N\text{-}C,\ norm} + 8.7\ (\pm\ 4.5) * am_{2N} + 8.6\ (\pm\ 4.6) * 2Trl_{C\text{-}N} \quad (1)$$
$$R^2 = 0.63,\ n = 23.$$

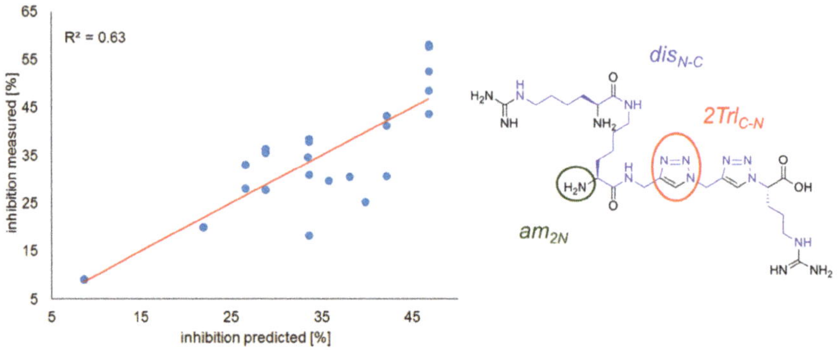

Figure 5. Correlation of observed vs. predicted (Model 2) inhibitory activity with marked variables.

The high coefficient of $dis_{N\text{-}C,\ norm}$ once again stresses the importance of the guanidines' separation. Some positive influence on activity is exerted by triazole unit at the second position counting from C to N ($2Trl_{C\text{-}N}$) and by a free amine at the second position counting from N to C (am_{2N}).

2.3. Molecular Modelling

In order to rationalize the obtained activity trends in structural terms, we have attempted to model complex of neuropilin-1 with compound **3** by means of molecular dynamics simulations. The starting binding mode was chosen by superimposing the compounds' arginine residue on the arginine residue of tuftsin in 2ORZ crystallographic structure [43]. The remaining elements of compound **3** (Lys(Har)-GlyΨ[Trl]GlyΨ[Trl]-) were added manually so that they were in an all-extended conformation (pointing to the solvent bulk). Three simulations (SIM-I, SIM-II, and SIM-III) with production runs of 420 ns in length were carried out with the expectation of finding a reliable binding mode for the compound.

In all three simulations, the guanidine group of the C-terminal arginine kept an ionic interaction with Asp320 (Figure 6A and SM-SIM-1, Table SM-SIM-1). In SIM-I, it has also maintained the hydrogen bonds of the free carboxylate with Ser346 and Thr349 (Figure 6B). In the other two (SIM-II—Figure SM-SIM-4-F-H and SIM-III—Figure SM-SIM-4-I-J), the arginine rotated in the manner that, while keeping the ionic contact with Asp320, the carboxylate was exposed to the solvent (Figure SM-SIM-2).

The 'linker' and the 'arm' parts of the inhibitor molecule perambulated over the protein surface, forming short-lived contacts with diverse residues. Several interaction patterns were more stable or appeared more than once. In SIM-I, the 'arm' tended to interact with the residues of the conventional 'north' of the binding site, while in SIM-II and SIM-III, the Har residue was directed to the 'south-east' (Figure 7A for explanation of the convention, Figures SM-SIM-4-F-J for representative examples from SIM-II and SIM-III).

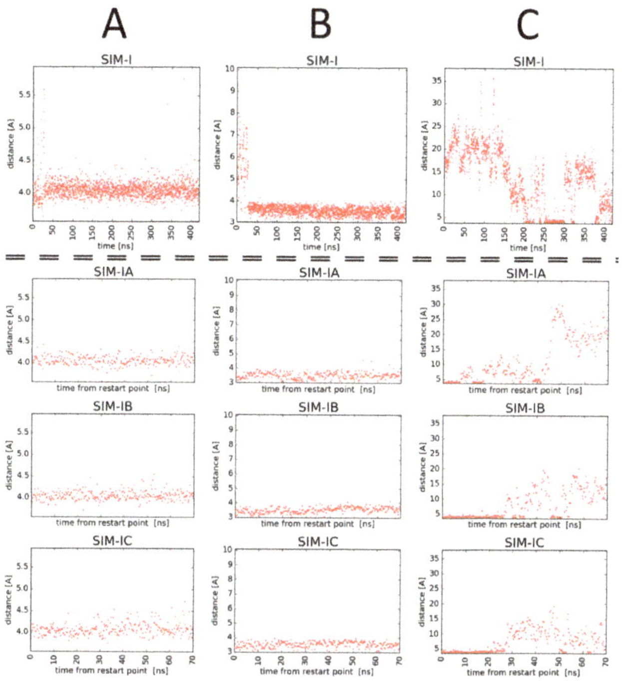

Figure 6. Time evolution of distances between (**A**) Cγ atom of Asp320 and Cζ of Arg residue in compound **3**; (**B**) Oγ atom of Ser346 and C of Arg residue in compound **3**; (**C**) Cδ atom of Glu319 and Cζ of Har residue in compound **3**. Data come from simulations SIM-I, SIM-IA, SIM-IB, and SIM-IC.

According to the crystallographic [43–45], mutagenetic [21], and molecular modelling studies (including our previous contributions [24,26,28–30]), three contacts of Arginine residue with Asp320, Ser346, and Thr349 are particularly important for binding of inhibitors with NRP1; therefore, we have decided to focus on SIM-I in which all three of these were maintained.

Three other replicas were run starting from the snapshot of SIM-I at t = 220.0 ns, because around this time point, there appeared a relatively stable binding pose (Figure 7B,C). In this configuration, the ligand formed the following contacts with the NRP1:

- Ionic interaction of C-terminal Arg guanidine with Asp320;
- Hydrogen bonds of C-terminal Arg carboxylate with Ser346 and Thr349;
- Dispersive contacts of C-terminal Arg aliphatic portion with the residue lining the binding cleft Tyr353, Tyr 297, Trp301, Thr316, Gly414, Ile415, and Ser416;
- Ionic interaction of Har guanidine with Glu319 or an H-bond of this moiety with carbonyl group of Gly318.

Additionally, hydrogen of the amide bond joining Har and Lys formed an H-bond with the phenolic function of Tyr297 or an intra-molecular hydrogen bond with $2Trl_{C\text{-}N}$. Furthermore, this triazole had transient H-bond interactions with Glu348 (via C5H). Another transient contact included H-bond between carbonyl of the peptide bond between Lys and Gly[Trl] and the phenol moiety of Tyr297.

It seems that this binding mode could be useful for explaining some of the SAR trends for our triazolopeptides. First, the stereochemistry of the Lys residue is roughly neutral to activity. The amine moiety does not form interactions with the protein. Configuration inversion at Lys Cα could be compensated by rotations of the arm's flexible bonds so that the Har interactions with Glu319/Gly318 are preserved.

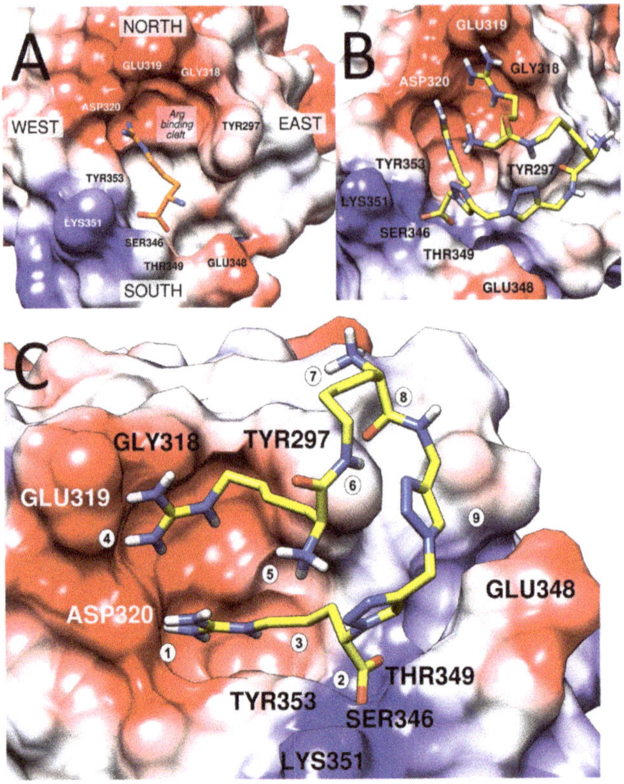

Figure 7. Binding site at the neuropilin-1. The protein is depicted as an electrostatic colour-coded surface (red: negative charges, white: neutral, blue: positive). (**A**) The binding site presented with the conventional assignment of directions as introduced in our previous contributions [28–30]. C-terminal arginine residue (orange, found in our inhibitors, but also in VEGF (4DEQ [44]) or tuftsin (2ORZ [43]) or arginine derivatives (5JGI, 5IYY, 5J1X, 5JGQ, 5JHK [45]) is shown in the cleft it occupies in crystal structures as well in simulations. (**B**) Compound **3** (yellow) at the NRP-1 binding site. A representative snapshot from SIM-I showing the discussed binding mode. Top projection. (**C**) Compound **3** (yellow) at the NRP-1 binding site. A representative snapshot from SIM-I showing the discussed binding mode. Rotated top projection. Marked are characteristic elements of the binding mode. 1—ionic interaction of Arg guanidine with Asp320; 2—hydrogen bonds of free carboxylate with Ser346 and Thr349; 3—Arg chain buried within the cleft, extended between Tyr353 and Tyr297, further apolar interactions with Trp301, Thr316, Gly414, Ile415, and Ser416; 4—Har interacts with Glu319 and Gly318; 5—Har free amine exposed to the solvent; 6—H of the amide bond interacts either with phenolic function of Tyr297 or forms an intramolecular hydrogen bond with triazole ring (N3); 7—Lys free amine exposed to the solvent; 8—carbonyl of the peptide bond forms an H-bond to the phenolic function of Tyr297; 9—C5H of the triazole ring is able to be involved in the H-bond with Glu348 depending on the rotameric state of this residue.

Second, masking of Har α-amine by Fmoc moiety (**14**, **15**) also does not affect activity, as the amine interacts neither with the protein, nor with any elements of the peptide.

Further, exchanging Lys for 5Ava/Dab/Dap (shorter, cmpds **17**, **18**, **20**) changes the position of the amide bond in the branched side-chain. In this way, formation of the intramolecular H-bond (Figure 7; characteristic element 6) or interaction with Tyr297 is distorted.

Assuming that the presented interaction mode is optimal for the compounds reported here, it is clear why Har is preferably attached by the side-chain rather than the main chain. Side-chain attachment allows for a more facile reaching of the negatively charged elements at the 'northern' wall of the binding cleft.

Still, the presented interaction mode was stable for only 20%, 32%, 52%, and 45% of simulation times of SIM-I, SIM-IA, SIM-IB, and SIM-IC, respectively (note that the latter three are shorter and restarted from a snapshot with this very configuration). This relative instability of the binding mode found in molecular dynamics (MD) simulations seems consistent with only moderate inhibitory activity of the compound **3**. The simulations reveal that even when the arginine residue sits tight in the cleft, the triazole-based linker and the Lys(Har) arm retain significant mobility, which compete against stable inhibitor–protein interactions. Thus, improving the inhibitory activity for peptidomimetics of the type presented here could be presumably achieved by introducing elements decreasing the conformational freedom and/or enabling additional interactions with the protein.

2.4. *In Vitro Proteolysis of Triazolopeptides*

Two of the most potent triazolopeptides, compounds **3** and **4**, were investigated as to their proteolytic resistance by incubation in human plasma at 37 °C. The samples of the incubated solutions were taken at constant time intervals (every 8 h) and analyzed with the use of HPLC-MS. This technique allows for determination of the proteolysis rate, and enables finding the cleavage sites by structural determination of appearing metabolites. To this aim, we used a previously established protocol [29].

Figure 8 shows the results of the measurements. During the monitored experiment time, both compounds were stable toward proteolytic cleavage and not fully degraded. In the case of **3**, after 48 h of incubation, ca. 70% of compound remained in the solution and **4** was almost non-degraded. The experiments were stopped after 48 h because of water evaporation/condensation processes in the Eppendorf tube, as these might affect the sample concentration and assay readouts.

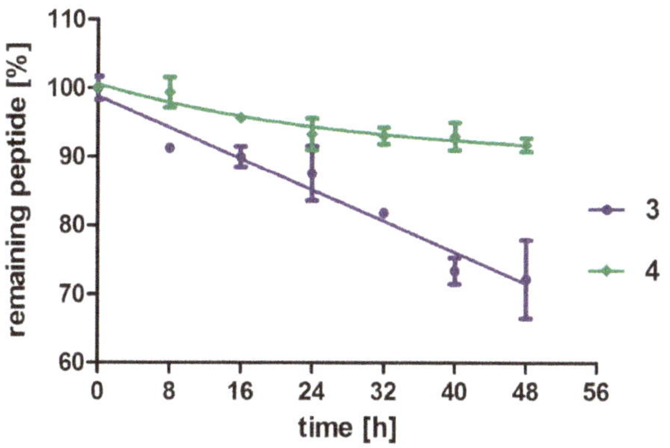

Figure 8. In vitro stability toward proteolysis of two triazolopeptides **3** violet line and **4** green line. Each point is an average result ± SD calculated from three independent experiments.

The only observed cleavage occurs at the "arm" site of the molecule (Lys(Har)-XXX) between lysine side chain and homo-arginine residue. The difference between stability of these two compounds is related to exchange of L-Lys (**3**) into D-Lys (**4**). Triazole rings were not metabolized within the monitored time of the experiment.

The compounds **3** and **4** exhibit improved stability ($t_{1/2}$ >> 48 h) as compared with our previously reported Lys(Har)-Dab/Dap-Pro-Arg ($t_{1/2}$ = 34 h/41 h) and Lys(Har)-Pro-Ala/Dab-Arg ($t_{1/2}$ = 39 min/44 min) [29]. Thus, it can be concluded that introducing triazole isosteres of the peptide bonds is a good way for improving the proteolytic stability of NRP-1/$VEGF_{165}$ interaction inhibitors.

Within the studied series, the best stability with optimal inhibitory activity is achieved when two triazole ring segments and D-Lys at the N-terminal position are simultaneously present.

2.5. In Vitro Cell Survival Test

Because of the fact that **4** was observed to be relatively resistant toward proteolysis, one should consider a scenario when the compound stays in the circulation for a prolonged time. For this reason, we carried out a preliminary cytotoxicity assay on murine progenitor cells (myeloblast-like cell line derived from long term cultures of bone marrow 32D) to investigate the impact of **4** at different concentrations on their viability.

According to the results shown in Figure 9, compound **4** does not exhibit any significant impact on cell survivability at relatively high (100 μM—one order of magnitude higher than IC_{50} value) dose and long-term (48 h) incubation. This might give some indication that the triazolopeptides are safe for normal cells; however, further research on a number of different cell types should be undertaken.

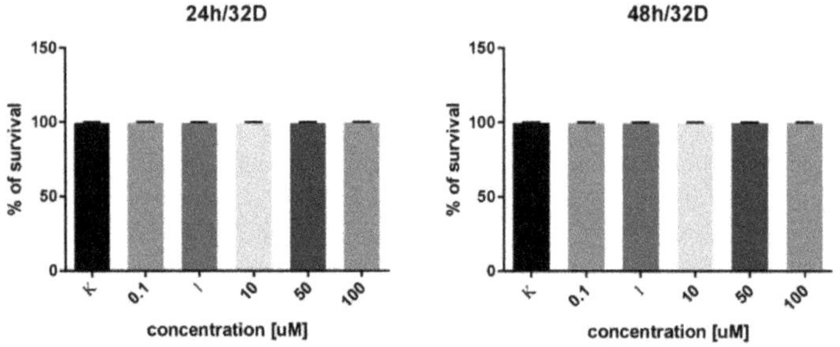

Figure 9. Survivability of myeloblast-like cell line derived from bone marrow at different concentrations of **4**. No significant differences in cell survival using a *t*-test were shown.

3. Materials and Methods

3.1. Synthesis

All solvents were purchased from local commercial suppliers: DMF, DCM, MeOH, and Et_2O (puriss) were used without further purification; THF (puriss) was freshly distilled before the use according to the standard protocols. Fmoc protected amino acids and coupling reagents were purchased from Iris Biotech GmbH. Wang resin with preloaded Fmoc-Arg(Pbf) with a capacity of 0.57 mmol/g was obtained from Activotec (Comberton, Cambridge, UK). Propargylamine was purchased from Sigma-Aldrich and Fmoc-OSu was obtained from Merck. HPLC grade solvents can and MeOH were purchased from Merck.

All compounds **1–23** were obtained manually using mixed solid phase peptide synthesis and solution phase according to standard coupling procedures for Fmoc/tBu strategy. The quantity of Wang polystyrene resin was fixed to carry out the synthesis in a scale of 0.15 mmol.

3.1.1. Wong Diazotransfer

During a typical reaction procedure, 1 mL of distilled H_2O sodium azide (98 mg, 1.5 mmol) was dissolved followed by the addition of 1.5 mL of DCM. The mixture was cooled in an ice bath, following which trifluoromethanesulfonic anhydride (85 mg, 53 μL, 0.3 mmol) was added dropwise for approximately five minutes. The reaction was carried out in an ice bath for two hours. After this time, the reaction mixture was transferred to a separatory funnel and the DCM phase was removed. The aqueous phase was extracted twice with 1 mL of DCM. The organic phase was then combined and washed once with saturated sodium carbonate solution and used for diazotransfer on solid support without any further purification. For this purpose, to the reaction vessel with resin beads, a previously described organic phase with 15 was added followed by 1 mL of MeOH and potassium carbonate (21 mg, 0.15 mmol) and copper (II) sulfate pentahydrate (0.25 mg, 1.0 μmole) dissolved in 1 mL of distilled water. The reaction was left overnight. ompletion of the reaction was determined with standard Kaiser test, and we observed a negative result.

3.1.2. Fmoc-Propargylamine (**24**) Preparation

A suspension of N-(9H-fluoren-9-ylmethoxycarbonyloxy) succinimide (338 mg, 1.0 mmol) in 4 mL of freshly dried and distilled THF was cooled with an ice bath, and propargylamine (44 mg, 54 μL, 0.8 mmol) was added dropwise. The reaction mixture was stirred and allowed to warm to room temperature over 2 h. The solvent was removed under reduced pressure to give a residue. The residue was dissolved in 20 mL of EtOAc, transferred to a separatory funnel, and washed a few times with 10 mL of distilled water. The organic layer was dried and the solvent was evaporated, affording 155 mg (0.56 mmol, yield 70%) of white/pale yellow needles.

Fmoc-Propargylamine (24): 1H NMR (DMSO, 400 MHz) δ A 7.89 (2H, d, *J* = 7.6 Hz, Fmoc H4 and H5), B 7.79 (1H, t, *J* = 5.8 Hz, NH), C 7.69 (2H, d, *J* = 7.4 Hz, Fmoc H1 and H8), D 7.33 (2H, td, *J* = 7.6, 1.3, Fmoc H2 and H7), E 7.41 (2H, td, *J* = 7.6, 1.2 Hz, Fmoc H3 and H6), F 4.31 (2H, d, *J* = 7.0 Hz, Fmoc CH2), G 4.22 (1H, t, *J* = 6.9 Hz, Fmoc H9), H 3.77 (2H, dd, *J* = 5.8, 2.5 Hz, H3), I 3.11 (1H, t, *J* = 2.5 Hz, H1); 13C NMR (DMSO, 100 MHz) δ 156.02 (C), 143.87 (C), 143.87 (C), 140.80 (C), 140.80 (C), 127.73 (CH), 127.73 (CH), 127.17 (CH), 127.17 (CH), 125.23 (CH), 125.23 (CH), 120.23 (CH), 120.23 (CH), 81.46 (C), 73.14 (CH), 65.74 (CH2), 46.66 (CH), 29.84 (CH2).

3.1.3. Click Reaction on Solid Support

In 4 mL of THF, a Fmoc-propargylamine (83 mg, 0.3 mmol) was dissolved and the mixture was transferred to the reaction vessel filled with resin beads. In the next step, the copper (II) sulfate pentahydrate (7.5 mg, 0.03 mmol) was added to 2 mL of distilled water. Both aqueous and organic solutions were combined with the resin and a portion of sodium ascorbate (20 mg, 0.1 mmol) was poured to the reaction vessel, after which the color of the solution changed from pale blue to bright yellow. The reaction was left for at least 10 h in an argon atmosphere. Completion of reaction was determined by a modified Kaiser test [40]. A few drops of 5% solution of triphenyl phosphine in THF and distilled water were added to the resin sample and heated in a closed vessel on a hot plate. After that, the standard Kaiser test solution was placed inside the vial, gently heated, and shaken. After cooling down, the negative result was noticed.

3.1.4. Common Procedures for Peptide Chain Elongation on Solid Support

Standard Fmoc deprotection was carried out stepwise with 20% piperidine in DMF through resin shaking for 5 min and a further 20 min with a fresh portion of reagent. For amino acids' coupling, a three-fold excess of Fmoc-protected amino acid, three-fold excess of OxymaPure, and three-fold excess of DIC were mixed in DMF and added to the solid support. After 60 min of shaking, completion of the reaction was confirmed by a negative result for the Kaiser test.

3.1.5. Guanylation Reaction of Lys to Gain Har

Guanylation reaction was carried out according to the protocol described in the literature [41]. The peptidyl resin with the deprotected ε-amino group was treated with 10 eq. of 3,5-dimethylpyrazole-1-carboxamidine nitrate dissolved in DMF and adjusted pH to ca. 10–11 by means of DIPEA. The reaction was left under constant shaking for 72 h to fully convert lysine into homoarginine.

3.1.6. Peptidotriazole Cleavage from Solid Support

After synthesis completion, the resin was washed trice with DCM, after that with MeOH, and finally with Et_2O. The resin was further dried under reduced pressure and treated with cleavage cocktail mixed from TFA/TIS/H_2O (0.95:2.5:2.5 in volume ratio). The reaction was left for at least 3 h and after that, the resin was filtered and washed trice with a fresh portion of TFA. The supernatants' volume was then reduced and a large excess of cold Et_2O (at least −20 °C) was added to the vessel to precipitate crude compound, which was centrifuged, decanted, washed trice with fresh Et_2O, and dried.

3.1.7. HPLC Analysis, Purification, and HRMS Characterization

The crude peptidotriazoles were analyzed and purified on RP-HPLC analytical column Jupiter Proteo I.D. 4.6 mm × 250 mm and preparative column Jupiter Proteo I.D. 21.2 mm × 250 mm. Phase A was ultrapure water + 0.1% volume TFA, phase B was gradient grade acetonitrile + 0.1% volume TFA. For all compounds, three types of linear gradient elution were used: [1]linear increase of phase B from 1% to 21% in 20 min; [2]linear increase of phase B from 10% to 40% in 20 min; and [3]linear increase of phase B from 20% to 40% in 20 min. Detection was carried out at 220 nm. Analytical flow = 1 mL/min, preparative flow = 20 mL/min. Fractions containing pure peptidotriazoles were freeze dried. Pure compounds were then analyzed using high-resolution mass spectrometry to confirm their general formula.

3.2. *ELISA Assays of Inhibitory Activity*

This assay was carried out according to a previously described method [29].

3.3. *Correlation Analysis*

The observed inhibitory activity at 10 µmol inhibitor concentration was correlated against several sets of structural descriptors. The sets included indicator variables, in which presence or absence of diverse structural elements was expressed as 1 or 0, respectively. Further, included was the topological distance between the guanidine groups at the N- and C-termini of the ligands ($dis_{N\text{-}C}$), that is, the number of atoms separating the two groups. If normalized, the variables were recalculated so that the smallest value of the set assumed 0 and the largest 1. The variable matrix is given in Supplementary Materials (Table SM-COR-1).

The multivariable linear correlations were performed using Microsoft Excel.

3.4. *Molecular Dynamics*

The complex of compound **3** with NRP-1 was studied by molecular dynamics (MD) in AMBER [46]. The starting structure was prepared by superposing C-terminal Arg of compound **3** onto the coordinates of Arg residue's atoms of tuftsin (TKPR), as found in 2ORZ crystallographic structure [43]. The remaining parts of compound **3** were added manually so that they were in all-extended conformation. AmberTools [46] was used to solvate the complex and to neutralize the system by adding Na^+ and Cl^- ions. The protonation states (in ligands and in the protein) were set as assumed in pH = 7. Ff14SB force field [47] was used with TIP3 water model. Parameters for triazole-based residues were taken from the work of Marion et al. [48].

The system was minimized and equilibrated (NVT). Then, the production step (NPT ensemble, T = 303.15 K, integration step = 2 fs, cut-off scheme Verlet, Nose–Hoover thermostat, Parrinello-Rahman barostat, LINCS H-bonds constraints) followed. In the first set, three independent simulations of 420 ns production were run (SIM-I, SIM-II, SIM-III). Another series included three simulations started from a SIM-I snapshot at t = 220.0 ns. These lasted 70 ns.

The analyses of the results were performed using AmberTools and in-house Python scripts (using MDAnalysis library [49]). The molecular graphics were prepared in UCSF Chimera [50].

3.5. *Stability*

The human plasma was provided by Mossakowski Medical Research Centre Polish Academy of Sciences (venous blood was obtained from three healthy donors and plasma samples were pooled in equal volumes). Triazolopeptide stock solution was prepared to achieve concentration ca. 1.4 mg/mL. Then, this solution was diluted two-fold into human plasma, affording a final concentration of ca. 1.1 μmol/mL. The samples were mixed on vortex mixer and incubated at 37 °C with 700 rpm mixing in thermoblock. Samples of 100 μL were taken every 8 h; the enzymatic cleavage was quenched by addition of 200 μL of 15% aqueos trichloroacetic acid and vortexed for a while. Precipitated proteins were then centrifuged at 14,000 rpm and 4 °C for 10 min to pellet them. After that, 150 μL of supernatant was taken and analyzed on HPLC-MS (quadrupole mass analyzer and electrospray ionization source). The system was equipped with Jupiter Proteo column I.D. 2.0 mm × 250 mm, phase A: ultrapure water + 0.05% TFA, phase B: gradient grade acetonitrile + 0.05% TFA, detection at 210 nm, quadrupole fixed on scan mode. Elution was with linear increase from 0% to 15% of phase B in 30 min, flow = 0.2 mL/min. All samples were analyzed trice in independent experiments.

3.6. *In Vitro Cell Survival Test*

For the cell survivability test, the myeloblast-like cell line derived from long term cultures of bone marrow (32D, ATCC #CRL-11346) was used. Experiments were carried out using Muse Count & Viability Kit and Muse Cell Analyzer (Merck Millipore) according to the procedure given. Cells were incubated for 24 or 48 h with given **4** concentration. Each experiment was performed in three technical replications in three independent experiments. Graphs were made with the use of GraphPad Prism.

4. Conclusions

In previous works, we disclosed several submicromolar (tetrapeptides and branched pentapeptides) inhibitors of the interaction between neuropilin-1 and vascular endothelial growth factor. In the present contribution, we describe follow-up research whose intent was to see whether the introduction of 1,4-disubstituted 1,2,3-triazole rings as peptide bond isosteres could give derivatives with improved proteolytic stability that still retain the inhibitory activity.

Thus, we report here 23 novel triazolopeptides along with their inhibitory activity. The structural variation within this set focused on modifying the "linker" part and the "arm" part of the molecules. The designed derivatives were obtained on solid support, mostly following typical procedures. Less usual, but very convenient was that the introduction of the triazole to the sequence went completely on solid support. By an adjustment of the Wong diazotransfer method, we were able to convert amines into azides directly on peptidyl-resin.

As to the activity, it spans from 9.2% to 58.1% at a concentration of 10 μM. The best three compounds include Lys(Har)-GlyΨ[Trl]GlyΨ[Trl]Arg (**3**, IC_{50} = 8.39 μM), D-Lys(Har)-GlyΨ[Trl]GlyΨ[Trl]Arg (**4**, IC_{50} = 10.22 μM), and D-Lys(D-Har)-GlyΨ[Trl]GlyΨ[Trl]Arg (**5**, IC_{50} = 9.11 μM)). None of the triazolopeptides are better than the reference A7R (ATWLPPR, IC_{50} = 5.86 μM). An analysis of the "linker" subseries allows for the conclusion that the best activity is obtained with -GlyΨ[Trl]GlyΨ[Trl]- in the middle part of the molecule. The stereochemistry at the N-terminal residue (Lys) is not critical. It seems to be more important that the "arm" construction, the derivatives in which Har is attached via the 'backbone', are worse than those where the residue is linked via a side-chain amide bond. The shortening of the 'arm' is adverse to activity. Thus, within the studied series, the optimal 'arm' is Lys(Har)- and other stereovariants thereof are not much worse.

Most of the observed trends in SAR can be explained by a binding mode based on molecular dynamics simulations of compound **3**. Further, the modelling points to large flexibility of the triazolopeptides studied herein. Its conformational freedom competes with the formation of stable protein–inhibitor interactions. Therefore, it seems that the introduction of elements decreasing the conformational space within the 'linker' part or forming additional interactions (e.g., branched or charged side-chains) may improve the affinity of NRP-1.

Compounds **3** and **4** were assayed for proteolytic stability. It turned out that both are remarkably stable. At 48 h after the start of the experiment, derivative **4** (with D-Lys(Har)- in the first position) was almost undigested, and in the case of derivative **3** (Lys(Har) in the first position), more than 70% of the substance remained in the sample. The only observed cleavage occurred at the N-terminal site of the molecule and the triazole rings were not metabolized. Thus, compounds **3** and **4** exhibit significantly improved stability compared with our previous inhibitors. Moreover, compound **4** does not exhibit any significant impact on normal cells' viability at a relatively high concentration (100 μmol) and long-term of incubation (48 h). Our results indicate that triazolopeptides 3 and 4 can be the starting structures for further modification to search for more active VEGF/NRP inhibitors.

Supplementary Materials: Supplementary Materials (SM) are available online, SM file is divided into sections that contain data pertaining to particular analysis subjects. Items in each section are independently numbered. The sections are as follows: **SM-SYN** (synthetic and analytical details for compounds **1–24**, 24 Figures a,b,c), **SM-INH** (dose-response curves for **3**, **4 and 5**, 3 Figures) **SM-COR** (input and results of correlational analysis, 1 Table and 1 Listing), **SM-SIM** (results of molecular dynamics simulations, 6 Figures and 1 table), **SM-RES** (TIC chromatograms and mass spectra 13 Figures, data sheet for linear graph 2 Tables), **SM-SUR** (datasheet from MUSE Cell Analyser, 1 Table).

Author Contributions: Conceptualization, B.F. and A.M.; Formal analysis, P.J.F.L.; Funding acquisition, R.W. and A.M.; Investigation, B.F., A.K.P., D.T., B.W., and W.D.; Supervision, R.W. and A.M.; Writing—original draft, B.F. and P.J.F.L.; Writing—review & editing, B.F., P.J.F.L., G.Y.P., R.W., and A.M.

Funding: This work was co-funded by National Science Centre of Poland [grant number N204 350940]; by the grant from National Centre for Research and Development #LIDER/35/0123/L-8/16/NCBR/2017; and co-financed by the EU from the European Regional Development Fund under the Operational Programme Innovative Economy, 2007–2013, and with the use of CePT infrastructure financed by the same EU program. Computational grant GB72-4 from Interdisciplinary Centre for Mathematical and Computational Modelling (ICM), Warsaw, Poland is gratefully acknowledged.

Acknowledgments: We would like to acknowledge the following: Andrzej Ziemba from Mossakowski Medical Research Centre, Polish Academy of Sciences for providing human plasma samples for stability assay; Katarzyna Piwocka, Head of Laboratory of Cytometry, Nencki Institute of Experimental Biology, Polish Academy of Sciences for sharing equipment and flow cytometry expertize; Kaja Harton for the help with cells survivability assay. Cell survival studies were performed at the Laboratory of Cytometry, Nencki Institute of Experimental Biology, Polish Academy of Sciences. On the occasion of his 80th birthday, Aleksandra Misicka wishes to thank Victor J. Hruby from University of Arizona, AZ, US for more than 20 years of most fruitful and enjoyable collaboration in the field of opioid research.

Conflicts of Interest: The authors declare no conflict of interest.

References

1. Fong, G.-H.; Rossant, J.; Gertsenstein, M.; Breitman, M.L. Role of the Flt-1 receptor tyrosine kinase in regulating the assembly of vascular endothelium. *Nature* **1995**, *376*, 66–70. [CrossRef]
2. Shay, S.; Hua-Quan, M.; Masashi, N.; Seiji, T.; Michael, K. VEGF165 mediates formation of complexes containing VEGFR-2 and neuropilin-1 that enhance VEGF165-receptor binding. *J. Cell. Biochem.* **2002**, *85*, 357–368.
3. Fuh, G. The interaction of Neuropilin-1 with Vascular Endothelial Growth Factor and its receptor Flt-1. *J. Biol. Chem.* **2000**, *275*, 26690–26695. [CrossRef]
4. Tordjman, R.; Lepelletier, Y.; Lemarchandel, V.; Cambot, M.; Gaulard, P.; Hermine, O.; Roméo, P.-H. A neuronal receptor, neuropilin-1, is essential for the initiation of the primary immune response. *Nat. Immunol.* **2002**, *3*, 477. [CrossRef]
5. Bruder, D.; Probst-Kepper, M.; Westendorf, A.M.; Geffers, R.; Beissert, S.; Loser, K.; von Boehmer, H.; Buer, J.; Hansen, W. Frontline: Neuropilin-1: A surface marker of regulatory T cells. *Eur. J. Immunol.* **2004**, *34*, 623–630. [CrossRef] [PubMed]
6. Mizui, M.; Kikutani, H. Neuropilin-1: The Glue between Regulatory T Cells and Dendritic Cells? *Immunity* **2008**, *28*, 302–303. [CrossRef] [PubMed]
7. Jubb, A.M.; Strickland, L.A.; Liu, S.D.; Mak, J.; Schmidt, M.; Koeppen, H.; Jubb M., A.; Strickland, A.L.; Liu, S.D.; Mak, J.; et al. Neuropilin-1 expression in cancer and development. *J. Pathol.* **2012**, *226*, 50–60. [CrossRef] [PubMed]
8. Soker, S.; Takashima, S.; Miao, H.Q.; Neufeld, G.; Klagsbrun, M. Neuropilin-1 Is Expressed by Endothelial and Tumor Cells as an Isoform-Specific Receptor for Vascular Endothelial Growth Factor. *Cell* **1998**, *92*, 735–745. [CrossRef]

9. Soker, S.; Fidder, H.; Neufeld, G.; Klagsbrun, M. Characterization of novel vascular endothelial growth factor (VEGF) receptors on tumor cells that bind VEGF165 via its exon 7-encoded domain. *J. Biol. Chem.* **1996**, *271*, 5761–5767. [CrossRef] [PubMed]
10. Goel, H.L.; Mercurio, A.M. VEGF targets the tumour cell. *Nat. Rev. Cancer* **2013**, *13*, 871. [CrossRef]
11. Bachelder, R.E.; Crago, A.; Chung, J.; Wendt, M.A.; Shaw, L.M.; Robinson, G.; Mercurio, A.M. Vascular Endothelial Growth Factor Is an Autocrine Survival Factor for Neuropilin-expressing Breast Carcinoma Cells. *Cancer Res.* **2001**, *61*, 5736–5740. [PubMed]
12. Hansen, W. Neuropilin 1 guides regulatory T cells into vegf-producing melanoma. *Oncoimmunology* **2013**, *2*. [CrossRef]
13. Djordjevic, S.; Driscoll, P.C. Targeting VEGF signalling via the neuropilin co-receptor. *Drug Discov. Today* **2013**, *18*, 447–455. [CrossRef]
14. Peng, K.; Bai, Y.; Zhu, Q.; Hu, B.; Xu, Y. Targeting VEGF–neuropilin interactions: A promising antitumor strategy. *Drug Discov. Today* **2019**, *24*, 656–664. [CrossRef] [PubMed]
15. Niland, S.; Eble, J.A. Neuropilins in the Context of Tumor Vasculature. *Int. J. Mol. Sci.* **2019**, *20*, 639. [CrossRef] [PubMed]
16. Powell, J.; Mota, F.; Steadman, D.; Soudy, C.; Miyauchi, J.T.; Crosby, S.; Jarvis, A.; Reisinger, T.; Winfield, N.; Evans, G.; et al. Small Molecule Neuropilin-1 Antagonists Combine Antiangiogenic and Antitumor Activity with Immune Modulation through Reduction of Transforming Growth Factor Beta (TGFβ) Production in Regulatory T-Cells. *J. Med. Chem.* **2018**, *61*, 4135–4154. [CrossRef] [PubMed]
17. Novoa, A.; Pellegrini-Moïse, N.; Bechet, D.; Barberi-Heyob, M.; Chapleur, Y. Sugar-based peptidomimetics as potential inhibitors of the vascular endothelium growth factor binding to neuropilin-1. *Bioorg. Med. Chem.* **2010**, *18*, 3285–3298. [CrossRef] [PubMed]
18. Liu, W.-Q.; Lepelletier, Y.; Montès, M.; Borriello, L.; Jarray, R.; Grépin, R.; Leforban, B.; Loukaci, A.; Benhida, R.; Hermine, O.; et al. NRPa-308, a new neuropilin-1 antagonist, exerts in vitro anti-angiogenic and anti-proliferative effects and in vivo anti-cancer effects in a mouse xenograft model. *Cancer Lett.* **2018**, *414*, 88–98. [CrossRef] [PubMed]
19. Borriello, L.; Montès, M.; Lepelletier, Y.; Leforban, B.; Liu, W.-Q.Q.; Demange, L.; Delhomme, B.; Pavoni, S.; Jarray, R.; Boucher, J.L.; et al. Structure-based discovery of a small non-peptidic Neuropilins antagonist exerting in vitro and in vivo anti-tumor activity on breast cancer model. *Cancer Lett.* **2014**, *349*, 120–127. [CrossRef]
20. Starzec, A.; Miteva, M.A.; Ladam, P.; Villoutreix, B.O.; Perret, G.Y. Discovery of novel inhibitors of vascular endothelial growth factor-A-Neuropilin-1 interaction by structure-based virtual screening. *Bioorg. Med. Chem.* **2014**, *22*, 4042–4048. [CrossRef]
21. Jarvis, A.; Allerston, C.K.; Jia, H.; Herzog, B.; Garza-Garcia, A.; Winfield, N.; Ellard, K.; Aqil, R.; Lynch, R.; Chapman, C.; et al. Small Molecule Inhibitors of the Neuropilin-1 Vascular Endothelial Growth Factor A (VEGF-A) Interaction. *J. Med. Chem.* **2010**, *53*, 2215–2226. [CrossRef] [PubMed]
22. Soker, S.; Gollamudi-Payne, S.; Fidder, H.; Charmahelli, H.; Klagsbrun, M. Inhibition of Vascular Endothelial Growth Factor (VEGF)-induced Endothelial Cell Proliferation by a Peptide Corresponding to the Exon 7-Encoded Domain of VEGF165. *J. Biol. Chem.* **1997**, *272*, 31582–31588. [CrossRef]
23. Jia, H.; Bagherzadeh, A.; Hartzoulakis, B.; Jarvis, A.; Löhr, M.; Shaikh, S.; Aqil, R.; Cheng, L.; Tickner, M.; Esposito, D.; et al. Characterization of a bicyclic peptide neuropilin-1 (NP-1) antagonist (EG3287) reveals importance of vascular endothelial growth factor exon 8 for NP-1 binding and role of NP-1 in KDR signaling. *J. Biol. Chem.* **2006**, *281*, 13493–13502. [CrossRef] [PubMed]
24. Grabowska, K.; Puszko, A.K.; Lipiński, P.F.J.; Laskowska, A.K.; Wileńska, B.; Witkowska, E.; Misicka, A. Design, synthesis and in vitro biological evaluation of a small cyclic peptide as inhibitor of vascular endothelial growth factor binding to neuropilin-1. *Bioorg. Med. Chem. Lett.* **2016**, *26*, 1–4. [CrossRef] [PubMed]
25. Getz, J.A.; Cheneval, O.; Craik, D.J.; Daugherty, P.S. Design of a Cyclotide Antagonist of Neuropilin-1 and -2 That Potently Inhibits Endothelial Cell Migration. *ACS Chem. Biol.* **2013**, *8*, 1147–1154. [CrossRef]
26. Grabowska, K.; Puszko, A.K.; Lipiński, P.F.J.; Laskowska, A.K.; Wileńska, B.; Witkowska, E.; Perret, G.Y.; Misicka, A. Structure-activity relationship study of a small cyclic peptide H-c[Lys-Pro-Glu]-Arg-OH: A potent inhibitor of Vascular Endothelial Growth Factor interaction with Neuropilin-1. *Bioorg. Med. Chem.* **2016**, *25*, 5–8. [CrossRef]

27. Binétruy-Tournaire, R.; Demangel, C.; Malavaud, B.; Vassy, R.; Rouyre, S.; Kraemer, M.; Plouët, J.; Derbin, C.; Perret, G.; Mazié, J.C. Identification of a peptide blocking vascular endothelial growth factor (VEGF)-mediated angiogenesis. *EMBO J.* **2000**, *19*, 1525–1533. [CrossRef] [PubMed]
28. Fedorczyk, B.; Lipiński, P.F.J.; Tymecka, D.; Puszko, A.K.; Wilenska, B.; Perret, G.Y.; Misicka, A. Conformational latitude—Activity relationship of KPPR tetrapeptide analogues toward their ability to inhibit binding of Vascular Endothelial Growth Factor 165 to Neuropilin-1. *J. Pept. Sci.* **2017**, *23*, 445–454. [CrossRef]
29. Tymecka, D.; Puszko, A.K.; Lipiński, P.F.J.; Fedorczyk, B.; Wilenska, B.; Sura, K.; Perret, G.Y.; Misicka, A. Branched pentapeptides as potent inhibitors of the vascular endothelial growth factor 165 binding to Neuropilin-1: Design, synthesis and biological activity. *Eur. J. Med. Chem.* **2018**, *158*, 453–462. [CrossRef]
30. Tymecka, D.; Lipiński, P.F.J.P.F.J.; Fedorczyk, B.; Puszko, A.; Wileńska, B.; Perret, G.Y.G.Y.; Misicka, A.; Lipi, P.F.J.; Puszko, A.; Wile, B.; et al. Structure-activity relationship study of tetrapeptide inhibitors of the Vascular Endothelial Growth Factor A binding to Neuropilin-1. *Peptides* **2017**, *94*, 25–32. [CrossRef]
31. Starzec, A.; Vassy, R.; Martin, A.; Lecouvey, M.; Di Benedetto, M.; Crépin, M.; Perret, G.Y. Antiangiogenic and antitumor activities of peptide inhibiting the vascular endothelial growth factor binding to neuropilin-1. *Life Sci.* **2006**, *79*, 2370–2381. [CrossRef]
32. Puszko, A.K.; Sosnowski, P.; Tymecka, D.; Raynaud, F.; Hermine, O.; Lepelletier, Y.; Misicka, A. Neuropilin-1 peptide-like ligands with proline mimetics, tested using the improved chemiluminescence affinity detection method. *Medchemcomm* **2019**, *10*, 332–340. [CrossRef]
33. Tron, G.C.; Pirali, T.; Billington, R.A.; Canonico, P.L.; Sorba, G.; Genazzani, A.A. Click chemistry reactions in medicinal chemistry: Applications of the 1,3-dipolar cycloaddition between azides and alkynes. *Med. Res. Rev.* **2008**, *28*, 278–308. [CrossRef]
34. Diness, F.; Schoffelen, S.; Meldal, M. Advances in Merging Triazoles with Peptides and Proteins. In *Peptidomimetics I.*; Lubell, W.D., Ed.; Springer International Publishing: Cham, Switzerland, 2017; pp. 267–304, ISBN 978-3-319-49119-6.
35. Tornøe, C.W.; Christensen, C.; Meldal, M. Peptidotriazoles on solid phase: [1,2,3]-Triazoles by regiospecific copper(I)-catalyzed 1,3-dipolar cycloadditions of terminal alkynes to azides. *J. Org. Chem.* **2002**, *67*, 3057–3064. [CrossRef]
36. Rostovtsev, V.V.; Green, L.G.; Fokin, V.V.; Sharpless, K.B. A Stepwise Huisgen Cycloaddition Process: Copper(I)-Catalyzed Regioselective "Ligation" of Azides and Terminal Alkynes. *Angew. Chemie Int. Ed.* **2002**, *41*, 2596–2599.
37. Ben Haj Salah, K.; Das, S.; Ruiz, N.; Andreu, V.; Martinez, J.; Wenger, E.; Amblard, M.; Didierjean, C.; Legrand, B.; Inguimbert, N. How are 1,2,3-triazoles accommodated in helical secondary structures? *Org. Biomol. Chem.* **2018**, *16*, 3576–3583. [CrossRef]
38. Nyffeler, P.T.; Liang, C.H.; Koeller, K.M.; Wong, C.H. The chemistry of amine-azide interconversion: Catalytic diazotransfer and regioselective azide reduction. *J. Am. Chem. Soc.* **2002**, *124*, 10773–10778. [CrossRef]
39. Lundquist IV, J.T.; Pelletier, J.C. Improved solid-phase peptide synthesis method utilizing α-azide-protected amino acids. *Org. Lett.* **2001**, *3*, 781–783. [CrossRef]
40. Punna, S.; Finn, M.G. A Convenient Colorimetric Test for Aliphatic Azides. *Synlett* **2004**, *2004*, 99–100.
41. Bernatowicz, M.S.; Youling, W.; Matsueda, G.R. 1H-Pyrazole-1-carboxamidine Hydrochloride: An Attractive Reagent for Guanylation of Amines and Its Application to Peptide Synthesis. *J. Org. Chem.* **1992**, *57*, 2497–2502. [CrossRef]
42. Starzec, A.; Ladam, P.; Vassy, R.; Badache, S.; Bouchemal, N.; Navaza, A.; du Penhoat, C.H.; Perret, G.Y. Structure-function analysis of the antiangiogenic ATWLPPR peptide inhibiting VEGF165 binding to neuropilin-1 and molecular dynamics simulations of the ATWLPPR/neuropilin-1 complex. *Peptides* **2007**, *28*, 2397–2402. [CrossRef] [PubMed]
43. Vander Kooi, C.W.; Jusino, M.A.; Perman, B.; Neau, D.B.; Bellamy, H.D.; Leahy, D.J. Structural basis for ligand and heparin binding to neuropilin B domains. *Proc. Natl. Acad. Sci. USA* **2007**, *104*, 6152–6157. [CrossRef] [PubMed]
44. Parker, M.W.; Xu, P.; Li, X.; Vander Kooi, C.W. Structural Basis for Selective Vascular Endothelial Growth Factor-A (VEGF-A) Binding to Neuropilin-1. *J. Biol. Chem.* **2012**, *287*, 11082–11089. [CrossRef]
45. Mota, F.; Fotinou, C.; Rhana, R.; Chan, A.W.E.; Yelland, T.; Arooz, M.T.; O'Leary, A.P.; Hutton, J.; Frankel, P.; Zachary, I.; et al. Architecture and hydration of the arginine-binding site of neuropilin-1. *FEBS J.* **2018**, *285*, 1290–1304. [CrossRef] [PubMed]

46. Case, D.A.; Babin, V.; Berryman, J.T.; Betz, R.M.; Cai, Q.; Cerutti, D.S.; Cheatham, T.E.I.; Darden, T.A.; Duke, R.E.; Gohlke, H.; et al. *Amber14*; University of California: San Francisco, CA, USA, 2014.
47. Maier, J.A.; Martinez, C.; Kasavajhala, K.; Wickstrom, L.; Hauser, K.E.; Simmerling, C. ff14SB: Improving the Accuracy of Protein Side Chain and Backbone Parameters from ff99SB. *J. Chem. Theory Comput.* **2015**, *11*, 3696–3713. [CrossRef] [PubMed]
48. Marion, A.; Góra, J.; Kracker, O.; Fröhr, T.; Latajka, R.; Sewald, N.; Antes, I. Amber-Compatible Parametrization Procedure for Peptide-like Compounds: Application to 1,4- and 1,5-Substituted Triazole-Based Peptidomimetics. *J. Chem. Inf. Model.* **2018**, *58*, 90–110. [CrossRef]
49. Michaud-Agrawal, N.; Denning, E.J.; Woolf, T.B.; Beckstein, O. MDAnalysis: A toolkit for the analysis of molecular dynamics simulations. *J. Comput. Chem.* **2011**, *32*, 2319–2327. [CrossRef] [PubMed]
50. Pettersen, E.F.; Goddard, T.D.; Huang, C.C.; Couch, G.S.; Greenblatt, D.M.; Meng, E.C.; Ferrin, T.E. UCSF Chimera—A Visualization System for Exploratory Research and Analysis. *J. Comput. Chem.* **2004**, *25*, 1605–1612. [CrossRef]

Sample Availability: Samples of the compounds **3** and **4** are available from the authors.

molecules

MDPI

Article

Rapid Discovery of Illuminating Peptides for Instant Detection of Opioids in Blood and Body Fluids

Shabnam Jafari [1], Yann Thillier [1], Yousif H. Ajena [1], Diedra Shorty [1], Jiannan Li [2], Jonathan S. Huynh [1], Bethany Ming-Choi Pan [1], Tingrui Pan [2], Kit S. Lam [1,*] and Ruiwu Liu [1,*]

1 Department of Biochemistry & Molecular Medicine, University of California Davis, Sacramento, CA 95817, USA; shjafari@ucdavis.edu (S.J.); Yann.Thillier@umassmed.edu (Y.T.); yousifajena5620@gmail.com (Y.H.A.); dshorty@ucdavis.edu (D.S.); jshuynh@ucdavis.edu (J.S.H.); bmpan@ucdavis.edu (B.M.-C.P.)

2 Department of Biomedical Engineering, University of California Davis, Davis, CA 95616, USA; jnli@stanford.edu (J.L.); trpan@ucdavis.edu (T.P.)

* Correspondence: kslam@ucdavis.edu (K.S.L.); rwliu@ucdavis.edu (R.L.); Tel.: +1-916-734-0910 (K.S.L.); +1-916-734-0905 (R.L.)

Received: 15 April 2019; Accepted: 5 May 2019; Published: 10 May 2019

check for updates

Abstract: The United States is currently experiencing an opioid crisis, with more than 47,000 deaths in 2017 due to opioid overdoses. Current approaches for opioid identification and quantification in body fluids include immunoassays and chromatographic methods (e.g., LC-MS, GC-MS), which require expensive instrumentation and extensive sample preparation. Our aim was to develop a portable point-of-care device that can be used for the instant detection of opioids in body fluids. Here, we reported the development of a morphine-sensitive fluorescence-based sensor chip to sensitively detect morphine in the blood using a homogeneous immunoassay without any washing steps. Morphine-sensitive illuminating peptides were identified using a high throughput one-bead one-compound (OBOC) combinatorial peptide library approach. The OBOC libraries contain a large number of random peptides with a molecular rotor dye, malachite green (MG), that are coupled to the amino group on the side chain of lysine at different positions of the peptides. The OBOC libraries were then screened for fluorescent activation under a confocal microscope, using an anti-morphine monoclonal antibody as the screening probe, in the presence and absence of free morphine. Using this novel three-step fluorescent screening assay, we were able to identify the peptide-beads that fluoresce in the presence of an anti-morphine antibody, but lost fluorescence when the free morphine was present. After the positive beads were decoded using automatic Edman microsequencing, the morphine-sensitive illuminating peptides were then synthesized in soluble form, functionalized with an azido group, and immobilized onto microfabricated PEG-array spots on a glass slide. The sensor chip was then evaluated for the detection of morphine in plasma. We demonstrated that this proof-of-concept platform can be used to develop fluorescence-based sensors against morphine. More importantly, this technology can also be applied to the discovery of other novel illuminating peptidic sensors for the detection of illicit drugs and cancer biomarkers in body fluids.

Keywords: OBOC; combinatorial chemistry; opioid; drug screen; molecular rotor dye; high throughput screening; sensor chip

1. Introduction

Opioid abuse is a rapidly growing epidemic, and according to data from the US Department of Health and Human Services, it caused more than 130 deaths per day in the US alone in 2017. Since the year 2000, the rate of deaths from drug overdoses has increased by 137%, including a 200% increase in the rate of overdose deaths involving opioids (specifically opioid pain relievers and heroin) [1–3].

There is a medical need to develop a portable point-of-care diagnostic device that allows paramedics to rapidly identify the opioid drug(s) taken by unconscious patients, thereby allowing treatment to begin in the field, and effectively saving more lives. Current approaches for opioid identification and quantification in body fluids include immunoassay and chromatographic methods (e.g., LC-MS, GC-MS), which require expensive instrumentation and extensive sample preparations [4–10]. The current homogeneous enzymatic immunoassays do not identify the opioid and often give false positive results if the patients are taking standard therapeutic doses of some antibiotics [11,12]. We proposed developing a straightforward and innovative fluorescence-based sensor chip to sensitively detect opioid drugs in the blood, using a homogeneous immunoassay without any washing steps. Illuminating peptides that specifically interact with a selected monoclonal antibody (mAb) can be discovered via high throughput screening of the one-bead one-compound (OBOC) combinatorial peptide library [13], that is covalently linked to a molecular rotor dye (MRD). Once identified and immobilized as peptide microarrays on a chip, the generated illuminating peptide spots function as activatable fluorescent probes to monitor the physical interactions with its target protein, which in this study was the anti-morphine mAb.

The term, molecular rotor, refers to a class of twisted intramolecular charge transfer complexes (TICT), with photophysical characteristics that depend on their environment. This class of fluorophores is characterized by their formation of twisted states through the rotation of various segments of the structure with respect to the rest of the molecule. The aforementioned intramolecular rotation changes the ground state and the excited-state energies, whilst the molecular rotors de-excited from the twisted state either through emission of a red-shifted emission band or by non-radiative relaxation. Since this rotation and thus the twisted state formation rate are strongly dependent on the solvent, parameters such as solvent polarity, hydrogen bond formation, isomerization, and steric hindrance, which are the predominant forms of the solvent–fluorophore interactions, can all affect the emission properties. Of these, steric hindrance is of high importance because it links the solvents micro-viscosity to the formation rate of the twisted intramolecular charge transfer state, which in turn determines the spectral emission [14–16]. Molecular rotor dyes (MRDs) have become increasingly popular as molecular imaging probes, since they exhibit very unique properties and they offer the possibility of imaging target biomolecules with minimal background [17,18]. MRDs have already been used as probes for ligand-receptor binding, guest fluorophores that turn on fluorescence with a target RNA aptamer or labels of biomolecules [19–21].

Malachite green (MG) is a triarylmethane MRD that has been extensively used in live cell imaging, as it exhibits low fluorescence in its unbound state, but has very high fluorescence (>2000-fold) when bound specifically to macromolecules (Figure 1A) [22,23]. The fluorescent-activation property of MG makes it an ideal candidate for the development of illuminating peptide-dye conjugates, which enables the dynamic detection of target–ligand interactions in the near infra-red range, whilst minimizing the background autofluorescence. Covalently attached molecular rotors are a widely applicable tool to study supramolecular protein assembly, and they can reveal the microrheological features of aggregating protein systems both in vitro and in cellulo, which are not otherwise observable through classical fluorescent probes operating in the light switch mode [24]. However, it is important to emphasize that the direct conjugation of MRDs to known protein ligands has not been well explored. To date, there have been few reports in the literature on using MRD-conjugated ligands to probe living cells. An example is using covalently attached molecular rotors as fluorogenic probes for monitoring peptide binding to class II MHC proteins in living cells [25]. A series of novel fluorogenic probes incorporating 4-*N*,*N*-dimethylaminophthalimidoalanine and 6-*N*,*N*-dimethylamino-2-3-naphthalimidoalanine have been developed to visualize these processes. These fluorophores show large changes in the emission spectra upon binding to class II MHC proteins. Peptides incorporating these fluorophores bind specifically to the class II MHC proteins on antigen-presenting cells and can be used to follow peptide binding in vivo. These probes have been used to track a developmentally regulated cell-surface peptide-binding activity in primary human monocyte-derived dendritic cells [25]. Another example is the successful imaging of the oxytocin G receptor using carbetocin peptide linked to an MRD [19]. MRDs have also been used as an exogenous probe to detect a single chain antibody against MG, that has been genetically grafted to the host protein for protein tracking in living cells [26].

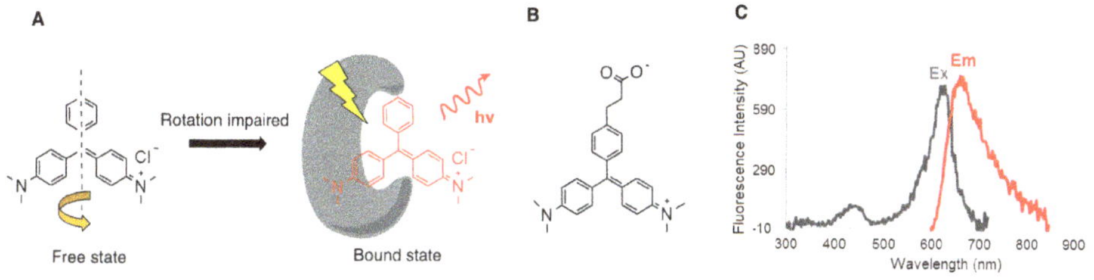

Figure 1. (**A**) Molecular rotor dye (MRD) malachite green (MG) in free and bound states. (**B**) Structure of the carboxyethyl malachite green (CEMG). (**C**) CEMG excitation, emission spectra were obtained in glycerol:PBS (80:20, *v*/*v*) at pH 7.4.

The OBOC combinatorial library method has proven to be a powerful tool for identifying bioactive molecules, including peptides, peptidomimetics, and small molecules [13,27]. Using a "split-and-pool" solid-phase synthesis strategy [13,28], the OBOC combinatorial libraries can be rapidly prepared such that each bead displays 10^{13} copies of a single chemical entity [13]. This approach allows millions of compounds to be synthesized and screened simultaneously within a few weeks. Solid-phase peptide synthesis (SPPS), which allows for a rapid peptide synthesis on solid support with high efficiency and reduced side reactions [13,28,29], was employed in the synthesis of OBOC illuminating peptide libraries. These OBOC combinatorial libraries contain a large number of random peptides while incorporating a MRD, carboxyethyl malachite green (CEMG, Figure 1B), to the lysine side chain amino group at different positions of the peptide sequences. A subsequent three-step fluorescent screening assay (Figure 2) using a confocal microscope was employed to track the beads that exhibited: (i) little to no fluorescence when plasma was added; (ii) an increase in fluorescence when bound to the anti-morphine mAb, due to its direct interaction with the illuminating peptide present on the bead; and (iii) a decrease in fluorescence upon the addition of a defined opioid through competitive binding with the antibody. Positive beads (bead C in Figure 2) meeting the desired criteria, i.e., displaying a noticeable change in the fluorescence intensity upon addition of the morphine, were isolated for decoding. The azido-modified illuminating peptides were then synthesized in soluble form and immobilized onto a microarray chip using efficient Cu-free click chemistry, to form a fluorescence-activatable sensor chip which was evaluated for its ability to detect morphine in plasma.

Peptide microarrays have been used for a variety of research and clinical applications, such as the identification of xenobiotic autoantigens in patients with biliary cirrhosis [30], profiling of cytotoxic T-lymphocyte activity [31], and serodiagnosis of *Burkholderia* infections in cystic fibrosis patients [32]. Unlike our fluorescent-activatable illuminating peptide microarray sensing platform, which utilizes a homogeneous assay, all these microarray platforms use heterogeneous assays that require multiple washing steps.

In this paper, we reported the discovery of novel morphine-sensitive illuminating peptides using the high throughput OBOC library approach [13] and the development of a fluorescence-based sensor-chip for the detection of morphine in blood. Applying the OBOC platform to the synthesis and detection of MRD-based sensing molecules against morphine is new and unique. This detection platform utilizes a homogeneous immunoassay; therefore, it is fast, simple, and straightforward. In principle, an array of multiple different illuminating peptide sensors can be printed on the chip, such that multiple drugs or disease biomarkers can be detected concurrently in a multiplex manner, using only a minute amount of body fluids, such as blood and urine.

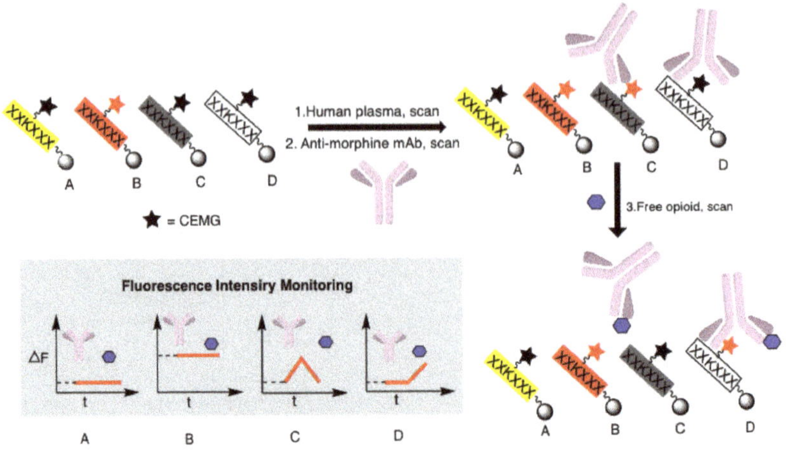

Figure 2. Three-step fluorescent screening assay of the illuminating peptide libraries.

2. Results

2.1. *Selection of the Polymer Beads for Construction of the OBOC Illuminating Peptide Libraries*

To identify an appropriate resin polymer for illuminating peptide discovery, different commercially available beads, including TentaGel, Chematrix, and acrylamide-polyethylene glycol (PEGA) beads were treated with increasing concentrations of MRDs, whilst the dye fluorescent activation was monitored using confocal fluorescence microscopy (CFM) over a period of 1 h. For the PEGA beads, no noticeable activation at the highest MRD concentration (5 μM) was detected (Figure 3). Therefore, to minimize the background fluorescent activation during screening, all the OBOC combinatorial libraries for illuminating peptide discovery were prepared using hydrophilic PEGA beads.

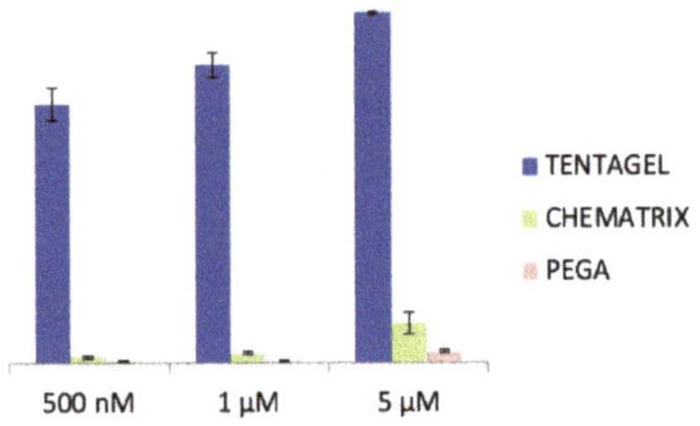

Figure 3. MRD concentrations: 500 nM, 1 μM, and 5 μM. Data collected for six random beads per resin.

2.2. *Design and Synthesis of the CEMG*

In order to effectively conjugate the MRDs to the peptide library, we first needed to functionalize the MRD with a carboxyl group. Consequently, CEMG was successfully synthesized in two steps (Figure 4), and its fluorescence excitation-emission spectra were then characterized (Figure 1C).

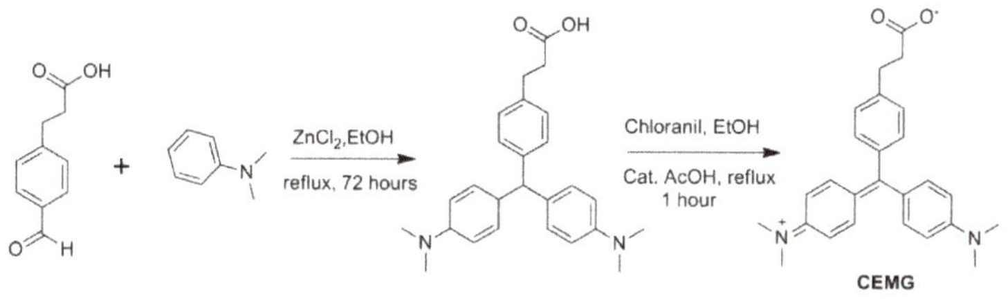

Figure 4. Synthetic scheme of the CEMG.

2.3. *Design and Synthesis of the OBOC Combinatorial Peptide Libraries*

The OBOC combinatorial peptide library method was used to discover the small cyclic illuminating peptides that specifically fluoresce upon binding to an anti-morphine antibody. Two disulfide cyclic OBOC libraries (Figure 5) containing 19^5 and 19^6 permutations, respectively, were synthesized on the bi-layer beads [33] via a "split-and-pool" strategy employing fluorenylmethyloxycarbonyl (Fmoc) chemistry [13,34]. In these libraries, the illuminating peptides were displayed on the surface of the beads and the coding tags, without MRD, and they were confined to the bead interior, such that they would not interfere with the screening. In order to speed up the library synthesis, we used the heating method for coupling of the Fmoc-amino acid (90 °C for 2 min) and Fmoc-deprotection (90 °C for 90 s) as described in Reference [35]. The two flanking D-cysteines in the peptides were coupled at room temperature for 2 h to avoid racemization. The synthetic scheme for library L1 is shown in Figure 6 as an example of the library synthesis.

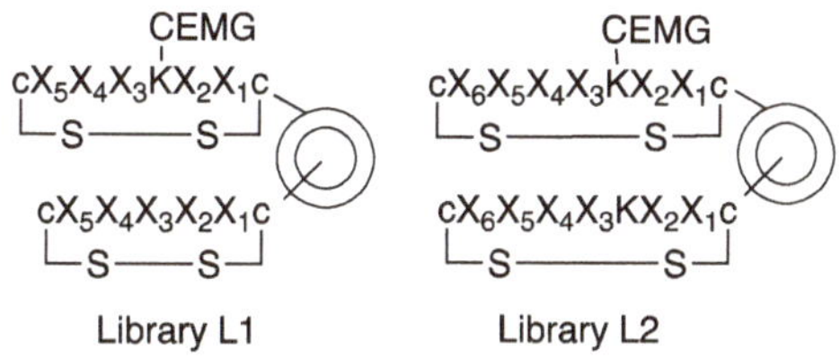

Figure 5. Structures of two OBOC illuminating peptide libraries, where the MRD moiety is introduced within the library onto an amino group of the lysine (K) side chain. X stands for 19 natural amino acids except L-cysteine.

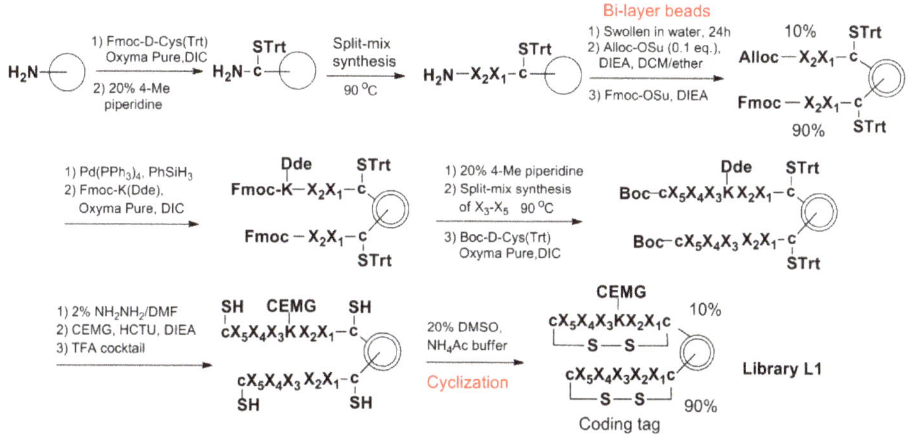

Figure 6. Synthetic scheme of OBOC library L1.

2.4. High-Throughput Screening of the OBOC Illuminating Peptide Library Beads

Library beads were successfully immobilized on a polystyrene plate by submersion in 90% *N,N*-dimethylformamide (DMF) in water. The plate, containing ~100,000 immobilized beads, (where each displayed a unique illuminating peptide) was scanned within 50 min using a confocal microscope. The library screening was achieved via a three-step strategy as described above and as shown in Figure 2. Changes in the fluorescent intensity ($\Delta F/F_0$) after each addition were analyzed using a customized algorithm written in MATLAB (Supplemental Figure S1). One strong positive bead from library L1 and three strong positive beads from library L2 were picked up for the Edman microsequencing. The result is shown in Table 1. Some sequence homology was observed between P1 and P2: where both contained 3 tryptophans and an additional hydrophobic amino acid, with two of the tryptophans lined up at the amino side of the Lys(CEMG). The four peptides were resynthesized on the PEGA beads via a similar method as used in the library synthesis. The fluorescence activation of the beads with the anti-morphine mAb and deactivation with the morphine were confirmed with beads P1, P2, and P3 (Supplemental Figure S2). Peptide P4 was excluded in making the sensor chip due to its high background fluorescence.

Table 1. Sequences of cyclic positive illuminating peptide hits.

	c	X_6	X_5	X_4	X_3	K(CEMG)	X_2	X_1	c
P1	c	F	Y	W	W	K(CEMG)	W	Q	c
P2	c		I	W	W	K(CEMG)	R	W	c
P3	c	T	S	Q	G	K(CEMG)	F	A	c
P4	c	N	V	G	N	K(CEMG)	Q	P	c

2.5. Preparation of the Sensor Chip

We recently reported the use of photolithography to generate arrays of microdiscs of polymerized PEG functionalized with amino groups for microfluidic assisted in situ peptide print-synthesis of the peptide microarrays [36]. In this study, we utilized the same microdisc arrays as the platform for the sensor chip, but we used the Cu-free dibenzocyclooctyne (DBCO)—azide click chemistry to ligate the illuminating peptides to the chip. DBCO was first introduced to the chip using DBCO-NHS in the presence of DIEA. Three individual azido-illuminating peptides (Figure 7) were synthesized on a TentaGel XV RAM, using the same chemistry used for the OBOC library synthesis. Fmoc-Lys(N_3)-OH, an unnatural amino acid to introduce an azide group to the peptide, was first coupled to the beads. The linear azido-illuminating peptides were cleaved off the bead, cyclized with CLEAR-OX resins [37,38], and then purified by HPLC. The illuminating peptides were then conjugated to the DBCO-modified micro-chip using the efficient Cu-free click chemistry (Figure 8). The resulting chip was then evaluated for the detection of morphine in human plasma (Figure 9). All three illuminating peptides were found to be able to detect morphine in the plasma at a concentration of 0.35 μM (100 ng/mL).

P1-azide

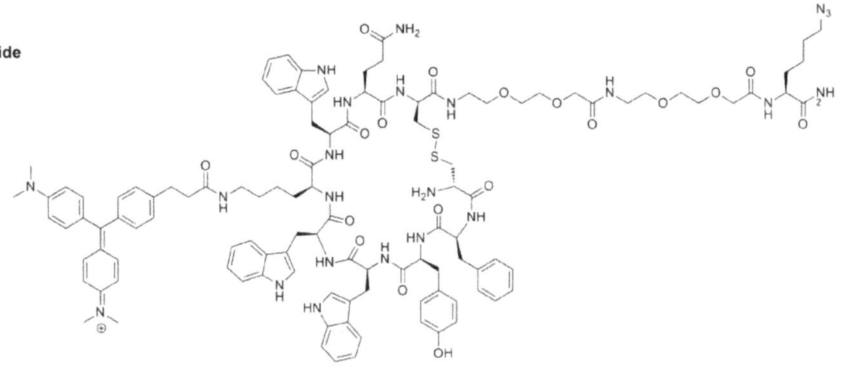

P2-azide

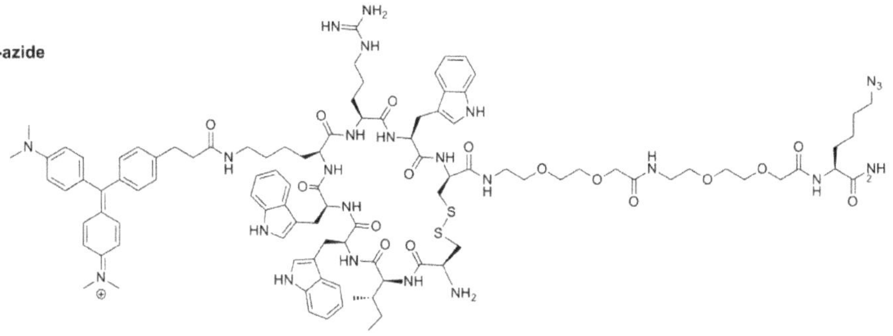

P3-azide

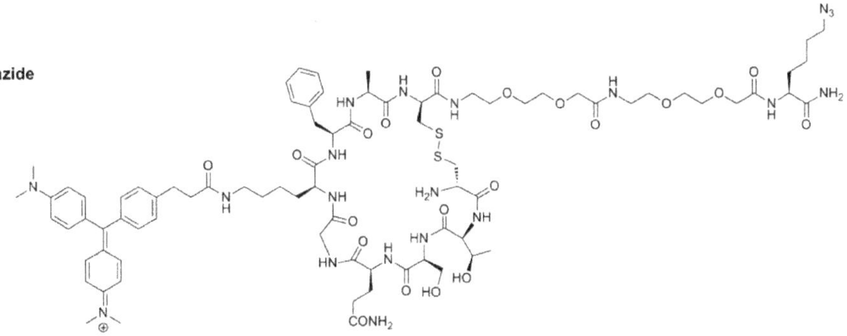

Figure 7. Structures of three azido-illuminating peptides from Table 1.

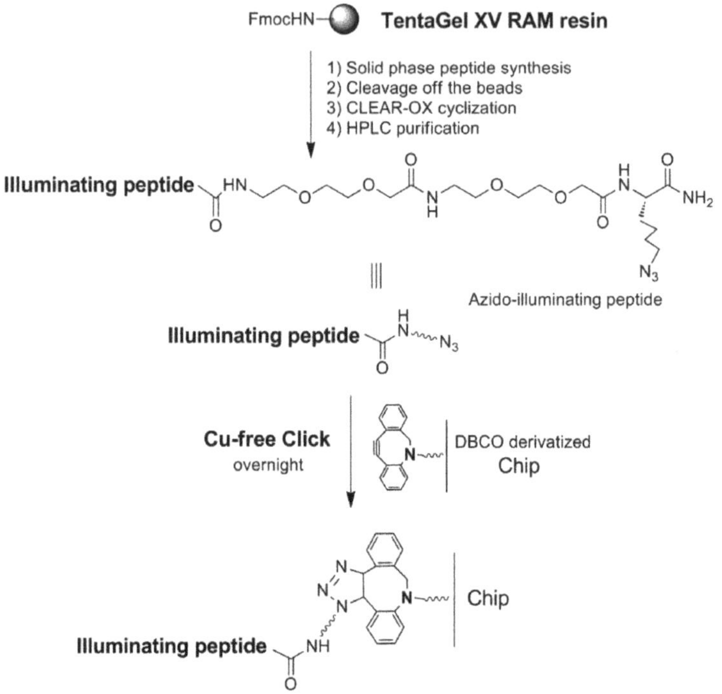

Figure 8. Immobilize illuminating peptides onto a microarray chip using efficient Cu-free click chemistry.

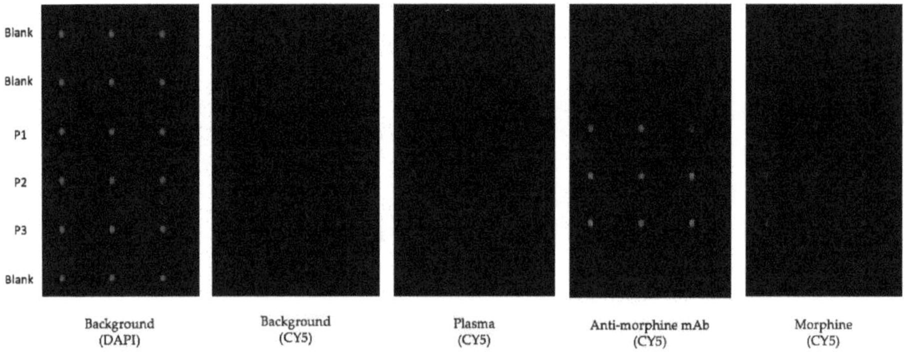

Figure 9. Testing the illuminating peptide sensor chip for morphine detection, after 20 min of incubation. The background picture was taken in PBS. Plasma picture was taken in 10% human blood plasma in PBS. Anti-morphine mAb concentration was 3.5 nM and morphine concentration was 0.35 μM. Rows number 1, 2, and 6 are blank spots without illuminating peptides.

3. Discussion

We aimed to develop a sensor chip that depended solely on the binding specificity between the anti-opioid mAb and the corresponding illuminating peptides, without the need of washing steps. Such illuminating peptides were easily discovered through the OBOC combinatorial library approach. PEGA beads were chosen as a solid support for the construction of the OBOC libraries because of their low autofluorescence and low propensity to activate MG. MRD CEMG was used to construct the

OBOC illuminating peptide libraries because of its ability to be easily conjugated to the lysine side chain of the peptide sequence.

The OBOC libraries were synthesized on bi-layer beads wherein the coding tag resided inside the bead to avoid interference with the screening probe [33]. In order to speed up the library synthesis, we used the heating method for coupling of the Fmoc-amino acid and Fmoc-deprotection [35]. To the best of our knowledge, this is the first report that applied the heating method to the synthesis of the OBOC library. Each library contains millions of beads, where each bead displays a unique illuminating peptide. The disulfide cyclic library yields conformational constrained peptides, which provide an ideal molecule for MRD activation upon the antibody binding. The simple method for immobilizing the library beads on polystyrene plates [39,40] enabled us to perform a sequential three-step screening, such that the fluorescent image of each and every library bead could be easily tracked and recorded. Beads that fulfilled the following three criteria were considered positive beads: (i) They did not fluoresce in the presence of plasma, (ii) they fluoresced when the anti-morphine mAb was added, and (iii) the fluorescent signal diminished greatly upon addition of the free morphine to the screening medium. Of the four positive beads isolated (Table 1), only three of them (P1, P2, and P3) were confirmed to be true positive upon resynthesis of the peptides on the PEGA beads (Supplemental Figure S2). P1 and P2 had significant sequence homology. Based on the homology, focused OBOC libraries can be developed to discover more sensitive illuminating peptides for morphine. Without further optimization, the three illuminating peptides can already easily detect 0.35 μM of morphine in the plasma. The lethal intoxication concentration of free morphine in the blood is about 170 ng/mL (median, equal to 0.6 μM) [41]. For other opioid drugs, such as fentanyl, which is much more potent and has lower blood and urine levels in addicts, their detection will require more sensitive fluorescent-activating peptides. Since plasma exposure was incorporated into one of the early screening steps, and the beads that fluoresced in plasma were eliminated from further consideration, the identified illuminating peptides were free of interference by the plasma proteins.

The antibody-based homogeneous assay reported here, after optimization, can potentially be used as an inexpensive point-of-care test for instant detection, identification, and quantification of specific opioids in bodily fluids. Although morphine was used as an example, the illuminating peptides against other opioid drugs and other street drugs (e.g., amphetamines) can also be discovered using this novel approach. We envision that the illuminating peptides against a range of controlled substances can be printed on microarrays for the concurrent screening of a large number of drugs.

It is noteworthy that during the course of the screening, we found a few beads that did not fluoresce in neither the plasma nor the addition of anti-morphine mAb but fluoresced upon the addition of morphine. This indicated that these cyclic peptides interacted with morphine directly. Work is currently underway to characterize these peptides. If interaction is specific and with high affinity, these morphine sensing peptides could potentially be used to develop an inexpensive sensor chip for the direct detection of opiates without the use of antibodies.

In summary, we have successfully developed a morphine-sensitive sensor chip and demonstrated that this proof-of-concept platform can be used to develop fluorescence-based sensors against morphine in a straightforward homogeneous immunoassay. The ultimate application of this platform is to develop a point-of-care device using a portable smartphone-based fluorescent reader (e.g., DxCELL fluorescent reader), for the instant and sensitive detection of opioids in body fluids, which is not currently available in the market. This fluorescent-activating peptide concept can potentially be applied to the development of sensor chips against not only illicit drugs, but also biomarkers for cancer and other diseases.

4. Materials and Methods

4.1. General Experiment Procedures

The OBOC library screening was done on a confocal microscope ZEISS LSM 800 (Carl Zeiss Microscopy, Thornwood, NY, USA). Data analysis was conducted using the Fiji and MATLAB programs. Matrix-assisted laser desorption/ionization time of flight mass spectrometry (MALDI-TOF MS) analysis was performed on a Bruker UltraFlextreme mass spectrometer (Billerica, MA, USA). The analytical HPLC was performed on a Waters 2996 HPLC system equipped with a 4.6 × 150 mm Waters Xterra MS C18 5.0 μm column, and it employed a 20 min gradient from 100% aqueous H_2O (0.1% TFA) to 100% CH_3CN (0.1% TFA), at a flow rate of 1.0 mL/min. Preparative HPLC was performed on a System Gold 126NMP solvent module (Beckman), with a C18 column (Vydac, 10 μm, 2.2 cm i.d. × 25 cm). A gradient elution of 0–60% B over 45 min, then 60–100% B over 5 min, followed by 100% B for 5 min, was used at a flow rate of 5 mL/min (solvent A, H_2O/0.1% TFA; B, acetonitrile/0.1% TFA).

PEGA beads (0.4 mmol/g, 150–300 μm) were purchased from Agilent Technologies (Santa Clara, CA, USA). TentaGel XV RAM resin (0.28 mmol/g) was purchased from Rapp Polymere GmbH (Tübingen, Germany). 1-[Bis(dimethylamino)methylene]-1*H*-1,2,3-triazolo[4,5-b]pyridinium 3-oxid hexafluorophosphate (HATU) and Fmoc-amino acids were purchased from P3BioSystems (Louisville, KY, USA). CLEAR-OX^{TM} resin was purchased from Peptide International Inc. (Louisville, KY, USA). *O*-(1*H*-6-Chlorobenzotriazole-1-yl)-1,1,3,3-tetramethyluronium hexafluorophosphate (HCTU), Boc-D-Cys(Trt)-OH and ethyl cyanohydroxy-iminoacetate (Oxyma Pure) were purchased from Chem-Impex International Inc. (Wood Dale, IL, USA). Fmoc-Lys(Dde)-OH was purchased from AAPPTec (Louisville, KY, USA). Fmoc-AEEA linker and Fmoc-Lys(N_3)-OH were purchased from ChemPep Inc. (Wellington, FL, USA). DBCO-NHS was obtained from BroadPharm (San Diego, CA, USA). 1,3-Diisopropylcarbodiimide (DIC), trifluoroacetic acid (TFA), *N*,*N*-diisopropylethylamine (DIEA), triisopropylsilane (TIS), dimethyl sulfoxide (DMSO), morphine sulfate salt pentahydrate, all solvents, and other chemical reagents were purchased from Sigma-Aldrich (St. Louis, MO, USA), and they were of analytical grade. The anti-morphine monoclonal antibody was purchased from MyBioSource (San Diego, CA, USA).

4.2. Synthesis of the CEMG

Under an atmosphere of nitrogen, 0.3 g of 3-(4-formylphenyl)propanoic acid (1.7 mmol, 1 eq) and 0.5 g of $ZnCl_2$ (3.7 mmol, 2.2 eq) were added in 18 mL of anhydrous ethanol. Then, 0.47 mL of *N*,*N*-dimethylaniline (3.7 mmol, 2.2 eq) was injected into the reaction mixture, which was allowed to stir under reflux overnight. The solvent was removed under reduced pressure and the crude product was purified by flash column chromatography, using a gradient from 0–5% methanol (MeOH) in dichloromethane (DCM) to yield 0.51 g (y = 75%) of leucomalachite green as a pale green solid. 1H NMR (400 MHz, $CDCl_3$): δ 7.07 (4H, q, *J* = 8.0 Hz), 6.97 (4H, d, *J* = 8.5 Hz), 6.71–6.62 (4H, d, *J* = 8.4 Hz), 5.34 (1H, s), 2.93 (2H, t, *J* = 8.6 Hz), 2.90 (12H, s), 2.65 (2H, t, *J* = 7.9 Hz). ^{13}C-NMR (101 MHz, $CDCl_3$): δ 178.33, 148.82, 143.26, 137.70, 133.34, 129.84, 129.37, 127.92, 112.98, 54.62, 40.90, 35.67, 30.24. HRMS (ESI): $[M + H]^+$ *m*/*z* calcd 403.2380, found 403.2371.

Thereafter, 0.30 g of leucomalachite green was dissolved in 15 mL of hot 95% ethanol (EtOH) in a reaction flask. Then, 0.275 g (1.5 eq.) of chloranil and a catalytic amount of acetic acid were added to the EtOH solution, and the mixture was refluxed for 1 h. The solution turned dark green within the first few minutes. The solvent was removed under vacuum and the residue was purified by flash column chromatography using a gradient from 0 to 6% MeOH in DCM to yield 245 mg (y = 82%) of CEMG zwitterion. ^{1}H-NMR (400 MHz, $CDCl_3$): δ 7.42 (2H, d, *J* = 7.8 Hz), 7.36 (4H, d, *J* = 8.9 Hz), 7.17 (2H, d, *J* = 7.8 Hz), 6.91 (4H, d, *J* = 8.9 Hz), 3.34 (12H, s), 3.08 (2H, t, *J* = 7.5 Hz), 2.96 (2H, t, *J* = 7.5 Hz). ^{13}C-NMR (101 MHz, $CDCl_3$): δ 178.64, 174.26, 156.79, 148.33, 141.00, 137.02, 135.16, 129.12, 127.19, 113.49, 41.00, 36.03, 31.15. HRMS (ESI): $[M + H]^+$ *m*/*z* calcd 401.2224, found 401.2220.

4.3. Synthesis of the OBOC Libraries

Figure 6 describes the library synthesis scheme. One gram of PEGA resin beads were swollen in DMF for 1 h before washing with DMF, MeOH, and DMF. Fmoc-D-Cys(Trt) was coupled to the beads in the presence of Oxyma Pure and DIC using 6 eq excess. The coupling proceeded at room temperature for 2 h. After the liquid was drained, the beads were washed with DMF, MeOH, and DMF. Fmoc-deprotection was achieved using 20% 4-methyl piperidine in DMF, for 5 min, and then 15 min. The beads were washed and separated into 19 aliquots, each aliquot was reacted with 6-fold molar excess of one of 19 Fmoc-amino acids (X_1). Coupling was initiated by the addition of 6 eq excess of Oxyma Pure and DIC. The coupling reactions were performed at 90 °C for 2 min as in Reference [35] in a 20-well heating block, and then monitored using the ninhydrin test. After the liquid was drained, the beads were washed with DMF and then deprotected using 20% 4-methyl piperidine in DMF at 90 °C for 90 s in a 20-well heating block. The beads were then combined and washed with DMF, MeOH, DMF, and re-divided for the next cycle of coupling (X_2). After the beads were combined and Fmoc-deprotected, the beads were washed with DMF, MeOH, and DCM. The beads were then dried in vacuum. The bi-layer beads were prepared using our previous bi-phasic solvent approach [33]. Then, the beads were swollen in water for 24 h. The water was removed by filtration, and the solution of Alloc-OSu (0.1 eq to the bead loading) in DCM/diethyl ether (*v/v*, 55/45) mixture was added to the wet beads, followed by the addition of DIEA. The mixture was shaken vigorously at room temperature for 45 min. After removal of the liquid by filtration, the beads were washed with DMF to remove water from inside the beads, followed by MeOH and DMF. A solution of Fmoc-OSu (3 eq) and DIEA (6 eq) in DCM was then added to the beads. The beads were shaken at room temperature for 1 h. Alloc was deprotected with $Pd(PPh_3)_4$ (0.2 eq) and $PhSiH_3$ (20 eq) in DCM, for 45 min twice. Following de-protection, the beads were washed sequentially with DCM, DMF, 0.5% DIEA in DMF, 0.5% sodium diethyldithiocarbamate in DMF, 50% DCM in DMF, MeOH, and DMF. Fmoc-Lys(Dde)-OH was coupled to the outer of beads using Oxyma Pure and DIC. The Fmoc on both the outer layer and inner layer was removed as described above. After the beads were washed, the beads were then used for the remaining cycles of split-and-pool synthesis of X_3–X_6 using the heating method. The Boc-D-Cys(Trt)-OH was coupled at the last cycle of the peptide assembling using HCTU and DIEA at room temperature for 2 h, until the ninhydrin test was negative. Then, Dde was removed with 2% hydrazine in DMF at room temperature, 3 times, each time for 3 min. After washing with DMF, MeOH, and DMF, the CEMG was coupled to the beads in the presence of HATU and DIEA overnight. After thorough washing with DMF, MeOH, and DCM, the beads were dried in vacuum. The side chain protecting groups were removed with a cocktail containing phenol/thioanisole/water/TIS/TFA (7.5:5:5:2.5:82.5, *w/v/v/v/v*). The cleavage solution was drained, and the bead-supported library was washed with DMF, MeOH, DCM, DMF, 50% DMF/water, and water. The libraries were then cyclized via disulfide bond linkage of the two flanking D-cysteines in 500 mL oxidation solution: water/acetic acid/DMSO (75:5:20, *v/v/v*), where the pH was adjusted to 6 with ammonium hydroxide before adding DMSO, for 2–3 days. Finally, the library beads were washed thoroughly with water, 50% DMF/water, DMF, and then stored in 90% DMF/water.

4.4. High-Throughput Screening of the Immobilized OBOC Illuminating Peptide Libraries

The library beads were suspended in 90% DMF/water, and then added onto a polystyrene plate (120 mm × 80 mm) and allowed to sit still for 30 min. Afterwards the DMF solution was gently removed with a pipette and the immobilized library beads were washed with 50% DMF/water, water, PBS, and then incubated with 10% plasma in PBS for 20 min, followed by scanning with a confocal fluorescence microscope. The fluorescent activation from the peptide bound to plasma proteins was then recorded. Next, the plate was incubated with 3.5 nM of anti-morphine antibody for 20 min, and the fluorescent activation from the illuminating peptide bound antibody was monitored. Thereafter, 0.35 μM morphine solution was added to the plate followed by measurement of the fluorescent intensity. Changes in the fluorescent intensity ($\Delta F/F_0$) after each addition were analyzed using a customized algorithm written in MATLAB. Then, positive beads were selected based on the largest fluorescence changes, and they were retrieved for decoding using Edman microsequencing.

4.5. Resynthesis of the Azido-Illuminating Peptides in Soluble Form

The three azido-illuminating peptides (Figure 7) were synthesized in soluble form using TentaGel XV RAM resin beads. After removal of the Fmoc from the beads with 20% 4-methyl piperidine in DMF (for 5 min, and then 15 min), Fmoc-Lys(N_3)-OH and two AEEA were coupled using 5 molar excess of [2-(2-(Fmoc-amino)ethoxy)ethoxy]acetic acid (Fmoc-AEEA-OH), Oxyma pure and DIC in DMF, respectively. The coupling reaction was conducted at room temperature for 2 h and monitored using the ninhydrin test. The resin was then washed, and deprotected using 20% 4-methyl piperidine in DMF at room temperature (for 5 min, and then 15 min). They were then washed again, and the first step was repeated to couple the second AEEA spacer. The coupling and deprotection cycles were repeated until the desired cycles of coupling were completed. The CEMG was then coupled to the lysine side chain after Dde deprotection as described in the library synthesis. To cleave the peptide from the resin, as well as to remove the side chain protecting groups, the resins were soaked in the cleavage solution, phenol/thioanisole/water/TIS/TFA (7.5:5:5:2.5:82.5, *w*/*v*/*v*/*v*) for 4 h. The liquid was then collected and the peptide was precipitated with cold diethyl ether. The disulfide bridge was then successfully made using CLEAR-OX resins as in Reference [37] and the peptides were purified using reversed phase HPLC. The purity was determined to be >90%. The identity of the compounds was confirmed using the MALDI-TOF MS. P1 *m/z* calcd 2174.00, found 2175.25; P2 *m/z*: calcd 2004.99, found 2004.97; P3 *m/z*: calcd 1767.83, found 1767.67.

4.6. Preparation of Sensor-Chip and Testing for Morphine-Binding

The PET sheet was chemically modified using silane coating, which allowed PDMS polymerization on the PET surface to support covalent bond formation. The silane modified PET was then treated with oxygen plasma to form hydroxy groups on the surface, and then uncured PDMS was spin coated onto the PET sheet and it underwent polymerization in a heated oven. Microdisc carriers were fabricated using our published photolithography technology [36]. Polyethylene glycol (PEG) was chosen as the structural material due to its long-term biocompatibility, ability to conjugate other functional derivatives, optical clarity, and most importantly, its excellent swelling property in both polar and non-polar solvents. The polymer composite included: 200 μL of PEG-diacrylate (MW 700 Da), 112 μL of trimethylolpropane ethoxylate triacrylate (cross-linker), 8 μL of 2-hydroxyl-2-methylpropiophenone (photo initiator), and 300 μL of 2-aminoethyl methacrylate·HCl (7.2 mg) solution in deionized water. Under ultraviolet exposure, the acrylate molecules can be polymerized to form a highly insoluble matrix. The addition of 2-aminoethyl methacrylate hydrochloride forms an amine-terminated end group of the matrix for the subsequent peptide synthesis [36]. Then, two Fmoc-AEEA spacers were coupled to the free amine groups on the chip using HCTU/DIEA coupling, following by Fmoc-deprotection and the addition of DBCO-OSu in the presence of DIEA. Illuminating peptides were dissolved in DMF, and then added to the corresponding spots on the chip and incubated at 4 °C overnight. After thorough washing with DMF, MeOH, DMF, 50% DMF/H_2O, and H_2O, the chip was ready for testing.

The chip was then placed in a polystyrene plate and PBS was added to the plate to cover all the microdiscs on the chip. Then, the chip was scanned by a confocal microscope to obtain the background image (Figure 9-background). To eliminate the non-specific positive hits, it was then incubated with 10% plasma in PBS for 20 min and the fluorescent activation from the illuminating peptide bound plasma proteins was monitored using a confocal microscope (Figure 9-plasma). The chip was then incubated with 3.5 nM of anti-morphine mAb for 20 min, and the fluorescent activation from the illuminating peptide bound antibody was monitored (Figure 9-anti-morphine mAb). Finally, 0.35 μM morphine solution was added to the plate and it was incubated for 20 min, followed by measurement of the fluorescent intensity (Figure 9-morphine).

Supplementary Materials: The following are available online at. Figure S1, Automated analysis of the illuminating peptide library beads; Figure S2, Binding confirmation of the resynthesized illuminating peptides on beads.

Author Contributions: Conceptualization, Y.T.; K.S.L.; and R.L.; experimental procedure, S.J.; Y.T.; Y.H.A.; D.S.; J.L.; J.S.H.; B.M.-C.P.; and R.L.; data analysis, S.J.; Y.T.; and R.L.; Investigation, S.J.; Y.T.; K.S.L.; and R.L.; Methodology, S.J.; Y.T.; J.L.; T.P.; and R.L.; Validation, S.J.; writing—original draft preparation, S.J.; R.L.; writing—review and editing, S.J.; Y.T.; D.S.; K.S.L.; and R.L.; supervision, K.S.L.; R.L.; and T.P.; funding acquisition, R.L. and K.S.L.

Funding: This project was supported by the NSF- and industry-funded I/UCRC Center for Biophotonic Sensors and Systems, NSF grant # 1650588 (R.L.), and it was partially supported by NIH 1R33CA196445-01A1 (K.S.L.).

Acknowledgments: The authors would like to acknowledge the UC Davis Pathology Biorepository for providing human plasma, and the Combinatorial Chemistry and Chemical Biology shared resource at UC Davis in assisting with the OBOC library synthesis and screening. Both resources are funded by the UC Davis Comprehensive Cancer Center Support Grant (CCSG) awarded by the National Cancer Institute (NCI P30CA093373). The authors also acknowledge the Campus Mass Spectrometry facility at UC Davis.

Conflicts of Interest: The authors declare no conflict of interest.

References

1. Rudd, R.A.; Aleshire, N.; Zibbell, J.E.; Gladden, R.M. Increases in Drug and Opioid Overdose Deaths—United States, 2000–2014. *MMWR Morb. Mortal. Wkly. Rep.* **2016**, *64*, 1378–1382. [CrossRef] [PubMed]
2. Paulozzi, L.J. Vital Signs: Overdoses of Prescription Opioid Pain Relievers—United States, 1999–2008. *MMWR Morb. Mortal. Wkly. Rep.* **2011**, *60*, 1487–1492.
3. Overdose Death Rates. Available online: https://www.drugabuse.gov/related-topics/trends-statistics/overdose-death-rates (accessed on 30 January 2019).
4. Rana, S.; Garg, R.K.; Singla, A. Rapid analysis of urinary opiates using fast gas chromatography–mass spectrometry and hydrogen as a carrier gas. *Egypt. J. Forensic Sci.* **2014**, *4*, 100–107. [CrossRef]
5. Strayer, K.E.; Antonides, H.M.; Juhascik, M.P.; Daniulaityte, R.; Sizemore, I.E. LC-MS/MS-Based Method for the Multiplex Detection of 24 Fentanyl Analogues and Metabolites in Whole Blood at Sub ng mL^{-1} Concentrations. *ACS Omega* **2018**, *3*, 514–523. [CrossRef] [PubMed]
6. Sofalvi, S.; Schueler, H.E.; Lavins, E.S.; Kaspar, C.K.; Brooker, I.T.; Mazzola, C.D.; Dolinak, D.; Gilson, T.P.; Perch, S. An LC-MS-MS Method for the Analysis of Carfentanil, 3-Methylfentanyl, 2-Furanyl Fentanyl, Acetyl Fentanyl, Fentanyl and Norfentanyl in Postmortem and Impaired-Driving Cases. *J. Anal. Toxicol.* **2017**, *41*, 473–483. [CrossRef] [PubMed]
7. Neerman, M.F. Drugs of Abuse: Analyses and Ingested Agents That Can Induce Interference or Cross-Reactivity. *Lab. Med.* **2006**, *37*, 358–361. [CrossRef]
8. Thevis, M.; Opfermann, G.; Schänzer, W. Urinary Concentrations of Morphine and Codeine after Consumption of Poppy Seeds. *J. Anal. Toxicol.* **2003**, *27*, 53–56. [CrossRef] [PubMed]
9. Marchei, E.; Pacifici, R.; Mannocchi, G.; Marinelli, E.; Busardò, F.P.; Pichini, S. New synthetic opioids in biological and non-biological matrices: A review of current analytical methods. *TrAC Trends Anal. Chem.* **2018**, *102*, 1–15. [CrossRef]
10. Chen, B.-G.; Wang, S.-M.; Liu, R.H. GC-MS analysis of multiply derivatized opioids in urine. *J. Mass Spectrom.* **2007**, *42*, 1012–1023. [CrossRef] [PubMed]
11. Baden, L.R.; Horowitz, G.; Jacoby, H.; Eliopoulos, G.M. Quinolones and false-positive urine screening for opiates by immunoassay technology. *JAMA* **2001**, *286*, 3115–3119. [CrossRef]
12. Keary, C.J.; Wang, Y.; Moran, J.R.; Zayas, L.V.; Stern, T.A. Toxicologic Testing for Opiates: Understanding False-Positive and False-Negative Test Results. *Prim. Care Companion CNS Disord.* **2012**, *14*, PCC.12f01371. [CrossRef] [PubMed]
13. Lam, K.S.; Salmon, S.E.; Hersh, E.M.; Hruby, V.J.; Kazmierski, W.M.; Knapp, R.J. A new type of synthetic peptide library for identifying ligand-binding activity. *Nature* **1991**, *354*, 82–84. [CrossRef]
14. Haidekker, M.A.; Theodorakis, E.A. Environment-sensitive behavior of fluorescent molecular rotors. *J. Biol. Eng.* **2010**, *4*, 11. [CrossRef]
15. Lacowiks, J.R. Probe Design and Chemical Sensing. In *Topics in Fluorescence Spectroscopy*; Springer: New York, NY, USA, 1994; ISBN 978-0-306-44784-6.

16. Rotkiewicz, K.; Grellmann, K.H.; Grabowski, Z.R. Reinterpretation of the anomalous fluorescense of p-n,n-dimethylamino-benzonitrile. *Chem. Phys. Lett.* **1973**, *19*, 315–318. [CrossRef]
17. Li, X.; Gao, X.; Shi, W.; Ma, H. Design Strategies for Water-Soluble Small Molecular Chromogenic and Fluorogenic Probes. *Chem. Rev.* **2014**, *114*, 590–659. [CrossRef]
18. Grimm, J.B.; Heckman, L.M.; Lavis, L.D. Chapter One—The Chemistry of Small-Molecule Fluorogenic Probes. Fluorescence-Based Biosensors. In *Progress in Molecular Biology and Translational Science*; Morris, M.C., Ed.; Academic Press: Cambridge, MA, USA, 2013; Volume 113, pp. 1–34.
19. Karpenko, I.A.; Kreder, R.; Valencia, C.; Villa, P.; Mendre, C.; Mouillac, B.; Mély, Y.; Hibert, M.; Bonnet, D.; Klymchenko, A.S. Red Fluorescent Turn-On Ligands for Imaging and Quantifying G Protein-Coupled Receptors in Living Cells. *ChemBioChem* **2014**, *15*, 359–363. [CrossRef] [PubMed]
20. Karpenko, I.A.; Collot, M.; Richert, L.; Valencia, C.; Villa, P.; Mély, Y.; Hibert, M.; Bonnet, D.; Klymchenko, A.S. Fluorogenic Squaraine Dimers with Polarity-Sensitive Folding As Bright Far-Red Probes for Background-Free Bioimaging. *J. Am. Chem. Soc.* **2015**, *137*, 405–412. [CrossRef]
21. Nadler, A.; Schultz, C. The Power of Fluorogenic Probes. *Angew. Chem. Int. Ed.* **2013**, *52*, 2408–2410. [CrossRef]
22. Babendure, J.R.; Adams, S.R.; Tsien, R.Y. Aptamers Switch on Fluorescence of Triphenylmethane Dyes. *J. Am. Chem. Soc.* **2003**, *125*, 14716–14717. [CrossRef]
23. Xu, S.; Hu, H.-Y. Fluorogen-activating proteins: Beyond classical fluorescent proteins. *Acta Pharm. Sin. B* **2018**, *8*, 339–348. [CrossRef] [PubMed]
24. Kubánková, M.; López-Duarte, I.; Bull, J.A.; Vadukul, D.M.; Serpell, L.C.; de Saint Victor, M.; Stride, E.; Kuimova, M.K. Probing supramolecular protein assembly using covalently attached fluorescent molecular rotors. *Biomaterials* **2017**, *139*, 195–201. [CrossRef]
25. Venkatraman, P.; Nguyen, T.T.; Sainlos, M.; Bilsel, O.; Chitta, S.; Imperiali, B.; Stern, L.J. Fluorogenic probes for monitoring peptide binding to class II MHC proteins in living cells. *Nat. Chem. Biol.* **2007**, *3*, 222–228. [CrossRef]
26. Szent-Gyorgyi, C.; Schmidt, B.F.; Schmidt, B.A.; Creeger, Y.; Fisher, G.W.; Zakel, K.L.; Adler, S.; Fitzpatrick, J.A.J.; Woolford, C.A.; Yan, Q.; et al. Fluorogen-activating single-chain antibodies for imaging cell surface proteins. *Nat. Biotechnol.* **2008**, *26*, 235–240. [CrossRef]
27. Liu, R.; Li, X.; Lam, K.S. Combinatorial chemistry in drug discovery. *Curr. Opin. Chem. Biol.* **2017**, *38*, 117–126. [CrossRef]
28. Furka, A.; Sebestyén, F.; Asgedom, M.; Dibó, G. General method for rapid synthesis of multicomponent peptide mixtures. *Int. J. Pept. Protein Res.* **1991**, *37*, 487–493. [CrossRef]
29. Merrifield, R.B. Solid Phase Peptide Synthesis. I. The Synthesis of a Tetrapeptide. *J. Am. Chem. Soc.* **1963**, *85*, 2149–2154. [CrossRef]
30. Rieger, R.; Leung, P.S.C.; Jeddeloh, M.R.; Kurth, M.J.; Nantz, M.H.; Lam, K.S.; Barsky, D.; Ansari, A.A.; Coppel, R.L.; Mackay, I.R.; et al. Identification of 2-nonynoic acid, a cosmetic component, as a potential trigger of primary biliary cirrhosis. *J. Autoimmun.* **2006**, *27*, 7–16. [CrossRef] [PubMed]
31. Hoff, A.; Bagû, A.C.; André, T.; Roth, G.; Wiesmüller, K.H.; Gückel, B.; Brock, R. Peptide microarrays for the profiling of cytotoxic T-lymphocyte activity using minimum numbers of cells. *Cancer Immunol. Immunother. CII* **2010**, *59*, 1379–1387. [CrossRef]
32. Peri, C.; Gori, A.; Gagni, P.; Sola, L.; Girelli, D.; Sottotetti, S.; Cariani, L.; Chiari, M.; Cretich, M.; Colombo, G. Evolving serodiagnostics by rationally designed peptide arrays: The *Burkholderia* paradigm in Cystic Fibrosis. *Sci. Rep.* **2016**, *6*, 32873. [CrossRef]
33. Liu, R.; Marik, J.; Lam, K.S. A Novel Peptide-Based Encoding System for "One-Bead One-Compound" Peptidomimetic and Small Molecule Combinatorial Libraries. *J. Am. Chem. Soc.* **2002**, *124*, 7678–7680. [CrossRef]
34. Peng, L.; Liu, R.; Marik, J.; Wang, X.; Takada, Y.; Lam, K.S. Combinatorial chemistry identifies high-affinity peptidomimetics against α 4 β 1 integrin for in vivo tumor imaging. *Nat. Chem. Biol.* **2006**, *2*, 381. [CrossRef] [PubMed]
35. Collins, J.M.; Porter, K.A.; Singh, S.K.; Vanier, G.S. High-Efficiency Solid Phase Peptide Synthesis (HE-SPPS). *Org. Lett.* **2014**, *16*, 940–943. [CrossRef]

36. Li, J.; Carney, R.P.; Liu, R.; Fan, J.; Zhao, S.; Chen, Y.; Lam, K.S.; Pan, T. Microfluidic Print-to-Synthesis Platform for Efficient Preparation and Screening of Combinatorial Peptide Microarrays. *Anal. Chem.* **2018**, *90*, 5833–5840. [CrossRef]
37. Darlak, K.; Wiegandt Long, D.; Czerwinski, A.; Darlak, M.; Valenzuela, F.; Spatola, A.F.; Barany, G. Facile preparation of disulfide-bridged peptides using the polymer-supported oxidant CLEAR-OX. *J. Pept. Res. Off. J. Am. Pept. Soc.* **2004**, *63*, 303–312. [CrossRef]
38. Annis, I.; Chen, L.; Barany, G. Novel Solid-Phase Reagents for Facile Formation of Intramolecular Disulfide Bridges in Peptides under Mild Conditions1,2. *J. Am. Chem. Soc.* **1998**, *120*, 7226–7238. [CrossRef]
39. Xiao, W.; Bononi, F.C.; Townsend, J.; Li, Y.; Liu, R.; Lam, K.S. Immobilized OBOC combinatorial bead array to facilitate multiplicative screening. *Comb. Chem. High Throughput Screen.* **2013**, *16*, 441–448. [CrossRef] [PubMed]
40. Shih, T.-C.; Liu, R.; Fung, G.; Bhardwaj, G.; Ghosh, P.M.; Lam, K.S. A Novel Galectin-1 Inhibitor Discovered through One-Bead Two-Compound Library Potentiates the Antitumor Effects of Paclitaxel in vivo. *Mol. Cancer Ther.* **2017**, *16*, 1212–1223. [CrossRef]
41. Meissner, C.; Recker, S.; Reiter, A.; Friedrich, H.J.; Oehmichen, M. Fatal versus non-fatal heroin "overdose": Blood morphine concentrations with fatal outcome in comparison to those of intoxicated drivers. *Forensic Sci. Int.* **2002**, *130*, 49–54. [CrossRef]

Sample Availability: Samples of the compounds P1–P4 are available from the authors.

molecules

MDPI

Article

Aza-Amino Acids Disrupt β-Sheet Secondary Structures

Michael A. McMechen †, Evan L. Willis †, Preston C. Gourville and Caroline Proulx *

Department of Chemistry, North Carolina State University, Raleigh, NC 27695-8204, USA; mamcmech@ncsu.edu (M.A.M.); elwilli5@ncsu.edu (E.L.W.); pcgourvi@ncsu.edu (P.C.G.)
* Correspondence: cproulx@ncsu.edu; Tel.: +1-919-515-9534
† These authors contributed equally to this work.

Academic Editors: Henry Mosberg, Tomi Sawyer and Carrie Haskell-Luevano
Received: 1 May 2019; Accepted: 17 May 2019; Published: 18 May 2019

Abstract: Cα to N substitution in aza-amino acids imposes local conformational constraints, changes in hydrogen bonding properties, and leads to adaptive chirality at the nitrogen atom. These properties can be exploited in mimicry and stabilization of peptide secondary structures and self-assembly. Here, the effect of a single aza-amino acid incorporation located in the upper β-strand at a hydrogen-bonded (HB) site of a β-hairpin model peptide (H-Arg-Tyr-Val-Glu-Val-D-Pro-Gly-Orn-Lys-Ile-Leu-Gln-NH_2) is reported. Specifically, analogs in which valine^3 was substituted for aza-valine^3 or aza-glycine^3 were synthesized, and their β-hairpin stabilities were examined using Nuclear Magnetic Resonance (NMR) spectroscopy. The azapeptide analogs were found to destabilize β-hairpin formation compared to the parent peptide. The aza-valine^3 residue was more disruptive of β-hairpin geometry than its aza-glycine^3 counterpart.

Keywords: peptidomimetics; azapeptides; aza-amino acids; β-hairpin; β-sheet

1. Introduction

β-sheets are common protein secondary structures that are often involved in protein-protein interactions and protein aggregation [1,2]. To understand factors governing folding, stability, and molecular recognition events involving β-sheets, water soluble β-hairpin model systems that are partially folded have been developed, consisting of two antiparallel β-strands connected by a reverse turn unit [3]. In the pursuit of protein-protein interaction (PPI) inhibitors, β-strand and β-sheet peptidomimetics have been explored using a variety of unnatural scaffolds [4]. When mimicking β-strands in particular, the hydrogen bonding pattern of a natural peptide is ideally replicated by the artificial templates to maintain cross-strand interactions, yet surface exposed hydrogen bonding sites should be minimized to prevent uncontrolled aggregation, creating a so-called "blocking strand" [5–7]. Here, we describe the effect of a single Cα substitution for a nitrogen at the Val^3 position of a model β-hairpin peptide. The aza-amino acid residue was envisioned to provide two distinct faces with divergent hydrogen bonding capabilities, while retaining side chain position and chemistry (Figure 1).

Aza-amino acids [8] have been used to promote β-turn secondary structures and hyperstable collagen peptide mimics [9,10] via a combination of hydrogen bonding and backbone dihedral angle modulation. Their effect on β-hairpin stability has yet to be quantified within β-strand regions. In aza-amino acids, perpendicular lone pair orientation between adjacent nitrogen and urea planarity typically reinforce backbone dihedral angles that fall within the range of β-turns and polyproline type II secondary structures [8]. Although this may prevent adoption of extended β-strand geometry [11], computational studies have set the energy barrier for rotation from the twisted conformer (φ = 90°) to the extended conformer (φ = 180°) to be < 1 kcal/mol within 1,2-diformylhydrazine in the *Z,Z* configuration as an azaGly model [12]. Two favorable intramolecular hydrogen bonds are proposed to stabilize the 180°

orientation. Although addition of side chain chemistry in aza-amino acids removes an intramolecular hydrogen bond with a neighboring residue, cross-strand hydrogen bonding and side chain; side chain interactions in a β-hairpin may provide added stability to the extended conformer. Substitution of Val[3] for aza-valine[3] was thus examined in a well-studied β-hairpin model system for which Nuclear Magnetic Resonance (NMR)-based quantification of β-hairpin folding have been established, first reported by Gellman et al. [13,14]: H-Arg-Tyr-Val-Glu-Val-D-Pro-Gly-Orn-Lys-Ile-Leu-Gln-NH_2 (**1a**). Valine[3] is situated in the middle of the upper β-strand at a hydrogen bonded (HB) site (Figure 2, in blue), equally removed from the D-Pro-Gly turn region and the *N*-terminus. In addition to azaVal[3] analog **1b**, D-Val[3] control **1c**, azaGly[3] analog **1d**, and previously described [14] positive control cyclic peptide **1e**, and negative control L-Pro[6]-Gly[7] peptide **1f**, all were synthesized and studied (Figure 2). Since the first incorporation of azaVal to give an azapeptide angiotensin analog [15], considerable interest has been generated in the synthesis and conformational properties of this aza-amino acid.

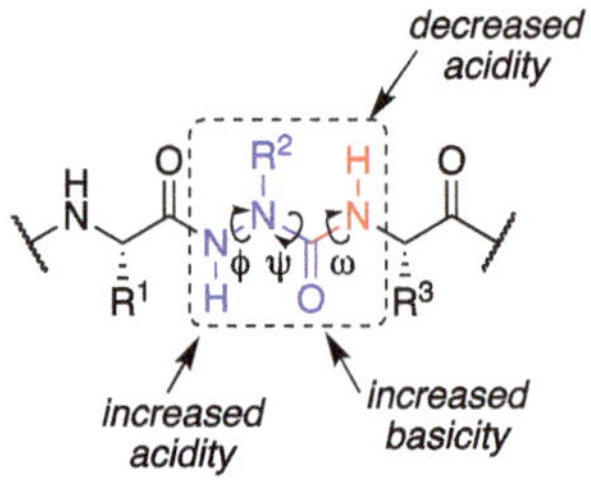

Figure 1. Aza-amino acid (in blue) creates one face with increased hydrogen bonding properties and one with reduced hydrogen bonding capacity.

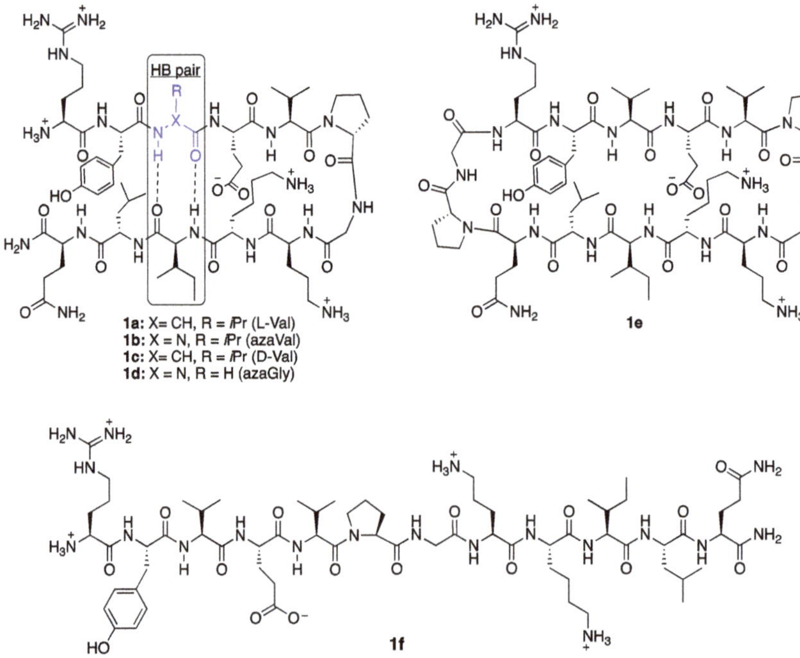

Figure 2. β-hairpin model peptide **1a** [8], derivatives **1b–d**, and controls **1e–f** [8] under study.

2. Results and Discussion

2.1. Synthesis

Solid-phase peptide synthesis was performed on Rink amide resin, using standard Fmoc procedures for all L- and D-amino acid coupling and deprotection cycles [16]. Incorporation of azaVal[3] for the synthesis of **1b** was accomplished via activation of *N*′-isopropyl-fluorenylmethyl carbazate [17] using bis-(trichloromethyl)carbonate (BTC) as the activating agent (Scheme 1) and as a safer alternative to phosgene. Although submonomer azapeptide synthesis protocols [18] were considered for the installation of aza-valine to circumvent the solution-phase synthesis and activation of hydrazine building blocks, *N*-alkylation of resin-bound semicarbazone intermediates with sterically hindered secondary alkyl halides has typically resulted in lower conversions [19]. In our hands, incorporation of aza-valine via *N*′-alkyl fluoren-9-ylmethyl carbazate activation with triphosgene afforded azapeptide **6** as the major product in 77% crude purity after a single overnight coupling reaction. In contrast, in accordance with previous literature, coupling to the aza-amino acid to give **9** was challenging due to the decreased nucleophilicity of semicarbazides [8] and steric hindrance from the branched aza-valine side chain. In the past, coupling to aza-valine and other aza-amino acids with branched side chains has been accomplished using *N*,*N*′-dicyclohexylcarbodiimide (DCC) [15], diisoproylcarbodiimide (DIC) [19,20], and BTC [21]. Here, the coupling of Fmoc-Tyr(^{t}Bu) to resin-bound azaV-EVpGOKILQ using BTC and 2,4,6-collidine in tetrahydrofuran (THF) provided **9** in only 33% conversion by liquid chromatography-mass spectrometry (LC-MS) analysis, with 21% uncoupled semicarbazide and 28% isocyanate or hydantoin byproduct [22] (Table 1, entry 1). In the context of β-hairpin synthesis, the already difficult coupling to aza-Val may be rendered even more challenging by folding or aggregation on-resin [23]. Attempts employing a LiCl salt additive to the BTC coupling solution to disrupt possible on-resin aggregation [24] were less successful than efforts to optimize the coupling reagent (Table 1, entries 2–5).

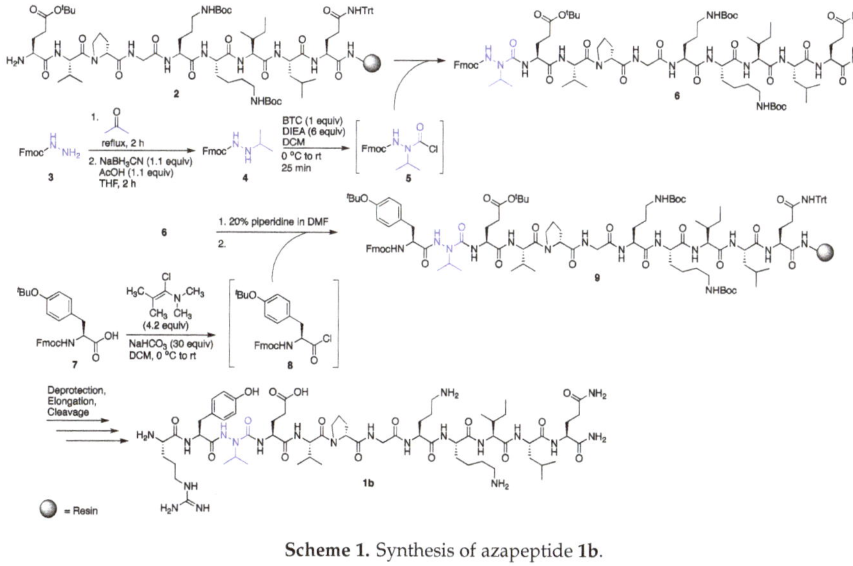

Scheme 1. Synthesis of azapeptide **1b**.

Recent successes using benzotriazol-1-yloxytris(pyrrolidinophosphonium-hexafluorophosphate (PyBOP)/*N*,*N*-diisopropylethylamine (DIEA) [25] and (1-cyano-2-ethoxy-2-oxoethylidenaminooxy) dimethylaminomorpholino-carbenium hexafluorophosphate (COMU)/DIEA [26,27] in difficult couplings to aza-amino acids led us to try these activating agents; however, **9** was obtained in low conversions in both cases (6–13%, Table 1, entries 2 and 3). We next investigated *N*,*N*,*N*′,*N*′-tetramethylchloroformamidinium hexafluorophosphate (TCFH)/*N*-methylimidazole (NMI) (Table 1, entry 4), which was recently developed [28] to couple sterically hindered carboxylic acids with non-nucleophilic aniline derivatives and sterically hindered amino acids, including valine. Gratifyingly, these conditions provided **9** in high conversion (89%) with little byproduct formation and no detectable starting material (Table 1, entry 4), although appearance of two peaks with identical masses by LC-MS suggested possible epimerization. Alternatively, the use of 1-chloro-*N*,*N*,2-trimethyl-1-propenylamine (Ghosez's reagent) [29] (Table 1, entry 5) provided the desired elongated azapeptide **9** as a single peak by LC-MS analysis in 67% conversion, with no uncoupled semicarbazide detected. Using this procedure for coupling onto azaVal, azapeptide **1b** was obtained in 53% crude purity, following deprotection, elongation, and cleavage from the resin. Purification of the crude azapeptide by reverse phase – high performance liquid chromatography (RP-HPLC) afforded **1b** in 8% yield (see Supporting Information).

Table 1. Optimization of coupling to resin-bound aza-VEVpGOKILQ.

Entry	Coupling Reagent	Equiv.	Base	Equiv.	Solvent	% Coupled	% Uncoupled	% Isocyanate/ Hydantoin Byproduct [22]
1	BTC	1	2,4,6-collidine	10	THF	33	21	28
2	PyBOP	3	DIEA	6	DMF	6	35	41
3	COMU	5	DIEA	10	DMF	13	17	53
4	TCFH [a]	3	NMI	9	CH_2Cl_2	89 [a]	0	10
5	Ghosez	4.2	$NaHCO_3$	30	CH_2Cl_2	67	0	22

[a] Possible epimerization was detected by LC-MS analysis.

Activation of *N*-Fmoc-hydrazine with phosgene equivalents was previously shown to lead to the formation of a cyclic oxadiazolone [30]. Although ring-opening of this heterocycle to afford the desired Fmoc-protected azaGly-terminated peptides may be possible [30], activation and coupling of aza-glycine using these conditions has been reported to be problematic in certain cases [31]. Here, aza-glycine installation was accomplished by activating fluoren-9-methyl carbazate with *N*,*N*′-disuccinimidyl carbonate (DSC) as the activating agent instead of BTC, which afforded the desired azapeptide in higher yields [32]. Fmoc-Tyr(^{t}Bu)-OH activation and coupling to the resin-bound aza-glycine-terminated peptide was accomplished using BTC/2,4,6-collidine in THF and required no further optimization.

2.2. *Conformational Analysis*

β-Hairpin folding was first assessed by measuring the extent of diastereotopic Gly^7 Hα splitting in the turn region for each analog and comparing it to the fully folded cyclic control (Equation (1)), as previously described [33]. Using this method, the relative stability of each β-hairpin analog can be quickly compared as the glycine signals lie in a distinct region of the spectra (Figure 3, Table 2).

$$\text{Fraction folded} = (\Delta\delta_{\text{Gly Obs}})/(\Delta\delta_{\text{Gly 100}}) \quad (1)$$

Replacing valine^3 for an aza-valine residue in analog **1b** caused a significant decrease in β-hairpin stability, reflected by the much smaller Gly^7 δHα–δHα′ value (Figure 3). Potential cross-strand hydrogen bonding and side chain - side chain interactions between azaVal^3 and Ile^{10} appear to be insufficient to stabilize the extended conformation in aza-valine^3, which likely adopts a twisted conformation (φ = 90°) that disrupts β-hairpin formation. Because aza-amino acids may exhibit adaptive chirality at Nα, the aza-valine residue could be achiral or exhibit either L or D-like chirality [34], which could in turn affect β-hairpin stability. We synthesized D-Val^3 analog **1c** as a control and found its Gly^7 δHα–δHα′ value to be larger than that of aza-Val^3 analog **1b**, yet smaller than the parent peptide **1a**. While changing the stereochemistry of the valine^3 residue from L to D decreased β-hairpin stability overall, this substitution was found to be less disruptive than the backbone Cα to Nα substitution in the aza-valine residue. As such, the destabilizing effect of the aza-valine residue cannot be solely attributed to the loss of a defined stereocenter.

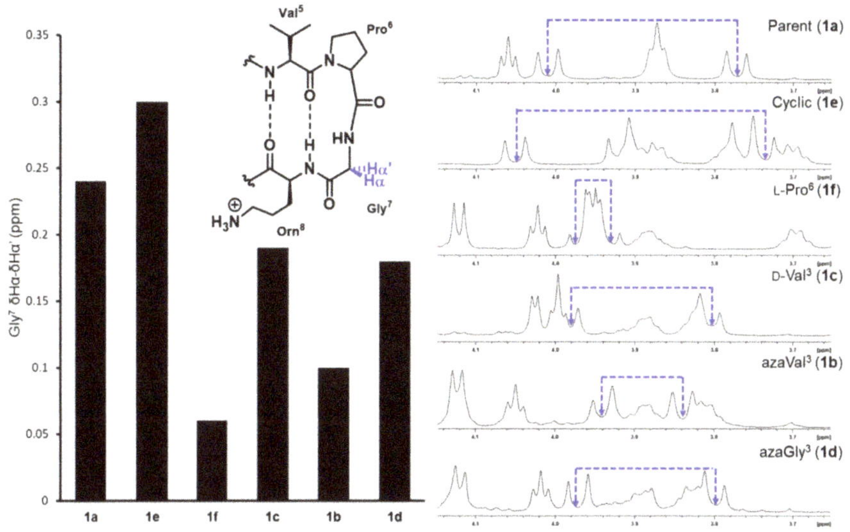

Figure 3. Diastereotopic splitting of Gly^7 Hα chemical shifts.

Given that the extended conformation in aza-glycine vs. aza-valine residues may be more favorable due to additional intramolecular hydrogen-bonding interactions (*vide supra*), the synthesis and conformational analysis of azaGly^3 analog **1d** was also pursued. Despite the absence of an isopropyl side chain, the aza-glycine substitution was found to be less detrimental to β-hairpin stability compared to the aza-Val^3 analog **1b**; however, β-hairpin folding was still decreased relative to the parent peptide **1a**. The disruptive effects of the azaGly^3 substitution are similar those observed in the D-Val^3 analog using Gly^7 diastereotopic Hα splitting measurements (Figure 3) [35].

It should be noted that glycine splitting measurements have been found to overestimate β-hairpin folding in sequences that use D-Pro-Gly turn units [36]. Downfield chemical shifts in CHα protons relative to unfolded peptide for residues away from the turn region, especially those situated at HB sites, can be used to quantify the degree of β-hairpin folding more reliably according to Equation (2), where δ_0 and δ_{100} are the chemical shift values for the unfolded analog **1f** and the cyclic control **1e**, respectively.

$$\text{Fraction folded} = (\delta_{Obs} - \delta_0)/(\delta_{100} - \delta_0) \tag{2}$$

Specifically, the downfield chemical shifts of Val^3, Ile^{10}, and Orn^8 have been found to be more reliable and are typically used to measure folded fractions for this β-hairpin model peptide and its derivatives [14]. Here, because the Cα of Val^3 is substituted by a nitrogen in our azapeptide analogs, we omitted this residue from our studies (Table 2). The CHα chemical shift values for Ile^{10} are particularly informative because this residue sits in the middle of the lower strand and is positioned to form hydrogen bonds with the variable residue in the third position; Orn^8 is situated closer to the turn region. Based on the chemical shift values for Ile^{10}, aza-Val^3 peptide 1b is completely unfolded, in contrast to the partially folded structure predicted based on glycine^7 Hα splitting measurements (Figure 3, Table 2). Considering that diastereotopic splitting of Gly^7 Hα overestimate folding in β-hairpin model peptides that have D-Pro-Gly turn units, incorporation of azaVal^3 is likely completely disrupting the β-hairpin fold. In contrast, the azaGly^3 analog 1d which lacks side chain functionality was ~50% folded based on the Ile^{10} downfield Hα chemical shifts, and exhibited a greater percentage of folding relative to both the aza-valine (1a) and D-valine (1c) analogs. The additional potential for azaGly to intra- and/or inter-strand hydrogen-bond may stabilize the extended conformer. The % folding values calculated from Orn^8 chemical shifts reinforced the conclusion that the aza-Valine analog 1b was the least folded of all analogs, yet suggested similar degrees of folding for the D-Val (1c) and the azaGly (1d) analogs.

Table 2. % folding based on glycine^7 splitting and Hα chemical shifts for Orn^8 and Ile^{10}.

Peptide	% Folding			
	Gly^7 δHα–δHα'	Orn^8	Ile^{10}	Average from Orn^8/Ile^{10}
1a	75	72	64	68
1b	17	36	0	18
1c	54	56	15	35.5
1d	50	50	49	49.5

3. Materials and Methods

3.1. General

Polystyrene Rink Amide resin (0.78 mmol/g) and Fmoc-glycine-2-chlorotrityl resin (200–400 mesh, 0.493 mmol/g) were purchased from Protein Technology Inc™ and Chem-Impex Int'l, Inc, respectively, and the manufacturer's reported loading of the resin was used in the calculation of the yields of the final products. Solid phase peptide synthesis was performed using an automated Biotage Syro Wave™ peptide synthesizer in 10 mL parallel reactors with polytetrafluoroethylene (PTFE) frits. Incorporation of aza-amino acids and further elongations were performed manually in disposable filter columns with 20 µM polyethylene (PE) frit filters and caps purchased from Applied Separations (cat # 2413 and 2416 for 3 mL and 6 mL filter columns, respectively) with gentle agitation on a Thermo Fisher vortex mixer equipped with a microplate tray. Solution draining and washing of the resin was accomplished by connecting the filter columns to a water aspirator vacuum via a waste trap. Analytical LC-MS analyses were performed using an Agilent Technologies 1260 Infinity II series LC-MS Single Quad instrument with ESI ion-source and positive mode ionization, equipped with a 5 µM, 150 × 4.6 mm C18 Vydac column purchased from Mac-Mod Analytical, Inc (cat # 218TP5415). A flow rate of 0.5 mL/min and 5–95%, 20–80%, or 12–60% gradients of CH_3CN [0.1% trifluoroacetic acid (TFA)] in water (0.1% TFA) over 12 min (total run time = 22 min) were used for all LC-MS analyses. Peptides were purified on a preparative HPLC (Agilent 218 purification system) using a preparative column (10–20 µM, 250 mm × 22 mm, C18 Vydac column, cat # 218TP101522) at a flow rate of 10 mL/min with gradients of CH_3CN [0.1% trifluoroacetic acid (TFA)] in water (0.1% TFA) over 30 min (total run time = 60 min).

3.2. Reagents

Amino acids, *N,N'*-diisopropylethylamine (DIEA), *N,N'*-Disuccinimidyl carbonate (DSC), Fmoc chloride, (1-cyano-2-ethoxy-2-oxoethylidenaminooxy)dimethylamino-morpholino-carbenium hexafluorophosphate (COMU), chloro-*N,N,N',N'*-tetramethylformamidinium hexafluorophospate (TCFH) and triphosgene (BTC) were purchased from Chem Impex Int'l, Inc. Reagents such as piperidine, lithium chloride, sodium cyanoborohydride ($NaBH_3CN$), triisopropylsilane (TIPS), sodium acetate-d$_3$, acetic acid-d$_4$, and D_2O were purchased from Sigma Aldrich. Reagents such as hydrazine monohydrate and 2,4,6-collidine were purchased from Alfa Aesar. Trifluoroacetic acid, glacial acetic acid, sodium bicarbonate, and solvents were purchased from Fisher. Reagents including HBTU and PyBOP were purchased from Oakwood Chemical. 1-Methylimidazole (NMI) and 1-chloro-*N,N*,2-trimethylpropenylamine (Ghosez's Reagent) were purchased from Acros Organics.

3.3. 9-Fluorenylmethoxycarbonyl (Fmoc)-Based Solid Phase Peptide Synthesis (SPPS): Fmoc Deprotection and HBTU Couplings

Peptide syntheses were performed under standard manual conditions on an automated shaker or using a Biotage Syro Wave^{TM} peptide synthesizer using Polystyrene Rink Amide resin (0.78 mmol/g). Couplings of amino acids (3 equiv) were performed in DMF using HBTU (3 equiv) as coupling reagent and DIEA (6 equiv) as base. Fmoc deprotections were performed initially by treating the resin with 20% piperidine in DMF (*v/v*) for 5 min, followed by treatment with a fresh solution of 20% piperidine in DMF (*v/v*) for 15 min. Resin was washed after each coupling with DMF (3 × 1 mL) and deprotection reaction with DMF, MeOH, and CH_2Cl_2 (2 × 1 mL). Prior to cleavage from the resin or storage, resin was washed with CH_2Cl_2 (3 × 1 mL).

3.4. Test Cleavages of Resin-Bound Peptides

A small amount of resin (1–5 mg) was washed with CH_2Cl_2 to remove traces of DMF, drained, and treated with a freshly made solution of TFA/H_2O/TIPS (90:5:5, *v/v/v*, 0.5 mL) for 2 h at room temperature. The cleavage solution was collected by filtering the resin through a disposable, PE fritted cartridge. The filtrate was evaporated to dryness and the crude peptide was precipitated twice with cold ether (4 mL) followed by decanting. The pellet (crude peptide sample) was dissolved in 1:1 MeCN/H_2O *v/v* (1 mg/mL) and subjected to LC-MS analysis.

3.5. N′-Isopropyl-fluoren-9-ylmethyl Carbazate (4)

Synthesized according to literature procedures [12,16]. Briefly, a solution of Fmoc-Cl (2.00 g, 7.73 mmol) in 120 mL of CH_3CN was added dropwise over 2 h at 0 °C to a solution of excess hydrazine hydrate (3.8 mL, 78.0 mmol, 10 equiv) in 26 mL of CH_3CN/H_2O (1:1, *v/v*). The solution was warmed to room temperature and left stirring for 12 h, prior to being concentrated in vacuo and filtered. The resulting solid was washed with water, followed by hexanes, to give 1.92 g of white solid in 98% yield. The resulting 9H-fluoren-9-ylmethyl hydrazinecarboxylate **3** (1.92 g, 7.55 mmol) was suspended in acetone (50 mL) and heated at reflux for 2 h. Acetone was evaporated in vacuo and the hydrazone intermediate was dissolved in THF (50 mL), treated with acetic acid (0.48 mL, 8.39 mmol, 1.1 equiv) and $NaBH_3CN$ (521 mg, 8.31 mmol, 1.1 equiv), and stirred for 2 h. The volatiles were removed and the crude was dissolved in EtOAc (100 mL), washed with 1 M aqueous $KHSO_4$ (4 × 50 mL) and brine (2 × 50 mL), dried over Na_2SO_4, and concentrated to give a white solid. The obtained product was dissolved in EtOH and heated for 1 h, followed by evaporation of EtOH to yield *N′*-isopropyl-fluoren-9-ylmethyl carbazate **4** as a white solid (1.32 g, 59% yield) after column chromatography using a 20–100% gradient of EtOAc in hexanes. NMR ($CDCl_3$) spectra matched literature values [12].

3.6. Incorporation of Aza-Valine on the Solid Phase

N′-isopropyl-fluoren-9-ylmethyl carbazate **4** (138 mg, 0.466 mmol, 3 equiv) was dissolved in dry CH_2Cl_2 (1 mL) and cooled to 0 °C. A solution of bis(trichloromethyl)carbonate (BTC, 46.4 mg, 0.156 mmol, 1 equiv) dissolved in dry CH_2Cl_2 (1 mL) and cooled to 0 °C was added dropwise to the *N′*-isopropyl-fluoren-9-ylmethyl carbazate suspension. The reaction mixture was left stirring at 0 °C for 5 min, allowed to warm to room temperature, and stirred for another 25 min. DIEA (0.163 mL, 0.930 mmol, 6.0 equiv) was added to the solution and the solution was stirred for 5 min prior to being transferred to a SPPS cartridge containing resin-bound peptide **2** (200 mg, 0.156 mmol) swollen in CH_2Cl_2. The SPPS cartridge was left shaking for 12 h, after which the solution was drained, and the resin was washed with CH_2Cl_2 (3 × 2 mL).

3.7. Coupling to AzaV-EVpGOKILQ

3.7.1. BTC Coupling

Fmoc-Tyr(^{t}Bu)-OH (53.8 mg, 0.117 mmol, 3.0 equiv) was dissolved in dry THF (0.3 mL), cooled to 0 °C, and treated dropwise with a cold solution of BTC (11.5 mg, 0.039 mmol, 1.0 equiv) in dry THF (0.3 mL). The reaction mixture was left stirring at 0 °C for 15 min, before adding 2,4,6-collidine (0.052 mL, 0.39 mmol, 10.0 equiv). The solution was stirred at 0 °C for 2 min, allowed to warm to room temperature, and stirred another 5 min. The activated amino acid was then transferred to a SPPS cartridge containing the resin-bound azapeptide (50 mg, 0.039 mmol), previously swollen in dry THF. The resin was left shaking at room temperature overnight, then washed with DMF (2 × 0.5 mL), MeOH (2 × 0.5 mL), and THF (2 × 0.5 mL).

3.7.2. PyBOP Coupling

Fmoc-Tyr(^{t}Bu)-OH (53.8 mg, 0.117 mmol, 3.0 equiv) and PyBOP (60.9 mg, 0.117 mmol, 3.0 equiv) were each dissolved in DMF (0.3 mL) and cooled to 0 °C separately. The PyBOP solution was then added dropwise to the solution of Fmoc-Tyr(^{t}Bu)-OH and the reaction mixture was stirred at 0 °C for 5 min. DIEA (0.0408 mL, 0.234 mmol, 6.0 equiv) was added to the solution and the reaction was allowed to warm to room temperature before being transferred to a SPPS cartridge containing the resin-bound azapeptide (50 mg, 0.039 mmol), previously swollen in DMF. The resin was shaken at room temperature overnight, then washed with DMF (2 × 0.5 mL), MeOH (2 × 0.5 mL), and CH_2Cl_2 (2 × 0.5 mL).

3.7.3. COMU Coupling

Fmoc-Tyr(^{t}Bu)-OH (89.6 mg, 0.195 mmol, 5.0 equiv) and COMU (83.5 mg, 0.195 mmol, 5.0 equiv) were each dissolved in 0.3 mL of DMF and cooled to 0 °C separately. The COMU solution was added dropwise to the solution of Fmoc-Tyr(^{t}Bu)-OH and the reaction mixture was stirred at 0 °C for 5 min. DIEA (0.0504 mL, 0.39 mmol, 10.0 equiv) was added and the reaction was warmed to room temperature before being transferred to a SPPS cartridge containing the resin-bound azapeptide (50 mg, 0.039 mmol), previously swollen in DMF. The resin was shaken at room temperature overnight, then washed with DMF (2 × 0.5 mL), MeOH (2 × 0.5 mL), and CH_2Cl_2 (2 × 0.5 mL).

3.7.4. NMI/TCFH Coupling

Fmoc-Tyr(^{t}Bu)-OH (53.8 mg, 0.117 mmol, 3.0 equiv) was dissolved in dry CH_2Cl_2 (0.3 mL), to which *N*-methyl imidazole (0.028 mL, 0.351 mmol, 9 equiv) was added before cooling the solution to 0 °C. A solution of TCFH (32.8 mg, 0.117 mmol, 3 equiv) in dry CH_2Cl_2 (0.3 mL), cooled to 0 °C, was added to the Fmoc-Tyr(^{t}Bu)-OH and NMI solution in a single portion and the reaction was immediately transferred to a SPPS cartridge containing the resin-bound azapeptide (50 mg, 0.039 mmol), previously swollen in dry CH_2Cl_2. The resin was shaken at room temperature overnight, then washed with DMF (2 × 0.5 mL), MeOH (2 × 0.5 mL), and CH_2Cl_2 (2 × 0.5 mL).

3.7.5. Ghosez Coupling

$NaHCO_3$ (98.3 mg, 1.17 mmol, 30 equiv) was added to the resin-bound azapeptide (50 mg, 0.039 mmol) pre-swelled in dry CH_2Cl_2 (0.2 mL) and shaken for 15 min. During that time, Fmoc-Tyr(^{t}Bu)-OH (53.8 mg, 0.117 mmol, 3.0 equiv) was dissolved in dry CH_2Cl_2 (0.4 mL) and cooled to 0 °C. Ghosez's reagent (0.0217 mL, 0.164 mmol, 4.2 equiv) was added dropwise to the cooled solution of Fmoc-Tyr(^{t}Bu)-OH and stirred for 5 min. The reaction was allowed to warm to room temperature for 5 min, prior to being transferred to the SPPS cartridge containing $NaHCO_3$ in CH_2Cl_2. The resin was shaken at room temperature overnight. The resin was washed with DMF (2 × 0.5 mL), MeOH (2 × 0.5 mL), and CH_2Cl_2 (2 × 0.5 mL).

3.8. *Incorporation of Aza-Glycine on the Solid Phase*

N,N'-Disuccinimidyl carbonate (DSC) (120 mg, 0.466 mmol, 3.0 equiv) was added to a solution of 9H-fluoren-9-ylmethyl hydrazinecarboxylate **3** (123 mg, 0.484 mmol, 3.1 equiv) in DMF and stirred for 5 min. The solution was then transferred to resin-bound peptide **2** (200 mg, 0.156 mmol) swollen in DMF and left shaking for 12 h. The solution was drained and the resin was washed with DMF (3 × 2 mL).

3.9. *Coupling to azaG-EVpGOKILQ*

Fmoc-Tyr(^{t}Bu)-OH (22.2 mg, 0.0484 mmol, 3.1 equiv) was dissolved in dry THF (0.3 mL), cooled to 0 °C, and treated dropwise with a cold solution of BTC (4.63 mg, 0.0156 mmol, 1.0 equiv) in dry THF (0.2 mL). The reaction mixture was left stirring at 0 °C for 15 min before adding 2,4,6-collidine (0.0206 mL, 0.156 mmol, 10.0 equiv). The solution was stirred at 0 °C for 5 min. The reaction was allowed to warm to room temperature prior to transferring the activated amino acid to a SPPS cartridge containing the resin-bound azapeptide (20 mg, 0.0156 mmol) previously swollen with dry THF. The reaction was left shaking at room temperature overnight, then washed with DMF (2 × 0.5 mL), MeOH (2 × 0.5 mL), and THF (2 × 0.5 mL).

3.10. *Synthesis of Cyclic Peptide 1e*

The linear precursor H_2N-Arg(Pbf)-Tyr(^{t}Bu)-Val-Glu(O^{t}Bu)-Val-pro-Gly-Orn(Boc)-Lys(Boc)-Ile-Leu-Gln(Trt)-pro-Gly-OH was synthesized on Fmoc-glycine-2-chlorotrityl resin (200–400 mesh, 0.493 mmol/g loading) according to standard SPPS protocols described above. Liberation of the side chain protected peptide from solid support was conducted using a freshly prepared solution of hexafluoroisopropanol in CH_2Cl_2 (20% *v/v*), the procedure was repeated, solutions were combined, and volatiles were removed in vacuo. The protected linear peptide was dissolved in DMF (15 mL) and a solution of HBTU (41.2 mg, 0.109 mmol, 6 equiv) and HOBt•H_2O (16.6 mg, 0.109 mmol, 6 equiv) in DMF (1 mL) was added dropwise, followed by an addition of DIEA (0.0494 mL, 0.283 mmol, 15 equiv) in DMF (1 mL). The reaction was allowed to proceed overnight under N_2 atmosphere. DMF was removed in vacuo and the cyclic side chain protected peptide was carried forward to global deprotection. A fresh 90:5:5 (v/v/v) solution of TFA: H_2O: TIPS was prepared and ~10 mL were added to the dried peptide. The reaction was stirred for 2 h at room temperature, followed by the removal of all volatiles in vacuo. Cold ether precipitation was performed followed by dissolution of the cyclic peptide in 20% MeCN in water (3 mL). The crude peptide sample was purified by RP-HPLC according to protocols described in General Methods.

3.11. *Full Cleavage and Purification of (Aza)Peptides*

The resin-bound (aza)peptide was washed with CH_2Cl_2 to remove traces of DMF, drained, transferred into a 20 mL scintillation glass vial, and treated a freshly made solution of TFA/H_2O/TIPS (90:5:5, v/v/v, 5 mL). The vial was capped and agitated for 2 h at room temperature on an orbital shaker. The cleavage mixture was filtered through a disposable, PP fritted cartridge into a 50 mL falcon tube containing cold ether (~20 mL). The ether was decanted following centrifugation at 8000 rpm for 2 min. The peptide pellet was suspended in 1:9 MeCN/H_2O *v/v* (5 mL). The sample was frozen and lyophilized. The crude (aza)peptpide was redissolved in a MeCN/H_2O solvent mixture and purified using reverse-phase HPLC. See Supporting Information for characterization data.

3.12. *NMR Spectroscopy*

Lyophilized (aza)peptides were diluted to concentrations of 3–4 mM in D_2O buffered with 50 mM NaOAc-d3 buffer at pH 4.2 (uncorrected), pH adjusted with AcOH-d3 [36]. All NMR spectra were collected at the Molecular Education, Technology, and Research Innovation Center (METRIC) at NC State University on a Bruker NEO 700 MHz instrument with a TCI cryoprobe at 5 °C. 1D spectra were collected with 32K data points and at least 32 scans and water suppression with a pre-saturation pulse or with a 1D-1H NOESY. 2D-experiments were collected on the same instrumentation, using the standard Bruker ROESY, COSY, and TOCSY pulse sequences with presaturation. All 2D experiments were done with eight scans, 2048 points in the first dimension, and 256 or 512 in the indirect dimension. TOCSY spectra were collected with 80 ms spin-lock and ROESY spectra were collected with a mixing time of 200 ms. Spectral analysis was performed with TopSpin 4.0.5 software.

4. Conclusions

Aza-amino acids have previously been shown to stabilize β-turn secondary structures and impart hyperstability to self-assembling collagen peptide mimics. Here, we expand the folding rules for aza-amino acids beyond turns and polyproline type II helices and characterize their effect on β-hairpin stability when incorporated into the β-strand region. Using NMR spectroscopy, we demonstrate that a valine to aza-valine substitution significantly disrupts β-hairpin folding, based on both glycine splitting measurements and CHα proton shifts at the Orn^8 and Ile^{10} residues relative to cyclic and unfolded controls. Aza-glycine incorporation at the same position was found to retain some folding, despite loss of side chain chemistry, which may be due to additional hydrogen bonding. Overall, our findings support earlier computational hypothesis that aza-amino acids are not well tolerated within β-sheet secondary structures.

Supplementary Materials: The following are available online: peptide and aza(peptide) characterization data; LC-MS chromatograms; tabulated ^{1}H NMR data for all peptide and aza(peptide) analogs.

Author Contributions: Conceptualization, C.P. and M.A.M.; Methodology and Analysis, M.A.M., E.L.W., P.C.G.; Writing-Original Draft Preparation, C.P.; Writing-Review and Editing, C.P., M.A.M., E.L.W., P.C.G.; Supervision, C.P.; Project Administration, C.P.

Funding: This research received no external funding.

Acknowledgments: The authors thank Peter Thompson for assistance with NMR spectroscopy and North Carolina State University for startup support. All NMR measurements were made in the Molecular Education, Technology, and Research Innovation Center (METRIC) at North Carolina State University.

Conflicts of Interest: The authors declare no conflict of interest.

References and Notes

1. Cheng, P.N.; Pham, J.D.; Nowick, J.S. The Supramolecular Chemistry of beta-Sheets. *J. Am. Chem. Soc.* **2013**, *135*, 5477–5492. [CrossRef] [PubMed]
2. Watkins, A.M.; Arora, P.S. Anatomy of beta-Strands at Protein-Protein Interfaces. *ACS Chem. Biol.* **2014**, *9*, 1747–1754. [CrossRef]
3. Hughes, R.M.; Waters, M.L. Model systems for beta-hairpins and beta-sheets. *Curr. Opin. Struct. Biol.* **2006**, *16*, 514–524. [CrossRef]
4. Loughlin, W.A.; Tyndall, J.D.A.; Glenn, M.P.; Fairlie, D.P. Beta-strand mimetics. *Chem. Rev.* **2004**, *104*, 6085–6117. [CrossRef]
5. Doig, A.J. A three stranded beta-sheet peptide in aqueous solution containing N-methyl amino acids to prevent aggregation. *Chem. Commun.* **1997**, *22*, 2153–2154. [CrossRef]
6. Nowick, J.S.; Chung, D.M.; Maitra, K.; Maitra, S.; Stigers, K.D.; Sun, Y. An unnatural amino acid that mimics a tripeptide beta-strand and forms beta-sheet like hydrogen-bonded dimers. *J. Am. Chem. Soc.* **2000**, *122*, 7654–7661. [CrossRef]
7. Sarnowski, M.P.; Kang, C.W.; Elbatrawi, Y.M.; Wojtas, L.; Del Valle, J.R. Peptide N-Amination Supports beta-Sheet Conformations. *Angew. Chem. Int. Ed.* **2017**, *56*, 2083–2086. [CrossRef]
8. Proulx, C.; Sabatino, D.; Hopewell, R.; Spiegel, J.; Ramos, Y.G.; Lubell, W.D. Azapeptides and their therapeutic potential. *Future Med. Chem.* **2011**, *3*, 1139–1164. [CrossRef]
9. Zhang, Y.T.; Malamakal, R.M.; Chenoweth, D.M. Aza-Glycine Induces Collagen Hyperstability. *J. Am. Chem. Soc.* **2015**, *137*, 12422–12425. [CrossRef] [PubMed]
10. Zhang, Y.T.; Herling, M.; Chenoweth, D.M. General Solution for Stabilizing Triple Helical Collagen. *J. Am. Chem. Soc.* **2016**, *138*, 9751–9754. [CrossRef]

11. Thormann, M.; Hofmann, H.J. Conformational properties of azapeptides. *J. Mol. Struct. THEOCHEM* **1999**, *469*, 63–76. [CrossRef]
12. Reynolds, C.H.; Hormann, R.E. Theoretical study of the structure and rotational flexibility of diacylhydrazines: Implications for the structure of nonsteroidal ecdysone agonists and azapeptides. *J. Am. Chem. Soc.* **1996**, *118*, 9395–9401. [CrossRef]
13. Stanger, H.E.; Gellman, S.H. Rules for antiparallel beta-sheet design: D-Pro-Gly is superior to L-Asn-Gly for beta-hairpin nucleation. *J. Am. Chem. Soc.* **1998**, *120*, 4236–4237. [CrossRef]
14. Syud, F.A.; Espinosa, J.F.; Gellman, S.H. NMR-based quantification of beta-sheet populations in aqueous solution through use of reference peptides for the folded and unfolded states. *J. Am. Chem. Soc.* **1999**, *121*, 11577–11578. [CrossRef]
15. Hess, H.J.; Moreland, W.T.; Laubach, G.D. N- [2-Isopropyl-3-(L-Aspartyl-L-Arginyl)-Carbazoyl]-L-Tyrosyl-L-Valyl-L-Histidyl-L-Prolyl-L-Phenylalanine, an Isostere of Bovine Angiotensin Ii. *J. Am. Chem. Soc.* **1963**, *85*, 4040–4041. [CrossRef]
16. Meienhofer, J.; Waki, M.; Heimer, E.P.; Lambros, T.J.; Makofske, R.C.; Chang, C.D. Solid-Phase Synthesis without Repetitive Acidolysis. *Int. J. Pept. Prot. Res.* **1979**, *13*, 35–42. [CrossRef]
17. Boeglin, D.; Lubell, W.D. Aza-amino acid scanning of secondary structure suited for solid-phase peptide synthesis with Fmoc chemistry and aza-amino acids with heteroatomic side chains. *J. Comb. Chem.* **2005**, *7*, 864–878. [CrossRef]
18. Chingle, R.; Proulx, C.; Lubell, W.D. Azapeptide Synthesis Methods for Expanding Side-Chain Diversity for Biomedical Applications. *Acc. Chem. Res.* **2017**, *50*, 1541–1556. [CrossRef]
19. Sabatino, D.; Proulx, C.; Klocek, S.; Bourguet, C.B.; Boeglin, D.; Ong, H.; Lubell, W.D. Exploring Side-Chain Diversity by Submonomer Solid-Phase Aza-Peptide Synthesis. *Org. Lett.* **2009**, *11*, 3650–3653. [CrossRef]
20. Kurian, L.A.; Silva, T.A.; Sabatino, D. Submonomer synthesis of azapeptide ligands of the Insulin Receptor Tyrosine Kinase domain. *Bioorg. Med. Chem. Lett.* **2014**, *24*, 4176–4180. [CrossRef]
21. Spiegel, J.; Mas-Moruno, C.; Kessler, H.; Lubell, W.D. Cyclic Aza-peptide Integrin Ligand Synthesis and Biological Activity. *J. Org. Chem.* **2012**, *77*, 5271–5278. [CrossRef] [PubMed]
22. Isocyanate and/or hydantoin byproducts likely arise from activation of the resin-bound semicarbazide with the carbonyl donor, followed by intramolecular attack by the nitrogen of the preceding amino acid residue. See: Quibell, M.; Turnell, W.G.; Johnson, T., Synthesis of Azapeptides by the Fmoc Tert-Butyl Polyamide Technique. *J. Chem. Soc. Perk. Trans 1* **1993**, *22*, 2843–2849. [CrossRef]
23. Paradis-Bas, M.; Tulla-Puche, J.; Albericio, F. The road to the synthesis of "difficult peptides". *Chem. Soc. Rev.* **2016**, *45*, 631–654. [CrossRef]
24. Murray, J.K.; Farooqi, B.; Sadowsky, J.D.; Scalf, M.; Freund, W.A.; Smith, L.M.; Chen, J.D.; Gellman, S.H. Efficient synthesis of a beta-peptide combinatorial library with microwave irradiation. *J. Am. Chem. Soc.* **2005**, *127*, 13271–13280. [CrossRef]
25. Chingle, R.; Ratni, S.; Claing, A.; Lubell, W.D. Application of Constrained aza-Valine Analogs for Smac Mimicry. *Biopolymers* **2016**, *106*, 235–244. [CrossRef] [PubMed]
26. Arujoe, M.; Ploom, A.; Mastitski, A.; Jarv, J. Comparison of various coupling reagents in solid-phase aza-peptide synthesis. *Tetrahedron Lett.* **2017**, *58*, 3421–3425. [CrossRef]
27. Arujoe, M.; Ploom, A.; Mastitski, A.; Jarv, J. Influence of steric effects in solid-phase aza-peptide synthesis. *Tetrahedron Lett.* **2018**, *59*, 2010–2013. [CrossRef]
28. Beutner, G.L.; Young, I.S.; Davies, M.L.; Hickey, M.R.; Park, H.; Stevens, J.M.; Ye, Q.M. TCFH-NMI: Direct Access to N-Acyl Imidazoliums for Challenging Amide Bond Formations. *Org. Lett.* **2018**, *20*, 4218–4222. [CrossRef] [PubMed]
29. Devos, A.; Remion, J.; Frisquehesbain, A.M.; Colens, A.; Ghosez, L. Synthesis of Acyl Halides under Very Mild Conditions. *J. Chem. Soc. Chem. Comm.* **1979**, *24*, 1180–1181. [CrossRef]
30. Gibson, C.; Goodman, S.L.; Hahn, D.; Ho¨lzemann, G.; Kessler, H. Novel Solid-Phase Synthesis of Azapeptides and Azapeptoides via Fmoc-Strategy and Its Application in the Synthesis of RGD-Mimetics. *J. Org. Chem.* **1999**, *64*, 7388–7394. [CrossRef]
31. Bourguet, C.B.; Sabatino, D.; Lubell, W.D. Benzophenone Semicarbazone Protection Strategy for Synthesis of Aza-Glycine Containing Aza-Peptides. *Biopolymers* **2008**, *90*, 824–831. [CrossRef] [PubMed]

32. Chingle, R.; Mulumba, M.; Chung, N.N.; Nguyen, T.M.; Ong, H.; Ballet, S.; Schiller, P.W.; Lubell, W.D. Solid-Phase Azopeptide Diels-Alder Chemistry for Aza-Pipecolyl Residue Synthesis to Study Peptide Conformation. *J. Org. Chem.* **2019**, *84*, 6006–6016. [CrossRef] [PubMed]
33. Searle, M.S.; Griffiths-Jones, S.R.; Skinner-Smith, H. Energetics of weak interactions in a beta-hairpin peptide: Electrostatic and hydrophobic contributions to stability from lysine salt bridges. *J. Am. Chem. Soc.* **1999**, *121*, 11615–11620. [CrossRef]
34. Bouayad-Gervais, S.H.; Lubell, W.D. Examination of the potential for adaptive chirality of the nitrogen chiral center in aza-aspartame. *Molecules* **2013**, *18*, 14739. [CrossRef]
35. It should be noted that replacement of valine for an aza-glycine residue results in an overall decrease in chiral environment, which may affect diastereotopic glycine splitting.
36. Kiehna, S.E.; Waters, M.L. Sequence dependence of beta-hairpin structure: Comparison of a salt bridge and an aromatic interaction. *Protein Sci.* **2003**, *12*, 2657–2667. [CrossRef] [PubMed]

Sample Availability: Samples of the compounds are available from the authors.

molecules

Article

The Characteristics of PD-L1 Inhibitors, from Peptides to Small Molecules

Yanwen Zhong, Xuanyi Li, Hequan Yao * and Kejiang Lin *

Department of Medicinal Chemistry, China Pharmaceutical University, Nanjing 210009, China; yhysjysypt@163.com (Y.Z.); 15261483658@163.com (X.L.)
* Correspondence: hyao@cpu.edu.cn (H.Y.); link@cpu.edu.cn (K.L.); Tel.: +86-25-83271445 (K.L.)

Academic Editors: Henry Mosberg, Tomi Sawyer and Carrie Haskell-Luevano
Received: 25 April 2019; Accepted: 19 May 2019; Published: 20 May 2019

Abstract: The programmed cell death ligand protein 1 (PD-L1) is a member of the B7 protein family and consists of 290 amino acid residues. The blockade of the PD-1/PD-L1 immune checkpoint pathway is effective in tumor treatment. Results: Two pharmacophore models were generated based on peptides and small molecules. Hypo 1A consists of one hydrogen bond donor, one hydrogen bond acceptor, two hydrophobic points and one aromatic ring point. Hypo 1B consists of one hydrogen bond donor, three hydrophobic points and one positive ionizable point. Conclusions: The pharmacophore model consisting of a hydrogen bond donor, hydrophobic points and a positive ionizable point may be helpful for designing small-molecule inhibitors targeting PD-L1.

Keywords: programmed cell death ligand protein 1; pharmacophore; peptide; small molecule

1. Introduction

Under normal circumstances, the immune system can identify and remove tumor cells in the tumor microenvironment [1]. However, to survive and grow, tumor cells can adopt different strategies to escape from the immune system. Immune checkpoints such as CTLA-4 (cytotoxic T lymphocyte-associated antigen-4) and PD-1 (programmed cell death protein 1), which regulate the activation of lymphocytes and balance immune responses, can protect tumor cells from the immune response. Immune checkpoint inhibitors, as one of focus of tumor immunotherapy, can be targeted in the immune system instead of tumor cells to stimulate an immune response [2,3]. Programmed cell death 1 (PD-1) is one of the best-studied immune checkpoints [4].

PD-1 is a member of the B7 superfamily which consists of 288 amino acid residues and acts as an inhibitory receptor. PD-1 is one of the death receptors which have been identified as a subgroup of the tumor necrosis factor (TNF)-receptor superfamily, which can induce apoptosis via a conserved cytoplasmic signaling module called the death domain, including TNF-R1, Fas, DR3 (death receptor 3) and so on [5,6]. PD-L1 and PD-L2 are the two ligands of PD-1 which are expressed on immune cells such as NK (natural killer) cells, active T cells and B cells [7]. The programmed cell death ligand protein 1 (PD-L1) is a member of the B7 protein family and consists of 290 amino acid residues. The PD-1/PD-L pathway plays a crucial role in immunotherapy. The binding of PD-1 and PD-L1 or PD-L2 results in the phosphorylation of the immune receptor tyrosine-based inhibition motif and the immune receptor tyrosine-based switch motif, which can recruit phosphatases SHP (Src homology 2 domain-containing tyrosine phosphatase)-1 and SHP-2 to the PD-1 intracellular domain; the phosphatases from the SHP family are mainly responsible for the effect caused by PD-1 intracellularly. After the phosphorylation of the SHP family, the downstream signaling pathways of T-cell receptors such as the phosphoinositide 3-kinase (PI3K)/Akt pathway will be inhibited, leading to the inhibition of the activity and proliferation of T cells. The binding of PD-1 and ligands will also result in a decrease in phosphorylation of the

CD3ζ (cluster of differentiation 3ζ) chains and ZAP-70 (Zeta-associated protein-70) [8]. This process can be blocked through the use of PD-1 or PD-L1 inhibitors [9,10].

Inhibitors of PD-1 may lead to the blockade of both the PD-1/PD-L1 pathway and the PD-1/PD-L2 pathway. However, inhibitors of PD-L1 can only block the PD-1/PD-L1 pathway, not the PD-1/PD-L1 pathway. Compared to PD-1 inhibitors, PD-L1 inhibitors can reduce the incidence of side effects resulting from immune disorders [11–13]. The FDA has approved three humanized monoclonal IgG4 antibodies targeting PD-L1, Atezolizumab, Avelumab and Durvalumab [14]. In addition to their great success in clinical trials, the problems of mAbs are very obvious, including higher production costs, lower oral bioavailability, poor tumor penetration, immune-related adverse events, etc. [15,16]. Moreover, compared to peptides and small molecules, the immunogenicity of mAbs can result in severe immune-related adverse events (irAEs) in a few cases. Due to the long half-lives and strong target occupancy of mAbs, the target inhibition is sustained, and irAEs are intractable [14]. In comparison with monoclonal antibodies, small-molecule and peptide inhibitors targeting PD-L1 have smaller molecular weights and more controllable pharmacokinetic and pharmacological profiles [17]. However, the development of small-molecule inhibitors of the PD-1/PD-L1 pathway is slow; only a few small-molecule and peptide inhibitors have been reported. In 2016, CA-170 became the only small-molecule inhibitor targeting PD-L1 in phase I clinical trials [18,19]. AUNP-12 (Aurigene NP-12) is the first peptide targeting PD-L1. Compared to peptides, small molecules have advantages in terms of their oral and plasma stability. Moreover, the oral bioavailability of small molecules is higher, and the synthesis of small molecules is easier [17,20]. The study of small-molecule PD-L1 inhibitors has attracted attention; because of the complexity and plasticity of the PD-L1 surface, it is difficult to design active small-molecule inhibitors targeting PD-L1. Therefore, many efforts have been made to develop small-molecule inhibitors, but only a few small-molecule inhibitors have been reported and patented [21,22].

In 2015, the crystal holo-structure of hPD-1 (human PD-1) with hPD-L1 (human PD-L1) was solved by the team of Zak (Protein Data Bank (PDB) ID: 4ZQK). This result resolved the uncertainty brought by the mPD-1 (mouse PD-1)/hPD-L1 crystal structure [23]. The crystal structure shows the interaction between PD-1 and PD-L1, in which three hydrophobic regions are thought to be major hot spots on the interaction surface of PD-L1. The discovery of the crystal structure of PD-1/PD-L1 provides a basis for designing non-antibody-based inhibitors of PD-L1. In 2016, three classes of peptide inhibitors of PD-L1 were published by Bristol–Myers–Squibb (BMS). Crystal structures of these peptides and PD-L1 were reported by Zak in 2017 (PDB ID: 5O45 and 5O4Y) [24], which can be helpful in designing peptide inhibitors targeting PD-L1. In 2016, a series of small-molecule inhibitors of PD-L1 was discovered by scientists at BMS. The team of Krzysztof M. Zak studied the interaction between these compounds and PD-L1 and provided a series of crystal structures of PD-L1 and its small-molecule ligands (PDB ID: 5J89, 5J8O, 5N2D, 5N2F, 5NIU, 5NIX) [25–27]. These crystal structures show that the interaction of PD-1/PD-L1 was blocked by the small molecules, which induced PD-L1 dimerization, and then the interaction surface of PD-1 could be occupied by another PD-L1 protein [25]. This information may be beneficial in designing small-molecule inhibitors targeting PD-L1.

It is challenging to design small-molecule inhibitors targeting the surface in protein–protein interactions because of the flexibility of proteins [28,29]. The disclosure of the crystal structures of PD-1/PD-L1 provides the possibility of designing small-molecule inhibitors targeting PD-L1 via computer-aided drug design (CADD). In this study, we built two pharmacophore models based on the crystal structures of peptides and small molecules, respectively (Supplementary Materials). Two models were compared to investigate the characteristics of PD-L1 inhibitors. These characteristics of peptides and small molecules are important in future efforts to discover and optimize PD-L1 inhibitors.

2. Results

2.1. Pharmacophore Model Hypo 1A Hypotheses and Validation

We built seven pharmacophore models based on the crystal structure of peptide-71 and PD-L1 (Table 1).

Table 1. Seven generated pharmacophore models.

Pharmacophore	Number of Features	Feature Set	Selectivity Score	Sensitivity *	Specificity *
Pharmacophore01	5	DHHHR	8.8639	0.703	0.993
Pharmacophore02	5	ADHHR	8.8639	0.703	0.919
Pharmacophore03	5	ADHHR	8.8639	0.741	0.993
Pharmacophore04	5	ADHHR	8.8639	0.667	0.980
Pharmacophore05	5	ADHHR	8.8639	0.889	0.966
Pharmacophore06	5	ADHHR	8.8639	0.741	0.993
Pharmacophore07	5	AHHHR	7.9504	0.778	0.838

* Sensitivity = true positives/(true positives + false negatives), specificity = true negatives/(true negatives + false positives).

Based on the selectivity score, sensitivity and specificity, Pharmacophore03 is the best choice. Pharmacophore03 is chosen as the best mainly because it seems that it is more important to effectively remove the inactive compound; in the case of the current example, most PD-L1 inhibitors are macromolecules. Compared to Pharmacophore06, Pharmacophore03 not only predicts active small molecules but also has good predictive power for active peptides, although the two pharmacophores have the same specificity and sensitivity to small-molecule active compounds. Pharmacophore03 was selected as the pharmacophore model (Hypo 1A) for the peptide targeting of PD-L1. Hypo 1A consists of one hydrogen bond donor, one hydrogen bond acceptor, two hydrophobic points and one aromatic ring point (Figure 1).

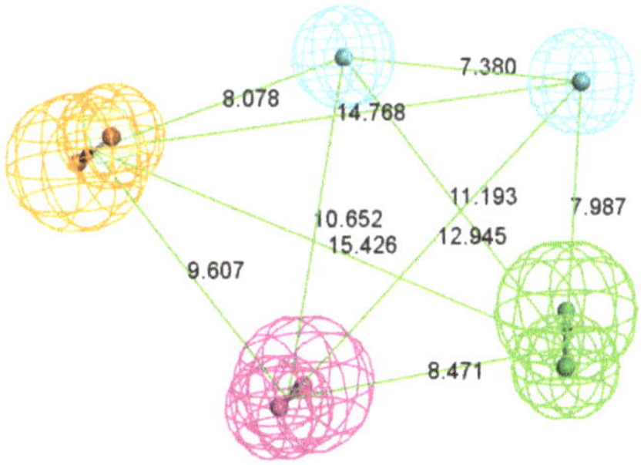

Figure 1. Pharmacophore model Hypo 1A. As the figure shows, the aromatic ring point is orange, the hydrophobic point is blue, the hydrogen bond acceptor is green, and the hydrogen bond donor is purple. The distance between the pharmacophore features is reported in angstroms.

2.2. Decoy Set of Hypo 1A

The specificity and sensitivity were calculated to evaluate the quality of the generated model. The resulting sensitivity was 0.741, and the specificity was 0.993 (Table 2).

Table 2. Results of the decoy set.

Parameter	Values
The number of molecules in the database	175
The number of actives in the database	27
The number of hit molecules from the database	21
The number of active molecules in the hit list	20
False negatives	6
False positives	1
% Yield of actives	74.1
% Sensitivity	74.1
% Specificity	99.3

2.3. *ROC Curve of Hypo 1A*

The AUC value of the model was 0.906, and Hypo 1A was thought to have the ability to distinguish active molecules from inactive molecules (Figure 2).

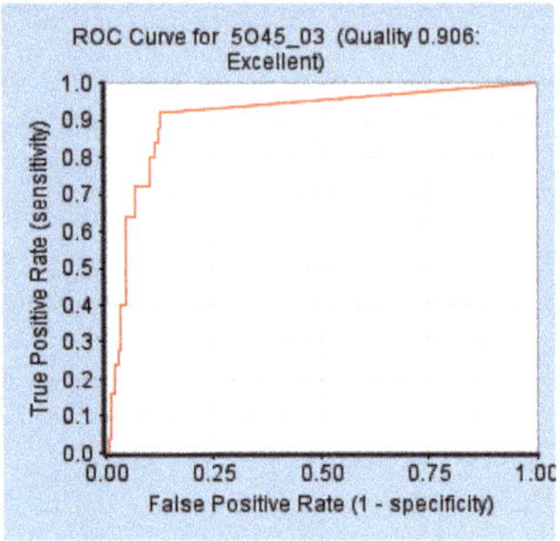

Figure 2. Receiver operating characteristics (ROC) curve of Hypo 1A.

2.4. *Pharmacophore Model Hypo 1B Hypotheses and Validation*

We built 10 pharmacophore models based on the crystal structure of BMS-1001 and PD-L1. The fit value is a predictor of the activity of the compound and reflects the degree of matching of the compound to the pharmacophore model (Table 3).

Table 3. Compound experimental IC_{50} values and predicted fit values of 10 pharmacophore models.

Compounds	BMS-1166	BMS-1001	BMS-202	28131141	BMS-200	28131140	BMS-242	BMS-37	28131145	28131143	R *
IC_{50} (nM)	1.4	2.25	18	43	80	6-100	6–100	6–100	110–1000	110–1000	
Model01 Fit Value	3.81036	4.48433	none	3.71533	3.80462	2.80741	none	none	1.56344	none	0.655
Model02 Fit Value	4.16447	3.93019	2.68308	3.7521	2.98747	2.73383	2.6811	2.67567	3.04527	2.58668	0.819
Model03 Fit Value	4.42391	4.52196	3.53526	3.90221	3.99688	3.30513	3.6466	3.95454	4.30285	4.01664	0.565
Model04 Fit Value	4.14129	4.63203	1.71529	2.9739	4.17607	2.10849	2.35671	1.76556	4.33115	2.77859	0.47
Model05 Fit Value	4.1626	4.4831	3.1851	3.27722	3.38762	3.0444	3.51356	2.73352	3.67542	3.56603	0.781
Model06 Fit Value	4.12881	4.49658	1.69069	3.43773	3.9225	2.71941	1.94917	1.82323	3.79388	2.59189	0.529
Model07 Fit Value	4.5101	4.72431	2.82402	3.79522	2.07746	3.38077	3.46818	3.61272	3.98516	3.93575	0.539
Model08 Fit Value	4.47768	4.73352	3.58699	4.03414	3.35641	3.77544	4.08634	4.03562	3.35984	4.07816	0.679
Model09 Fit Value	3.82049	4.05292	0.09738	4.00387	4.45517	2.82319	1.18001	0.17939	2.31305	0.11979	0.428
Model10 Fit Value	3.30267	4.09233	1.80806	3.41994	4.28178	2.67542	2.27937	1.80307	3.69411	2.88655	0.28

* The correlation coefficient (R) is a numerical measure of the correlation between experiments and predictions.

Model02 was selected as the pharmacophore model (Hypo 1B) with the highest correlation. Hypo 1B consists of one hydrogen bond donor, three hydrophobic points and one positive ionizable point (Figure 3).

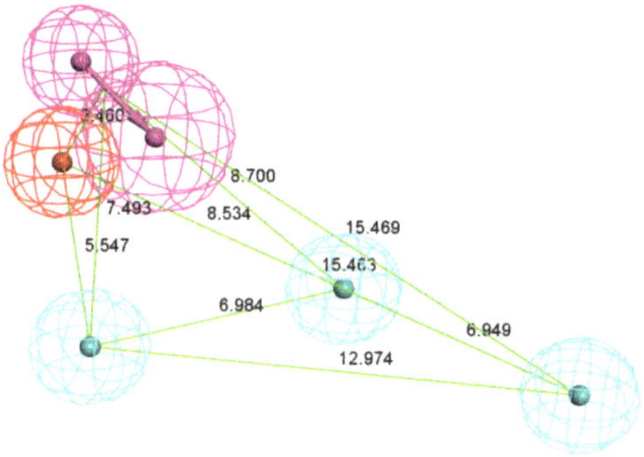

Figure 3. Pharmacophore model 1B. As the figure shows, the positive ionizable point is red, the hydrophobic point is blue, and the hydrogen bond donor is purple.

2.5. Decoy Set of Hypo 1B

Specificity and sensitivity were calculated to evaluate the quality of the generated model Hypo 1B. The resulting sensitivity was 0.709, and the specificity was 1 (Table 4).

Table 4. Results of the decoy set.

Parameter	Values
The number of molecules in the database	260
The number of actives in the database	110
The number of hit molecules from the database	78
The number of active molecules in the hit list	78
False negatives	32
False positives	0
% Yield of actives	70.9
% Sensitivity	70.9
% Specificity	100

2.6. ROC Curve of Hypo 1B

The AUC value of the model was 0.985, and Hypo 1B was thought to have the ability to distinguish active molecules from inactive molecules (Figure 4).

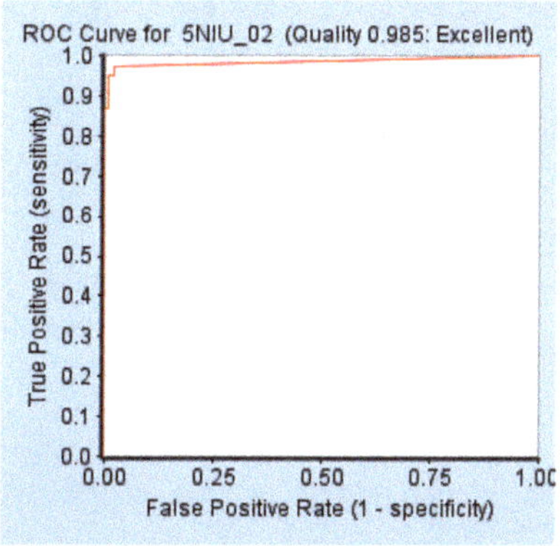

Figure 4. ROC curve of Hypo 1B.

2.7. *Molecular Docking Study*

We docked BMS compounds to PD-L1 (PDB ID: 5NIX) based on CHARMM using CDOCKER in DS. The interaction energy of BMS-1166, BMS-1001, BMS-37, BMS-202, BMS-8, BMS-200, BMS-242 and PD-L1 were 76.614, 67.602, 65.688, 63.355, 59.252, 70.329, 65.587 respectively.

3. Materials and Methods

The computational molecular modelling studies were carried out using Discovery Studio (DS, Accelrys, San Diego, CA, USA).

3.1. *Generation and Validation of the Pharmacophore Model Based on Peptides*

Since the crystal structures of PD-1/PD-L1 were published, more and more peptides targeting PD-L1 have been disclosed. Generating pharmacophore models based on peptide inhibitors can be helpful in designing non-antibody inhibitors of PD-L1. The structures of two macrocyclic peptides targeting PD-L1 disclosed by BMS were published in 2017 [24], of which peptide-57 contains 15 residues (PDB ID:5O4Y) and peptide-71 contains 14 residues (PDB ID:5O45). Pharmacophore models based on peptides were generated using the crystal structure of peptide-71 and PD-L1 (PDB ID: 5O45) because the IC_{50} of peptide-71 is 7 nM, indicating that it is more active than peptide-57 (Figure 5). The "receptor–ligand pharmacophore generation" protocol was used to identify a set of features from the binding ligand. Features of the ligands were identified by receptor–ligand interactions, and hydrogen bond acceptors, hydrogen bond donors, hydrophobic points, negative ionizable points, positive ionizable points and aromatic rings were considered during pharmacophore generation. A maximum of five features was permitted in each pharmacophore. The "maximum pharmacophores" protocol was set to 10, while the "maximum features" and "minimum features" protocols were set to 5. Seven pharmacophore models were generated.

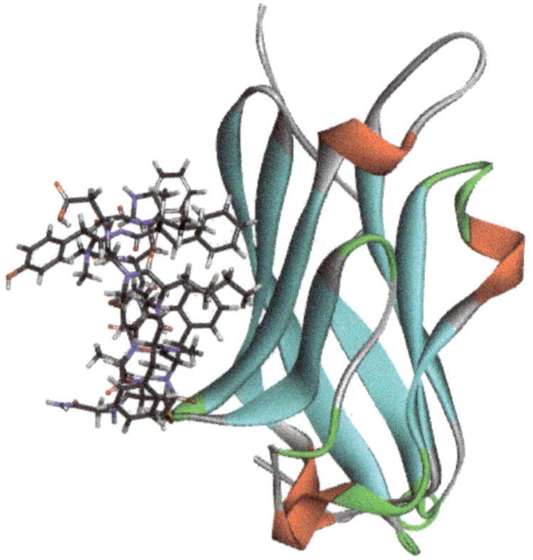

Figure 5. The crystal structure of peptide-71 and human programmed cell death ligand 1 (hPD-L1) (Protein Data Bank (PDB) ID: 5O45).

The decoy set, ROC (receiver operating characteristics) curve, sensitivity and specificity were used to evaluate the quality of the pharmacophore hypothesis. Sensitivity is defined as the power of a model to identify positives, and specificity is defined as the power of a model to determine negatives. These attributes were calculated as follows to validate the pharmacophore model:

$$\text{Sensitivity} = \text{true positives}/(\text{true positives} + \text{false negatives})$$

$$\text{Specificity} = \text{true negatives}/(\text{true negatives} + \text{false positives})$$

The decoy consists of positives and negatives. The 148 angiotensin-converting enzyme inhibitors used as negatives were selected from the database (http://dude.docking.org/) at random. The 27 active compounds used as positives were acquired from Integrity [30] or Reaxys [31]. The "build 3D database" protocol was applied to build the database, and the "search 3D database" protocol was applied to screen the database. The "build 3D database" protocol was used to generate the ligand database, which was indexed via sub-structures, pharmacophore features and shape information for database searching via the "search 3D database" protocol.

Active and inactive molecules were used to generate the ROC curve, which is used to evaluate the ability of a pharmacophore model to distinguish active molecules from inactive molecules. The area under the curve (AUC) value is the area under the ROC curve, which often ranges from 0 to 1. The model is thought to be better if the AUC value is closer to 1.

3.2. Generation and Validation of the Pharmacophore Model Based on Small Molecules

Scientists at Bristol–Myers–Squibb (BMS) have discovered a series of nonpeptidic small-molecule PD-L1 inhibitors, and the activities of these compounds were tested in a homogeneous time-resolved fluorescence (HTRF) binding assay [25–27]. In this study, the crystal structure of BMS-1001 and hPD-L1 (PDB ID: 5NIU) was chosen to generate and evaluate the inhibitor pharmacophore (Figure 6). The "receptor–ligand pharmacophore generation" protocol was used to identify a set of features from the binding ligand. A maximum of five features was permitted in each pharmacophore. Hydrogen bond acceptors, hydrogen bond donors, hydrophobic points, negative ionizable points, positive ionizable points and aromatic rings were selected for pharmacophore generation. The "maximum pharmacophores" protocol was set to 10, while the "maximum features" and "minimum features" protocols were set to 5. Ten pharmacophore models were generated.

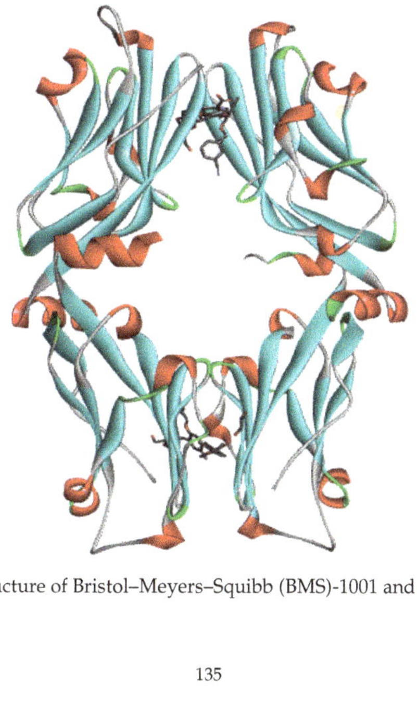

Figure 6. The crystal structure of Bristol–Meyers–Squibb (BMS)-1001 and hPD-L1 (PDB ID: 5NIU).

The decoy set and ROC curve were used to evaluate the quality of the pharmacophore hypothesis. The decoy set including 260 molecules was constructed from 150 negatives, which were angiotensin-converting enzyme inhibitors selected from the DUDE (A Database of Useful Decoys Enhanced) database at random, and 110 active molecules selected from Reaxys.

In addition to BMS-1001, which was used to generate the pharmacophore models, the BMS series contains six other small molecules: BMS-8, BMS-37, BMS-200, BMS-202, BMS-242, and BMS-1166. Additionally, 6 other small molecules with known activity values were selected in Reaxys (Table 5). "Ligand Pharmacophore Mapping" protocol was employed to screen 13 small molecules, in which "maximum omitted features" protocol was set to 0 and the "fitting method" protocol was set to Rigid. The "Fit Value" was used to measure how well the ligands fit the pharmacophore model. The ligands fit the model better when the fit value was higher.

Table 5. Structures of compounds showing IC_{50} values determined via the homogenous time-resolved fluorescence (HTRF) binding assay.

Name	Structure	IC_{50} (nM)
BMS-1166	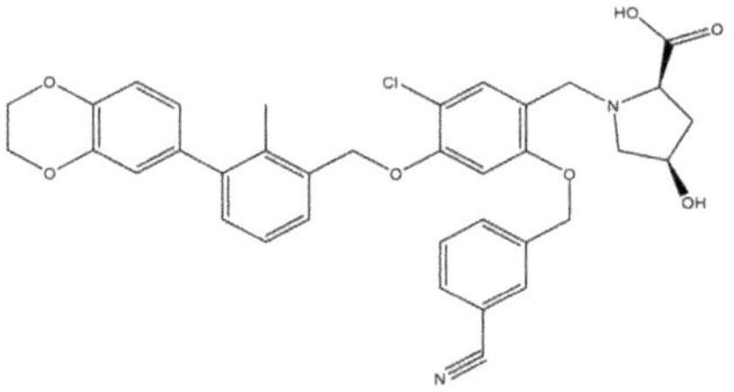	1.4
BMS-1001	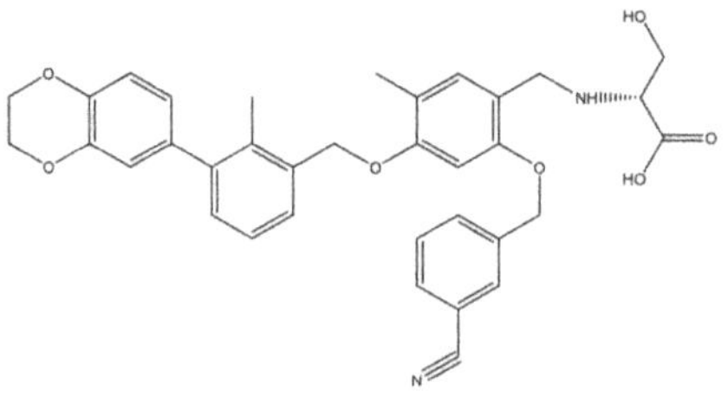	2.25
BMS-202	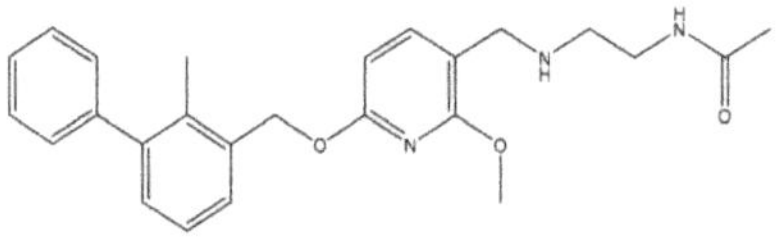	18
28131141	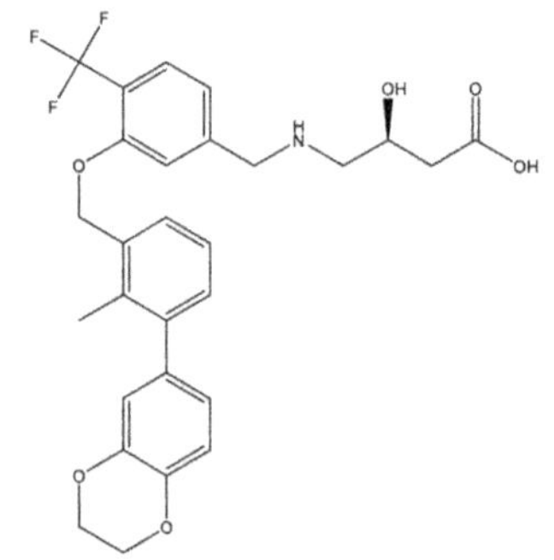	43

Table 5. *Cont.*

Name	Structure	IC_{50} (nM)
BMS-200	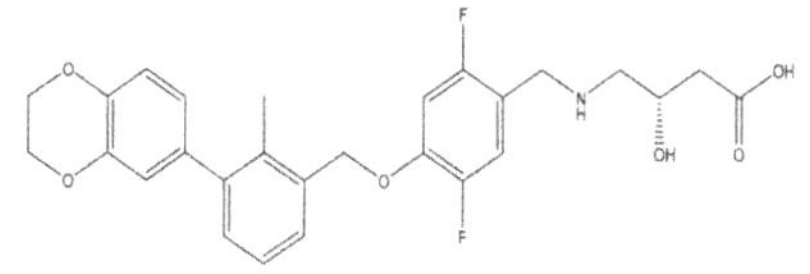	80
28131140	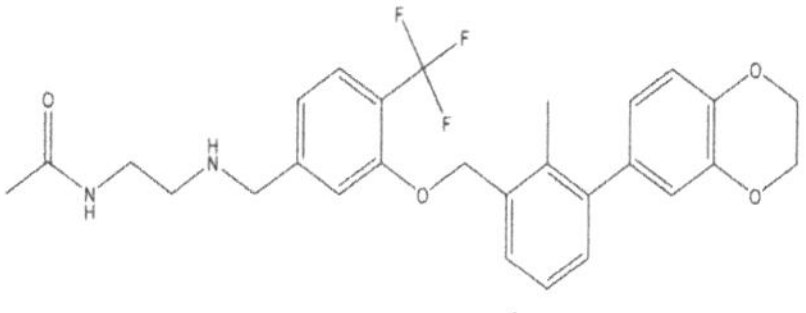	6-100
BMS-242	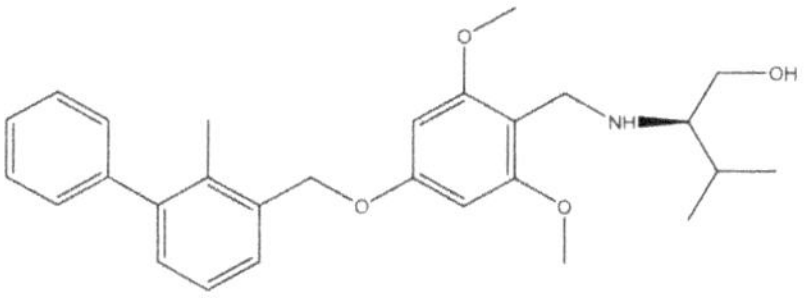	6-100
BMS-37	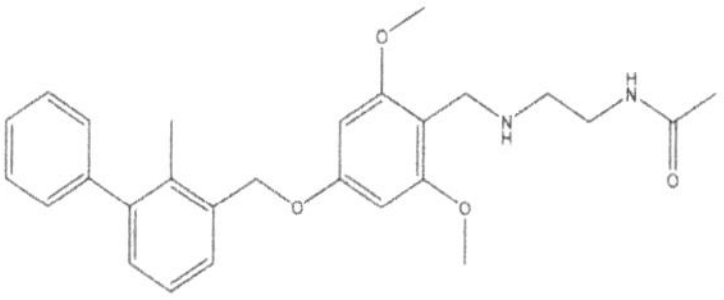	6-100
28131135	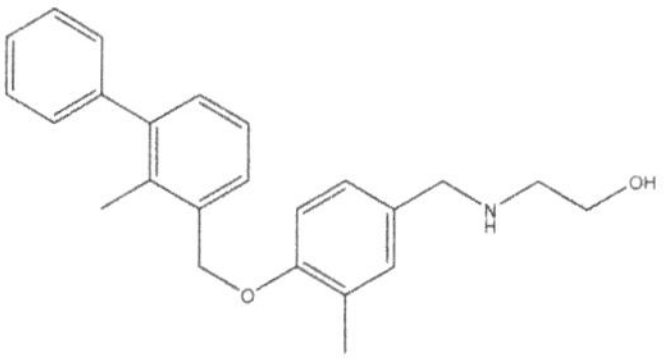	6-100
28131138	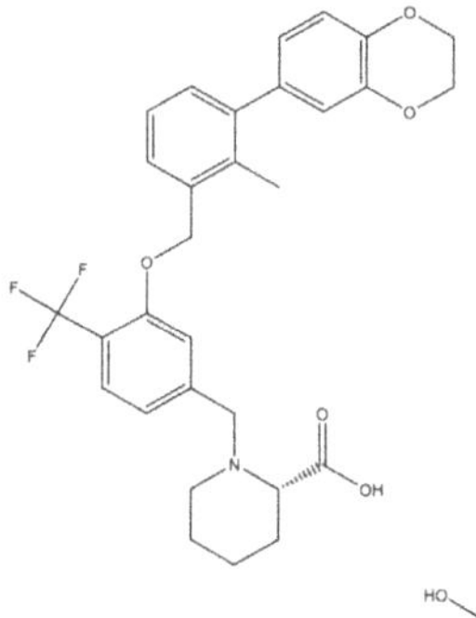	6-100
BMS-8	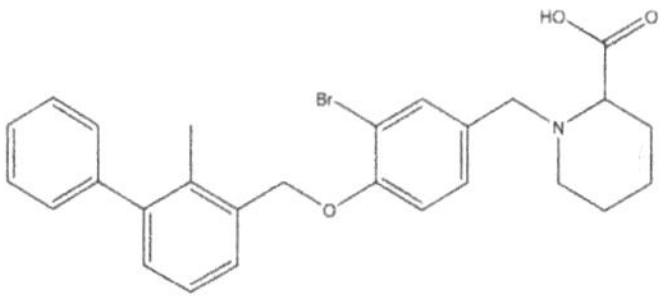	146

Table 5. *Cont.*

Name	Structure	IC_{50} (nM)
28131145	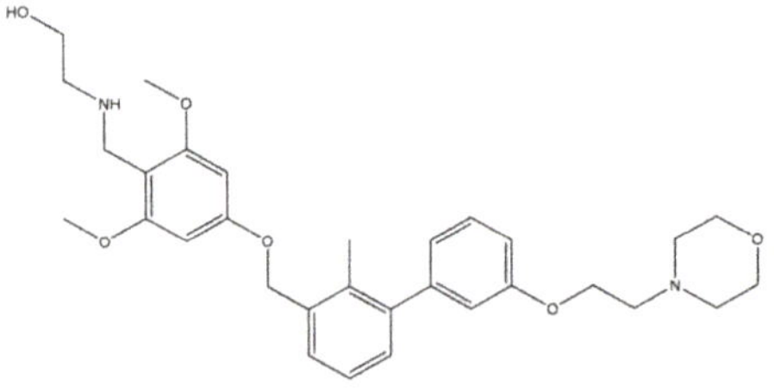	110-1000
28131143	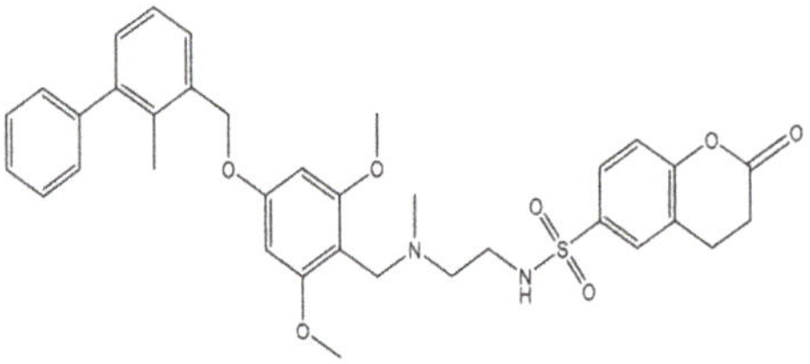	110-1000

3.3. Molecular Docking Study

According to reports [23], the hydrophobic pocket consisting of Tyr56, Glu58, Arg113, Met115, Tyr123 of PD-L1 is the optimal binding site for small molecules. The crystal structure of PD-L1 was downloaded from the Protein Data Bank (PDB). Water molecules were deleted and hydrogen atoms were added in the protein. The "clean protein" protocol was applied to prepare the protein. The "prepare ligands" protocol was applied to prepare BMS compounds. The space located at (−8.651, 60.227, −19.21) with a radius of 12 Angstrom was defined as the binding site. CDOCKER (a representative docking method in Discovery Studio) with default settings was used to dock the compounds to the protein based on the CHARMM (Chemistry at HARvard Macromolecular Mechanics) forcefield.

3.4. Analysing Interactions between PD-L1 and BMS Compounds

The crystal structures of PD-L1 and BMS-1166 (PDB ID: 5NIX), PD-L1 and BMS-1001 (PDB ID: 5NIU), PD-L1 and BMS-200 (PDB ID: 5N2F), PD-L1 and BMS-37 (PDB ID: 5N2D), PD-L1 and BMS-202 (PDB ID: 5J89), and PD-L1 and BMS-8 (PDB ID: 5J8O) were downloaded from the Protein Data Bank (PDB). Water molecules were deleted, and hydrogen atoms were added to the protein. The "display receptor–ligand interactions" and "analyze ligand poses" protocols were used to analyze the interactions between PD-L1 and the BMS compounds.

3.5. Comparing the Model Based on Peptides with the Model Based on Small Molecules

The "pharmacophore comparison" protocol was used to map and align the two models generated based on peptides and small molecules, respectively. The root mean squared error (RMSE) is an indicator of matching pharmacophore features.

4. Discussion

4.1. Features of Hypo 1A

Hypo 1A consists of one hydrogen bond donor, one hydrogen bond acceptor, two hydrophobic points and one aromatic ring point. The hydrophobic points were located at NMePhe7 and Val6, the aromatic ring point was located at Trp10, the hydrogen bond donor was located at Leu12, and the hydrogen bond acceptor was located at Asp5 (Figure 7). Peptide-57 can be well mapped with Hypo 1A. The two hydrophobic points were located at NMeNle12 and NMeNle11, the aromatic ring point was located at Trp10, the hydrogen bond donor was located at Arg13, and the hydrogen bond acceptor was located at Scc14 (Figure 8). The hydrophobic zone on peptide-57 consists of Phe1, Trp8, Trp10, NMeNle11 and NMeNle12. According to the report, if each of the residues responsible for interactions is replaced by a smaller amino acid, the activity will drop. The activity will drop from 9 nm to 3656 nm if Trp10 is lacking. Analyzing the interactions between PD-L1 and peptide-57, we can observe that residues located at the Arg13 and Scc14 provided solvent contact points [24]. The activity of peptide may not drop drastically if Arg13 and Scc14 are replaced by other hydrophilic amino acids.

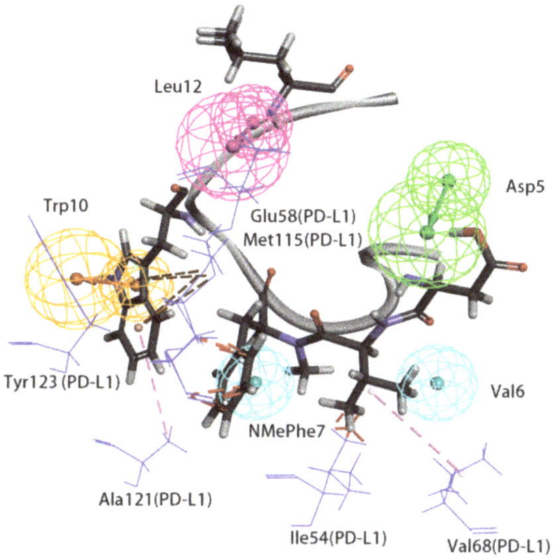

Figure 7. Superposition between Hypo 1A and peptide-71. As the figure shows, the hydrophobic point is blue, the hydrogen bond donor is purple, the hydrogen bond acceptor is green, and the aromatic ring point is orange. The interacted residues of PD-L1 are blue.

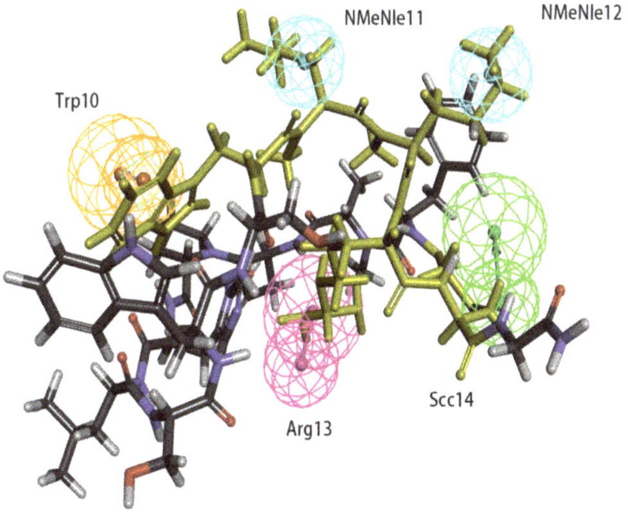

Figure 8. Superposition between Hypo 1A and peptide-57. As the figure shows, the hydrophobic point is blue, the hydrogen bond donor is purple, the hydrogen bond acceptor is green, and the aromatic ring point is orange. The labelled residues are yellow.

We can observe that Leu12 on peptide-71 interacts with Glu58 on PD-L1 via hydrogen bonds, and an intramolecular hydrogen bond can be generated between Asp5 and Tyr8 on peptide-71. Val6 on peptide-71 interacts with Ile54 on PD-L1 via hydrophobic bonds, Trp10 on peptide-71 interacts with Ala121 on PD-L1 via hydrophobic bonds, and NMePhe7 on peptide-71 interacts with Met115 on PD-L1 via hydrophobic bonds. Intramolecular hydrogen bonds can be generated between Arg13 and Trp8 and between Scc14 and Ser7 on peptide-57. Trp10 on peptide-57 interacts with Arg113, Met115, and Tyr123 on PD-L1 via hydrophobic bonds. In conclusion, Ile54, Arg113, Met115, Ala121, and Try123 of PD-L1 may be important in the hydrophobic interactions between peptides and PD-L1.

The binding surface of the peptide consists of hydrophobic regions and hydrophilic regions, and the hydrophobic interactions are essential for the binding of peptides to PD-L1 [24]. According to a report, the affinity between PD-L1 and peptide-71 is dominated by several interactions with low energy in shallow pockets instead of in any noticeable pockets [24,32]. The hydrophobic interaction is the major type of interaction involved in the binding of PD-L1 and peptide-71. The hydrophobic area consists mostly of Phe1, NMePhe7, and Trp10, supplemented with NMeNle3 and Val6. Phe1, Trp10 and Val6 were related to the hydrophobic interaction between peptide-71 and Tyr56, Ala121, and Ile54 on PD-L1, respectively. Moreover, Leu12 and Scc13 contributed to the formation of hydrogen bonds between peptide-71 and Glu58, Asp61, and Asn63 of PD-L1. The binding of PD-L1 and peptide-57 was also mainly guided by hydrophobic interactions. The hydrophobic pocket on the surface of PD-L1, which was filled with Trp10 on peptide-57, consists of Tyr56, Glu58, Arg113, Met115, and Tyr123. Moreover, NMeNle12 and NMeNle11 were related to weak hydrophobic interactions between peptide-57 and PD-L1. Additionally, Leu6 and Trp8 provided two hydrogen bonds with PD-L1. It is consistent with our pharmacophore that Ile54, Arg113, Met115, Ala121, and Try123 of PD-L1 are related to the hydrophobic interactions between peptides and PD-L1.

4.2. Features of Hypo 1B

The model consists of one hydrogen bond donor, three hydrophobic points and one positive ionizable point. According to the interactions between PD-L1 and its ligand, we can observe that the group of the ligand corresponding to the hydrophobic features interacts with Ile54, Tyr56, Val68, Met115 and Ala121 of PD-L1 via hydrophobic interactions, and the group of the ligand corresponding to the hydrogen bond donor interacts with Asp122 and Lys124 of PD-L1 via hydrophobic interactions. In addition, the group corresponding to the positive ionizable point interacts with Asp122 (Figure 9). The outcome concluded from the pharmacophore model is consistent with the conclusion from the analysis of interactions between PD-L1 and BMS compounds.

By analyzing the interactions between PD-L1 and BMS compounds, we observed that Ile54, Tyr56, Val68, Met115 and Ala121 of PD-L1 are important in generating hydrophobic bonds between PD-L1 and molecules; that Asp122 and Lys124 of PD-L1 are helpful in forming hydrogen bonds between molecules and PD-L1; and that the positive ionizable located at Asp122 of PD-L1 may be essential for the interactions between molecules and PD-L1. This outcome was consistent with Hypo 1B, which consists of one hydrogen bond donor, three hydrophobic points and one positive ionizable point.

An attempt was made to map peptide-57 and peptide-71 with Hypo 1B. Peptide-57 could be well mapped with the model (Figure 10). The positive ionizable point was located at Arg13, and the hydrogen bond donor was also located at Arg13. The three hydrophobic points were located at NMeNle12 and Trp10. Peptide-71 could be mapped with the pharmacophore model, except for a positive ionizable point (Figure 11). The hydrogen bond donor was located at Gly-$NH_2$14, and the three hydrophobic points were located at Phe1, NMeNle3, and Trp10.

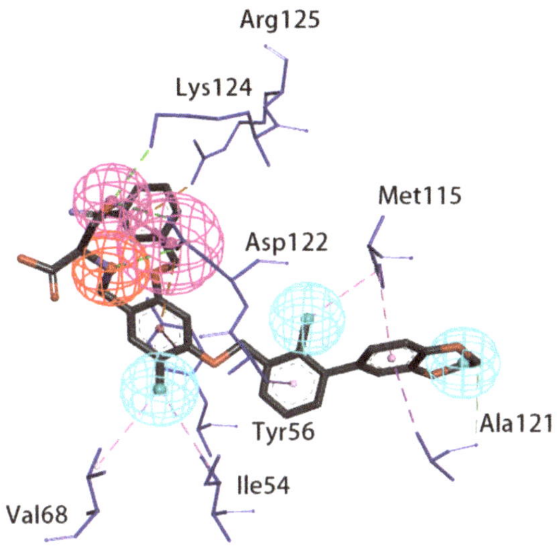

Figure 9. Superposition between BMS-1001 and the pharmacophore model. As the figure shows, the positive ionizable point is red, the hydrophobic point is blue, and the hydrogen bond donor is purple. The interacted residues of PD-L1 are blue.

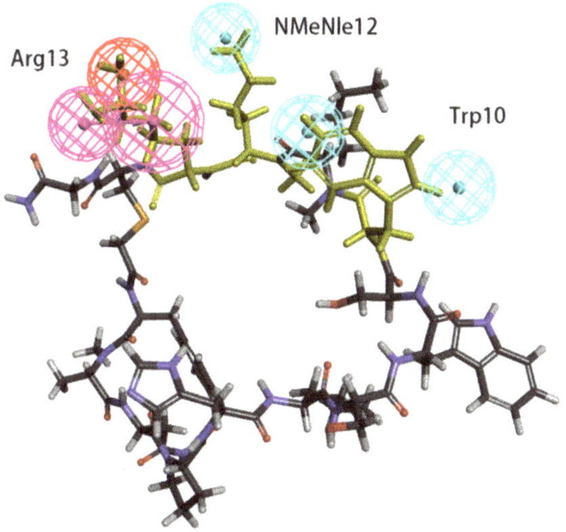

Figure 10. Superposition between Hypo 1B and peptide-57. As the figure shows, the positive ionizable point is red, the hydrophobic point is blue, and the hydrogen bond donor is purple. The labelled residues are yellow.

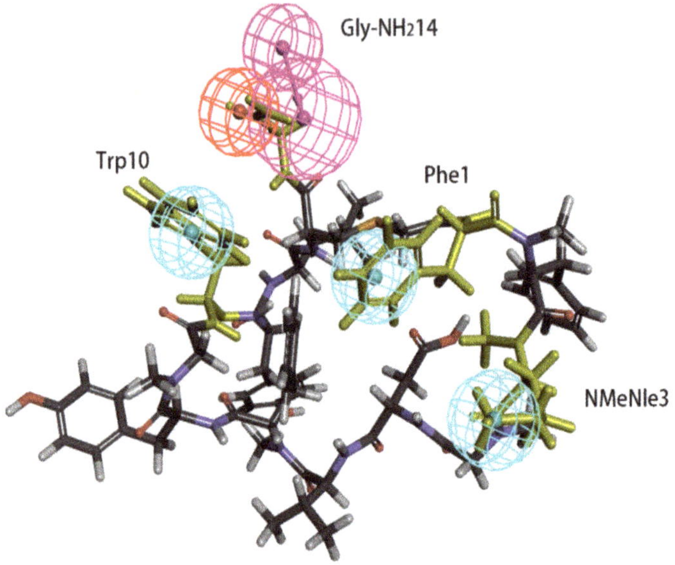

Figure 11. Superposition between Hypo 1B and peptide-71. As the figure shows, the positive ionizable point is red, the hydrophobic point is blue, and the hydrogen bond donor is purple. The labelled residues are yellow.

4.3. *Comparison between Hypo 1A and Hypo 1B*

The two models were superimposed using the pharmacophore comparison in DS, and the RMSE of Hypo 1A and 1B was 2.58. There were some common features between the two models; two hydrophobic points and one hydrogen bond donor could almost be matched. However, a hydrophobic point and a positive ionizable point of Hypo 1B and an aromatic ring point and a hydrogen bond acceptor of Hypo 1A were not in the same location (Figure 12).

There were some differences between Hypo 1A and Hypo 1B. First, a hydrophobic point of Hypo 1B and an aromatic ring point of Hypo 1A were not in the same location. The aromatic ring point of Hypo 1A located at Trp10 of peptide-71 interacted with Met115 and Ala121 of PD-L1 via hydrophobic interactions, and it was thought to play the same role as that of the hydrophobic point [24]. The hydrophobic and aromatic ring features of the two models were accommodated in the same hydrophobic pocket on PD-L1, which consists of Ile54, Tyr56, Met115, Ala121, and Tyr123. Second, the hydrogen bond acceptor did not exist in Hypo 1B. Residues located at the hydrogen bond acceptor provided solvent contact points [24] and didn't play a key role in the interaction between PD-L1 and ligands, so the hydrogen bond acceptor may be unnecessary in Hypo 1B. Third, the positive ionizable point was non-existent in Hypo 1A. The superposition between Hypo 1B and two peptides showed that the positive ionizable point matched peptide-57 well, of which the IC_{50} value is 9 nM. When peptide-57 was mapped with Hypo 1B, the positive ionizable point was located at Arg13 (Figure 13). This outcome meant that a positive ionizable point may be necessary for both small-molecule and peptide inhibitors. Though differences between the two models did exist, the model generated based on small-molecule inhibitors was more representative and may be helpful in the design of non-antibody-based PD-L1 inhibitors.

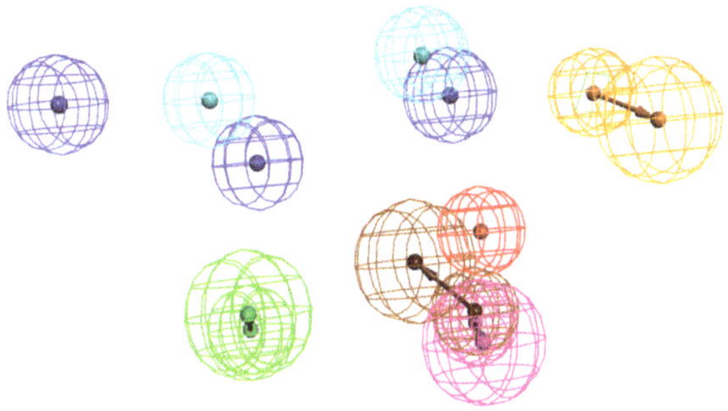

Figure 12. Superimposition of Hypo 1A and Hypo 1B. As the figure shows, in Hypo 1A, the hydrophobic point is light blue, the hydrogen bond acceptor is green, the hydrogen bond donor is purple, and the aromatic ring point is orange. In Hypo 1B, the hydrophobic point is Lyons blue, the positive ionizable point is red, and the hydrogen bond donor is brown.

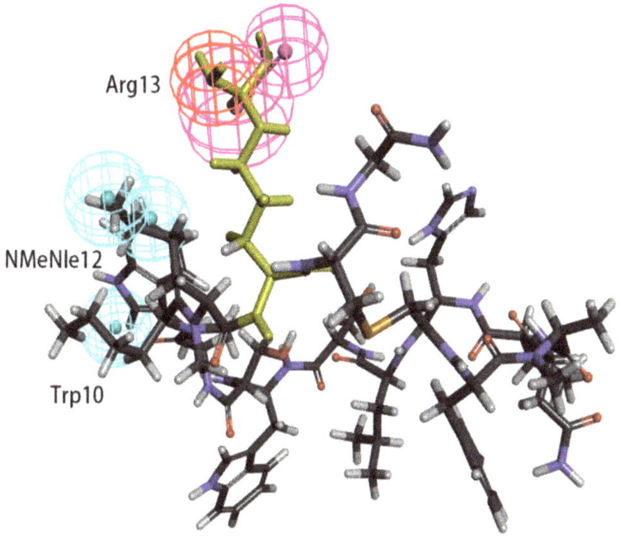

Figure 13. Superposition between Hypo 1B and peptide-57. As the figure shows, the positive ionizable point is red, the hydrophobic point is blue, and the hydrogen bond donor is purple. The yellow amino acid is Arg13.

5. Conclusions

In this study, the critical chemical features of PD-L1 inhibitors were found via pharmacophore models. Two pharmacophore models, Hypo 1A and Hypo 1B, were built based on small molecules and peptides, respectively. Hypo 1A consists of two hydrogen bond donors, three hydrophobic points and one positive ionizable point. Hypo 1B consists of one hydrogen bond donor, one hydrogen bond acceptor, two hydrophobic points and one aromatic ring point. The reliability of the pharmacophore models was validated by ROC curves and a decoy set. Hydrophobic features located in the same hydrophobic pocket are essential for both peptide and small-molecule inhibitors. The hydrogen bond donors of two models could be mapped. Though the positive ionizable point only exists in the pharmacophore model based on small-molecule inhibitors, it may be important for both small-molecule and peptide inhibitors. The similarity between Hypo1A and Hypo1B means that pharmacophore models consisting of a hydrogen bond donor, a hydrophobic point and a positive ionizable point may be helpful in designing small-molecule inhibitors targeting PD-L1.

Supplementary Materials: The supplementary materials are available online.

Author Contributions: Conceptualization, K.L.; methodology, K.L. and Y.Z.; formal analysis, X.L. and Y.Z.; validation, H.Y. and K.L.; investigation, Y.Z.; data curation, Y.Z. and X.L.; writing—original draft preparation, Y.Z.; writing—review and editing, K.L. and X.L.; supervision, H.Y. and K.L.

Funding: This research was funded by the National Key R&D Program of China (2018YFC0311003), the "Double First-Class" University Project, China (CPU2018GY15) and Key Laboratory of Spectrochemical Analysis & Instrumentation (Xiamen University), Ministry of Education, China (SCAI1802).

Acknowledgments: We thank American Journal Experts (AJE), Durham, North Carolina, USA, for their English language editing.

Conflicts of Interest: The authors declare no conflict of interest.

References

1. Massari, F.; Santoni, M.; Ciccarese, C.; Daniele, S. The Immunocheckpoints in Modern Oncology: The next 15 Years. *Expert Opin. Biol. Ther.* **2015**, *15*, 917–921. [CrossRef] [PubMed]
2. Bellmunt, J.; Powles, T.; Vogelzang, N.J. A Review on the Evolution of Pd-1/Pd-L1 Immunotherapy for Bladder Cancer: The Future is Now. *Cancer Treat. Rev.* **2017**, *54*, 58–67. [CrossRef]
3. Boussiotis, V.A. Molecular and Biochemical Aspects of The Pd-1 Checkpoint Pathway. *New Engl. J. Med.* **2016**, *375*, 1767–1778. [CrossRef] [PubMed]
4. Collin, M. Immune Checkpoint Inhibitors: A Patent Review (2010–2015). *Expert Opin. Ther. Patents* **2016**, *26*, 555–564. [CrossRef]
5. Wajant, H. Death Receptors. *Essays Biochem.* **2003**, *39*, 53–71. [CrossRef] [PubMed]
6. Schulze-Osthoff, K.; Ferrari, D.; Los, M.; Wesselborg, S.; Peter, M.E. Apoptosis Signaling by Death Receptors. *Eur. J. Biochem.* **1998**, *254*, 439–459. [CrossRef]
7. Ahmed, M.; Barakat, K. The Too Many Faces of Pd-L1: A Comprehensive Conformational Analysis Study. *Biochemistry* **2017**, *56*, 5428–5439. [CrossRef] [PubMed]
8. Dermani, F.K.; Samadi, P.; Rahmani, G.; Kohlan, A.K.; Najafi, R. Pd-1/Pd-L1 Immune Checkpoint: Potential Target for Cancer Therapy. *J. Cell Physiol.* **2019**, *234*, 1313–1325. [CrossRef] [PubMed]
9. Gong, J.; Chehrazi-Raffle, A.; Reddi, S.; Salgia, R. Development of Pd-1 And Pd-L1 Inhibitors as A form of Cancer Immunotherapy: A Comprehensive Review of Registration Trials and Future Considerations. *J. Immunother Cancer* **2018**, *6*, 8. [CrossRef] [PubMed]
10. Sun, C.; Mezzadra, R.; Schumacher, T.N. Regulation and Function of the Pd-L1 Checkpoint. *Immunity* **2018**, *48*, 434–452. [CrossRef]
11. Khunger, M.; Rakshit, S.; Pasupuleti, V.; Hernandez, A.V.; Mazzone, P.; Stevenson, J.; Pennell, N.A.; Velcheti, V. Incidence of Pneumonitis with Use of Programmed Death 1 and Programmed Death-Ligand 1 Inhibitors in Non-Small Cell Lung Cancer: A Systematic Review and Meta-Analysis of Trials. *Chest* **2017**, *152*, 271–281. [CrossRef] [PubMed]
12. Kythreotou, A.; Siddique, A.; Mauri, F.A.; Bower, M.; Pinato, D.J. Pd-L1. *J. Clin. Pathol.* **2018**, *71*, 189–194. [CrossRef]
13. Spagnuolo, A.; Gridelli, C. "Comparison of the Toxicity Profile of Pd-1 Versus Pd-L1 Inhibitors in Non-Small Cell Lung Cancer": Is There a Substantial Difference or not? *J. Thorac. Dis.* **2018**, *10*, S4065. [CrossRef] [PubMed]
14. Chen, T.; Li, Q.; Liu, Z.; Chen, Y.; Feng, F.; Sun, H. Peptide-Based and Small Synthetic Molecule Inhibitors on Pd-1/Pd-L1 Pathway: A New Choice for Immunotherapy? *Eur. J. Med. Chem.* **2019**, *161*, 378–398. [CrossRef] [PubMed]
15. Patil, S.P.; Fink, M.A.; Enley, E.S.; Fisher, J.E.; Herb, M.C.; Klingos, A.; Proulx, J.T.; Fedorky, M.T. Identification of Small-Molecule Inhibitors of Pd-1/Pd-L1 Protein-Protein Interaction. *Chemistryselect* **2018**, *3*, 2185–2189. [CrossRef]
16. Mondanelli, G.; Volpi, C.; Orabona, C.; Grohmann, U. Challenges in the Design of Reliable Immuno-Oncology Mouse Models to Inform Drug Development. *Future Med. Chem.* **2017**, *9*, 1313–1317. [CrossRef]

17. Yang, J.; Hu, L. Immunomodulators Targeting The Pd-1/Pd-L1 Protein-Protein Interaction: From Antibodies To Small Molecules. *Med. Res. Rev.* **2019**, *39*, 265–301. [CrossRef]
18. Sasikumar, P.G.; Ramachandra, M. Small-Molecule Antagonists of the Immune Checkpoint Pathways: Concept to Clinic. *Future Med. Chem.* **2017**, *9*, 1305–1308. [CrossRef]
19. Powderly, J.; Patel, M.R.; Lee, J.J.; Brody, J.; Meric-Bernstam, F.; Hamilton, E.; Aix, S.P.; Garcia-Corbacho, J.; Bang, Y.J.; Ahn, M.J.; et al. Ca-170, A First in Class Oral Small Molecule Dual Inhibitor of Immune Checkpoints Pd-L1 and Vista, Demonstrates Tumor Growth Inhibition in Pre-Clinical Models and Promotes T Cell Activation in Phase 1 Study. *Ann. Oncol.* **2017**, *28*. [CrossRef]
20. Li, K.; Tian, H. Development of Small-Molecule Immune Checkpoint Inhibitors of Pd-1/Pd-L1 as A New Therapeutic Strategy for Tumor Immunotherapy. *J. Drug Target.* **2019**, *27*, 244–256. [CrossRef]
21. Kopalli, S.R.; Kang, T.B.; Lee, K.H.; Koppula, S. Novel Small Molecule Inhibitors of Programmed Cell Death (Pd)-1, And Its Ligand, Pd-L1 in Cancer Immunotherapy: A Review Update of Patent Literature. *Recent Pat. Anticancer Drug Discov.* **2018**. [CrossRef]
22. Cheng, B.; Yuan, W.E.; Su, J.; Liu, Y.; Chen, J. Recent Advances in Small Molecule Based Cancer Immunotherapy. *Eur. J. Med. Chem.* **2018**, *157*, 582–598. [CrossRef]
23. Zak, K.M.; Kitel, R.; Przetocka, S.; Golik, P.; Guzik, K.; Musielak, B.; Domling, A.; Dubin, G.; Holak, T.A. Structure of the Complex of Human Programmed Death 1, Pd-1, and Its Ligand Pd-L1. *Structure* **2015**, *23*, 1348–2341. [CrossRef]
24. Magiera-Mularz, K.; Skalniak, L.; Zak, K.M.; Musielak, B.; Rudzinska-Szostak, E.; Berlicki, L.; Kocik, J.; Grudnik, P.; Sala, D.; Zarganes-Tzitzikas, T.; et al. Bioactive Macrocyclic Inhibitors of the Pd-1/Pd-L1 Immune Checkpoint. *Angew Chem. Int. Ed. Engl.* **2017**, *56*, 13732–13735. [CrossRef]
25. Zak, K.M.; Grudnik, P.; Guzik, K.; Zieba, B.J.; Musielak, B.; Domling, A.; Dubin, G.; Holak, T.A. Structural Basis For Small Molecule Targeting of The Programmed Death Ligand 1 (Pd-L1). *Oncotarget* **2016**, *7*, 30323–30335. [CrossRef]
26. Guzik, K.; Zak, K.M.; Grudnik, P.; Magiera, K.; Musielak, B.; Torner, R.; Skalniak, L.; Domling, A.; Dubin, G.; Holak, T.A. Small-Molecule Inhibitors of the Programmed Cell Death-1/Programmed Death-Ligand 1 (Pd-1/Pd-L1) Interaction via Transiently Induced Protein States and Dimerization of Pd-L1. *J. Med. Chem.* **2017**, *60*, 5857–5867. [CrossRef]
27. Skalniak, L.; Zak, K.M.; Guzik, K.; Magiera, K.; Musielak, B.; Pachota, M.; Szelazek, B.; Kocik, J.; Grudnik, P.; Tomala, M.; et al. Small-Molecule Inhibitors of Pd-1/Pd-L1 Immune Checkpoint Alleviate The Pd-L1-Induced Exhaustion of T-Cells. *Oncotarget* **2017**, *8*, 72167–72181. [CrossRef]
28. Perry, E.; Mills, J.J.; Zhao, B.; Wang, F.; Sun, Q.; Christov, P.P.; Tarr, J.C.; Rietz, T.A.; Olejniczak, E.T.; Lee, T.; et al. Fragment-Based Screening of Programmed Death Ligand 1 (Pd-L1). *Bioorg. Med. Chem. Lett.* **2019**. [CrossRef]
29. Zhan, M.M.; Hu, X.Q.; Liu, X.X.; Liu, X.X.; Ruan, B.F.; Xu, J.; Liao, C. From Monoclonal Antibodies to Small Molecules: The Development of Inhibitors Targeting the Pd-1/Pd-L1 Pathway. *Drug Discov. Today* **2016**, *21*, 1027–1036. [CrossRef] [PubMed]
30. Integrity. Available online: Https://Integrity.Clarivate.Com/ (accessed on 20 January 2019).
31. Reaxys. Available online: Https://Integrity.Clarivate.Com/ (accessed on 20 January 2019).
32. Villar, E.A.; Beglov, D.; Chennamadhavuni, S.; Porco, J.A., Jr.; Kozakov, D.; Vajda, S.; Whitty, A. How Proteins Bind Macrocycles. *Nat. Chem. Biol.* **2014**, *10*, 723–731. [CrossRef] [PubMed]

Sample Availability: Not available.

molecules

MDPI

Article

ACPred: A Computational Tool for the Prediction and Analysis of Anticancer Peptides

Nalini Schaduangrat [1], Chanin Nantasenamat [1], Virapong Prachayasittikul [2] and Watshara Shoombuatong [1,*]

[1] Center of Data Mining and Biomedical Informatics, Faculty of Medical Technology, Mahidol University, Bangkok 10700, Thailand; nalini.schaduangrat@gmail.com (N.S.); chanin.nan@mahidol.edu (C.N.)

[2] Department of Clinical Microbiology and Applied Technology, Faculty of Medical Technology, Mahidol University, Bangkok 10700, Thailand; virapong.pra@mahidol.ac.th

* Correspondence: watshara.sho@mahidol.ac.th; Tel.: +66-2-441-4371 (ext. 2715)

Received: 1 April 2019; Accepted: 17 May 2019; Published: 22 May 2019

Abstract: Anticancer peptides (ACPs) have emerged as a new class of therapeutic agent for cancer treatment due to their lower toxicity as well as greater efficacy, selectivity and specificity when compared to conventional small molecule drugs. However, the experimental identification of ACPs still remains a time-consuming and expensive endeavor. Therefore, it is desirable to develop and improve upon existing computational models for predicting and characterizing ACPs. In this study, we present a bioinformatics tool called the ACPred, which is an interpretable tool for the prediction and characterization of the anticancer activities of peptides. ACPred was developed by utilizing powerful machine learning models (support vector machine and random forest) and various classes of peptide features. It was observed by a jackknife cross-validation test that ACPred can achieve an overall accuracy of 95.61% in identifying ACPs. In addition, analysis revealed the following distinguishing characteristics that ACPs possess: (i) hydrophobic residue enhances the cationic properties of α-helical ACPs resulting in better cell penetration; (ii) the amphipathic nature of the α-helical structure plays a crucial role in its mechanism of cytotoxicity; and (iii) the formation of disulfide bridges on β-sheets is vital for structural maintenance which correlates with its ability to kill cancer cells. Finally, for the convenience of experimental scientists, the ACPred web server was established and made freely available online.

Keywords: anticancer peptide; therapeutic peptides; support vector machine; random forest; machine learning; classification

1. Introduction

Cancer remains one of the leading causes of death worldwide, accounting for an estimated 18.1 million new cases and resulting in 9.6 million deaths in 2018 [1]. Of these, the most common cancer types causing mortality worldwide include lung, colorectal, stomach, liver and breast cancer, respectively [1,2]. The global burden of cancer has risen dramatically in the last few decades thereby making the prevention of cancer the most significant and challenging public health concern of the 21st century [3]. In spite of the many advanced clinical methods available for the treatment of cancer (e.g., chemotherapy, radiation therapy, hormonal therapy, etc.) their recurrence rate still remains high. In addition, anti-cancer drugs are known to exert their therapeutic effects by killing off normal cells and tissues, which exacerbates the immunodeficiency of patients. Thus, the discovery and development of novel anti-cancer drugs are crucial for decreasing premature death as well as for increasing the survival of many populations. In this regard, peptide-based therapeutics have gained much attention as a new drug class since they are considered to be relatively safe, highly selective, possess good tolerability, lower production cost, easy to modify and synthesize while also exhibiting promising pharmacological profiles [4–7]. In the last decade, more than 7000 naturally occurring peptides have been discovered and they are found to exhibit a wide range of bioactivities including tumor homing, antihypertensive, antiparasitic, antiviral, antiangiogenic, antibiofilm, antimicrobial and anticancer [8–10]. Currently, 60 peptide-based drugs have been FDA-approved [11] with preclinical and clinical studies in the pipeline for another 150 peptides [6].

Anticancer peptides (ACPs) are a subset of antimicrobial peptides (AMPs) that are have been shown to exhibit anticancer activities. These peptides are typically made up of short (5–30 amino acids) cationic residues that mostly adopts the -helical structure (e.g., BMAP-27, BMAP-28, Cecropin A and B, LL-37, Magainins etc.) or folds into a β-sheet (e.g., Defensins, Lactoferricin and Tachylepsin I) while extended linear forms (e.g., Tritrpticin and Indolicidin) have also been reported [12,13], as shown in Figure 1.

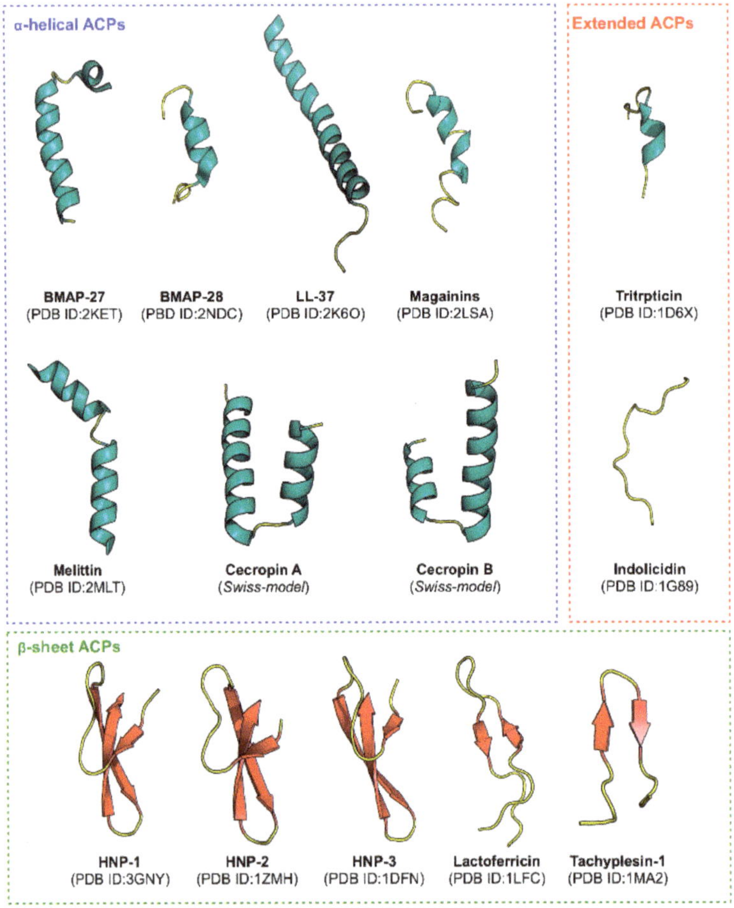

Figure 1. Overview of the structural diversity of three classes of anticancer peptides. Each structure is labeled by its common name followed by the Protein Data Bank (PDB ID) in parenthesis on the subsequent line. In cases where the PDB ID was not available, the SWISS-MODEL server (available at: https://swissmodel.expasy.org/) was used to construct the structure.

In comparison to normal cells, the cancer cell membrane exhibits different properties (i.e., larger surface area due to the higher number of microvili, high negative charge of the cell membrane, higher membrane fluidity, etc.) [14–17]. Thus, the inherent cationic property of ACPs is responsible for the electrostatic interactions between ACPs and the anionic cell membrane of cancer cells, and hence allow the selective killing of cancer cells [18]. Previously, many studies have reported that ACPs display several advantages over small molecule drugs. For instance, they exhibit a shorter half-life that consequently leads to decreased probability of resistance, lowered toxicity (not harming normal cells as much), higher specificity, good solubility as well as good tumor penetration capabilities thereby indicating their great potential in cancer therapy [19–22].

Accurate prediction of ACPs is of great importance for the exploration of their mechanism of action and for the development of therapeutic ACPs. As the experimental identification and development of novel ACPs is a very time-consuming and labor-intensive process, therefore bioinformatics tools are needed for effective analysis of the available big data on existing peptides so as to allow the identification of novel ACPs while also shedding light about their mechanism of action.

Recently, many sequence-based computational methods, for example, AntiCP [23], Hajisharifi et al.'s method [24], ACPP [25], iACP [26], Li and Wang's method [27], iACP-GAEnsC [28], MLACP [29], SAP [30] and TargetACP [31], have been developed using a wide range of machine learning methods and peptide features as summarized in Table 1. In 2014, Hajisharifi et al. [24] established a benchmark dataset spanning 138 experimentally confirmed ACPs (positive dataset) and 227 non-AMPs (negative dataset). In their method, support vector machine (SVM) with pseudo amino acid composition were used for model building and an accuracy of 92.68% were attained. As noticed in Table 1, iACP [26] was the first computational method based on informative features. In this method, Chen et al. utilized a feature selection technique for obtaining an informative feature set subsequently followed by encoding them for constructing an ACP predictor known as iACP [26] via the use of SVM. This method yielded better prediction accuracy (95.06%) than the two previous methods [23,24]. Thusfar, state-of-the-art ACP predictors includes iACP-GAEnsC [28] and TargetACP [31] in which both afforded high prediction accuracies of 96.45% and 98.78%, respectively. The iACP-GAEnsC [28] method follows the concept of evolutionary intelligent genetic algorithm-based ensemble model for improving the true classification rate. iACP-GAEnsC was developed using various classification algorithms (e.g., random forest, *k*-nearest neighbor, support vector machine, generalized neural network and probabilistic neural network) and three types of peptide features (e.g., pseudo g-gap dipeptide composition, amphiphilic pseudo amino acid composition and reduced amino acid alphabet). More recently, Kabir et al. developed the TargetACP [31] for solving the problem of class imbalance presented in the previously described benchmark dataset [24] by integrating sequential and evolutionary-profile information as input features and using SVM as the classifier. In addition, the authors utilized the synthetic minority oversampling technique (SMOTE) to solve the imbalance phenomenon between minority (ACPs) and majority (non-ACPs) samples.

Table 1. Summary of existing methods for predicting anticancer peptides.

Method (Year)	Classifier [a]	Sequence Features [b]	Interpretable	Web Server
AntiCP (2013)	SVM	AAC, DPC, BP	No	✓
Hajisharifi et al. (2014)	SVM	PseACC, LAK	No	
ACPP (2015)	SVM	PRM	No	✓[c]
iACP (2016)	SVM	g-gap DPC	**Yes**	✓
Li and Wang (2016)	SVM	AAC, RACC, acACS	No	
iACP-GAEnsC (2017)	Ensemble method	Pse-g-gap DPC, Am-PseAAC, RACC	No	
MLACP (2017)	RF	AAC, ATC, DPC, PCP	**Yes**	✓
SAP (2018)	SVM	g-gap DPC	No	
TargetACP (2018)	SVM	CPSR, SAAC, PsePSSM	No	
ACPred (this study)	SVM	AAC, DPC, PCP, PseAAC, Am-PseAAC	**Yes**	✓

[a] RF: random forest, SVM: support vector machine. [b] AAC: amino acid composition, ATC: atomic composition, acACS: auto covariance of the average chemical shift, Am-PseAAC: amphiphilic pseudo amino acid composition, BP: binary profile, CPDR: composite protein sequence representation, DPC: dipeptide composition, g-gap DPC: G-Gap dipeptide composition, LAK: local alignment kernel, PCP: Physicochemical properties, PseACC: Pseudo amino acid composition, Pse-g-gap DPC: Pseudo G-Gap dipeptide composition, PRM: protein relatedness measure, RACC: reduce amino acid composition, SAAC: split amino acid composition. [c] The web server is not accessible.

Although, iACP-GAEnsC and TargetACP yielded encouraging performances with reasonably high prediction accuracies, the overall utility of these two methods is limited in terms of interpretability and practical utility thereby warranting further improvements [32]. One of the major limitations of iACP-GAEnsC and TargetACP was that there was no web server provided for these two methods. Therefore, their utility is limited to researchers with informatics background who can develop in-house prediction models. In addition, the underlying mechanisms of the investigated bioactivity for these two methods affords limited interpretability for experimental scientists. Owing to the heterogeneous computational architecture and design of the study as well as differences in the benchmark dataset used, it is not easy to identify and assess which methods and features provided the greatest contribution to good prediction. Motivated by aforementioned issues presented in previous models [32–36], in order to establish an interpretable ACP predictor we propose a systematic effort for the prediction and analysis of anticancer activities of peptides called the ACPred. Firstly, ACPred was built using various types of peptide features and two powerful machine learning algorithms including random forest (RF) and support vector machine (SVM). Secondly, insights into the ACP mechanism of action were attained via the identified important interpretable features and subsequent in-depth analysis pertaining to the underlying biophysical and biochemical properties of anticancer activities of peptides [33,34,36–38]. Thirdly, if-then interpretable rules were extracted using the RF model (IR-ACP). Our prediction results on the benchmark dataset showed that the proposed ACPred achieved an accuracy and MCC of 95.61% and 0.91, respectively, which outperforms most of the existing sequence-based computational methods including Hajisharifi et al.'s method [24], iACP [26], Li and Wang's method [27], iACP-GAEnsC [28], MLACP [29] and SAP [30]. As previously noted, although iACP-GAEnsC and TargetACP boasts good predictive performances but their interpretability and practical utility prompted the development of ACPred. Thus, ACPred is a user-friendly and publicly accessible web server that allow robust predictions to be made without the need to develop in-house prediction models.

2. Materials and Methods

The overall framework of ACPred is illustrated in Figure 2. It can be seen that four major steps are involved in the development of this method as follows: (i) data preparation, (ii) model construction (feature extraction and feature combination), (iii) feature importance analysis and (iv) web server construction. The first step prepares the benchmark dataset, the second step extracts and combines peptide features and the third step analyzes the important features governing ACP prediction via the RF model. Finally, the fourth step involves the construction of a publicly accessible web server using the best model.

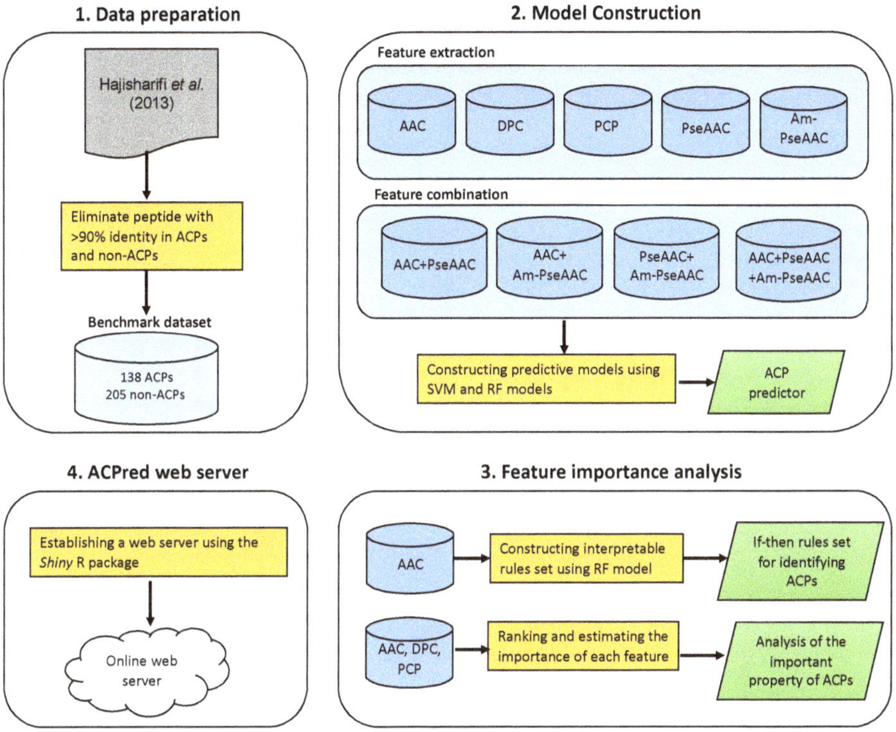

Figure 2. Schematic framework of ACPred.

2.1. Benchmark Dataset

A high-quality benchmark dataset can ensure the reliability of the proposed method. Therefore, the investigated dataset was retrieved from the work of Hajisharifi et al. [24], which contains 192 ACPs and 215 non-ACP. As to guarantee the quality of the benchmark dataset, the following steps were considered. Firstly, in order to avoid a dataset containing redundant peptides, the CD-HIT program was used to eliminate ACPs and non-ACPs with >90% identity. Secondly, ACPs and non-ACP containing special characters, such as X and U, were removed. After such screening procedures, a set of 138 ACPs and 205 non-ACPs was attained for prediction and analysis of ACPs.

2.2. Feature Representation

In order to build an effective prediction model, it is necessary to represent each peptide as numerical vectors that can encompass the perspective of its biophysical and biochemical properties. For peptide or protein sequences, the most classical and interpretable features are amino acid composition (AAC), dipeptide composition (DPC) and physicochemical property (PCP).

According to the classical definition, AAC and DPC are the proportions of each amino acid and dipeptide in a peptide sequence **P** that are expressed as fixed lengths of 20 and 400, respectively. Thus, in terms of AAC and DPC features, a peptide **P** can be expressed by vectors with 20D and 400D (dimension) spaces, respectively, as formulated by the following two equations:

$$\mathbf{P} = [aa_1, aa_2, \ldots, aa_{20}]^T \tag{1}$$

$$\mathbf{P} = [dp_1, dp_2, \ldots, dp_{400}]^T \tag{2}$$

where T is the transpose operator, while $aa_1, aa_2, \ldots, aa_{20}$ and $dp_1, dp_2, \ldots, dp_{400}$ are occurrence frequencies of the 20 and 400 native amino acids and dipeptides, respectively, in a peptide sequence **P**. PCP is one of the most intuitive features associated with biophysical and biochemical reactions. In fact, there are 544 PCPs of amino acids extracted from the amino acid index database (AAindex) [39], which is a collection of published literature as well as different biochemical and biophysical properties of amino acids. Each physicochemical property consists of a set of 20 numerical values for amino acids. After removing 13 PCPs with not applicable (NA) as their amino acid indices, a total of 531 PCPs were further used in this study.

As mentioned in the study of [40–42], the sequence order information of AAC and DPC would be lost. To deal with such a dilemma, the pseudo amino acid composition (PseAAC) and amphiphilic pseudo amino acid composition (Am-PseAAC) approaches were proposed. According to Chou's PseAAC [41], the general form of PseAAC for a peptide **P** is formulated by: where the subscript Ω is an integer to reflect the feature's dimension. The value of Ω and the component of Ψ_u, where $u = 1, 2, \ldots, \Omega$ depends on the protein or peptide sequences. In this study, the parameters of PseAAC, i.e., the discrete correlation factor λ and weight of the sequence information ϖ, were set by default in the protr R package [43]. The dimension of PseAAC feature is 20 + $\lambda \times \varpi$. Since the hydrophobic and hydrophilic properties of proteins play an important role in its folding and interaction of proteins, Am-PseAAC was introduced by Chou [40]. The dimension of Am-PseAAC feature is 20 + 2λ whereby, the first 20 components are the 20 basic AAC ($p_1, p_2, \ldots, p_{20}$) and the next 2λ ones are a set of correlation factors that reveal the physicochemical properties such as hydrophobicity and hydrophilicity along a protein or peptide sequence as formulated by:

$$\mathbf{P} = [\Psi_1, \Psi_2, \ldots, \Psi_u, \ldots, \Psi_\Omega]^T \tag{3}$$

where the subscript Ω is an integer to reflect the feature's dimension. The value of Ω and the component of Ψ_u, where $u = 1, 2, \ldots, \Omega$ depend on the protein or peptide sequences. In this study, the parameters of PseAAC, i.e., the discrete correlation factor λ and weight of the sequence information ϖ, were set by defaults using the protr R package [43]. The dimension of PseAAC feature is $20 + \lambda \times \varpi$. Since hydrophobic and hydrophilic properties play an important role in the folding and interaction of proteins, Am-PseAAC was introduced by Chou [40] for representing such features. The dimension of Am-PseAAC feature is $20 + 2\lambda$ whereby the first 20 components are the 20 basic AAC ($p_1, p_2, \ldots, p_{20}$) while the next 2λ ones are a set of correlation factors that pertains to physicochemical properties namely hydrophobicity and hydrophilicity along a protein or peptide sequence as formulated by:

$$\mathbf{P} = [p_1, p_2, \ldots, p_{20}, p_{20+\lambda}, p_{20+\lambda+1}, \ldots p_{20+2\lambda}]^T \tag{4}$$

In this study, the five aforementioned features of peptide sequences were calculated using the protr package in the R software [43].

2.3. Dataset Modelability

The prediction performances of QSAR models are directly influenced by the dataset and the types of feature used. Recently, the concept of dataset modelability has been proposed by Golbraikh et al. [32,35,44,45] for evaluating the feasibility of developing a robust and predictive model for a given dataset of interest. In this study, the MODI score for each type of peptide features and their combinations were calculated using an in-house developed R code. Prediction models are recommended for further analysis if the MODI score is greater than 0.65; otherwise, prediction models are not recommended. Further details pertaining to the calculation of the MODI score can be found elsewhere [44].

2.4. Classifier Selection

In this study, we employed two successful machine learning algorithms namely random forest (RF) and support vector machine (SVM). Previously, these approaches have been successfully used in the prediction of various functions and properties of peptides and proteins [33,36,38,46–51] as well as other biological or chemical entities [35,45,52–55]. Herein, the basic concepts and associated parameter optimizations for the two classifiers are briefly described hereafter.

RF models were constructed according to the described original RF algorithm [56]. These models were developed by growing many weak classification and regression tree (CART) classifiers where each classifier is generated using a random vector sampled independently from the input vector as to enhance the prediction performance of CART [56,57]. In the RF method, the out-of-bag (OOB) approach is used for evaluating the feature importance as follows: (1) two-thirds of the training data was utilized to construct the predictive classifier while the remaining was used for evaluating the performance of such classifier and (2) the feature importance of each feature can be evaluated by measuring the decrease in the prediction performance. It should be noted that the performance evaluation of the model can be either accuracy or Gini index. Herein, the RF classifier was established using the *randomForest* package in the R software [58]. To enhance the performance of the RF model, two parameters namely, *ntree* (i.e., the number of trees used for constructing the RF classifier) and *mtry* (i.e., the number of random candidate features) were determined using the *caret* package in the R software [59] via a 5-fold cross-validation (5-fold CV) approach. The search space of *ntree* and *mtry* were [100, 500] and [1, 10] using steps of 100 and 1, respectively.

SVM is a supervised learning model based on the principles of structure risk minimization and kernel method as proposed by Vapnik [60–62]. SVM model can deal with the problem of over-fitting arising with the use of a small training dataset by mapping the input samples to a higher dimension space and then searching for the maximum-margin hyperplane for constructing the classifier [63,64]. Previously, SVM models were used in many applications because of their predictive performance capabilities when applied to classification, prediction, and regression problems. In the optimization process, the regularization parameter $C \in \{0.25, 0.50, 1, 2, 4\}$ was determined with a 5-fold CV approach using the *caret* package in the R software [59].

2.5. Identification of Important Features

The analysis and identification of feature importance can provide a better understanding on the underlying biophysical and biochemical properties governing anticancer activities of peptides. Herein, the efficient and effective built-in feature importance estimator of the RF method was used to reveal and characterize differences between ACPs and non-ACPs. As mentioned above, the RF method provides two measures for ranking feature importance, i.e., the mean decrease of the Gini index (MDGI) and the mean decrease of prediction accuracy. Since Calle and Urrea [65] demonstrated that the MDGI provided more robust results when compared with the mean decrease of prediction accuracy, we utilized the MDGI to rank the importance of interpretable features that included AAC, DPC and PCP. Until now, these three features have been used to characterize many peptides and proteins such as for predicting HIV-1 CRF01-AE co-receptor usage [46], predicting protein crystallization [51,66], predicting the oligomeric states of fluorescent proteins [38], predicting the bioactivity of host defense peptides [47], prediction of human leukocyte antigen gene [37,49], predicting antifreeze proteins [33], predicting the hemolytic activity of peptides [34] and predicting the antihypertensive activity of peptides [36].

The MDGI is an impurity measure that corresponds to the ability of each feature in discriminating the sample classes. The Gini index can be defined as follows:

$$1 - \sum_{c=1}^{2} p^2(c|t) \tag{5}$$

where denotes the estimated class probability for node t in a tree classifier and c is the class label (i.e., either ACPs or non-ACPs). Features with the largest MDGI value is considered to be an important feature as it significantly contributes to the prediction performance.

2.6. Rule Extraction

This work presented an interpretable rule extraction of ACPs (IR-ACP) based on the RF method cooperating with AAC features for determining how the features work in combination within the learning process. A set of rules from an individual tree is derived from the root to the leaves. In this study, only 100 decision trees were used to extract if-then interpretable rules for explaining the prediction results by means of the *RRF*, *inTrees* and *xtable* packages in the R software [56,57,67]. More details of the rule extraction process can be found in previous related works [67,68].

2.7. Performance Evaluation

Three testing methods consisting of (i) sub-sampling test (2-, 5- or 10-fold cross-validation), (ii) jackknife test or also known as leave-one-out cross-validation (LOO-CV), and (iii) independent (or external) testing dataset are often used to evaluate the prediction performance. The sub-sampling test is one of the popular cross-validation methods for assess the predictive capability of a model. As elucidated in [41,69] and demonstrated by Equation (50) of [70], among the three cross-validation methods, the jackknife test is considered as one of the most rigorous and objective methods for cross-validation in statistics and can provide a unique result for a given benchmark dataset. Thus, in this study, the 5-fold cross-validation (5-fold CV) and jackknife test were used to evaluate the prediction performance of our models. The former set (5-fold CV) makes use of data from the training set where the data set is separated into five subsets. Practically, one subset from a total of five subsets is left out as the testing set while the remaining are used for training the model. This process is repeated iteratively until all data samples have had the chance to be left out as the testing set. During the jackknifing process, each sample in the dataset (N samples) is left out as an independent sample (one sample) and the remaining sequences (N-1 samples) are used for training the model. This process is repeated iteratively until all samples have had the chance to be left out as the independent sample.

In order to evaluate the prediction ability of the model, the following sets of four metrics are used:

$$Ac = \frac{TP + TN}{(TP + TN + FP + FN)} \tag{6}$$

$$Sn = \frac{TP}{(TP + FN)} \tag{7}$$

$$Sp = \frac{TN}{(TN + FP)} \tag{8}$$

$$MCC = \frac{TP \times TN - FP \times FN}{\sqrt{(TP + FP)(TP + FN)(TN + FP)(TN + FN)}} \tag{9}$$

where Ac, Sn, Sp and MCC represent accuracy, sensitivity, specificity and Matthews coefficient correlation, respectively. TP, TN, FP, and FN represent the instances of true positive, true negative, false positive and false negative, respectively. Moreover, in order to evaluate the prediction performance of models using threshold-independent parameters, receiver operating characteristic (*ROC*) curves were plotted using the pROC package in the R software [71]. The area under the ROC curve (*auAUC*) was used to measure the prediction performance, where *AUC* values of 0.5 and 1 are indicative of perfect and random models, respectively.

2.8. Reproducible Research

To ensure the reproducibility of models proposed herein, all R codes and the benchmark dataset used in the construction of the predictive models, graphical figures and the ACPred web server are available on GitHub at https://github.com/Shoombuatong2527/acpred and https://github.com/chaninlab/acpred-webserver.

3. Results and Discussion

3.1. Prediction Performance

In this study, effort is directed toward the determination of feature types that are beneficial for the prediction of APCs. This was performed by comparing the performance of different feature types as constructed using SVM and RF by means of 5-fold CV and jackknife test. The five basic features consisting of AAC, DPC, PCP, PseAAC and Am-PseAAC were considered as well as their combinations: AAC + PseACC, AAC + Am-PseACC, PseACC + Am-PseACC and AAC + PseACC + Am-PseACC, which were also utilized to investigate the complementarity of the five aforementioned features.

Prior to the development of the predictive model, the assessment of modelability of the benchmark dataset was performed by computing the MODI index. This index helps modelers to estimate the feasibility of obtaining robust and reliable predictive models. For the binary classification problem, if the value of MODI index is greater than 0.65, the feature is considered to be reliable for classification modelling; otherwise, the feature is not recommended for classification modelling.

As shown in Table A1, all feature types and their combinations from the benchmark dataset met these criteria. Thus, it could be stated that our proposed features are reliable and efficient for constructing ACP predictor.

Tables 2 and 3 shows the performance comparison amongst different feature types with RF and SVM on the benchmark dataset via 5-fold CV and jackknife test, respectively. In addition, Figure 3 shows the receiver operating characteristic (*ROC*) curve of the five considered feature sets obtained from RF (top and bottom left) and SVM (top and bottom right) as evaluated by 5-fold CV (top left and right) and jackknife test (bottom left and right). As seen in Tables 2 and 3, SVM model with the Am-PseAAC feature afforded the highest accuracy of 95.03% as evaluated by the jackknife test. Meanwhile, RF model with PseACC feature and SVM model with AAC feature performed well with the second and third the highest accuracy of 93.28% and 92.98%, respectively. These results showed that ACC, PseACC and Am-PseAAC were effective for ACP prediction. Since using a combination of various features might yield better prediction performance, four combinations of the three effective features were also considered. The highest accuracy and *MCC* of 95.61% and 0.91, respectively, was achieved by using SVM model cooperating with the combination feature of AAC and Am-PseAAC, while using the combination of the three effective features, i.e., ACC, PseACC and Am-PseAAC, performed slightly worse than the combination feature of AAC and Am-PseAAC with an accuracy and *MCC* of 94.74% and 0.89, respectively. In addition, our prediction results were well consistent with previous studies [27–29] and related studies [33,34,36,72].

Table 2. Performance comparison of SVM and RF with various types of sequence features over five-fold cross-validation.

Feature	Classifier	*Ac* (%)	*Sn* (%)	*Sp* (%)	*MCC*	*auROC*
AAC	SVM	92.69	83.94	98.54	0.850	0.977
	RF	91.23	92.80	90.32	0.817	0.958
DPC	SVM	83.92	100.00	78.85	0.687	0.942
	RF	87.14	91.89	84.85	0.733	0.944
PCP	SVM	84.80	63.50	99.02	0.698	0.938
	RF	83.63	90.10	80.91	0.661	0.872
PseAAC	SVM	92.98	84.67	98.54	0.856	0.990
	RF	92.11	93.65	91.20	0.835	0.959
Am-PseAAC	SVM	95.03	87.59	100.00	0.899	0.995
	RF	92.40	100.00	88.75	0.848	0.974
AAC + PseAAC	SVM	93.57	85.40	99.02	0.869	0.991
	RF	92.98	96.69	90.95	0.855	0.964
AAC + Am-PseAAC	SVM	95.32	89.05	99.51	0.904	0.994
	RF	93.28	97.50	90.99	0.862	0.969
PseAAC + Am-PseAAC	SVM	94.44	86.86	99.51	0.887	0.994
	RF	92.69	98.28	89.82	0.851	0.967
AAC + PseAAC + Am-PseAAC	SVM	94.15	86.13	99.51	0.881	0.993
	RF	92.98	98.29	90.22	0.857	0.972

Table 3. Performance comparison of SVM and RF with various types of sequence features over jackknife test.

Feature	Classifier	*Ac* (%)	*Sn* (%)	*Sp* (%)	*MCC*	*auROC*
AAC	SVM	92.98	83.94	99.02	0.857	0.978
	RF	91.23	92.80	90.32	0.817	0.959
DPC	SVM	85.09	98.86	80.32	0.706	0.941
	RF	86.84	89.66	85.40	0.725	0.947
PCP	SVM	84.80	63.50	99.02	0.698	0.937
	RF	83.63	88.57	81.44	0.659	0.868
PseAAC	SVM	92.98	84.67	98.54	0.856	0.990
	RF	93.28	97.50	90.99	0.862	0.960
Am-PseAAC	SVM	95.03	87.59	100.00	0.899	0.995
	RF	92.40	99.12	89.08	0.847	0.969
AAC + PseAAC	SVM	93.57	85.40	99.02	0.869	0.990
	RF	93.28	98.31	90.63	0.863	0.962
AAC + Am-PseAAC	SVM	95.61	89.78	99.51	0.910	0.994
	RF	93.57	98.32	91.03	0.869	0.967
PseAAC + Am-PseAAC	SVM	93.86	85.40	99.51	0.875	0.992
	RF	93.57	99.15	90.67	0.870	0.959
AAC + PseAAC + Am-PseAAC	SVM	94.74	87.59	99.51	0.893	0.994
	RF	92.98	99.13	89.87	0.858	0.973

Furthermore, observations pertaining to the performance comparisons from Tables 2 and 3 and Figure 3, it can be briefly summarized as follows. Tables 2 and 3 shows that both RF and SVM models afforded improved prediction performances when using the Am-PseACC feature while the best prediction performance on the benchmark dataset via both 5-fold CV and jackknife test were achieved by the SVM model trained using the combination of AAC and Am-PseAAC features.

For the convenience of subsequent descriptions, we will refer to this method as ACPred as it represents the best model that will be used for further comparisons with other tools.

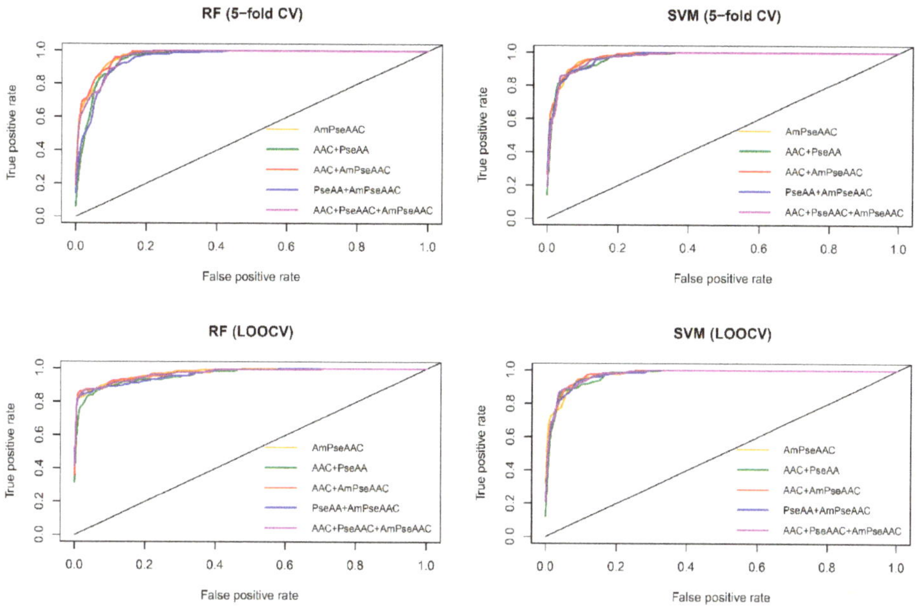

Figure 3. ROC curve of RF (top and bottom left) and SVM (top and bottom right) models as assessed by 5-fold cross-validation (top left and right) and jackknife test or leave-one-out cross-validation (bottom left and right).

3.2. Comparison with Other Methods

To indicate the effectiveness of the proposed method, we compared the performance of our selected model (named ACPred) with other popular ACP predictors. Since Hajisharifi et al. [24] were the first group to establish the benchmark dataset, and iACP [26], iACP-GAEnsC [28] and TargetACP [31] were state-of-the-art ACP predictors that provided prediction results as assessed by the jackknife test, therefore these predictors were used for performance comparisons. Table 4 lists the performance comparisons of ACPred with the three ACP predictors. As noticed from Table 4, prediction results were obtained from two different experimental designs: (i) the prediction model was performed on the benchmark dataset as derived from the work of [24] as well as those of Hajisharifi et al.'s method, iACP, iACP-GAEnsC, TargetACP and ACPred, (ii) the prediction model was built using the balanced dataset including TargetACP and ACPred. The reported results from aforementioned methods as summarized in Table 4 was obtained directly from the work of iACP-GAEnsC [28].

Table 4. Performance comparison of the proposed ACPred model with existing methods.

Method [a]	*Ac (%)*	*Sn (%)*	*Sp (%)*	*MCC*
Hajisharifi et al. [b]	92.68	89.70	85.18	0.78
iACP [b]	95.06	89.86	98.54	0.90
iACP-GAEnsC [b]	96.45	95.36	97.54	0.91
TargetACP [b]	96.22	94.20	97.57	0.92
TargetACP [c]	98.78	99.02	98.54	0.97
ACPred [b]	95.61	89.78	99.51	0.91
ACPred-modified [c]	97.56	96.08	99.02	0.95

[a] Results were reported from the work of TargetACP. [b] Results were performed on the benchmark dataset consisting of 138 ACPs and 205 non-ACPs. [c] Results were performed on the balanced dataset consisting of 205 ACPs and 205 non-ACPs by using the SMOTE technique on the benchmark dataset.

As for performance comparisons on the benchmark dataset, it was found that ACPred was comparable with that of iACP-GAEnsC and TargetACP as indicated by four statistical parameters. Moreover, ACPred yielded a greater prediction performance than the method proposed by Hajisharifi et al. and iACP. To the best of our knowledge, iACP-GAEnsC is the only method that utilizes the synthetic minority oversampling technique (SMOTE) [73] technique for constructing a balanced dataset from the original benchmark dataset [24]. From the perspectives of machine learning, it is not fair to directly compare prediction results between TargetACP and ACPred because TargetACP was trained and tested on the balanced dataset consisting of 205 ACPs and 205 non-ACPs. In order to perform a fair comparison, the herein proposed ACPred method was applied on the balanced dataset (called ACPred-modified), which was generated by means of the SMOTE technique. Herein, the oversampling method was used to add synthetic samples for the minority class (i.e., ACPs) presented in the benchmark dataset by setting the parameters of the number of nearest neighbours (k), the number of extra cases (oversampling) to add to the minority class (perc.over) and the number of cases to reduce (undersampling) from the majority class (perc.under) were set to 9, 50 and 300, respectively. As seen in Table 4, ACPred-modified was found to outperform Hajisharifi et al.'s method, iACP and iACP-GAEnsC with an improvement of 2%–4% and 3%–7% on *Ac* and *MCC*, respectively. However, it was observed that ACPred-modified performed slightly worse than TargetACP by approximately 2%–3% where ACPred-modified and TargetACP provided 97.56% *Ac*/0.95 *MCC* and 98.78% *Ac*/0.97 *MCC*, respectively. Nevertheless, TargetACP was constructed with a sophisticated design thus, it is not easy to identify and assess which features offer the most contribution to the prediction improvement. On the other hand, ACPred was designed in a systematic manner for prediction and characterization of anticancer activities of peptides. In addition, a user-friendly web server ACPred was developed to facilitate high-throughput prediction of ACP. Therefore, the proposed ACPred model could become a practical tool for predicting and interpreting the anticancer activity of peptides, or at least as a complementary tool to existing methods in the field.

Thinking to the future, some possible improvements that could enhance the prediction performance for predicting anticancer activity of peptides are described hereafter. Firstly, it is worthy to explore the separation of peptides according to their sequence lengths (e.g., peptides having 4, 5 or 6 amino acids, peptides having 7–12 amino acids, and peptides having more than 12 amino acids) followed by the development of separate predictive models for each of the five sequence range [36,74]. Secondly, extract 5, 10 and 15 amino acids from the N or C terminus for the development of predictive QSAR models, which has successfully been demonstrated by the group of P.S. Raghava [23] Thirdly, explore the modelability of the dataset using the approach of Golbraikh et al. [44] such that robust models could be developed. Fourthly, the currently employed non-anticancer peptides [24] are not based on true experimentally-determined inactive peptides but are random peptides obtained from the UniProt database therefore, if such true inactive peptides could be determined they may aid in the development of robust models.

Aside from the aforementioned methodological improvements that have been witnessed from the literature in the development of anticancer peptide classifiers, however, the underlying origin of anticancer activity of investigated peptides as rationalized by peptide features is an area that deserves more attention. Current predictive models used for the prediction of anticancer activity of peptides are primarily based on sequence order-independent descriptors that does not consider the order of amino acids in a peptide sequence (e.g., AAC and DPC), which hampers the identification of motifs from peptides. Such limitation has been addressed by the group of KC Chou [41,75,76] in which they developed PseAAC and Am-PseAAC descriptors that take into account sequence order information based on physicochemical properties. However, the interpretability of these descriptors is limited and thus, existing approaches for rationalizing biological interpretation from these predictive models are resorted back to the sequence order-independent descriptors such as AAC and DPC. Analysis of the literature revealed that interpretable descriptors such as the z-scale descriptors [77,78] have been successful for predicting robust and interpretable models, however the flaw of this approach is that the peptides used in the development of the model should be of equal length so as to conduct sequence alignment. Methodological tweaks addressing such limitation have been made via the use of autocorrelation such that sequence alignment is not needed and would allow the models to be built on peptides of varied lengths. In spite of this, this method is not applicable in this study field in which the prepared dataset removes peptides having high similarity of greater than 90% therefore, rendering the removal of a large number of peptides that is normally needed when using *z*-scale descriptors. As such, there is ample room for the discovery of new and interpretable descriptors for the development of predictive models of peptides, which is an important area for further driving the field of anticancer peptide prediction.

3.3. Biological Space

The identification of feature importance from AAC and DPC descriptors can provide a better understanding on the biochemical and biophysical properties of anticancer activities of peptides. Previously, AAC and DPC features have been analyzed as to further gain insights on how to characterize therapeutic peptides [29,34,36,47] and protein functions [33,51,79]. In this study, the value of MDGI was adopted to rank and estimate the importance of each AAC and DPC feature. Such information is derived from the analysis of the benchmark dataset that consists of 138 ACPs and 205 non-ACPs. Table 5 lists the percentage values of the 20 amino acids for both ACPs and non-ACPs along with amino acid composition difference between the two classes as well as their MDGI values. In addition, a heatmap showing the feature importance for DPC features is shown in Figure 4. From Table 5, it can be observed that the ten informative amino acids with the highest MDGI values are Lys, Cys, Gln, Arg, Ile, Leu, His, Pro, Glu and Gly (29.54, 19.71, 15.89, 11.42, 10.13, 7.84, 7.80, 7.37, 6.88 and 6.56, respectively). Meanwhile, Figure 4 shows that the 20 top-ranked dipeptides according to their MDGI value are KK, KI, CY, IK, AK, KV, IP, LK, TC, SC, CG, LF, FK, GL, FL, LR, PP, LG, IG and AQ. Interestingly, among the 5 top-ranked informative amino acids, 3 of these are polar (i.e., Lys, Gln and Arg), while 2 are non-polar (i.e., Cys and Ile) and hydrophobic residues. In addition, Lys and Arg are also positively-charged residues, which may support the anti-cancer cell penetrating properties of peptides (i.e., that is required for targeting tumors with specificity and low toxicity) [80]. Although the percentage compositions differentiating ACPs from non-ACPs as presented in Table 5 highlight that ACPs a have higher percentage of polar residues and lower percentage of basic residues as compared to non-ACPs, cell surface binding and internalization are critical for specific targeting of cells with anti-cancer activities. According to the membrane of cancer cells presenting anionic molecules such as phosphatidyl serine (PS), heparin sulfate and O-glycosylated mucins, the ACPs that contain positive charge are critical for endocytosis and selectively killing cancer cells. While hydrogen bonds that appear on ACPs were designed for improving the solubilization of hydrophobic molecules on ACPs. However, positively charged amino acids alone are not enough to completely neutralize cancer cells but rather aid in rapid internalization of cancer cells for selective killing with low toxicity to normal cells. Moreover, hydrogen bonded interactions to encapsulate anti-cancer drugs has been utilized for increasing the oral efficiency and drug-controlled release. Therefore, only hydrogen bond on ACPs are not adequate to resist cancer cells. Thus, the combination between crucial amino acids and physicochemical properties could provide a synergistic effect that enhances the efficiency of ACPs [81]. As such, results from the analysis of the top ranked informative AAC are discussed below.

Table 5. Amino acid compositions (%) of anticancer and non-anticancer peptides along with their difference as well as MDGI values. The rank of each amino acid amongst their 20 amino acids are shown in parenthesis for AAC difference and MDGI.

Amino Acid	ACP (%)	Non-ACP (%)	Difference	*p*-Value	MDGI
A-Ala	7.623	11.005	−3.383 (7)	<0.05	6.41 (11)
C-Cys	3.906	8.015	−4.109 (5)	<0.05	19.71 (2)
D-Asp	2.417	3.418	−1.002 (15)	<0.05	3.85 (15)
E-Glu	1.707	3.523	−1.816 (12)	<0.05	6.88 (9)
F-Phe	6.823	2.41	4.413 (2)	<0.05	6.12 (12)
G-Gly	1.975	4.123	−2.148 (11)	<0.05	6.56 (10)
H-His	1.536	5.798	−4.262 (4)	<0.05	7.80 (7)
I-Ile	10.072	6.98	3.092 (9)	<0.05	10.13 (5)
K-Lys	2.542	1.651	0.892 (17)	0.086	29.54 (1)
L-Leu	8.099	3.739	4.36 (3)	<0.05	7.84 (6)
M-Met	9.831	13.888	−4.057 (6)	<0.05	4.34 (14)
N-Asn	11.497	3.964	7.533 (1)	<0.05	4.98 (13)
P-Pro	0.905	2.224	−1.319 (13)	<0.05	7.37 (8)
Q-Gln	5.385	2.711	2.674 (10)	<0.05	15.89 (3)
R-Arg	4.211	7.495	−3.283 (8)	<0.05	11.42 (4)
S-Ser	6.537	5.832	0.705 (19)	0.245	3.50 (16)
T-Thr	3.781	4.704	−0.923 (16)	0.098	3.13 (17)
V-Val	2.258	1.560	0.698 (20)	0.083	2.96 (18)
W-Trp	2.244	1.423	0.821 (18)	<0.05	2.51 (20)
Y-Tyr	6.65	5.539	1.111 (14)	0.091	2.90 (19)

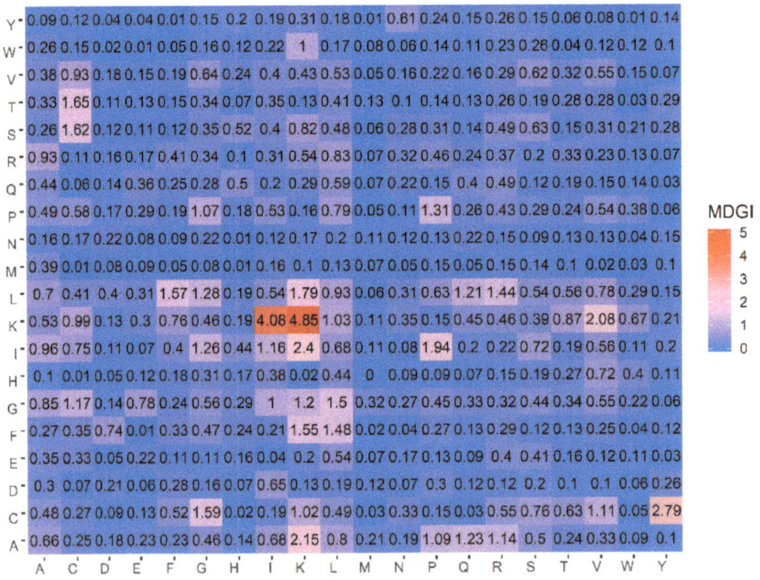

Figure 4. Heat map of the mean decrease of Gini index of dipeptide compositions.

To roughly analyze the characteristics of ACPs, a few studies have shed light on important amino acids and dipeptides commonly found in ACPs by using simple composition analysis approaches without the use of experimental methods. For instance, Tyagi et al. [23] reported results of residue preference at 10 N-terminus and 10 C-terminus by using the sequence logos. Their analysis revealed that Leu and Lys were typically found at the N-terminus while Cys, Leu and Lys were typically found at the C-terminus. Chen et al. [26] also confirmed that amino acids including Lys, Ile, Cys, Glu, and Gly were abundant in ACPs as compared to non-ACPs. Recently, Manavalan et al. [29] revealed that the three top-ranked informative dipeptides consisted of KK, AK and KL. As can be noticed in Table 5 and Figure 4, our analysis results derived from the MDGI values of AAC and DPC were quite consistent with the three aforementioned studies.

As mentioned above, amongst the five top-ranked informative amino acids, Lys had the highest MDGI value of 29.54. Such feature with the highest MDGI is considered to be the most important factor governing the anticancer activity. As a basic residue, Lys is highly conserved in the composition of therapeutic peptides as it enhances the formation of electrostatic interactions between the peptide and the plasma membrane owing to its cationicity [82]. The role of cationicity in ACPs have been previously investigated by the study of Gopal et al. [83]. The authors modified a synthetic AMP known as HPA3NT3 (FKRLKKLFKKIWNWK), which was derived from Helicobacter pylori by substituting Arg and Asn with Lys at positions 3 and 13, respectively. Gopal et al. reported that the Lys-modified peptide increased the peptide selectivity toward negatively-charged membrane surface, which could allow for endocytosis and specificity of the APC in killing cancer cells. In addition, Wang et al. [84] has shown that the cell-penetrating ability is critical for specifically targeting cationic cancer cells. The authors observed that a Lys-rich peptide, L-K6 (IKKILSKIKKLLK-NH2) could internalize into MCF-7 cells without significant cell surface disruption. Interestingly, the authors also found that the internalized L-K6 could induce MCF-7 cell death without significant cytoskeleton disruption and mitochondrial impairment. Moreover, these findings indicated that the negatively-charged phosphatidylserine (PS) reported to be abundantly exposed on cancer cell surfaces [85,86] might contribute to the preferential binding of L-K6 to MCF-7 cancer cells. Furthermore, defensins are a large subfamily of natural cationic human AMP showing anticancer properties. Their roles in the immunomodulation of the innate and adaptive immune system have extensively been studied in previous works [87,88]. Defensins are categorized as either α-defensins or β-defensins, depending on their sequence homology and Cys connectivity (Figure 1), they are found to be rich in cationic residues (e.g., Lys and Arg) that enhances their immunomodulatory effects [89]. Papo et al. [90] constructed a short 15 amino acid peptide consisting of D- or L- amino acids (D-K_6L_9; LKLLKKLLKKLLKLL-NH2) and observed that D-K_6L_9 specifically targets and lyses cancer cells as well as inhibiting the growth of primary and metastatic tumors in in vivo models. The ability of D-K_6L_9 in selectively targeting cancer cells can be attributed to its cationicity whereby the peptide can bind to highly enriched surface-exposed PS in cancer cells as compared to non-cancer cells [91]. Similarly, Arg, which is a positively-charged residue that differs from Lys by its side chain, was shown to be the fourth informative amino acid form our analysis thus, reiterating the importance of the cationic property of APCs.

The second most important amino acid was Cys that afforded an MDGI value of 19.71. Cys is a highly reactive amino acid in which it contains a thiol group that is oxidized to form a dimer thus creating a disulfide bridge between two spatially adjacent Cys residues. The significance of disulfide bridges are seen in their strong, hydrophobic nature which are extremely important for the overall structural fold of the peptide, while also increasing the peptide stability against proteolytic degradation [92]. Almost a decade ago, GO-201 ($[R]_9$CQCRRKNYGQLDIFP) achieved in facilitating the inhibition of mucin-1 cytoplasmic domain (MUC1-CD) [93]. Thus far, many studies have established the function of the GO-201 peptide whereby its anticancer activity was demonstrated both in vitro and in vivo against human breast cancer, prostate cancer, chronic myelogenous leukemia and pancreatic cancer [93–96]. From these aforementioned studies, the researchers were able to determine key motifs responsible for the anticancer activity of GO-201 as CxC, thus reiterating the crucial role of Cys disulfide bridges [97]. Furthermore, Tyuryaeva et al. [98] explored the molecular mechanism of Cys-induced cytotoxicity and the resulting apoptosis of cancer cells by designing and testing peptide sequences containing the key CxC ($[R]_9$KCGCFF; named DIL) or CxxC ($[R]_9$FF**C**PH**C**YQ; named DOL) motifs. The results obtained from this study suggests that the disulfide oxidoreductase is responsible for the effective cytotoxic action of Cys. Therefore, it can be inferred that peptides containing the CxC or CxxC motifs form disulfide bridges that pilot a partial loss of protein function and the rapid onset of apoptosis. It can therefore be anticipated that such peptide sequences could help to create a potentially valuable new class of ACPs. Similarly, Schroeder et al. [99] ascertained a novel peptide GKAKCCK having pronounced antimicrobial activity. The authors discovered that the efficiency of this peptide was critically dependent on the two continuous cysteines and that upon mutating these residues to Ala or Ser, its activity was completely abrogated. Hence, given the well-established connection between antimicrobial and anticancer peptides [13,100], it is likely that the GKAKCCK peptide is able to induce antitumorigenic effects.

3.4. Mechanistic Interpretation of Informative PCP

The physicochemical properties of amino acids play an essential role as effective features for identifying and characterizing protein or peptide functions from their primary sequences [33,34,36,51,79]. It is well known that PCPs [39], such as molecular volume, exposure or accessible surface, polarity (hydrophobicity/hydrophilicity), charge/pK, hydrogen-bonding potential and so forth are correlated with the structure and function of the amino acid sequence [101]. Herein, we have obtained the ten top-ranked informative PCPs corresponding to their MDGI values as shown in Table 6.

Table 6. Ten top-ranked physiocochemical properties from the AAindex having the highest MDGI values.

Rank	AAindex	Categorized Property	Description	MDGI
1	ARGP820101	Hydrophobicity	Hydrophobicity index (Argos et al., 1982)	1.51
2	ARGP820102	Hydrophobicity	Signal sequence helical potential (Argos et al., 1982)	1.40
3	BHAR880101	Hydrophobicity	Average flexibility indices (Bhaskaran-Ponnuswamy, 1988)	1.08
4	ARGP820103	Hydrophobicity	Membrane-buried preference parameters (Argos et al., 1982)	1.04
5	BEGF750102	Beta propensity	Conformational parameter of beta-structure (Beghin-Dirkx, 1975)	1.00
6	BEGF750101	Alpha and turn propensities	Conformational parameter of inner helix (Beghin-Dirkx, 1975)	0.92
7	BIGC670101	Physicochemical properties	Residue volume (Bigelow, 1967)	0.91
8	BEGF750103	Alpha and turn propensities	Conformational parameter of beta-turn (Beghin-Dirkx, 1975)	0.87
9	BIOV880102	Hydrophobicity	Information value for accessibility; average fraction 23% (Biou et al., 1988)	0.85
10	ISOY800107	Hydrophobicity	Normalized relative frequency of double bend (Isogai et al., 1980)	0.83

The most important PCP is seen to be 'hydrophobicity' with an MDGI value of 1.51, which corresponds to the AAindex ARGP820101. In addition, from the analysis, 4 of the 10 top-ranked informative PCPs are related to α-helix properties of peptides consisting of ARGP820102, BEGF750101, ISOY800106 and CHOP780201 with corresponding MDGI values of 1.40, 0.92, 0.64 and 0.61, respectively. Furthermore, 3 of 10 top-ranked informative PCPs including the AAindices of BEGF750102, BEGF750103 and CHOP780101 are related to β-sheet properties with MDGI values of 1.00, 0.87 and 0.83, respectively. Consequently, it could be inferred that the hydrophobicity of a peptide along with its structural orientation (i.e., α-helix or β-sheet) are significant in determining the anticancer properties of peptides. The important PCPs of ACPs are analyzed and discussed below.

3.4.1. Hydrophobic Residues on α-Helical Structure Enhances Cell Penetrating Properties of Anticancer Peptides

It is commonly known that the hydrophobicity property is critical for the 3D structure of a protein. Many descriptors have been developed for measuring the hydrophobicity of proteins, depending on the presence of hydrophobic residues at specific locations in the peptide sequence. These indices are usually based on the 3D crystal structure of proteins coupled with the physicochemical properties of their side chains [102,103]. For instance, Argos et al. [104] utilized the hydrophobic index as measured by Nozaki and Tanford [105] for the 20 canonical amino acids for determining the role of hydrophobicity on the structure of amino acids. As mentioned above, the property of ARGP820101 with an MDGI value of 1.51 pertained to the hydrophobicity property. This result suggests that the presence of hydrophobic amino acid residues on the α-helix might be important for governing the anticancer activity of peptides. Moreover, the property of ARGP820103 (the fourth most important PCPs) is also associated with hydrophobicity property. Many previous studies have described the need for symbiosis between hydrophobicity and cationicity of peptides in order to enhance its cell penetrating property and its ability to reach target cell as to exert its effects [106–109]. In addition, researchers have made efforts to assess the influence of hydrophobicity on anticancer effects. For instance, Huang et al. [108] systematically altered the hydrophobicity of a 26-residue α-helical peptide (peptide **P**; KWKSFLKTFKSAKKTVLHTALKAISS) by replacing Ala residues with the more hydrophobic Leu residues as to increase its hydrophobicity or by changing Leu residues to Ala residues as to decrease its hydrophobicity. On the basis of these results, the authors observed a correlation between higher hydrophobic variants whereby the Leu-substituted peptides (A12L and A20L) exhibited greater anticancer activity against cancer cells with higher IC_{50} values than peptide P. Thus, peptides with higher hydrophobicity are assumed to penetrate deeper into the hydrophobic core of the cell membrane, thereby causing pores or channels on the cancer cell membrane and exhibiting greater anticancer activity. From these results, it can be inferred that the presence of hydrophobic residues on the α-helical structure of ACPs can enhance its anticancer properties.

3.4.2. Peptides Forming an Amphipathic α-Helix Contributes to Anticancer Activity

Interestingly, four of the ten top-ranked informative PCPs consisting of ARGP820102, BEGF750101, ISOY800106 and CHOP780201 described helical properties of peptides such as helical potential [104], inner helix [110], frequency of helix end [111] and frequency of α-helix [112], respectively, as shown in Table 6. This supports the notion that the helical structure plays a principal role in governing the anticancer property of peptides. In addition, the α-helical conformation as adopted by many ACPs in biological membranes, is now regarded as a key determinant of anticancer activity [113]. BMAP-27 (GRFKRFRKKFKKLFKKLSPVIPLLHL) and BMAP-28 (GGLRSLGRKILRAWKKY GPIIVPIIRI) are well-known peptides derived from bovine sources having a cationic NH_2 terminal that forms an amphipathic α-helix. They exert their cytotoxic activity against human leukemia cells by enhancing membrane permeability, which allows for an influx of Ca++ ions, thereby leading to apoptosis via DNA fragmentation [114]. In addition, the structures of Cecropin A (KWKLFKKIEKVGQNIRDGIIKAGPAVAVVGQATQIAK) and Cecropin B (KWKVFKKIEKMGRNIRNGIVKAGPAIAVLGEAKAL), which were first derived from insects, primarily consisted of two α-helix [115,116] while its amphipathic N-terminal (i.e., that is capable of interacting with anionic membrane components) is responsible for mediating the cytotoxic activity against cancer cells. On the other hand, the C-terminal is hydrophobic and it is postulated to facilitate peptide entry into the membrane thereby enabling oligomerization to occur, which subsequently leads to leakage of cell components due to pore formation and eventual cell death [117]. In addition, Srisailam et al. [118] designed a custom lytic peptide by modifying the cecropin B (CB) to contain two identical hydrophobic segments on both the N and the C terminals, thus disrupting its normal α-helical structure. The resulting peptide CB-3, was unable to effectively lyse cell membranes on cancer cells as well as bacterial cells as compared to the control peptide, therefore highlighting the significance of the peptide structure on its function. Interestingly, Moore et al. [119] uncovered that CB exhibited anticancer activities when tested against colon adenocarcinoma cells in vivo and cytotoxicity against multidrug-resistant breast and ovarian cancer cell lines in vitro.

Similarly, Magainins isolated from the skin of *Xenopus laevis* is comprised of a α-helical secondary structure with separate cationic and hydrophobic faces. Magainin-2 (GIGKFLHSAKKFGKAFVGEIMNS) causes lysis of both hematopoietic and solid tumor cell lines as while observing selective cytotoxic activity against several human bladder cell lines [120]. In addition, it was perceived using florescence spectrometry that magainins could lyse tumor cells by forming ion-conducting α-helical channels in the cancer cell membrane [121]. Melittin (GIGAVLKVLTTGLPALISWIKRKRQQ) is another well-known ACP that is derived from the venom of European honeybee (*Apis mellifera*) [122]. The N-terminal region of melittin is largely hydrophobic whereas the C-terminal contains positively-charged amino acid residues.

Melittin form channels in lipid bilayers and is lytic against both cancer cells and normal cells [123]. Self-association of amphipathic α-helical monomers of melittin is largely suggested to be responsible for perturbations of membrane integrity thereby leading to cellular lysis via the barrel stave mechanism [124]. Furthermore, the only human cathelicidin-derived cationic ACP to date, LL-37 (LLGDFFRKSKEKIGKEFKRIVQRIKDFLRNLVPRTES) is present throughout the body and assumes a α-helical conformation that is comprised of both cationic and hydrophobic faces oriented in a parallel manner with lipid membranes. As such these peptides are suggested to engage in a carpet-like mechanism for its cytotoxicity [125]. However, unlike other ACPs, LL-37 is toxic to eukaryotic cells at slightly higher concentrations and thus lacks the selectivity of an ACP. Nevertheless, Okumura et al. [126] showed that a C-terminal fragment of LL-37 (hCAP18) was able to induce mitochondrial depolarization and apoptosis in human oral squamous carcinoma cells but not in healthy human gingival fibroblasts and human keratinocyte cells. In summary, it is evident that the amphipathicity associated with certain α-helical structures is pivotal for the elicitation of peptide anticancer activities.

3.4.3. Peptides Forming β-Sheet Are Vital to Peptide Structure and Contribute to Anticancer Activity

As seen in Table 6, 3 out of the 20 top-ranked informative PCPs pertain to β-sheet structure (i.e., BEGF750102, BEGF750103 and CHOP78010) which correspond to properties such as conformational parameter of β-structure, conformational parameter of β-turn and normalized frequency of β-turn [110], respectively. Although, most of the well-known APCs are α-helical structures, some β-sheet ACPs have also been extensively studied. Many studies showed that defensins contain a group of closely related Cys-Arg rich cationic peptides. Out of these, human α- and β-defensins remain the most studied, comprising of six conserved Cys residues that form three intramolecular disulfide bridges between the N-terminal and the C-terminal regions of the peptide [127,128]. In the studies of [129,130], human neutrophil peptides (HNPs) -1 (ACYCRIPACIAGERRYGTCIYQGRLWAFCC), -2 (CYCRIPACIAGERRYGTCIYQGRLWAFCC) and -3 (DCYCRIPACIAGERRYGTCIY QGRLWAFCC) were shown to possess cytotoxic effects against several human and mouse tumor cells such as human B-lymphoma cells, human oral squamous carcinoma cells, and mouse teratocarcinoma cells. HNPs were also shown to kill cancer cells through membrane binding mediated by electrostatic interactions, followed by rapid collapse of the membrane potential and loss of membrane integrity [130,131]. In addition, Mader et al. [100,132] reported that bovine lactoferricin (LfcinB; FKCRRWQWRMKKLGAPSITCVRRAF) isolated from cow's milk, represents a cationic ACP with amphipathic β-sheet configuration displaying anticancer activity against leukemia cells and various other carcinomas [100,132]. Moreover, LfcinB not only exerts its action by inducing apoptosis through direct disruption of the mitochondrial membrane, but is also capable of lysing the membrane itself, depending on the cancer cell type [133,134].

Furthermore, isolated from the hemocytes of horseshoe crab (*Tachypleus tridentatus*), the ACP tachyplesin I (KWCFRVCYRGICYRRCR) is arranged in two anti-parallel β-sheets that are held in place by two disulfide bonds [135]. Chen et al. [136] discovered that tachyplesin I killed cancer cells in a unique way by binding to hyaluronan on human prostate carcinoma cells, as well as to the C1q complement component in human serum, leading to the activation of the classical immune complement pathway. As a result, complement-mediated lysis of tachyplesin I-coated cancer cells was achieved. In a separate study, Adamia et al. [137] observed that the binding activity of tachyplesin I to C1q was dependent on its secondary structure which consists of two disulfide bonds formed by Cys residues at positions 3–16 and 7–12. Previously it has also been demonstrated that, the deletion of Cys residues from tachyplesin I altered its β-sheet structure to that of a linear form thus, disrupting its activity [138]. Therefore, from the aforementioned studies, it can be postulated that β-sheet is vital for maintaining the stability of peptide structures. As noticed in Table 5, our result of informative amino acids is consistent with the above-mentioned studies, where Cys is the second most important amino acid having a MDGI value of 19.71.

Nevertheless, further research is necessary to determine the key amino acids that could transform non-ACPs into ACPs and thus, allow the generation of a library of potentially novel ACPs. The design of effective ACPs from non-ACPs could possibly be based on the improvement of physicochemical properties, like hydrophobicity, positive charge, replacing the amino acid used or adding a functional motif with better activity towards the targeted cancer cells. In that regard, Tada et al. [139] revealed that the replacement of amino acid His to Arg in epidermal growth factor receptor (EGFR) binding peptide increased its anti-tumor activity via stronger binding affinity to the EGFR on cancer cells. Furthermore, the utilization of a motif containing the amino acids Trp, Met and Trp (WMW) was able to sensitize apoptosis and reduce the migratory effect on cancer cells which in turn could synergize the anti-cancer activity of peptides [140]. Therefore, it is of paramount importance to explore this area further.

3.5. Interpretable Rules Acquisition Obtained from the RF Model

Interpretable rules crucial for discriminating ACPs from non-ACPs were derived from the RF model built using AAC features on the benchmark dataset known as IR-ACP. The main advantages of these constructed rules are two folds: (i) to demonstrate which amino acid or which combination of amino acids are effective for ACP prediction, and (ii) to simply discriminate ACPs from non-ACPs without the need to go through the mathematical and computational details. Tables 7 and A2 shows the twenty interpretable rules that were important for ACPs and eleven that were important for non-ACPs.

Table 7. Eight if-then rules for the prediction of anticancer peptides using random forest and amino acid composition.

No.	Rule	Covered Samples	Misclassified Sample	Ac (%)
1	$G > 0.041$ and $I > 0.0615$ and $L \leq 0.1715$ and $K > 0.0385$ and $M \leq 0.027$	48	1	97.92
2	$R \leq 0.0515$ and $Q \leq 0.026$ and $K > 0.094$	48	1	97.92
3	$C > 0.1145$ and $P \leq 0.073$	35	0	100.00
4	$L \leq 0.093$ and $F > 0.0715$ and $S \leq 0.152$	33	4	87.88
5	$A \leq 0.0145$ and $Q \leq 0.026$	26	4	84.62
6	$R \leq 0.0665$ and $E \leq 0.044$ and $H > 0.052$	21	4	80.95
7	$I > 0.108$ and $K > 0.055$	42	6	85.71
8	$E \leq 0.0545$ and $G > 0.0365$ and $K > 0.108$ and $M \leq 0.04$	49	1	97.96

Table 7 presents eight interpretable rules that were important for identifying ACPs and each rule comprises a different number of criteria. If a query peptide meets all of the criteria in at least one of the eight rules, then it will be predicted as an ACP. As observed in Table 7, four rules afforded a prediction accuracy larger than 95%, namely rules #1, #2, #3 and #8, while the remaining rules provided acceptable results with accuracy ranging between 80.79% and 87.88%. These results indicated that the constructed rules are robust, both in terms of their accuracy and interpretability for predicting and characterizing ACPs.

3.6. ACPred Web Server

In order to make the prediction model presented herein a practical tool that can be widely used by the scientific community, we have constructed a web server called the ACPred using the best model as described in previous sections. The web interface has been established using the Shiny package under the R programming environment. The web server is freely accessible at http://codes.bio/acpred/. Screenshots of the ACPred web server is shown in Figure 5 in which panel A shows the web server prior to submission of input data and panel B shown the web server after the prediction has been made.

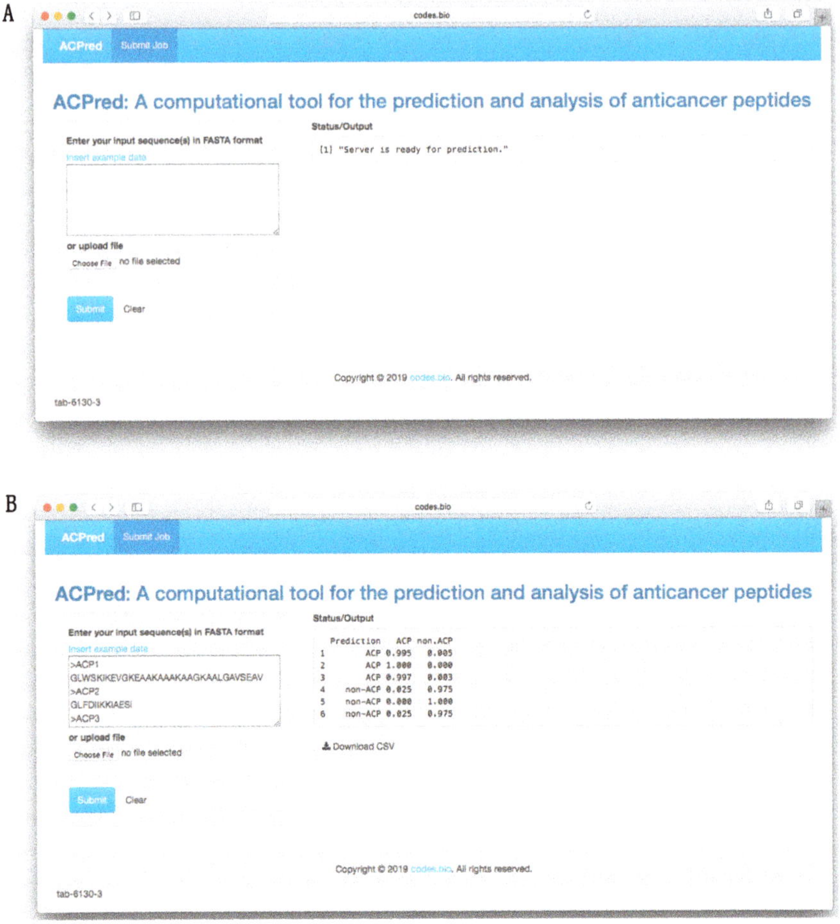

Figure 5. Screenshots of the ACPred web server before (**A**) and after (**B**) submission of sequence data for prediction.

Briefly, a step-by-step guide on using the web server is given below:

- Step 1. Enter the following URL into the web browser, http://codes.bio/acpred/.
- Step 2. Either enter the query peptide sequence into the Input box or upload the sequence file by clicking on the "Choose file" button (i.e., found below the "Enter your input sequence(s) in FASTA format heading").
- Step 3. Click on the "Submit" button to initiate the prediction process.
- Step 4. Prediction results are automatically displayed in the grey box found below the "Status/Output" heading. Typically, it takes a few seconds for the server to process the task. Users can also download the prediction results as a CSV file by pressing on the "Download CSV button".

Additionally, users can also run a local copy of ACPred on their own computer by using the following one-line code in an R environment:

shiny::runGitHub('acpred-webserver', 'chaninlab')

However, prior to running the aforementioned code, it is recommended that users first install the prerequisite R packages. This can be performed by using the following code:

```
install.packages(c('shiny', 'shinyjs', 'shinythemes', 'protr', 'seqinr', 'caret', 'markdown'))
```

4. Conclusions

There is increasing evidence indicating that ACPs could be a potential, valuable therapeutic agent for cancer treatment. With the avalanche of peptide sequences generated from many sources, there is significant demand for computational methods that can support the timely discrimination of ACPs from other peptides, as well as offer insights from analysis using only their primary sequences. In this study, we have developed a the ACPred model in a systematic manner by taking advantage of two powerful machine learning methods consisting of support vector machine (SVM) and random forest (RF) for the prediction and characterization of anticancer activities of peptides. The best model for further development of ACPred was achieved by using the SVM method coupled with the combination of amino acid composition and pseudo amino acid composition features. By comparing with the state-of-the-art method, the TargetACP, it was found that the performance of ACPred was comparable to that of TargetACP (95.61% vs. 96.22% accuracies) as assessed by the rigorous jackknife test. Moreover, the feature importance analysis and interpretable rules extraction were carried out by using the RF model to identify which feature was the most important in predicting ACPs while also providing a better understanding of the anticancer activities of investigated peptides. Results from model interpretation revealed that the hydrophobic residues on the α-helical structure, Cys residues on the β-sheet structure and the formation of amphipathic α-helix played a crucial role in the anticancer activity of the investigated peptides. Finally, a web server named ACPred was established and made freely available online at https://codes.bio/acpred/.

Author Contributions: W.S. conceived, designed, performed and analyzed the experiments. N.S. and C.N. analyzed the data. W.S., N.S. and V.P. drafted the manuscript. W.S. and C.N. contributed the code for constructing the web server. C.N. vetted the manuscript. All authors read and approved the manuscript.

Funding: This work is supported by the Office of Higher Education Commission and the Thailand Research Fund (No. MRG6180226); the New Researcher Grant (A31/2561) from Mahidol University; and the Center of Excellence on Medical Biotechnology (CEMB), the S&T Postgraduate Education and Research Development Office (PERDO) and the Office of Higher Education Commission (OHEC), Thailand.

Acknowledgments: We thank the reviewers for their great comments.

Conflicts of Interest: The authors declare no conflict of interest.

Appendix A

Table A1. Summary of MODI index as derived from various types of peptide features on the benchmark dataset.

Feature	MODI
AAC	0.868
DPC	0.836
PCP	0.722
PseAAC	0.859
Am-PseAAC	0.859
AAC + PseAAC	0.859
AAC + Am-PseAAC	0.859
PseAAC + Am-PseAAC	0.856
AAC + PseAAC + Am-PseAAC	0.856

Table A2. Twenty if-then rules for discriminating ACP from non-ACP using random forest and amino acid composition.

% Covered Samples	Rule	Prediction Result
14.33	R > 0.017 and C ≤ 0.1145 and H ≤ 0.0645 and L > 0.1605 and K ≤ 0.1035	non-ACP
13.74	G > 0.041 and I > 0.0615 and L ≤ 0.1715 and K > 0.0385 and M ≤ 0.027	ACP
9.65	E > 0.058 and G ≤ 0.068	non-ACP
7.89	R ≤ 0.0515 and Q ≤ 0.026 and K > 0.094	ACP
7.89	C ≤ 0.1145 and H ≤ 0.0645 and K ≤ 0.1055 and W > 0.028	non-ACP
5.26	C > 0.1145 and P ≤ 0.073	ACP
4.97	N > 0.019 and K ≤ 0.1705 and M > 0.037	non-ACP
4.09	Q > 0.098 and K ≤ 0.0575	non-ACP
3.22	C > 0.015 and C ≤ 0.043	non-ACP
3.80	L ≤ 0.093 and F > 0.0715 and S ≤ 0.152	ACP
6.43	R > 0.013 and R ≤ 0.1345 and C ≤ 0.1205 and H ≤ 0.0465 and F ≤ 0.1345	non-ACP
2.63	A ≤ 0.0145 and Q ≤ 0.026	ACP
3.22	I ≤ 0.0335 and P > 0.074	non-ACP
2.34	R ≤ 0.0665 and E ≤ 0.044 and H > 0.052	ACP
1.75	N ≤ 0.0565 and H ≤ 0.0415 and K≤ 0.0335	non-ACP
1.46	I > 0.108 and K > 0.055	ACP
1.17	E ≤ 0.0545 and G > 0.0365 and K > 0.108 and M ≤ 0.04	ACP
2.05	I ≤ 0.0665 and F ≤ 0.006	non-ACP
2.05	S ≤ 0.04	non-ACP
2.05	Else	ACP

References

1. WHO Cancer. Available online: https://www.who.int/news-room/fact-sheets/detail/cancer (accessed on 30 January 2019).
2. Bray, F.; Ferlay, J.; Soerjomataram, I.; Siegel, R.L.; Torre, L.A.; Jemal, A. Global cancer statistics 2018: GLOBOCAN estimates of incidence and mortality worldwide for 36 cancers in 185 countries. *CA Cancer J. Clin.* **2018**, *68*, 394–424. [CrossRef] [PubMed]
3. Ferlay, J.; Colombet, M.; Soerjomataram, I.; Mathers, C.; Parkin, D.M.; Pineros, M.; Znaor, A.; Bray, F. Estimating the global cancer incidence and mortality in 2018: GLOBOCAN sources and methods. *Int. J. Cancer* **2018**, *144*, 1941–1953. [CrossRef]
4. Craik, D.J.; Fairlie, D.P.; Liras, S.; Price, D. The future of peptide-based drugs. *Chem. Biol. Drug Des.* **2013**, *81*, 136–147. [CrossRef] [PubMed]
5. Vlieghe, P.; Lisowski, V.; Martinez, J.; Khrestchatisky, M. Synthetic therapeutic peptides: Science and market. *Drug Discov. Today* **2010**, *15*, 40–56. [CrossRef]
6. Lau, J.L.; Dunn, M.K. Therapeutic peptides: Historical perspectives, current development trends, and future directions. *Bioorg. Med. Chem.* **2018**, *26*, 2700–2707. [CrossRef] [PubMed]
7. Fosgerau, K.; Hoffmann, T. Peptide therapeutics: Current status and future directions. *Drug Discov. Today* **2015**, *20*, 122–128. [CrossRef]
8. O'Brien-Simpson, N.M.; Hoffmann, R.; Chia, C.S.B.; Wade, J.D. Editorial: Antimicrobial and Anticancer Peptides. *Front. Chem.* **2018**, *6*, 13. [CrossRef]
9. Jin, G.; Weinberg, A. Human antimicrobial peptides and cancer. *Semin. Cell Dev. Biol.* **2018**, *88*, 156–162. [CrossRef] [PubMed]
10. Karpinski, T.M.; Adamczak, A. Anticancer Activity of Bacterial Proteins and Peptides. *Pharmaceutics* **2018**, *10*, 54. [CrossRef]
11. Usmani, S.S.; Bedi, G.; Samuel, J.S.; Singh, S.; Kalra, S.; Kumar, P.; Ahuja, A.A.; Sharma, M.; Gautam, A.; Raghava, G.P.S. THPdb: Database of FDA-approved peptide and protein therapeutics. *PLoS ONE* **2017**, *12*, e0181748. [CrossRef]
12. Deslouches, B.; Di, Y.P. Antimicrobial peptides with selective antitumor mechanisms: Prospect for anticancer applications. *Oncotarget* **2017**, *8*, 46635–46651. [CrossRef]
13. Gaspar, D.; Veiga, A.S.; Castanho, M.A. From antimicrobial to anticancer peptides. A review. *Front. Microbiol.* **2013**, *4*, 294. [CrossRef]
14. Ran, S.; Downes, A.; Thorpe, P.E. Increased exposure of anionic phospholipids on the surface of tumor blood vessels. *Cancer Res.* **2002**, *62*, 6132–6140.
15. Yoon, W.H.; Park, H.D.; Lim, K.; Hwang, B.D. Effect of *O*-glycosylated mucin on invasion and metastasis of HM7 human colon cancer cells. *Biochem. Biophys. Res. Commun.* **1996**, *222*, 694–699. [CrossRef]
16. Sok, M.; Sentjurc, M.; Schara, M. Membrane fluidity characteristics of human lung cancer. *Cancer Lett.* **1999**, *139*, 215–220. [CrossRef]

17. Chaudhary, J.; Munshi, M. Scanning electron microscopic analysis of breast aspirates. *Cytopathology* **1995**, *6*, 162–167. [CrossRef]
18. Dobrzynska, I.; Szachowicz-Petelska, B.; Sulkowski, S.; Figaszewski, Z. Changes in electric charge and phospholipids composition in human colorectal cancer cells. *Mol. Cell. Biochem.* **2005**, *276*, 113–119. [CrossRef]
19. Domalaon, R.; Findlay, B.; Ogunsina, M.; Arthur, G.; Schweizer, F. Ultrashort cationic lipopeptides and lipopeptoids: Evaluation and mechanistic insights against epithelial cancer cells. *Peptides* **2016**, *84*, 58–67. [CrossRef]
20. Gaspar, D.; Freire, J.M.; Pacheco, T.R.; Barata, J.T.; Castanho, M.A. Apoptotic human neutrophil peptide-1 anti-tumor activity revealed by cellular biomechanics. *Biochim. Biophys. Acta* **2015**, *1853*, 308–316. [CrossRef]
21. Figueiredo, C.R.; Matsuo, A.L.; Massaoka, M.H.; Polonelli, L.; Travassos, L.R. Anti-tumor activities of peptides corresponding to conserved complementary determining regions from different immunoglobulins. *Peptides* **2014**, *59*, 14–19. [CrossRef]
22. Riedl, S.; Zweytick, D.; Lohner, K. Membrane-active host defense peptides–challenges and perspectives for the development of novel anticancer drugs. *Chem. Phys. Lipids* **2011**, *164*, 766–781. [CrossRef] [PubMed]
23. Tyagi, A.; Kapoor, P.; Kumar, R.; Chaudhary, K.; Gautam, A.; Raghava, G. In silico models for designing and discovering novel anticancer peptides. *Sci. Rep.* **2013**, *3*, 2984. [CrossRef]
24. Hajisharifi, Z.; Piryaiee, M.; Beigi, M.M.; Behbahani, M.; Mohabatkar, H. Predicting anticancer peptides with Chou' s pseudo amino acid composition and investigating their mutagenicity via Ames test. *J. Theor. Biol.* **2014**, *341*, 34–40. [CrossRef] [PubMed]
25. Vijayakumar, S.; Lakshmi, P. ACPP: A web server for prediction and design of anti-cancer peptides. *Int. J. Pept. Res. Ther.* **2015**, *21*, 99–106. [CrossRef]
26. Chen, W.; Ding, H.; Feng, P.; Lin, H.; Chou, K.-C. iACP: A sequence-based tool for identifying anticancer peptides. *Oncotarget* **2016**, *7*, 16895. [CrossRef] [PubMed]
27. Li, F.-M.; Wang, X.-Q. Identifying anticancer peptides by using improved hybrid compositions. *Sci. Rep.* **2016**, *6*, 33910. [CrossRef]
28. Akbar, S.; Hayat, M.; Iqbal, M.; Jan, M.A. iACP-GAEnsC: Evolutionary genetic algorithm based ensemble classification of anticancer peptides by utilizing hybrid feature space. *Artif. Intell. Med.* **2017**, *79*, 62–70. [CrossRef]
29. Manavalan, B.; Basith, S.; Shin, T.H.; Choi, S.; Kim, M.O.; Lee, G. MLACP: Machine-learning-based prediction of anticancer peptides. *Oncotarget* **2017**, *8*, 77121. [CrossRef]
30. Xu, L.; Liang, G.; Wang, L.; Liao, C. A Novel Hybrid Sequence-Based Model for Identifying Anticancer Peptides. *Genes* **2018**, *9*, 158. [CrossRef]
31. Kabir, M.; Arif, M.; Ahmad, S.; Ali, Z.; Swati, Z.N.K.; Yu, D.-J. Intelligent computational method for discrimination of anticancer peptides by incorporating sequential and evolutionary profiles information. *Chemom. Intell. Lab. Syst.* **2018**, *182*, 158–165. [CrossRef]
32. Shoombuatong, W.; Schaduangrat, N.; Nantasenamat, C. Unraveling the bioactivity of anticancer peptides as deduced from machine learning. *EXCLI J.* **2018**, *17*, 734.
33. Pratiwi, R.; Malik, A.A.; Schaduangrat, N.; Prachayasittikul, V.; Wikberg, J.E.; Nantasenamat, C.; Shoombuatong, W. CryoProtect: A Web Server for Classifying Antifreeze Proteins from Nonantifreeze Proteins. *J. Chem.* **2017**, *2017*. [CrossRef]
34. Win, T.S.; Malik, A.A.; Prachayasittikul, V.; S Wikberg, J.E.; Nantasenamat, C.; Shoombuatong, W. HemoPred: A web server for predicting the hemolytic activity of peptides. *Future Med. Chem.* **2017**, *9*, 275–291. [CrossRef]
35. Shoombuatong, W.; Schaduangrat, N.; Nantasenamat, C. Towards understanding aromatase inhibitory activity via QSAR modeling. *EXCLI J.* **2018**, *17*, 688.
36. Win, T.S.; Schaduangrat, N.; Prachayasittikul, V.; Nantasenamat, C.; Shoombuatong, W. PAAP: A web server for predicting antihypertensive activity of peptides. *Future Med. Chem.* **2018**, *10*, 1749–1767. [CrossRef]
37. Shoombuatong, W.; Mekha, P.; Chaijaruwanich, J. Sequence based human leukocyte antigen gene prediction using informative physicochemical properties. *Int. J. Data Min. Bioinform.* **2015**, *13*, 211–224. [CrossRef]
38. Simeon, S.; Shoombuatong, W.; Anuwongcharoen, N.; Preeyanon, L.; Prachayasittikul, V.; Wikberg, J.E.; Nantasenamat, C. osFP: A web server for predicting the oligomeric states of fluorescent proteins. *J. Cheminform.* **2016**, *8*, 72. [CrossRef]

39. Kawashima, S.; Kanehisa, M. AAindex: Amino acid index database. *Nucleic Acids Res.* **2000**, *28*, 374. [CrossRef]
40. Chou, K.-C. Using amphiphilic pseudo amino acid composition to predict enzyme subfamily classes. *Bioinformatics* **2004**, *21*, 10–19. [CrossRef]
41. Chou, K.-C. Some remarks on protein attribute prediction and pseudo amino acid composition. *J. Theor. Biol.* **2011**, *273*, 236–247. [CrossRef]
42. Shen, H.-B.; Chou, K.-C. PseAAC: A flexible web server for generating various kinds of protein pseudo amino acid composition. *Anal. Biochem.* **2008**, *373*, 386–388. [CrossRef]
43. Xiao, N.; Cao, D.-S.; Zhu, M.-F.; Xu, Q.-S. protr/ProtrWeb: R package and web server for generating various numerical representation schemes of protein sequences. *Bioinformatics* **2015**, *31*, 1857–1859. [CrossRef] [PubMed]
44. Golbraikh, A.; Muratov, E.; Fourches, D.; Tropsha, A. Data set modelability by QSAR. *J. Chem. Inf. Model.* **2014**, *54*, 1–4. [CrossRef]
45. Shoombuatong, W.; Prathipati, P.; Prachayasittikul, V.; Schaduangrat, N.; Malik, A.A.; Pratiwi, R.; Wanwimolruk, S.; Wikberg, J.E.; Gleeson, M.P.; Spjuth, O. Towards Predicting the Cytochrome P450 Modulation: From QSAR to Proteochemometric Modeling. *Curr. Drug Metab.* **2017**, *18*, 540–555. [CrossRef]
46. Shoombuatong, W.; Hongjaisee, S.; Barin, F.; Chaijaruwanich, J.; Samleerat, T. HIV-1 CRF01_AE coreceptor usage prediction using kernel methods based logistic model trees. *Comput. Biol. Med.* **2012**, *42*, 885–889. [CrossRef]
47. Simeon, S.; Li, H.; Win, T.S.; Malik, A.A.; Kandhro, A.H.; Piacham, T.; Shoombuatong, W.; Nuchnoi, P.; Wikberg, J.E.; Gleeson, M.P. PepBio: Predicting the bioactivity of host defense peptides. *RSC Adv.* **2017**, *7*, 35119–35134. [CrossRef]
48. Shoombuatong, W.; Prachayasittikul, V.; Prachayasittikul, V.; Nantasenamat, C. Prediction of aromatase inhibitory activity using the efficient linear method (ELM). *EXCLI J.* **2015**, *14*, 452.
49. Shoombuatong, W.; Mekha, P.; Waiyamai, K.; Cheevadhanarak, S.; Chaijaruwanicha, J. Prediction of human leukocyte antigen gene using k-nearest neighbour classifier based on spectrum kernel. *ScienceAsia* **2013**, *39*, 42–49. [CrossRef]
50. Shoombuatong, W.; Traisathit, P.; Prasitwattanaseree, S.; Tayapiwatana, C.; Cutler, R.; Chaijaruwanich, J. Prediction of the disulphide bonding state of cysteines in proteins using Conditional Random Fields. *Int. J. Data Min. Bioinform.* **2011**, *5*, 449–464. [CrossRef]
51. Charoenkwan, P.; Shoombuatong, W.; Lee, H.-C.; Chaijaruwanich, J.; Huang, H.-L.; Ho, S.-Y. SCMCRYS: Predicting protein crystallization using an ensemble scoring card method with estimating propensity scores of P-collocated amino acid pairs. *PLoS ONE* **2013**, *8*, e72368. [CrossRef] [PubMed]
52. Anuwongcharoen, N.; Shoombuatong, W.; Tantimongcolwat, T.; Prachayasittikul, V.; Nantasenamat, C. Exploring the chemical space of influenza neuraminidase inhibitors. *PeerJ* **2016**, *4*, e1958. [CrossRef]
53. Shoombuatong, W.; Prachayasittikul, V.; Anuwongcharoen, N.; Songtawee, N.; Monnor, T.; Prachayasittikul, S.; Prachayasittikul, V.; Nantasenamat, C. Navigating the chemical space of dipeptidyl peptidase-4 inhibitors. *Drug Des. Dev. Ther.* **2015**, *9*, 4515.
54. Suvannang, N.; Preeyanon, L.; Malik, A.A.; Schaduangrat, N.; Shoombuatong, W.; Worachartcheewan, A.; Tantimongcolwat, T.; Nantasenamat, C. Probing the origin of estrogen receptor alpha inhibition via large-scale QSAR study. *RSC Adv.* **2018**, *8*, 11344–11356. [CrossRef]
55. Simeon, S.; Anuwongcharoen, N.; Shoombuatong, W.; Malik, A.A.; Prachayasittikul, V.; Wikberg, J.E.; Nantasenamat, C. Probing the origins of human acetylcholinesterase inhibition via QSAR modeling and molecular docking. *PeerJ* **2016**, *4*, e2322. [CrossRef]
56. Breiman, L. Random forests. *Mach. Learn.* **2001**, *45*, 5–32. [CrossRef]
57. Breiman, L. *Classification and Regression Trees*; Routledge: London, UK, 2017.
58. Breiman, L. randomForest: Breiman and Cutler's Random Forests for Classification and Regression. R Package Version. 2006. Available online: http://stat-www.berkeley.edu/users/breiman/RandomForests (accessed on 30 January 2019).
59. Kuhn, M. Building predictive models in R using the caret package. *J. Stat. Softw.* **2008**, *28*, 1–26. [CrossRef]
60. Cortes, C.; Vapnik, V. Support-vector networks. *Mach. Learn.* **1995**, *20*, 273–297. [CrossRef]
61. Drucker, H.; Burges, C.J.; Kaufman, L.; Smola, A.J.; Vapnik, V. Support Vector Regression Machines. In *Advances in Neural Information Processing Systems*; MIT Press: Cambridge, MA, USA, 1997; pp. 155–161.
62. Joachims, T. Svmlight: Support Vector Machine. SVM-Light Support. Vector Machine. University of Dortmund, 1999, 19. Available online: http://svmlight.joachims.org/ (accessed on 30 January 2019).

63. Lameski, P.; Zdravevski, E.; Mingov, R.; Kulakov, A. SVM parameter tuning with grid search and its impact on reduction of model over-fitting. In *Rough Sets, Fuzzy Sets, Data Mining, and Granular Computing*; Springer: Berlin, Germany, 2015; pp. 464–474.
64. Tung, C.-W.; Ziehm, M.; Kämper, A.; Kohlbacher, O.; Ho, S.-Y. POPISK: T-cell reactivity prediction using support vector machines and string kernels. *BMC Bioinform.* **2011**, *12*, 446. [CrossRef]
65. Calle, M.L.; Urrea, V. Letter to the editor: Stability of random forest importance measures. *Brief. Bioinform.* **2010**, *12*, 86–89. [CrossRef]
66. Shoombuatong, W.; Huang, H.-L.; Chaijaruwanich, J.; Charoenkwan, P.; Lee, H.-C.; Ho, S.-Y. Predicting Protein Crystallization Using a Simple Scoring Card Method. In Proceedings of the IEEE Symposium on Computational Intelligence in Bioinformatics and Computational Biology (CIBCB), Singapore, 16–19 April 2013; pp. 23–30.
67. Hasan, M.M.; Yang, S.; Zhou, Y.; Mollah, M.N.H. SuccinSite: A computational tool for the prediction of protein succinylation sites by exploiting the amino acid patterns and properties. *Mol. Biosyst.* **2016**, *12*, 786–795. [CrossRef]
68. Worachartcheewan, A.; Shoombuatong, W.; Pidetcha, P.; Nopnithipat, W.; Prachayasittikul, V.; Nantasenamat, C. Predicting metabolic syndrome using the random forest method. *Sci. World J.* **2015**, *2015*, 58150. [CrossRef] [PubMed]
69. Chou, K.-C.; Shen, H.-B. Cell-PLoc: A package of Web servers for predicting subcellular localization of proteins in various organisms. *Nat. Protoc.* **2008**, *3*, 153. [CrossRef] [PubMed]
70. Chou, K.-C.; Shen, H.-B. Recent progress in protein subcellular location prediction. *Anal. Biochem.* **2007**, *370*, 1. [CrossRef]
71. Robin, X.; Turck, N.; Hainard, A.; Tiberti, N.; Lisacek, F.; Sanchez, J.-C.; Müller, M. pROC: An open-source package for R and S+ to analyze and compare ROC curves. *BMC Bioinform.* **2011**, *12*, 77. [CrossRef]
72. Liaw, C.; Tung, C.-W.; Ho, S.-Y. Prediction and analysis of antibody amyloidogenesis from sequences. *PLoS ONE* **2013**, *8*, e53235. [CrossRef]
73. Chawla, N.V.; Bowyer, K.W.; Hall, L.O.; Kegelmeyer, W.P. SMOTE: Synthetic minority over-sampling technique. *J. Artif. Intell. Res.* **2002**, *16*, 321–357. [CrossRef]
74. Kumar, R.; Chaudhary, K.; Chauhan, J.S.; Nagpal, G.; Kumar, R.; Sharma, M.; Raghava, G.P. An in silico platform for predicting, screening and designing of antihypertensive peptides. *Sci. Rep.* **2015**, *5*, 12512. [CrossRef] [PubMed]
75. Shen, H.-B.; Chou, K.-C. Gneg-mPLoc: A top-down strategy to enhance the quality of predicting subcellular localization of Gram-negative bacterial proteins. *J. Theor. Biol.* **2010**, *264*, 326–333. [CrossRef]
76. Chou, K.-C.; Shen, H.-B. Plant-mPLoc: A top-down strategy to augment the power for predicting plant protein subcellular localization. *PLoS ONE* **2010**, *5*, e11335. [CrossRef]
77. Hellberg, S.; Sjoestroem, M.; Skagerberg, B.; Wold, S. Peptide quantitative structure-activity relationships, a multivariate approach. *J. Med. Chem.* **1987**, *30*, 1126–1135. [CrossRef]
78. Sandberg, M.; Eriksson, L.; Jonsson, J.; Sjöström, M.; Wold, S. New chemical descriptors relevant for the design of biologically active peptides. A multivariate characterization of 87 amino acids. *J. Med. Chem.* **1998**, *41*, 2481–2491. [CrossRef]
79. Huang, H.-L. Propensity scores for prediction and characterization of bioluminescent proteins from sequences. *PLoS ONE* **2014**, *9*, e97158. [CrossRef] [PubMed]
80. Borrelli, A.; Tornesello, A.L.; Tornesello, M.L.; Buonaguro, F.M. Cell Penetrating Peptides as Molecular Carriers for Anti-Cancer Agents. *Molecules* **2018**, *23*, 295. [CrossRef]
81. Benabdelouahab, Y.; Muñoz-Moreno, L.; Frik, M.; de la Cueva-Alique, I.; El Amrani, M.A.; Contel, M.; Bajo, A.M.; Cuenca, T.; Royo, E. Hydrogen Bonding and Anticancer Properties of Water-Soluble Chiral p-Cymene RuII Compounds with Amino-Oxime Ligands. *Eur. J. Inorg. Chem.* **2015**, *2015*, 2295–2307. [CrossRef]
82. Carlberg, C. Current understanding of the function of the nuclear vitamin D receptor in response to its natural and synthetic ligands. *Recent Results Cancer Res.* **2003**, *164*, 29–42.
83. Gopal, R.; Park, S.C.; Ha, K.J.; Cho, S.J.; Kim, S.W.; Song, P.I.; Nah, J.W.; Park, Y.; Hahm, K.S. Effect of Leucine and Lysine substitution on the antimicrobial activity and evaluation of the mechanism of the HPA3NT3 analog peptide. *J. Pept. Sci.* **2009**, *15*, 589–594. [CrossRef]
84. Wang, C.; Dong, S.; Zhang, L.; Zhao, Y.; Huang, L.; Gong, X.; Wang, H.; Shang, D. Cell surface binding, uptaking and anticancer activity of L-K6, a lysine/leucine-rich peptide, on human breast cancer MCF-7 cells. *Sci. Rep.* **2017**, *7*, 8293. [CrossRef] [PubMed]

85. Riedl, S.; Rinner, B.; Asslaber, M.; Schaider, H.; Walzer, S.; Novak, A.; Lohner, K.; Zweytick, D. In search of a novel target—Phosphatidylserine exposed by non-apoptotic tumor cells and metastases of malignancies with poor treatment efficacy. *Biochim. Biophys. Acta* **2011**, *1808*, 2638–2645. [CrossRef] [PubMed]
86. Wang, C.; Chen, Y.W.; Zhang, L.; Gong, X.G.; Zhou, Y.; Shang, D.J. Melanoma cell surface-expressed phosphatidylserine as a therapeutic target for cationic anticancer peptide, temporin-1CEa. *J. Drug Target.* **2016**, *24*, 548–556. [CrossRef] [PubMed]
87. Yang, D.; Biragyn, A.; Hoover, D.M.; Lubkowski, J.; Oppenheim, J.J. Multiple roles of antimicrobial defensins, cathelicidins, and eosinophil-derived neurotoxin in host defense. *Annu. Rev. Immunol.* **2004**, *22*, 181–215. [CrossRef] [PubMed]
88. Yang, D.; Oppenheim, J.J. Antimicrobial proteins act as "alarmins" in joint immune defense. *Arthritis Rheum.* **2004**, *50*, 3401–3403. [CrossRef]
89. Zou, G.; de Leeuw, E.; Li, C.; Pazgier, M.; Li, C.; Zeng, P.; Lu, W.Y.; Lubkowski, J.; Lu, W. Toward understanding the cationicity of defensins. Arg and Lys versus their noncoded analogs. *J. Biol. Chem.* **2007**, *282*, 19653–19665. [CrossRef]
90. Papo, N.; Seger, D.; Makovitzki, A.; Kalchenko, V.; Eshhar, Z.; Degani, H.; Shai, Y. Inhibition of tumor growth and elimination of multiple metastases in human prostate and breast xenografts by systemic inoculation of a host defense-like lytic peptide. *Cancer Res.* **2006**, *66*, 5371–5378. [CrossRef]
91. Zwaal, R.F.; Comfurius, P.; Bevers, E.M. Surface exposure of phosphatidylserine in pathological cells. *Cell. Mol. Life Sci.* **2005**, *62*, 971–988. [CrossRef]
92. Tanabe, H.; Ayabe, T.; Maemoto, A.; Ishikawa, C.; Inaba, Y.; Sato, R.; Moriichi, K.; Okamoto, K.; Watari, J.; Kono, T.; et al. Denatured human alpha-defensin attenuates the bactericidal activity and the stability against enzymatic digestion. *Biochem. Biophys. Res. Commun.* **2007**, *358*, 349–355. [CrossRef]
93. Raina, D.; Ahmad, R.; Joshi, M.D.; Yin, L.; Wu, Z.; Kawano, T.; Vasir, B.; Avigan, D.; Kharbanda, S.; Kufe, D. Direct targeting of the mucin 1 oncoprotein blocks survival and tumorigenicity of human breast carcinoma cells. *Cancer Res.* **2009**, *69*, 5133–5141. [CrossRef]
94. Joshi, M.D.; Ahmad, R.; Yin, L.; Raina, D.; Rajabi, H.; Bubley, G.; Kharbanda, S.; Kufe, D. MUC1 oncoprotein is a druggable target in human prostate cancer cells. *Mol. Cancer Ther.* **2009**, *8*, 3056–3065. [CrossRef]
95. Yin, L.; Ahmad, R.; Kosugi, M.; Kawano, T.; Avigan, D.; Stone, R.; Kharbanda, S.; Kufe, D. Terminal differentiation of chronic myelogenous leukemia cells is induced by targeting of the MUC1-C oncoprotein. *Cancer Biol. Ther.* **2010**, *10*, 483–491. [CrossRef]
96. Banerjee, S.; Mujumdar, N.; Dudeja, V.; Mackenzie, T.; Krosch, T.K.; Sangwan, V.; Vickers, S.M.; Saluja, A.K. MUC1c regulates cell survival in pancreatic cancer by preventing lysosomal permeabilization. *PLoS ONE* **2012**, *7*, e43020. [CrossRef]
97. Raina, D.; Ahmad, R.; Rajabi, H.; Panchamoorthy, G.; Kharbanda, S.; Kufe, D. Targeting cysteine-mediated dimerization of the MUC1-C oncoprotein in human cancer cells. *Int. J. Oncol.* **2012**, *40*, 1643–1649.
98. Tyuryaeva, I.I.; Lyublinskaya, O.G.; Podkorytov, I.S.; Skrynnikov, N.R. Origin of anti-tumor activity of the cysteine-containing GO peptides and further optimization of their cytotoxic properties. *Sci. Rep.* **2017**, *7*, 40217. [CrossRef]
99. Schroeder, B.O.; Wu, Z.; Nuding, S.; Groscurth, S.; Marcinowski, M.; Beisner, J.; Buchner, J.; Schaller, M.; Stange, E.F.; Wehkamp, J. Reduction of disulphide bonds unmasks potent antimicrobial activity of human beta-defensin 1. *Nature* **2011**, *469*, 419–423. [CrossRef]
100. Hoskin, D.W.; Ramamoorthy, A. Studies on anticancer activities of antimicrobial peptides. *Biochim. Biophys. Acta* **2008**, *1778*, 357–375. [CrossRef]
101. Tsai, C.S. *Biomacromolecules: Introduction to Structure, Function and Informatics*; John Wiley & Sons: Hoboken, NJ, USA, 2007.
102. Roseman, M.A. Hydrophilicity of polar amino acid side-chains is markedly reduced by flanking peptide bonds. *J. Mol. Biol.* **1988**, *200*, 513–522. [CrossRef]
103. Kyte, J.; Doolittle, R.F. A simple method for displaying the hydropathic character of a protein. *J. Mol Biol* **1982**, *157*, 105–132. [CrossRef]
104. Argos, P.; Rao, J.K.; Hargrave, P.A. Structural prediction of membrane-bound proteins. *Eur. J. Biochem.* **1982**, *128*, 565–575. [CrossRef]
105. Nozaki, Y.; Tanford, C. The solubility of amino acids and two glycine peptides in aqueous ethanol and dioxane solutions. Establishment of a hydrophobicity scale. *J. Biol. Chem.* **1971**, *246*, 2211–2217.

106. Mader, J.S.; Hoskin, D.W. Cationic antimicrobial peptides as novel cytotoxic agents for cancer treatment. *Expert Opin. Investig. Drugs* **2006**, *15*, 933–946. [CrossRef]
107. Chen, C.; Yang, C.; Chen, Y.; Wang, F.; Mu, Q.; Zhang, J.; Li, Z.; Pan, F.; Xu, H.; Lu, J.R. Surface Physical Activity and Hydrophobicity of Designed Helical Peptide Amphiphiles Control Their Bioactivity and Cell Selectivity. *ACS Appl. Mater. Interfaces* **2016**, *8*, 26501–26510. [CrossRef]
108. Huang, Y.B.; Wang, X.F.; Wang, H.Y.; Liu, Y.; Chen, Y. Studies on mechanism of action of anticancer peptides by modulation of hydrophobicity within a defined structural framework. *Mol. Cancer Ther.* **2011**, *10*, 416–426. [CrossRef]
109. Park, J.H.; Kim, H.A.; Cho, S.H.; Lee, M. Characterization of hydrophobic anti-cancer drug-loaded amphiphilic peptides as a gene carrier. *J. Cell. Biochem.* **2012**, *113*, 1645–1653. [CrossRef]
110. Chou, P.Y.; Fasman, G.D. Conformational parameters for amino acids in helical, beta-sheet, and random coil regions calculated from proteins. *Biochemistry* **1974**, *13*, 211–222. [CrossRef]
111. Isogai, Y.; Nemethy, G.; Rackovsky, S.; Leach, S.J.; Scheraga, H.A. Characterization of multiple bends in proteins. *Biopolymers* **1980**, *19*, 1183–1210. [CrossRef] [PubMed]
112. Chou, P.Y.; Fasman, G.D. Empirical predictions of protein conformation. *Annu. Rev. Biochem.* **1978**, *47*, 251–276. [CrossRef] [PubMed]
113. Vermeer, L.S.; Lan, Y.; Abbate, V.; Ruh, E.; Bui, T.T.; Wilkinson, L.J.; Kanno, T.; Jumagulova, E.; Kozlowska, J.; Patel, J.; et al. Conformational flexibility determines selectivity and antibacterial, antiplasmodial, and anticancer potency of cationic alpha-helical peptides. *J. Biol. Chem.* **2012**, *287*, 34120–34133. [CrossRef] [PubMed]
114. Risso, A.; Zanetti, M.; Gennaro, R. Cytotoxicity and apoptosis mediated by two peptides of innate immunity. *Cell. Immunol.* **1998**, *189*, 107–115. [CrossRef]
115. Holak, T.A.; Engstrom, A.; Kraulis, P.J.; Lindeberg, G.; Bennich, H.; Jones, T.A.; Gronenborn, A.M.; Clore, G.M. The solution conformation of the antibacterial peptide cecropin A: A nuclear magnetic resonance and dynamical simulated annealing study. *Biochemistry* **1988**, *27*, 7620–7629. [CrossRef]
116. Hung, S.C.; Wang, W.; Chan, S.I.; Chen, H.M. Membrane lysis by the antibacterial peptides cecropins B1 and B3: A spin-label electron spin resonance study on phospholipid bilayers. *Biophys. J.* **1999**, *77*, 3120–3133. [CrossRef]
117. Merrifield, R.B.; Merrifield, E.L.; Juvvadi, P.; Andreu, D.; Boman, H.G. Design and synthesis of antimicrobial peptides. *Ciba Found. Symp.* **1994**, *186*, 5–20, discussion 20-6.
118. Srisailam, S.; Kumar, T.K.; Arunkumar, A.I.; Leung, K.W.; Yu, C.; Chen, H.M. Crumpled structure of the custom hydrophobic lytic peptide cecropin B3. *Eur. J. Biochem.* **2001**, *268*, 4278–4284. [CrossRef]
119. Moore, A.J.; Devine, D.A.; Bibby, M.C. Preliminary experimental anticancer activity of cecropins. *Pept. Res.* **1994**, *7*, 265–269. [PubMed]
120. Lehmann, J.; Retz, M.; Sidhu, S.S.; Suttmann, H.; Sell, M.; Paulsen, F.; Harder, J.; Unteregger, G.; Stockle, M. Antitumor activity of the antimicrobial peptide magainin II against bladder cancer cell lines. *Eur. Urol.* **2006**, *50*, 141–147. [CrossRef]
121. Cruciani, R.A.; Barker, J.L.; Zasloff, M.; Chen, H.C.; Colamonici, O. Antibiotic magainins exert cytolytic activity against transformed cell lines through channel formation. *Proc. Natl. Acad. Sci. USA* **1991**, *88*, 3792–3796. [CrossRef] [PubMed]
122. Gauldie, J.; Hanson, J.M.; Shipolini, R.A.; Vernon, C.A. The structures of some peptides from bee venom. *Eur. J. Biochem.* **1978**, *83*, 405–410. [CrossRef] [PubMed]
123. Tosteson, M.T.; Alvarez, O.; Hubbell, W.; Bieganski, R.M.; Attenbach, C.; Caporales, L.H.; Levy, J.J.; Nutt, R.F.; Rosenblatt, M.; Tosteson, D.C. Primary structure of peptides and ion channels. Role of amino acid side chains in voltage gating of melittin channels. *Biophys. J.* **1990**, *58*, 1367–1375. [CrossRef]
124. Sui, S.F.; Wu, H.; Guo, Y.; Chen, K.S. Conformational changes of melittin upon insertion into phospholipid monolayer and vesicle. *J. Biochem.* **1994**, *116*, 482–487. [CrossRef]
125. Henzler Wildman, K.A.; Lee, D.K.; Ramamoorthy, A. Mechanism of lipid bilayer disruption by the human antimicrobial peptide, LL-37. *Biochemistry* **2003**, *42*, 6545–6558. [CrossRef]
126. Okumura, K.; Itoh, A.; Isogai, E.; Hirose, K.; Hosokawa, Y.; Abiko, Y.; Shibata, T.; Hirata, M.; Isogai, H. C-terminal domain of human CAP18 antimicrobial peptide induces apoptosis in oral squamous cell carcinoma SAS-H1 cells. *Cancer Lett.* **2004**, *212*, 185–194. [CrossRef]

127. Dhople, V.; Krukemeyer, A.; Ramamoorthy, A. The human beta-defensin-3, an antibacterial peptide with multiple biological functions. *Biochim. Biophys. Acta* **2006**, *1758*, 1499–1512. [CrossRef]
128. Selsted, M.E.; Harwig, S.S. Determination of the disulfide array in the human defensin HNP-2. A covalently cyclized peptide. *J. Biol. Chem.* **1989**, *264*, 4003–4007.
129. Lichtenstein, A.; Ganz, T.; Selsted, M.E.; Lehrer, R.I. In vitro tumor cell cytolysis mediated by peptide defensins of human and rabbit granulocytes. *Blood* **1986**, *68*, 1407–1410.
130. Lichtenstein, A.K.; Ganz, T.; Nguyen, T.M.; Selsted, M.E.; Lehrer, R.I. Mechanism of target cytolysis by peptide defensins. Target cell metabolic activities, possibly involving endocytosis, are crucial for expression of cytotoxicity. *J. Immunol.* **1988**, *140*, 2686–2694.
131. Lichtenstein, A. Mechanism of mammalian cell lysis mediated by peptide defensins. Evidence for an initial alteration of the plasma membrane. *J. Clin. Investig.* **1991**, *88*, 93–100. [CrossRef]
132. Mader, J.S.; Salsman, J.; Conrad, D.M.; Hoskin, D.W. Bovine lactoferricin selectively induces apoptosis in human leukemia and carcinoma cell lines. *Mol. Cancer Ther.* **2005**, *4*, 612–624. [CrossRef]
133. Furlong, S.J.; Ridgway, N.D.; Hoskin, D.W. Modulation of ceramide metabolism in T-leukemia cell lines potentiates apoptosis induced by the cationic antimicrobial peptide bovine lactoferricin. *Int. J. Oncol.* **2008**, *32*, 537–544. [CrossRef]
134. Eliassen, L.T.; Berge, G.; Leknessund, A.; Wikman, M.; Lindin, I.; Lokke, C.; Ponthan, F.; Johnsen, J.I.; Sveinbjornsson, B.; Kogner, P.; et al. The antimicrobial peptide, lactoferricin B, is cytotoxic to neuroblastoma cells in vitro and inhibits xenograft growth in vivo. *Int. J. Cancer* **2006**, *119*, 493–500. [CrossRef]
135. Nakamura, T.; Furunaka, H.; Miyata, T.; Tokunaga, F.; Muta, T.; Iwanaga, S.; Niwa, M.; Takao, T.; Shimonishi, Y. Tachyplesin, a class of antimicrobial peptide from the hemocytes of the horseshoe crab (*Tachypleus tridentatus*). Isolation and chemical structure. *J. Biol. Chem.* **1988**, *263*, 16709–16713.
136. Chen, J.; Xu, X.M.; Underhill, C.B.; Yang, S.; Wang, L.; Chen, Y.; Hong, S.; Creswell, K.; Zhang, L. Tachyplesin activates the classic complement pathway to kill tumor cells. *Cancer Res.* **2005**, *65*, 4614–4622. [CrossRef]
137. Adamia, S.; Maxwell, C.A.; Pilarski, L.M. Hyaluronan and hyaluronan synthases: Potential therapeutic targets in cancer. *Curr. Drug Targets Cardiovasc. Haematol. Disord.* **2005**, *5*, 3–14. [CrossRef]
138. Rao, A.G. Conformation and antimicrobial activity of linear derivatives of tachyplesin lacking disulfide bonds. *Arch. Biochem. Biophys.* **1999**, *361*, 127–134. [CrossRef]
139. Tada, N.; Horibe, T.; Haramoto, M.; Ohara, K.; Kohno, M.; Kawakami, K. A single replacement of histidine to arginine in EGFR-lytic hybrid peptide demonstrates the improved anticancer activity. *Biochem. Biophys. Res. Commun.* **2011**, *407*, 383–388. [CrossRef] [PubMed]
140. Barras, D.; Chevalier, N.; Zoete, V.; Dempsey, R.; Lapouge, K.; Olayioye, M.A.; Michielin, O.; Widmann, C. A WXW motif is required for the anticancer activity of the TAT-RasGAP317–326 peptide. *J. Biol. Chem.* **2014**, *289*, 23701–23711. [CrossRef] [PubMed]

Sample Availability: Not applicable.

molecules

Article

Novel pH Selective, Highly Lytic Peptides Based on a Chimeric Influenza Hemagglutinin Peptide/Cell Penetrating Peptide Motif

Bethany Algayer, Ann O'Brien, Aaron Momose, Dennis J. Murphy, William Procopio, David M. Tellers and Thomas J. Tucker *

Merck Research Laboratories, Merck and Co, Inc., West Point, PA 19486, USA; bethany_algayer@merck.com (B.A.); aobrien@incyte.com (A.O.); aam888010@icloud.com (A.M.); dennis.murphy@merck.com (D.J.M.); wmprocop@gmail.com (W.P.); david_tellers@merck.com (D.M.T.)

* Correspondence: tom_tucker@merck.com; Tel.: 215-652-5275

Academic Editors: Henry Mosberg, Tomi Sawyer and Carrie Haskell-Luevano
Received: 2 May 2019; Accepted: 24 May 2019; Published: 31 May 2019

Abstract: Delivery of macromolecular cargos such as siRNA to the cytosol after endocytosis remains a critical challenge. Numerous approaches including viruses, lipid nanoparticles, polymeric constructs, and various peptide-based approaches have yet to yield a general solution to this delivery issue. In this manuscript, we describe our efforts to design novel endosomolytic peptides that could be used to facilitate the release of cargos from a late endosomal compartment. These amphiphilic peptides, based on a chimeric influenza hemagglutinin peptide/cell-penetrating peptide (CPP) template, utilize a pH-triggering mechanism in which the peptides are protonated after acidification of the endosome, and thereby adopt an alpha-helical conformation. The helical forms of the peptides are lytically active, while the non-protonated forms are much less or non-lytically active at physiological pH. Starting from an initial lead peptide (INF7-Tat), we systematically modified the sequence of the chimeric peptides to obtain peptides with greatly enhanced lytic activity that maintain good pH selectivity in a red blood cell hemolysis assay.

Keywords: peptides; endosomolytic; amphiphilic; fusogenic; influenza hemagglutinin; RBC lysis

1. Introduction

The use of siRNA to treat various disorders remains a promising potential novel approach for future intervention [1]. Unfortunately, delivery remains a key unsolved issue. Following endocytosis, endosomal entrapment of siRNA-based cargos remains a critical unsolved barrier for efficient delivery of siRNA to the cytosol where it can engage RNA-induced silencing complex (RISC) and effect message knockdown [1,2]. Numerous approaches to enhancing endosomal escape have been tried or are currently under investigation [2], however to date none have solved the problem. Among these approaches, the use of cell penetrating (CPP) and/or endosomal escape peptides (EEP) has been featured in the literature [3]. The peptides have been used primarily as mixtures with siRNA [1], formulated into lipid nanoparticles (LNPs) [2], or in a few cases directly conjugated to the siRNA [4]. To date, none of these approaches has shown more than incremental improvement in cargo delivery.

As part of our investigation of siRNA delivery approaches, we decided to make use of small peptides as potential endosomal escape agents. Our initial strategy was to design novel, membrane lytic peptides that used a pH triggering mechanism as a potential safety margin. Similar approaches involving endolytic polymer scaffolds are also currently being investigated for the delivery of siRNA cargos [2]. Ideally, the small peptides would be delivered in a specific, targeted manner to the chosen target cell via conjugation to the cargo using an appropriate linker. After endocytosis, the peptide would be freed from the linker/cargo and concentrated in an endosome. Theoretically, as the endosome progressed through its life-cycle and the associated acidification process, one could take advantage of the pH drop to act as a trigger for the peptide. We hoped to design novel pH triggered peptides that were relatively inactive at physiological pH (7.4), but at late endosomal pH (5.5) were protonated and underwent a conformational change that conferred membrane lytic activity to the peptide. Such pH-triggered peptides are widely known in the literature and form the basis for the fusogenic peptides used by viruses to allow their genetic material to escape from endosomes and induce viral replication [5]. Since such viral processes are well evolved and quite efficient, we theorized that this would be an excellent mechanism to attempt to mimic for endosomal escape of siRNA-based cargos. Of course, the potential for toxicity would exist in such an endosomolytic process by releasing endosomal contents into the cytosol. Theoretically, any mechanism that results in the widespread leakage of endosomal contents into the cytoplasm could have this liability, and detailed studies to understand the limitations of these approaches and the potential for toxicity will clearly be needed. Despite this, it is possible that such a peptide might be useful for cytosolic delivery of endosomally-entrapped cargos, and such peptides have been studied in the literature and have in some cases been show to effect cargo delivery to the cytosol without inducing toxicity [6]. We were also interested in expanding our fundamental knowledge of the interaction of various classes of membrane active peptides with membranes, regardless of the potential for toxicity that is inherent in this mechanism. Extensive mechanistic studies in the literature with membrane active [7], lytic [8], fusogenic [9], and antimicrobial peptides [10] have demonstrated complex behavior and have shown diverse and often contradictory results based on the assay or system used to study the peptides. We wanted to avoid the complexity and diversity of these kinds of approaches, and instead chose to pursue an empirical, medicinal chemistry/structure-activity relationship approach to investigating and optimizing the lytic activity of this class of peptides. While numerous publications [11,12] have discussed the membrane disrupting properties of many peptides, there are no reports of highly systematic synthetic chemistry studies undertaken to optimize these peptides as potential endosomolytic agents. In this manuscript, we detail our efforts to design and systematically investigate the SAR of a series of novel, chimeric lytic peptides based on the influenza hemagglutinin peptide (HA2) and the well-characterized cell-penetrating/cargo delivery peptide Tat.

2. Results and Discussion

2.1. Generation of Lead Chimeric Peptides

The biology and mechanism of action of the influenza hemagglutinin peptide HA2 is well-known and has been described in detail [12]. Our approach was based on an initial study of the lytic properties of this peptide and some related literature analogs [12]. We also investigated a number of literature CPPs [13]. We initially hypothesized that fusion of a CPP sequence with the membrane active HA2 peptide sequence could provide a chimeric peptide with cellular uptake and endosomal escape properties combined in the same peptide. Simultaneous to our investigations, several other authors reported similar chimeric peptides that were shown to have lytic properties and effect intracellular delivery of cargos [14–19]. In addition, fusogenic peptides from this class have been reported to enhance endosomal escape [20]; whether this activity is mediated by direct endosomolysis or not remains uncertain but seems likely. In most cases these investigations focused on the biology of the cellular delivery processes associated with these peptides, but little or no medicinal chemistry was done to specifically investigate the structure –activity relationships required to drive and optimize this activity. We chose a different approach, using a systematic, synthetic analog-driven program to enhance the lytic properties of these peptides to understand and increase their efficiency as possible endosomal escape agents. Since our internal investigations had confirmed that endosomal escape was a highly inefficient process and a key barrier to intracellular delivery, we surmised that we could make the largest direct impact on delivery by enhancing this process.

Initially, we investigated the lytic activity of several CPPs, several influenza hemagglutinin derivatives, and their chimeric fusion peptides (Table 1). Peptides were synthesized using standard FMOC—solid phase synthesis protocols and were obtained as N-terminal amines/C-terminal amides unless otherwise noted (see Methods and Materials for full details). All peptides included a free cysteine reside in the peptide sequences to allow for possible direct conjugation to linkers and potential cargo molecules. To prevent dimerization of the cysteinylated peptides, small amounts of acetic acid and DTT were added to the stock solutions and assay buffer to ensure that the peptides were tested as monomers; the presence of monomers was randomly confirmed by LC/MS analysis of the assay solutions. All peptides were shown to be greater than 95% in purity by HPLC analysis and demonstrated the correct masses by HRMS analysis. Peptides were tested for lytic activity in a standard red blood cell hemolysis assay at pH 7.4 and 5.5 using a modified version of published protocols (see Methods and Materials). This assay is widely considered to be one of the better assays for evaluation of the lytic properties of synthetic peptides. All the peptides tested were freely soluble at up to 10 μM concentrations in the stock solutions and assay buffers, and only the most lipophilic peptides exhibited limited solubility at higher (>10 μM) concentrations. Consequently, solubility does not appear to have played a role in the observed behavior of most of the peptides.

Table 1. Lead Chimeric Peptides.

Number	Sequence	RBC Lysis IC_{50}, pH 5.5 (μM)	RBC Lysis IC_{50}, pH 7.4 (μM)	Comments
std	CGIGAVLKVLTTGLPALISWIKRKRQQ	0.8 ± 0.2 (*n* =25)	2.6 ± 0.6 (*n* = 25)	Melittin
1	CYGRKKRRQRR	>20	>20	Tat
2	CRQIKIWFQNRRMKWKK	>20	>20	Penetratin
3	CGLFEAIAGFIENGWEGMIDGWYG	>20	>20	HA2
4	CGLFEAIEGFIENGWEGMIDGWYG	16	>20	INF7
5	CGLFEAIAGFIENGWEGMIDGWYGYGRKKRRQRR	2.3 ± 0.5 (*n* = 10)	5.7 ± 1.1 (*n* = 10)	HA2-Tat
6	CGLFEAIEGFIENGWEGMIDGWYGYGRKKRRQRR	1.4 ± 0.4 (*n* = 10)	4.6 ± 1.2 (*n* = 10)	INF7-Tat
7	CGLFHAIAHFIHGGWHGLIHGWYGYGRKKRRQRR	5.9	0.3	H5WYG-Tat
8	CGLFKAIAKFIKGGWKGLIKGWYGYGRKKRRQRR	1.9	0.9	K5WYG-Tat
9	CGLFEAIAEFIEGGWEGLIEGWYGYGRKKRRQRR	>20	2.2	E5WYG-Tat
10	CGLFEAIAGFIENGWEGMIDGWYGRQIKIWFQNRRMKWKKGG	>20	>20	HA2-Penetratin
11	CGLFEAIEGFIENGWEGMIDGWYGRQIKIWFQNRRMKWKKGG	>20	>20	INF7-Penetratin

All peptides were >95% purity by HPLC analysis and demonstrated the correct HRMS profiles. Peptides were tested three times at each pH unless otherwise noted, and the values are reported as the mean. Standard Deviations are reported for peptides with larger *n* values to provide a reference for the reproducibility of the data. As solubility allowed, testing at pH 7.4 was pushed to the highest possible concentrations to determine as close as possible approximate IC_{50}.

We found that the literature cell penetrating cargo delivery peptides **1** (Tat) [21,22] and **2** (Penetratin) [22] were devoid of lytic activity at both pH 7.2 and 5.5. We also found that the parent influenza hemagglutinin peptide **3** (HA2) had weak but detectable lytic activity at either pH, while the HA2 analog **4** (INF7) [23] showed only a trace of lytic activity at pH 5.5. Given that these types of peptides have been shown in the literature to safely effect cargo delivery to the cytosol, we were encouraged by the potential of optimizing this inherent but weak lytic activity. When peptides **1** and **3** were fused together to create the chimeric peptide **5** (HA2-Tat) [14,15,18,19] a large increase in lytic potency was observed at both pH, with about 3-fold selectivity for the lower pH. This was a quite remarkable finding, indicating that something about the combination of the two peptide sequences was conferring potent lytic activity that was not present in either of the two individual peptides. We prepared several analogs (Table 1, **6**–**9**) of the lead chimeric peptide by combining several known HA2 analogs with Tat and found varying degrees of potent lytic activity with each of these peptides. We theorized that the selectivity of the peptide and its pH responsiveness was governed directly by the pKa of the protonatable groups in the peptide, with the mixture of protonatable sidechains in peptide **6** providing the best overall profile. Peptide **6** (INF7-Tat) [24,25] was the most potent of these analogs at pH 5.5, while also maintaining the 3-fold pH selectivity of the lead peptide, and this peptide also demonstrated far superior physical properties and solubility behavior versus the others, and as such became our lead peptide for further optimization. We also prepared the chimeric fusion peptides of HA2 and INF7 with Penetratin (Table 1, **10–11**), but surprisingly both were devoid of lytic activity, again confirming the uniqueness of the combination of Tat and the HA2—like peptides. A preliminary CD (circular dichroism) analysis (Figure 1) of **6** showed that the peptide had a random coil conformation at pH 7.4, however at pH 5.5 the peptide was strongly alpha-helical, suggesting that the pH switching mechanism that we hoped to build into the peptides and optimize was indeed present [26,27].

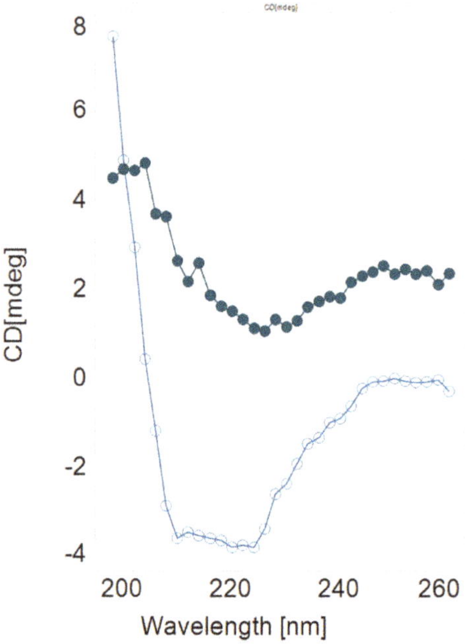

Figure 1. CD Spectrum of Peptide **6**. Filled circles = pH 7.4; open circles = pH 5.5.

2.2. *SAR and Optimization of Lytic Activity for Lead Peptide 6*

To fully examine the SAR surrounding the lead peptide **6**, as well as optimize the peptide for lytic activity and selectivity, we began a position-by-position amino acid walkthrough across the entire peptide sequence. Each amino acid in the INF7 portion of the sequence was varied individually, and selective changes were made to the Tat portion of the peptide as well. Positions were varied by charge, polarity, and lipophilicity based on their position on either the polar face or the lipophilic face of a helical wheel diagram of the lead peptide **6** (Figure 2). Table 2 summarizes the RBC lysis data for the position-by- position walkthrough of the INF7 portion of the chimeric peptide. The N-terminal residue (cysteine in most cases) was designated as position 1, moving from N-terminus to C-terminus across the peptides. The use of an N-terminal cysteine in the peptides was not in general detrimental for lytic activity. This is quite interesting in the context of previous publications that have suggested that the N-terminal residues of HA2-like peptides are critical for membrane insertion, with a glycine or other similar residues highly conserved and often a requirement for fusion activity [28,29]. In several cases, the cysteine was moved to other positions in the peptide sequence, and this had a minimal effect on lytic potency.

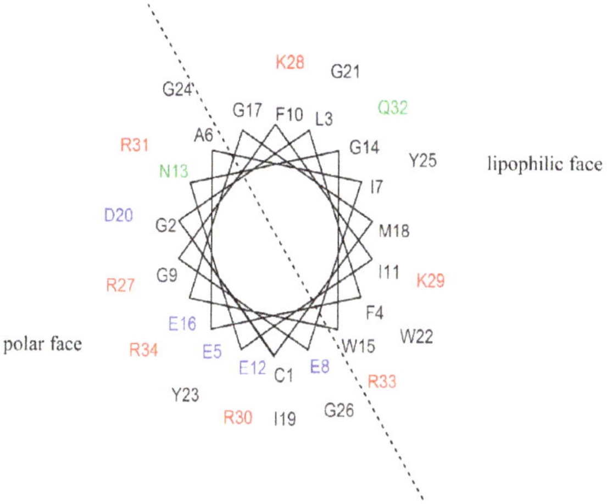

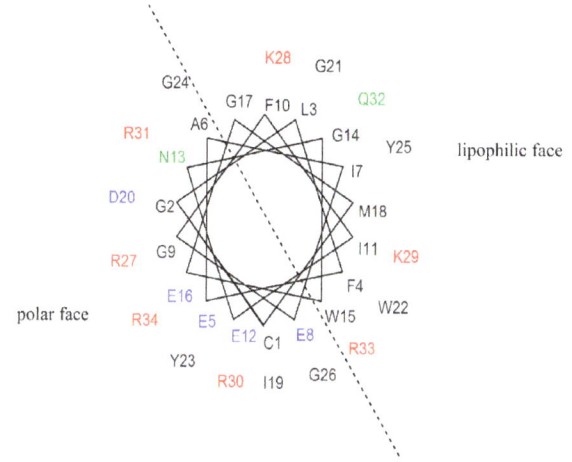

CGLFEAIEGFIENGWEGMIDGWYGYGRKKRRQRR
1 34

Figure 2. Helical wheel projection of HA-2 Tat.

Table 2. Modifications to the INF7 portion of the chimeric peptide.

Number	Sequence	RBC Lysis IC_{50}, pH 5.5 (μM)	RBC Lysis IC_{50}, pH 7.4 (μM)
12a	CRLFEAIEGFIENGWEGMIDGWYGYGRKKRRQRR	0.8	3.5
12b	CELFEAIEGFIENGWEGMIDGWYGYGRKKRRQRR	1.5	>20
12c	CGGGLFEAIEGFIENGWEGMIDGWYGYGRKKRRQRR	1	0.9
12d	C(Nle)LFEAIEGFIENGWEGMIDGWYGYGRKKRRQRR	0.8	2.4
12e	CVLFEAIEGFIENGWEGMIDGWYGYGRKKRRQRR	0.72	>20
12f	C(b-Ala)LFEAIEGFIENGWEGMIDGWYGYGRKKRRQRR	0.38 ± 0.17 (*n* = 5)	>20 (*n* = 5)
12g	CSLFEAIEGFIENGWEGMIDGWYGYGRKKRRQRR	0.66	>20
13a	CGFFEAIEGFIENGWEGMIDGWYGYGRKKRRQRR	0.35	1.16
13b	CGKFEAIEGFIENGWEGMIDGWYGYGRKKRRQRR	>20	>20
13c	CGEFEAIEGFIENGWEGMIDGWYGYGRKKRRQRR	>20	>20
13d	CGGFEAIEGFIENGWEGMIDGWYGYGRKKRRQRR	>10	>10
13e	CGNFEAIEGFIENGWEGMIDGWYGYGRKKRRQRR	>10	>10
14a	CGLNEAIEGFIENGWEGMIDGWYGYGRKKRRQRR	>100	>100
14b	CGLGEAIEGFIENGWEGMIDGWYGYGRKKRRQRR	>20	>20
14c	CGLKEAIEGFIENGWEGMIDGWYGYGRKKRRQRR	>10	>10
14d	CGLEEAIEGFIENGWEGMIDGWYGYGRKKRRQRR	2.5	>10
14e	CGLAEAIEGFIENGWEGMIDGWYGYGRKKRRQRR	1.3 (max. 65%)	>10
14f	CGLLEAIEGFIENGWEGMIDGWYGYGRKKRRQRR	0.93	3.67
15a	CGLFGAIEGFIENGWEGMIDGWYGYGRKKRRQRR	0.4	1
15b	CGLFAAIEGFIENGWEGMIDGWYGYGRKKRRQRR	1.26	0.75
15c	CGLFNAIEGFIENGWEGMIDGWYGYGRKKRRQRR	1.12	1.78
15d	CGLFLAIEGFIENGWEGMIDGWYGYGRKKRRQRR	>10	>10

Table 2. *Cont.*

Number	Sequence	RBC Lysis IC_{50}, pH 5.5 (μM)	RBC Lysis IC_{50}, pH 7.4 (μM)
15e	CGLFKAIEGFIENGWEGMIDGWYGYGRKKRRQRR	0.71	1.27
16a	CGLFENIEGFIENGWEGMIDGWYGYGRKKRRQRR	>10	>10
16b	CGLFELIEGFIENGWEGMIDGWYGYGRKKRRQRR	0.23	1.93
16c	CGLFEEIEGFIENGWEGMIDGWYGYGRKKRRQRR	0.26	>10
16d	CGLFEKIEGFIENGWEGMIDGWYGYGRKKRRQRR	0.04	1.11
17a	CGLFEAKEGFIENGWEGMIDGWYGYGRKKRRQRR	>10	>10
17b	CGLFEAEEGFIENGWEGMIDGWYGYGRKKRRQRR	4.74	>10
17c	CGLFEALEGFIENGWEGMIDGWYGYGRKKRRQRR	0.8	5
18a	CGLFEAIWGFIENGWEGMIDGWYGYGRKKRRQRR	0.9	1.2
18b	CGLFEAIKGFIENGWEGMIDGWYGYGRKKRRQRR	2.2	6.5
18c	CGLFEAIHGFIENGWEGMIDGWYGYGRKKRRQRR	7.7	>80
18d	CGLFEAIRGFIENGWEGMIDGWYGYGRKKRRQRR	1.2	2.8
18e	CGLFEAIDGFIENGWEGMIDGWYGYGRKKRRQRR	3.7	>100
18f	CGLFEAIGGFIENGWEGMIDGWYGYGRKKRRQRR	2.1	2.1
19a	CGLFEAIENFIENGWEGMIDGWYGYGRKKRRQRR	2.7	3.09
19b	CGLFEAIEKFIENGWEGMIDGWYGYGRKKRRQRR	2.32	>10
19c	CGLFEAIEEFIENGWEGMIDGWYGYGRKKRRQRR	0.41	>10
19d	CGLFEAIEGGIENGWEGMIDGWYGYGRKKRRQRR	2.52	>10
20a	CGLFEAIEGAIENGWEGMIDGWYGYGRKKRRQRR	0.88	4.71
20b	CGLFEAIEGLIENGWEGMIDGWYGYGRKKRRQRR	0.24	1.97
20c	CGLFEAIEGGIENGWEGMIDGWYGYGRKKRRQRR	2.52	>10
20d	CGLFEAIEGAIENGWEGMIDGWYGYGRKKRRQRR	0.88	4.71
20e	CGLFEAIEGLIENGWEGMIDGWYGYGRKKRRQRR	0.24	1.97
21a	CGLFEAIEGFGENGWEGMIDGWYGYGRKKRRQRR	>10	>10
21b	CGLFEAIEGFAENGWEGMIDGWYGYGRKKRRQRR	1.59	>10
21c	CGLFEAIEGFLENGWEGMIDGWYGYGRKKRRQRR	0.59	2.8
21d	CGLFEAIEGFWENGWEGMIDGWYGYGRKKRRQRR	0.35	>10
21e	CGLFEAIEGFKENGWEGMIDGWYGYGRKKRRQRR	>10	>10
21f	CGLFEAIEGFNENGWEGMIDGWYGYGRKKRRQRR	>100	>100
22a	CGLFEAIEGFILNGWEGMIDGWYGYGRKKRRQRR	1.06	1.1
22b	CGLFEAIEGFIWNGWEGMIDGWYGYGRKKRRQRR	0.44	0.95
22c	CGLFEAIEGFIKNGWEGMIDGWYGYGRKKRRQRR	4.27	>10
22d	CGLFEAIEGFIGNGWEGMIDGWYGYGRKKRRQRR	6.16	>10
23a	CGLFEAIEGFIEPGWEGMIDGWYGYGRKKRRQRR	>10	>10
23b	CGLFEAIEGFIEPGWEGMIDGWYGYGRKKRRQRR	>10	>10
23c	CGLFEAIEGFIEGGWEGMIDGWYGYGRKKRRQRR	1.11	6.55
23d	CGLFEAIEGFIELGWEGMIDGWYGYGRKKRRQRR	1.34	1.31
23e	CGLFEAIEGFIEWGWEGMIDGWYGYGRKKRRQRR	0.54	5.18
23f	CGLFEAIEGFIEKGWEGMIDGWYGYGRKKRRQRR	1.52	>10
24a	CGLFEAIEGFIENEWEGMIDGWYGYGRKKRRQRR	max. 45% @ 2.0 uM	>100
24b	CGLFEAIEGFIENKWEGMIDGWYGYGRKKRRQRR	>10	>10
24c	CGLFEAIEGFIENNWEGMIDGWYGYGRKKRRQRR	6.39	>10
24d	CGLFEAIEGFIENHWEGMIDGWYGYGRKKRRQRR	3.06	2.9

Table 2. *Cont.*

Number	Sequence	RBC Lysis IC_{50}, pH 5.5 (μM)	RBC Lysis IC_{50}, pH 7.4 (μM)
24e	CGLFEAIEGFIENPWEGMIDGWYGYGRKKRRQRR	1.71	4.72
24f	CGLFEAIEGFIENAWEGMIDGWYGYGRKKRRQRR	1.88	1.28
24g	CGLFEAIEGFIENWWEGMIDGWYGYGRKKRRQRR	1.1	>10
25a	CGLFEAIEGFIENGEEGMIDGWYGYGRKKRRQRR	1.55	0.31
24b	CGLFEAIEGFIENGKEGMIDGWYGYGRKKRRQRR	>10	>10
25c	CGLFEAIEGFIENGLEGMIDGWYGYGRKKRRQRR	0.66	4.43
26a	CGLFEAIEGFIENGWDGMIDGWYGYGRKKRRQRR	0.55	1.3
26b	CGLFEAIEGFIENGWRGMIDGWYGYGRKKRRQRR	0.19	3.3
26c	CGLFEAIEGFIENGWKGMIDGWYGYGRKKRRQRR	0.34	>10
26d	CGLFEAIEGFIENGWHGMIDGWYGYGRKKRRQRR	2.54	>10
26e	CGLFEAIEGFIENGWNGMIDGWYGYGRKKRRQRR	1.47	>10
26f	CGLFEAIEGFIENGWLGMIDGWYGYGRKKRRQRR	0.84	2.03
26g	CGLFEAIEGFIENGWAGMIDGWYGYGRKKRRQRR	1.3	>10
26h	CGLFEAIEGFIENGWGGMIDGWYGYGRKKRRQRR	3.1	>10
27a	CGLFEAIEGFIENGWEAMIDGWYGYGRKKRRQRR	0.12(max. 65%)	0.95
27b	CGLFEAIEGFIENGWENMIDGWYGYGRKKRRQRR	0.42	>10
27c	CGLFEAIEGFIENGWEKMIDGWYGYGRKKRRQRR	1.01	8.99
27d	CGLFEAIEGFIENGWEEMIDGWYGYGRKKRRQRR	3.76	>10
28a	CGLFEAIEGFIENGWEG(M sulfoxide)IDGWYGYGRKKRRQRR	>100	>100
28b	CGLFEAIEGFIENGWEG(M sulfone)IDGWYGYGRKKRRQRR	>100	>100
28c	CGLFEAIEGFIENGWEGNIDGWYGYGRKKRRQRR	>10	>10
28d	CGLFEAIEGFIENGWEGQIDGWYGYGRKKRRQRR	>10	>10
28e	CGLFEAIEGFIENGWEGTIDGWYGYGRKKRRQRR	>10	>10
28f	CGLFEAIEGFIENGWEGSIDGWYGYGRKKRRQRR	>10	>10
28g	CGLFEAIEGFIENGWEGLIDGWYGYGRKKRRQRR	0.71	2.9
28h	CGLFEAIEGFIENGWEG(Nle)IDGWYGYGRKKRRQRR	0.53	3.94
28i	CGLFEAIEGFIENGWEGYIDGWYGYGRKKRRQRR	2.56	>10
28j	CGLFEAIEGFIENGWEGFIDGWYGYGRKKRRQRR	0.52	9.65
28k	CGLFEAIEGFIENGWEGIDGWYGYGRKKRRQRR (delete)	50	>100
29a	CGLFEAIEGFIENGWEGMLDGWYGYGRKKRRQRR	10.2	>10
29b	CGLFEAIEGFIENGWEGMADGWYGYGRKKRRQRR	>10	>10
29c	CGLFEAIEGFIENGWEGMGDGWYGYGRKKRRQRR	2.53	>10
29d	CGLFEAIEGFIENGWEGMNDGWYGYGRKKRRQRR	1.04	>10
29e	CGLFEAIEGFIENGWEGMKDGWYGYGRKKRRQRR	1.17	9.1
29f	CGLFEAIEGFIENGWEGMEDGWYGYGRKKRRQRR	>10	>10
30a	CGLFEAIEGFIENGWEGMIEGWYGYGRKKRRQRR	4.4	>10
30b	CGLFEAIEGFIENGWEGMIAGWYGYGRKKRRQRR	>10	2.83
30c	CGLFEAIEGFIENGWEGMIWGWYGYGRKKRRQRR	>10	>10
30d	CGLFEAIEGFIENGWEGMILGWYGYGRKKRRQRR	>10	>10
31a	CGLFEAIEGFIENGWEGMIDAWYGYGRKKRRQRR	1.4	>10
31b	CGLFEAIEGFIENGWEGMIDLWYGYGRKKRRQRR	0.32	0.96
31c	CGLFEAIEGFIENGWEGMIDIWYGYGRKKRRQRR	1.68	>10
31d	CGLFEAIEGFIENGWEGMIDWWYGYGRKKRRQRR	0.55 ± 0.25 (n = 8)	7.14 ± 0.73 (n = 8)

Table 2. *Cont.*

Number	Sequence	RBC Lysis IC_{50}, pH 5.5 (μM)	RBC Lysis IC_{50}, pH 7.4 (μM)
31e	CGLFEAIEGFIENGWEGMIDNWYGYGRKKRRQRR	6.07	7.26
31f	CGLFEAIEGFIENGWEGMIDKWYGYGRKKRRQRR	2.86	>10
31g	CGLFEAIEGFIENGWEGMIDEWYGYGRKKRRQRR	1.5	>10
32a	CGLFEAIEGFIENGWEGMIDGYGRKKRRQRR	>10	>10
32b	CGLFEAIEGFIENGWEGMIDGGGGYGRKKRRQRR	>10	>10
33a	CGLFEAIEGFIENGWEGMIDGLYGYGRKKRRQRR	4.24	1.75
33b	CGLFEAIEGFIENGWEGMIDGAYGYGRKKRRQRR	4.07	>10
33c	CGLFEAIEGFIENGWEGMIDGGYGYGRKKRRQRR	>10	>10
33d	CGLFEAIEGFIENGWEGMIDGNYGYGRKKRRQRR	2.5	>10
33e	CGLFEAIEGFIENGWEGMIDGKYGYGRKKRRQRR	6.6	>10
33f	CGLFEAIEGFIENGWEGMIDGEYGYGRKKRRQRR	4.26	>10
34a	CGLFEAIEGFIENGWEGMIDGWAGYGRKKRRQRR	>10	>10
34b	CGLFEAIEGFIENGWEGMIDGWHGYGRKKRRQRR	5.04	>10
34c	CGLFEAIEGFIENGWEGMIDGWNGYGRKKRRQRR	0.13	1.72
34d	CGLFEAIEGFIENGWEGMIDGWEGYGRKKRRQRR	3.94	>10
35a	CGLFEAIEGFIENGWEGMIDGWYAYGRKKRRQRR	2	>10
35b	CGLFEAIEGFIENGWEGMIDGWYWYGRKKRRQRR	0.17 (max. 70%)	3.05
35c	CGLFEAIEGFIENGWEGMIDGWYEYGRKKRRQRR	1.04 (max. 60%)	>10

All peptides were >95% purity by HPLC analysis and demonstrated the correct HRMS profiles. Peptides were tested three times at each pH unless otherwise noted, and the values are reported as the mean. Standard Deviations are reported for peptides with larger *n* values to provide a reference for the reproducibility of the data. As solubility allowed, testing at pH 7.4 was pushed to the highest possible concentrations to determine as close as possible approximate IC_{50}.

A drastic effect on lytic potency is observed when the glycine at position 2 is modified. Substitution with charged residues **12a–b**, lipophilic residues **12d–e**, or a polar residue **12g** results in peptides with equal or improved lytic potency and in several cases much improved pH selectivity. In addition, the insertion of a larger "spacer" residue at this position such as a β–alanine (**12f**) provides a substantial increase in lytic potency at lower pH, while also providing much better pH selectivity. Even a large spacer like three glycines (**12c**) does not affect the lytic potency at pH 5.5; however, it does appear to affect the pH selectivity somewhat. As previously described above, the promiscuousness of the activity observed at this position contrasts with previous literature reports describing the N-terminal residues of HA2–like peptides [28,29]. This again points to the uniqueness of these peptides, and strongly suggests a highly disparate SAR for fusion activity and lytic activity, which is solidified by further data generated in our study.

SAR at position 3 (**13a–e**) clearly points to the requirement for a lipophilic residue at this position. This is not surprising given the position of this residue on the lipophilic face of the helical wheel projection of the peptide. A similar analysis can be made for position 4 (compounds **14a–f**), which also lies on the lipophilic face of the peptide. An interesting exception at this position is the glutamic acid analog **14d** which does appear to be tolerated in this position and appears to provide an improvement in pH selectivity.

Position 5 (compounds **15a–e**) appears tolerant to most polar and charged residues. Again, this is not surprising, given its location on the polar face of the helix, clustered among several charged residues.

The replacement of a glutamic acid at this position with a basic lysine residue (**15e**) confers increased potency, but compromises selectivity. This is a trend observed at multiple positions bearing glutamic acids across the peptide. Position 6 lies on the interface between the polar and lipophilic faces of the peptide, and as such analogs at this position demonstrate tolerability for both charged (compounds **16c–d**) and lipophilic (compound **16b**) residues. The glutamic acid analog at this position (**16c**) is especially noteworthy, providing a 5-fold enhancement of lytic potency at pH 5.5, and excellent pH selectivity. Figure 3 shows a comparison of the CD spectrum of **16c** at pH 7 and 5.5, providing clear conformational support for the high degree of selectivity observed with this peptide. This peptide is one of the best performing single amino acid modifications identified in this study and highlights the critical importance of this position for lytic activity. Interestingly, the asparagine analog at this position is not well tolerated and loses all lytic potency. This is an interesting observation and is somewhat difficult to rationalize given the other SAR at this position.

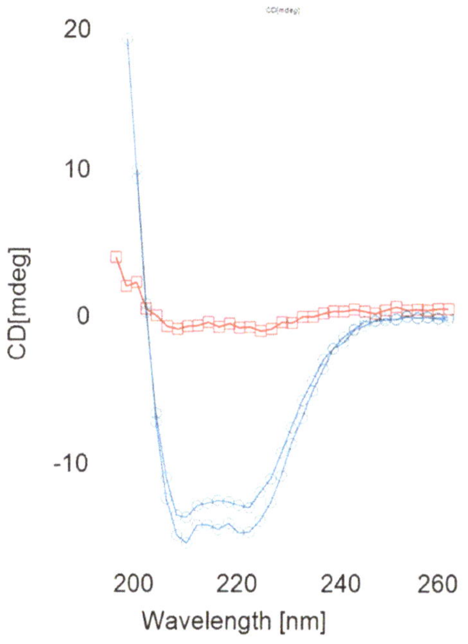

Boxes = pH 7.4; circles = pH 5.5

Figure 3. CD spectrum at pH 7 and 5.5 for peptide **16c**.

Position 7, occupied in the lead peptide by an isoleucine residue and lying in the center of the lipophilic face of the peptide helix would be expected to be highly intolerant of polar or charged residues, and the SAR directly confirms this. The leucine analog at this position **17c** provides a peptide with enhanced potency at lower pH, as well as improved pH selectivity. The charged, basic lysine analog **17a** loses all lytic potency at both pH. Once again, as seen with the similar position 4, a glutamic acid (compound **17b**) is somewhat tolerated in this position along the lipophilic face of the helix.

In a similar manner to position 6, position 8 lies along the interface between the polar and lipid faces of the peptide helix. As such, this position appears to be one of the most tolerant positions in the entire peptide, able to be replaced by lipophilic/aromatic (**18a**), charged (**18b–e**), or small/no sidechain (**18f, 5**) containing amino acid residues. Only the histidine analog (**18c**) at this position produced a reduction in lytic potency at pH 5.5. In terms of pH selectivity, there was no clear trend, but all the analogs were either balanced in terms of pH selectivity or showed improved selectivity versus the lead peptide.

Position 9 of the peptide lies along the polar face of the peptide helix and as such would be expected to tolerate polar and charged residues **19a–c**, and this is confirmed by our data. This position surprisingly is also tolerant of a lipophilic residue (**19d**), in a similar manner to the glycine 2 residue that is located close by on the peptide helix. Also, in a similar manner to glycine 2, a glutamic acid residue (compound **19c**) is well tolerated at this position and provides a 3-fold increase in lytic potency at pH 5.5 as well as an increase in pH selectivity. The fact that these two glycine residues are close to each other on the peptide helix and share some common SAR features may indicate that this region of the peptide is acting as a unit to govern overall peptide behavior.

Position 10 of the peptide lies on the lipophilic face of the peptide helix and our SAR analysis at this position indicates a strong preference for non-polar/non-charged residues. Glycine (**20a**), alanine (**20b**), and leucine (**20c**) each provide increasing lytic potency at pH 5.5 as the size/lipophilicity increases of the sidechain. Interestingly, a similar trend is seen at pH 7.4, with lytic activity increasing with sidechain size/lipophilicity. Unlike several other residues in this region, neither acidic (**20e**) nor basic (**20f**) amino acid sidechains are tolerated at this position.

SAR at position 11 of the lead peptide also appears to be largely governed by its position on the lipophilic face of the peptide helix. The glycine substitution (**21a**) at this position provides a peptide devoid of lytic activity, however gradually increasing the size of the substituent here from a methyl (alanine; **21b**) to a larger carbon chain (leucine; **21c**), to finally a large aromatic substituent (tryptophan; **21d**) results in concomitant increases in lytic potency at pH 5.5. In each case, selectivity is maintained or increased, indicating that this position may be an important handle for introducing increased pH selectivity into the peptide. Replacement with a polar sidechain (asparagine; **21e**) or a charged sidechain (lysine; **21f**) results in complete loss of lytic activity at both pH.

Position 12 of the parent peptide is located on the polar face of the helix, in an area that appears to be a cluster of glutamic acid residues. Interestingly, replacement of this glutamic acid residue with lipophilic residues such as a leucine (**22a**) or a tryptophan (**22b**) produces peptides with equal or improved lytic activity at lower pH; however, the peptides become equipotent at physiological pH as well. A basic lysine residue (**22c**) or an unsubstituted glycine residue (**22d**) at this position produced peptides that retain some lytic activity at pH 5.5, although the activity is diminished from the parent peptide.

Positions 13 and 14 define a region of the INF7 portion of the peptide that has been described by previous authors as a "hinge region" in HA2 peptides [30–32], providing flexibility between separate N-terminal and C-terminal helical regions and allowing the peptide to form a "boomerang" or U–shaped conformation that is theorized to aid the peptide in penetrating biological membranes for fusion activity [30–32]. We incorporated several amino acids at each of these positions that were designed to test this hypothesis. Theoretically, a proline at position 13 might serve as an excellent mimic of such a hinge; however, we found that substitution of proline (**23a**) at this position produced a complete loss of lytic potency. Substitution with glycine at this position (**23b**), which may also be able to support a hinge mechanism, was better tolerated and provided a profile equal to the parent peptide. Increasing the size of the amino acid sidechain at this position from leucine (**23c**) to tryptophan (**23d**) provided peptides with equal or better lytic potency at pH 5.5 versus parent. Charged residues such as lysine (**23e**) or glutamic acid (**23f**) also provided peptides with equal or better lytic potency at pH 5.5 with good selectivity versus physiological pH. Position 14 showed a somewhat different profile, with highly charged residues such as glutamic acid (**24a**) or lysine (**24b**) not well tolerated, but less charged/polar residues such as asparagine (**24c**) or histidine (**24d**) showing moderate lytic potency. In contrast to position 13, proline (**24e**) was well tolerated, showing a slight loss in potency at lower pH with only slight pH selectivity observed. Interestingly, replacement of the glycine with an alanine (**24f**) led to a peptide with a potent, balanced lytic profile, while replacement with the lipophilic/aromatic tryptophan (**24g**) produced a peptide with lytic potency similar to parent at acidic pH, with improved pH selectivity.

The tryptophan residue at position 15 lies on the lipophilic face of the peptide in a helical projection, very close to the interface/transition between the lipid and polar faces of the peptide. Interestingly, replacement of the tryptophan with a glutamic acid (**25a**) produces a peptide that exhibits an inverted pH profile. This peptide was one of the most lytically potent peptides we observed at physiological pH. Changing the charge at this position from negative to positive as in the lysine replacement (**25b**) provided a peptide that was inactive at both pH. This position appears to be quite important for pH selectivity as demonstrated by these two oppositely charged amino acid analogs. Simply replacing the tryptophan with a lipophilic but non-aromatic leucine residue (**25c**) provided an approximately two-fold increase in lytic potency at acidic pH while also improving the pH selectivity.

Position 16 appears to be one of the more tolerant positions along the peptide backbone and was largely tolerant of all amino acid changes that were made. Simple modification of the glutamic acid to an aspartic acid provided a peptide with several fold enhanced potency at pH 5.5 (**26a**). A positively charged residue at this position (**26b–d**) also maintained some level of potency and selectivity, with the lysine sidechain at this position (**26c**) providing one of the overall best profiles of all peptides in the study. A non-charged, polar residue such as asparagine maintained good potency at pH 5.5 with enhanced pH selectivity (**26e**). Small alkyl sidechains (compounds **26f–g**) at this position maintained some level of lytic potency and pH selectivity, while even a glycine (**26h**) maintained some level of potency at acidic pH with good pH selectivity. Several the modifications at this position demonstrated complete pH selectivity, confirming this residue as another key position for maintaining the desired pH balance.

Modification of the glycine residue at position 17 provided several interesting novel peptides. Substitution with an alanine residue at this position (**27a**) provided a peptide with enhanced potency at pH 5.5, but a blunted maximal lytic effect. Addition of a charged sidechain at this position, whether negative (**27b**) or positive (**27c**) provided peptides that maintained lytic potency at pH 5.5 but showed somewhat enhanced pH selectivity. Interestingly, the asparagine analog (**27d**) demonstrated a very nice overall profile, with enhanced potency at lower pH and improved pH selectivity.

The methionine residue at position 18 was of particular interest to us, since we had seen some propensity for oxidation to occur at this position on storage of the peptide in solution. Consequently, we were eager to explore alternative amino acid substitutions at this position. We prepared samples of both potential oxidation products at this position, and both the sulfoxide (**28a**) and sulfone (**28b**) were completely devoid of any lytic activity at either pH. Interestingly, if one looks at the helical projection of the peptide, this residue lies near the center of the lipophilic face of the peptide, and consequently polar substitutions would be likely to be detrimental to stability of the helix and in turn lytic activity. Confirming this hypothesis, replacement of this residue with polar, uncharged sidechains (**26c–f**) resulted in peptides that were lytically inactive at both pH. Intuitively, one would also expect that lipophilic sidechain modifications at this position would much better tolerated, and that does appear to be the case. Substitution with either a leucine (**28g**) of a norleucine (**28h**) provided peptides with enhanced lytic potency at pH 5.5 and similar selectivity to parent. Aromatic sidechain-containing residues such as tyrosine (**28i**) and phenylalanine (**28j**) were also well tolerated, providing equal or better lytic potency at pH 5.5 with somewhat enhanced pH selectivity. As expected, complete deletion of the residue (**28k**) provided a peptide with only very weak lytic activity, presumably due to the disruption of the overall amino acid sidechain arrangement of the helical form of the peptide.

Replacement of the isoleucine at position 19 provided a somewhat interesting SAR. Replacement of this highly lipophilic, branched residue with a very similar leucine residue (**29a**) surprisingly resulted in a loss in lytic potency. Shrinking the sidechain even more to an alanine (**29b**) resulted in a complete loss of lytic activity. However, completely removing the sidechain and substituting with a glycine residue (**29c**) restored the lytic activity to near the level of parent, with enhanced pH selectivity also observed. Substitution with an uncharged polar residue (**29d**) provided a peptide with improved lytic potency at pH 5.5 and improved pH selectivity. Substitution with a positively charged lysine residue (**29e**) provided a peptide with an almost identical profile; however, substitution with a negatively charged residue (**29f**) resulted in a complete loss of lytic activity. It is difficult to rationalize the observations made by changing the sidechain residues at this position, other than to speculate that if one looks at a helical projection of the peptide, this residue lies close to the interface between the lipophilic and polar faces of the amphiphilic helix, and this may in part help to explain the somewhat contrary SAR observed for this position.

Position 20 appears to be one of the least tolerant positions in the peptide sequence. Modification from glutamic to aspartic acid at this position (**30a**) resulted in a loss of lytic potency, and substitution with small (**30b**) or large (**30c-d**) lipophilic sidechains completely obliterated lytic activity.

Contrary to the observation for position 20, position 21 appeared highly tolerant of substitution and proved to be an excellent position for enhancing lytic potency at pH 5.5 as well as optimizing pH selectivity. Substitution with alanine at this position (**31a**) provided a peptide with equal lytic potency to parent at pH 5.5 but enhanced pH selectivity. Adding a larger lipophilic sidechain such as leucine (**31b**) provided enhanced lytic potency at low pH while maintaining a similar selectivity ratio to parent. Interestingly, substitution of isoleucine at this position (**31c**) provided similar lytic potency to parent at pH 5.5, but greatly enhanced pH selectivity. Substitution with the larger lipophilic/aromatic sidechain of tryptophan (**31d**) provided a peptide with enhanced lytic potency at pH 5.5 and improved pH selectivity; this individual peptide had one of the more favorable overall profiles of all the peptides tested. Substitution with a polar, uncharged asparagine residue (**31e**) resulted in a reduction of lytic potency and selectivity, however charged polar residues such as lysine (**31f**) or glutamic acid (**31g**) were tolerated with equal lytic potency at pH 5.5 and improved pH selectivity.

Positions 22–24 compose the "WYG addition" to the C-terminus of the INF7 portion of the chimeric peptide. Addition of the WYG residues that are present at the C-terminus of the native HA2 fusogenic peptide to numerous similar peptides has been reported in the literature [33] to provide increased membrane affinity and fusogenic potency, so we sought to incorporate this into our sequences from the beginning of our investigations. Indeed, two of the first peptide sequences that we prepared were the parent with and without the WYG addition. Interestingly, removal of the WYG insert from the parent chimeric peptide (**32a**) resulted in a complete loss in lytic potency, suggesting the critical importance of this small addition to the peptide. The uniqueness and specificity of this small insert into the parent chimeric sequence was confirmed by simply substituting a GGG spacer for this sequence. This peptide (**32b**) was also lytically inactive. It is difficult to infer why these three amino acid inserts are so critical to the activity of these peptides. If one compares the helical distribution of the peptides with and without these three amino acids, both peptides are remarkably similar in their amphiphilicity and amino acid distribution. The peptide with the WYG insert does add an additional tryptophan to the lipophilic face of the peptide in a region that is quite close to another tryptophan residue at position 15, and there has been some experimental evidence published [33] suggesting that this residue is a key residue for anchoring the HA-2 family peptides in the membrane. So, it is possible that the additional tryptophan may aid in this membrane anchoring process, however this remains highly speculative and there is no definitive experimental evidence to support this hypothesis.

The individual residues at positions 22–24 were also varied in an independent manner as with the rest of the peptide. Position 22 proved to be somewhat intolerant to various changes. Substitution with a smaller, non-aromatic but lipophilic leucine sidechain (**33a**) resulted in a peptide with an inverted pH profile, and further reduction of the size of the sidechain to a methyl (**33b**) resulted in lower in lytic potency at both pH. Completely removing the side chain (**33c**) by substitution of a glycine at this position eliminated lytic activity at both pH. Substitution with a polar, non-charged asparagine residue (**33d**) provided a peptide with reduced potency at both pH, but a favorable overall selectivity profile. Substitution with either a positively charged lysine residue (**33e**) of a negatively charged glutamic acid residue (**33f**) provided peptides with reduced lytic potency. In general, the tryptophan at this position does indeed appear to be very important for maintaining lytic activity.

Variation at position 23 also provided some interesting and somewhat surprising results. Shrinking the sidechain to a methyl (**34a**) resulted in a complete loss of lytic potency. Replacement of the aryl sidechain with a heteroaryl imidazole (**34b**) provided a peptide with reduced lytic potencies at both pH. Interestingly, substitution with an asparagine residue at this position (**34c**) resulted in a ten-fold increase in lytic potency at pH 5.5, and a corresponding three-fold increase at physiological pH. A glutamic acid substitution lowered lytic activity at both pH but provided a peptide with a favorable overall pH profile.

Several single amino acid variants at position 24 were also examined. Modification to an alanine at this position (**35a**) resulted in a peptide with similar lytic activity at pH 5.5 to parent but improved pH selectivity. Modification to a large lipophilic aromatic residue (**35b**) at this position provided a peptide with apparently enhanced lytic activity at both pH; however, the peptide did not provide maximum activity at lower pH. A similar profile was seen for substitution with a glutamic acid at this position (**35c**), with the peptide providing only 60% maximum lytic activity at lower pH.

Beyond the systematic single amino variants at each position of the INF7 portion of the chimeric peptide, we also investigated several other important peptide analogs. The results for these subsequent peptide analogs are summarized in Table 3. One series of analogs that we wanted to consider was the possibility of inserting a spacer between the INF7 and Tat portions of the chimeric peptide. Moving the position of the cysteine residue from the N-terminus to the center of the peptide (**36a**) provided a peptide with a balanced lytic profile. Inserting a GGG spacer between the two component peptides (**36b**) provided a peptide with two-fold enhanced lytic potency at pH 5.5, and improved pH selectivity versus physiological pH. Given this interesting result, we attempted to make the spacer between the two individual peptide chimeras larger by inserting amino/acid terminated peg spacers. Quite remarkably, good lytic potency and pH selectivity were maintained for (peg)3 (**36c**) and (peg)6 (**36d**) spacers, and even the (peg)11 (**36e**) spacer showed a reasonable overall profile. Pushing this to a larger (peg)27 (**36f**) spacer eliminated lytic activity.

Table 3. Modifications to the spacer between the peptide chimera, the Tat potion of the chimeric peptide, and miscellaneous modifications.

Number	Sequence	RBC Lysis IC_{50}, pH 5.5 (μM)	RBC Lysis IC_{50}, pH 7.4 (μM)
36a	GLFEAIEGFIENGWEGMIDGWYGCYGRKKRRQRR	2.09	2.1
36b	CGLFEAIEGFIENGWEGMIDGWYGGGGYGRKKRRQRR	0.7	7.9
36c	CGLFEAIEGFIENGWEGMIDGWYG(Peg 3)YGRKKRRQRR	1.92	>10
36d	CGLFEAIEGFIENGWEGMIDGWYG(Peg 6)YGRKKRRQRR	1.22	>10
36e	CGLFEAIEGFIENGWEGMIDGWYG(Peg11)YGRKKRRQRR	2.4	>100
36f	CGLFEAIEGFIENGWEGMIDGWYG(Peg 27)YGRKKRRQRR	28	>100
37a	CGLFEAIEGFIENGWEGMIDGWYGYGKKKKKQKK	7.78	>100
37b	CGLFEAIEGFIENGWEGMIDGWYGYGHKKHHQHH	0.90 ± 0.19 (*n* = 8)	>100 (*n* = 8)
37c	CGLFEAIEGFIENGWEGMIDGWYGYGRKKRRQRRR	1.77	6.82
37d	CGLFEAIEGFIENGWEGMIDGWYGYGRKKRRQR	0.75	>100
37e	CGLFEAIEGFIENGWEGMIDGWYGYGRKKRRQ	0.96	>100
37f	CGLFEAIEGFIENGWEGMIDGWYGYGRKKRR	1.61	>100
37g	CGLFEAIEGFIENGWEGMIDGWYGYGRKKR	7.8	>100
37h	CGLFEAIEGFIENGWEGMIDGWYGYGHKKHHQHR	0.58 ± 0.17 (*n* = 10)	>100 (*n* = 10)
38a	GLFEAIEGFIENGWEGMIDGWYGYGRKKRRQRRC	0.96	>10
38b	YGRKKRRQRRGLFEAIEGFIENGWEGMIDGWYGC	2.91	>100
38c	CYGRKKRRQRRGLFEAIEGFIENGWEGMIDGWYG	1.17	>20
38d	rrqrrkkrgygywgdimgewgneifgeiaeflgc	5	>100
38e	crrqrrkkrgygywgdimgewgneifgeiaeflg	0.1	1.51
38f	cglfeaiegfiengwegmidgwygygrkkrrqrr	2.3	>20

All peptides were >95% purity by HPLC analysis and demonstrated the correct HRMS profiles. Peptides were tested three times at each pH unless otherwise noted, and the values are reported as the mean. Standard Deviations are reported for peptides with larger *n* values to provide a reference for the reproducibility of the data. As solubility allowed, testing at pH 7.4 was pushed to the highest possible concentrations to determine as close as possible approximate IC_{50}.

While we did not individually vary the residues in the Tat portion of the chimeric peptide, we did make several interesting changes to this region of the peptide that resulted in favorable contributions to the overall SAR. To favorably alter the overall pH selectivity profile of the parent peptide, we focused on examining multiple changes to the basic, protonatable residues present in the Tat potion of the chimeric peptide. Replacement of all five of the arginine residues with lysines (**37a**) provided a peptide with reduced lytic potency at both pH. Similarly, replacement of all the arginines with histidines (**37b**) provided a peptide with slightly improved lytic potency at lower pH, but improved pH selectivity. Adding an additional arginine to the C-terminus of the parent (**37c**) sequence provided a peptide with a largely identical lytic profile. Interestingly, removal of one of the arginines from the C-terminus (**37d**) provided an increase in lytic potency at lower pH, along with an improvement in pH selectivity. Given this result, we systematically removed C-terminal residues one by one until we began to see a detrimental effect on lytic activity. Removal of two arginines (**37e**), or even of the last three residues (two arginines and a glutamine; **37f**) provided peptides that maintained good profiles. It was only when the four consecutive C-terminal residues were removed (**37g**) that a large drop off in lytic potency was observed. Replacing four of the five Tat arginine residues with histidine but maintaining the C-terminal arginine (**37h**) provided a peptide with one of the most favorable overall pH profiles that we saw in the entire study, exhibiting a three –fold increase in lytic potency at pH 5.5 and enhanced pH selectivity. This peptide was soluble enough that we were able to push the concentration up to as high as 100 μM at physiological pH and saw no lytic activity at this concentration. Once again as stated earlier, the pH responsiveness of the overall chimeric peptide can clearly be changed by altering the pKa and number of protonatable groups present in the peptide. However, being able to control this in a systematic, predictable manner proved to be quite challenging, and once again our efforts were driven primarily by intuition and empirically observed data.

We also examined several other overall variants of the parent chimeric peptide sequence. Simply moving the cysteine residue from the N-terminus of the peptide to the C-terminus of the peptide (**38a**) provided a peptide with a slightly improved overall pH profile over parent. Simple retro-analogs (**38b,c**) with the cysteine at either the C-or N-termini showed similar profiles to parent and **38a**. The all (D) version of the peptide (**38f**) once again showed a similar profile, while the retro-inverso peptides (**38d,e**) showed lower lytic potency at pH 5.5. Interestingly, the similar activity observed for the all (D) peptide strongly suggests that the lytic activity seen with these peptides is likely a function of the alpha-helical, amphiphilic nature of these peptides, is independent of the overall chirality of the peptide analogs and suggests that these effects are independent of direct interactions with any specific binding sites. This may also be important in terms of metabolic stability; the harsh environment of the late endosome is likely a very unfavorable environment for metabolically unstable peptides, and the all (D) versions likely offer substantial advantages in these regards.

Given that the membrane disruptive/lytic activity observed with these peptides strongly appeared to be driven by physiochemical properties such as helicity and amphiphilicity, we wanted to prepare some stapled analogs of these peptides to see if the incorporation of a hydrocarbon staple across the lipophilic face of these peptides would make the transition from a more random conformation to an alpha helical conformation more favorable (Table 4) and thus improve lytic potency and/or selectivity. By simply looking at the helical wheel representation of the parent peptide (Figure 2), several potential target stapled peptides were identified. We chose to initially try stapling between the following residues using *i,i+7* hydrocarbon staples: L3 and F10, F4 and Ill, and Ill and M18. We consistently used the same amino acid side-chain lengths for each analog (5 carbon terminal olefin for the more N-terminal residue, and 8 carbon terminal olefin residues for the more C-terminal residue of the staple) as suggested by the literature [34–36] and followed established literature guidelines [34–36] for stereochemistry at each residue. Hydrocarbon stapled peptides were synthesized using standard Fmoc-solid phase peptide chemistry, with the metathesis reaction performed on resin using Grubbs Gen. II catalyst [34–36], followed by deprotection and cleavage. All three hydrocarbon stapled analogs (**39a–c**) showed impressive lytic activity at pH 5.5 that was equal to or better than parent with good pH selectivity. However, compound **39b**, which had the hydrocarbon staple spanning from residue 4 to residue 11 showed one of the best overall profiles of all the peptides tested in this study. This result further strengthens our hypothesis regarding the critical importance of the amphiphilic, alpha-helical character of the peptides for achieving potent lytic activity. Unfortunately, these stapled derivatives proved quite difficult to work with due to inherent issues with solubility and aggregation, as well as poor synthetic yields coupled with difficult purifications. Nonetheless, the constraint of peptides in this class using hydrocarbon staples appears to be a promising strategy for enhancing lytic potency and pH selectivity, and further studies to take advantage of this strategy while also enhancing the physical properties of the peptides are in progress and will be reported in more depth in future publications.

Table 4. Stapled and lipidated peptide analogs.

Number	Sequence	RBC Lysis IC_{50}, pH 5.5 (μM)	RBC Lysis IC_{50}, pH 7.4 (μM)
39a	CGX$_{(R)}$FEAIEGZ$_{(S)}$IENGWEGMIDGWYGYGRKKRRQRR 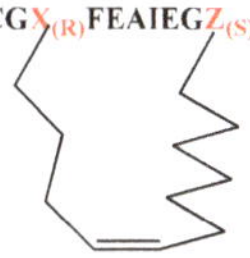	0.48	>10
39b	CGLX$_{(R)}$EAIEGFZ$_{(S)}$ENGWEGMIDGWYGYGRKKRRQRR 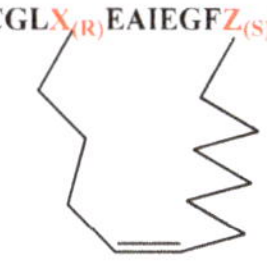	0.19	>10
39c	CGLFEAIEGFX$_{(R)}$ENGWEGZ$_{(S)}$IDGWYGYGRKKRRQRR 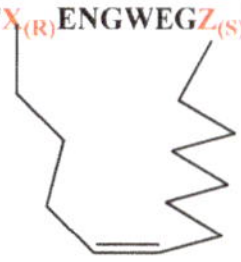	1.89	>10
39d	CGLFEAIEGFIENGWEGMIDGWYGYGRKKRRQRRK(Stearoyl)	0.58 ± 0.2 (*n* = 6)	0.94 ± 0.4 (*n* = 6)
39e	(stearoyl)GLFEAIEGFIENGWEGMIDGWYGYGRKKRRQRRC	0.7	>10

All peptides were >95% purity by HPLC analysis and demonstrated the correct HRMS profiles. Peptides were tested three times at each pH unless otherwise noted, and the values are reported as the mean. Standard Deviations are reported for peptides with larger *n* values to provide a reference for the reproducibility of the data. As solubility allowed, testing at pH 7.4 was pushed to the highest possible concentrations to determine as close as possible approximate IC_{50} values. For peptide **40a**, the stearoyl group was acylated onto the N-terminus of the peptide, and for peptide **40b**, a lysine was added to the C-terminus of the peptide and the epsilon amine was acylated with the steroyl group.

One other modification that we considered was the addition of lipid chains to the termini of the parent peptide (Table 4). Theoretically, the addition of a lipid to the peptide could aid in interaction with and insertion into lipid membranes. To add a lipid at the C-terminus, we added a lysine residue to the C-terminus of the parent peptide and acylated the sidechain amine of the lysine with stearic acid to provide peptide **39d** (Table 4). This peptide showed an interesting, highly lytic profile that was potent and balanced at both pH. Acylation of the N-terminus of the peptide directly with stearic acid and shifting the cysteine conjugation point to the C-terminus provided peptide **39e**, which showed two-fold better lytic potency at pH 5.5 and improved pH selectivity. Unfortunately, once again the extremely poor physical properties of the peptides limited the effort in this area.

Of course, after these extensive SAR studies, the clear question becomes how much of this SAR can be combined in an additive or synergistic manner to produce more lytically potent and pH selective peptides. There are literally thousands of possible permutations and combinations of the observed SAR, and we will highlight just a few of the most interesting combination analogs here. In general, we tried to combine some of the most interesting single amino acid changes to look for additivity or synergy.

From the results in Table 3, there are several interesting trends. In general, potency at pH 5.5 is in almost all cases enhanced, while pH selectivity in almost all cases is also better than parent. So, the overall trend is toward peptides with enhanced profiles. However, the specifics of the combined modifications are quite varied, and peptides with several very different profiles are observed by combining various amino acid changes. While the general trend was toward better peptides, the specific combinations were not always additive or even mutually tolerated. Interesting peptides were found by combining as few as two amino acid changes, or as many as nine amino acid changes (Table 5).

Table 5. Combination peptide analogs.

Number	Sequence	RBC Lysis IC_{50}, pH 5.5 (μM)	RBC Lysis IC_{50}, pH 7.4 (μM)
40	CELFEAIEGFIENGWEGLIDGWYGYGRKKRRQRR	2.12	>10
41	CGLFGAIEGFIENGWEGLIDGWYGYGRKKRRQRR	0.41	0.9
42	CGLFEAIEGFIENGWKGMIDWWYGYGRKKRRQRR	0.66	0.29
43	CGLFEAIEGFIENGWEGLIDAWYGYGRKKRRQRR	0.62	>10
44	CELFEAIWGFIENGWEGMIDGWYGGGGYGRKKRRQRR	1 (max.50%)	5 (max.60%)
45	CELFEAIEGFIENGWEGLIDGWYGYGRKKRRQRRR	2.98	4.32
46	CRLFEAIWGFIENGWEGMIDGWYGGGGYGRKKRRQRR	0.35	0.12
47	CGLFGAIEGFIENGWEGLIDGWYGYGRKKRRQRRR	1.55	3.97
48	CGLFEEIEGFIENGWEGLIDWWYGYGRKKRRQRR	0.72	>10
49	CELFGAIWGFIENGWEGLIDGWYGYGRKKRRQRR	>10	>10
50	CELFGAIEGFIENGWEGLIDGWYGYGRKKRRQRRR	2	max. 35% @ >10
51	CELFGAIEGFIENGWKGLIDWWYGYGRKKRRQRR	0.14	3.29
52	CGLFGAIEGFIENGWKGLIDAWYGYGRKKRRQRR	0.1	3.41
53	CGLFEAIEGFIENGLKGLIDAWYGYGRKKRRQRR	0.18	>10
54	CELFGAIEGFIENGWKGLIDWWYGYGRKKRRQRR	0.14	3.29
55	CELFGAIEGFIENGWKGLIDAWYGYGRKKRRQRR	0.71	3.19
56	CGIFGAIEGFIENGWWGLIDAWYGYGRKKRRQRR	0.07	2.35
57	CGFFEAIEGFIENGLKGLIDAWYGYGRKKRRQRR	0.17	3.99
58	CGLAEAIEGFIENGLKGLIDWWYGYGRKKRRQRR	0.06	2
59	CGLFEAIAEFIEGGWEGLIEGWYGYGRKKRRQRR	0.79	>10
60	C(b-Ala)GFEFIEEFIENGLKNLIDWWYGYGRKKRRQRR	1.14	12.8
61	CGLFGEIEELIEEGLKNLIDWWYGYGRKKRRQRR	0.97	8.07
62	CGLFGEIEELIEEGLKNLIDWWYGYGHKKHHQHR	1.28	>20
63	CGLFGEIEELIEEGLENLIDWWYGYGRKKRRQRR	3.6	>20
64	CGLFGEIEELIEEGLENLIDWWYGYGHKKHHQHR	3.91	>20
65	CGLFGEIEEFIEEGLENLIDWWYGYGRKKRRQRR	3.15	>20
66	CGLFGEIEEFIEEGWENFIDWWYGYGRKKRRQRR	4.08	>20
67	CGLFGEIEELIEEGWEGLIDWWYGYGRKKRRQRR	3.4	>20
68	CGLFEEIEELIEEGLENLIDWWYGYGRKKRRQRR	4.11	>20
69	CGLFEEIEELIEEGLENLIDWWYGYGHKKHHQHR	8.73	>20
70	CGLFEEIEELIEEGLKNLIDWWYGYGHKKHHQHR	2.28	>20

All peptides were >95% purity by HPLC analysis and demonstrated the correct HRMS profiles. Peptides were tested three times at each pH unless otherwise noted, and the values are reported as the mean. Standard Deviations are reported for peptides with larger *n* values to provide a reference for the reproducibility of the data. As solubility allowed, testing at pH 7.4 was pushed to the highest possible concentrations to determine as close as possible approximate IC_{50}.

One of the most interesting peptides in the entire study (compound **53**) was obtained by combining optimal modifications at positions 15, 16, 18, and 21; this peptide is among the most lytically potent peptides tested at pH 5.5, while demonstrating excellent pH selectivity. In terms of raw potency at pH 5.5, several peptides with five amino acid changes from parent were observed to possess sub-100 nM potency (compounds **56** and **58**), while maintaining respectable levels of pH selectivity. This represents a greater than 20-fold enhancement of lytic potency at pH 5.5 by simple substitution of five key amino acid residues. Even peptides with as many as nine (**62**) amino acid changes maintained respectable overall profiles that were better than parent.

We were intrigued by the sequence of peptide **61** (Table 5), which maintains good lytic potency at pH 5.5 and good pH selectivity despite having many anionic residues in the sequence. While the parent HA-2 type and other fusogenic peptides are anionic in nature, and there are known cell penetrating [37] or membrane active/antimicrobial peptides [38,39] that are largely anionic, most peptides in this space are typically highly cationic peptides. To further probe the relationship of charge to lytic activity and pH selectivity, we prepared a group of analogs based on the sequence of **61**, in which we made additional amino acid substitutions using the data gathered from our amino acid walk-through as a guide (Table 5). Combining the INF7 portion of **61** with the histidine-modified Tat from **37h** provided peptide **62**, which maintained lytic potency at pH 5.5 while providing full pH selectivity. This peptide is also noteworthy in that it has 14 amino acid positional changes from the original lead structure and maintains good lytic potency and pH selectivity. Substituting additional negatively charged residues into the sequences of **61** and **62** at position 16 provided peptides **63** and **64**. Although both peptides lost some lytic potency, they still retain a reasonable level of lytic activity. This is quite interesting in that peptides **63–64** both possess an overall net charge of zero, having 7 positively and seven negatively charged residues in their sequences. These peptides represent the first peptides that we have identified in this series that maintain lytic activity without having an overall positive charge. Similar analogs **64–67** which have slightly modified sequences maintain the overall net zero charge and exhibit quite similar potency and selectivity to **63** and **64**. Investigating this further to insert an additional negative charge provides peptide **68**, which continues the trend towards reduced lytic potency but remarkably still retains some level of lytic activity and selectivity even with an overall negative charge on the peptide. Again, combining the features of **68** with the histidine-modified Tat from **37h** provided peptide **69**, which showed an additional potency loss. However, simply removing one of the negatively charged residues at position **16** improved the lytic potency of the peptide at pH 5.5 back into a reasonable range while maintaining good pH selectivity. While the lytic activity of peptides **62–70** is diminished versus the most potent analogs observed in this study, the SAR clearly suggests that negatively charged residues can act in a similar manner to positively charged residues to help drive membrane disruption. This finding once again suggests that overall charge distribution and amphiphilicity likely play a greater role than the actual charge itself in the observed lytic activity. It is also noteworthy that peptides such as **61–70** may constitute novel and unique lytic/membrane active peptide space, and as such it may be possible to use these sequences as next generation leads for further reengineering or optimization.

To elucidate more information regarding the mechanistic aspects of the interaction of these peptides with membranes, we investigated the effects of peptide **38f** on extruded multilamellar vesicles in a liposomal leakage model where the liposomal membranes were designed to mimic either RBC or late endosomal membranes. Late endosomal model membranes were prepared using the combination of phosphocholine/phosphoethanolamine/phosphoinositol/BMP, while RBC-mimicking membranes were prepared using phosphocholine/sphingomyelin/cholesterol. We also prepared "shielded" (PEG coated; post-inserted 2 mol% PEG-2000 DMG) late endosomal liposomes designed to prevent fusion events between vesicles. Liposomes were constructed to contain an ANTS-dye and a DPX -quencher (Figure 4), and the liposomes were treated with a solution of the test peptide at pH 5.5 (late endosomal pH) and pH 7.4 (physiological). Upon lysis of the liposomal membrane, the ANTS dye is freed and on separation from the DPX quencher produces a fluorescent signal which can be quantified to provide the level of leakage observed. Figure 5 summarizes the results for peptide **38f.** A clear separation is seen between the leakage activity demonstrated against the late endosomal membrane (LEM) liposomes versus the RBC-mimicking liposomes, with the peptide demonstrating selectivity for the LEM-mimicking liposomes. Leakage from LEM is clearly evident with some observation of fusion/aggregation of these liposomes; coating the liposomes with PEG prevented the fusion and aggregation events but did not prevent leakage. This data suggests that the leakage event is primarily driven by peptide insertion and direct disruption of the endosomal membranes, rather than by "leaky" endosomal fusion events. As stated earlier, we believe that the peptides undergo a pH/protonation-driven conformational change at late endosomal pH, causing them to snap into an alpha -helical conformation, which we believe is the active species that inserts into the membrane leading to disruption and ultimately lysis of the endosomal membranes. Interestingly, we observed an almost "on-off" switch-like behavior for these peptides. The peptides remain inactive until they reach a threshold concentration, as which point leakage begins and rapidly increases. This mass-driven effect is seen often with various classes of membrane active peptides and is suggestive of a carpet-like mechanism of membrane disruption in which the peptides coat the membrane surface and insert into the membrane causing a generalized, detergent-like disruption of the membrane integrity. However, the observed selectivity for late endosome-like membranes is quite interesting. Most cationic, membrane disruptive peptides that behave in a carpet-like mechanism are known to be generalized membrane disruptors with little selectivity. It is likely that in the case of these peptides, the highly amphiphilic, alpha-helical conformation allows for efficient insertion into membranes while the sequence and display of the charged and lipophilic residues is perfect to induce a preference for direct interaction with the more negatively charged lipids of late endosomal membranes.

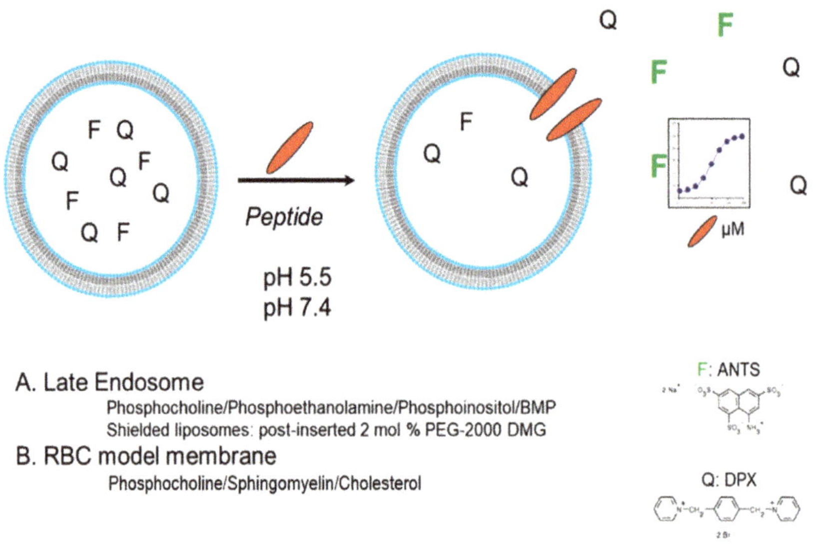

Figure 4. Liposomal leakage model.

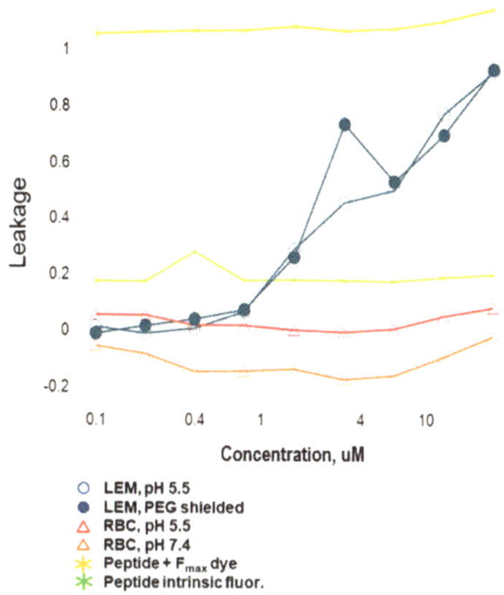

Figure 5. Liposomal leakage data for peptide **38f**.

One might ask if these peptides in general possess cell-penetrating/cargo delivery properties. While this was not the focus of our studies, and we will not detail specific data regarding this, in general we found that these peptides were quite inefficient as classical cell penetrating peptides/cargo delivery peptides. This is not surprising, given that the focus of our SAR studies was to design peptides with maximized membrane disruptive capabilities and was not focused on cargo delivery. Our in—house studies with these peptides and several other classical cell penetrating peptides suggests a huge diversity of properties and behaviors for this entire class of peptides. We have found in general that the cell lines and conditions under which many cell penetrating/cargo delivery peptides are tested largely govern the behavior observed with them and attempts to define the mechanisms of these peptides or to find general rules that could be applied across the board to new peptide design were largely inconclusive. By synthesizing a simple chimeric fusion of two very different membrane active peptides and systematically optimizing for lytic potency and selectivity, we obtained novel peptides with profiles quite disparate from that exhibited by the individual peptides. Our results suggest that that various classes of membrane active peptides likely have quite differing structure-activity relationships, and defining specific, sequence-based rules for novel peptide design would likely prove to be quite difficult. Instead, a more empirical approach employing general consideration of the overall properties and secondary structure of the peptides is likely a better way to optimize membrane interactions. Lipophilicity, charge, amphiphilicity, and helicity appear to be key drivers for these processes. Unfortunately, experimental tools that allow one to make scientifically proven conclusions about specific mechanisms are in general lacking, and results based on flawed models fuel widespread speculation in the field of membrane active peptide/CPP design.

3. Materials and Methods

3.1. Peptides

Peptides **1–10** were synthesized in-house on a CEM Liberty Microwave Peptide Synthesizer (Matthews, NC, USA), using standard Fmoc-chemistry. After cleavage and isolation all crude peptides were purified to >95% purity using reversed phase HPLC (C4, C8, or C18 columns). Stapled peptides **39a–c** were synthesized by CPC (Hangzhou, China). All other peptides were custom synthesized externally by Biopeptek (Malvern, PA, USA). Peptides were obtained as N-terminal amines/C-terminal amides unless otherwise noted. All internally and externally synthesized peptides were purified to >95% purity and demonstrated correct masses after HRMS analysis.

3.2. RBC Lysis Assay and Analysis

The human red blood cell hemolysis assay was by carried out as described previously [40] with modifications. Briefly, 5 mL aliquots of human blood from healthy individuals were dispensed into 50 mL centrifuge tubes and resuspended in 35 mL of buffer containing 150 mM NaCl and either 20 mM MES adjusted to pH 5.5 or 20 mM HEPES adjusted to pH 7.4. Red blood cells (RBCs) were washed 3 times via centrifugation with buffer and finally resuspended in a total of 50 mL of buffer. For the final assay, 175 µL of buffer solution was dispensed into each well of a clear-bottomed 96-well plate followed by 50 µL of final resuspended RBCs (approximately 2.5 × 107 cells). For transfers of RBCs, wide-bore pipet tips were used to avoid cell damage. Test peptides at the appropriate concentration were first diluted in 25 µL of buffer and then added to the cells. Small amounts of acetic acid and DTT were added to the stock solutions and assay buffer to ensure that the peptides were tested as monomers; the presence of monomers was randomly confirmed by LC/MS analysis of the assay solutions. Serial dilutions of peptides to be tested were prepared in an Easy-Wash (Costar 3368), 96 well plate, in water. Serial dilutions of peptides to be tested were prepared using a multichannel pipet. The standard assay uses a 10 point 2-fold dilution series. Compound dilutions typically are prepared at a 10× (200 µM) concentration in 25 µL final volume. The highest concentration tested was dependent on the material and its respective solubility. Buffer alone and 1% Triton X-100 in PBS were included as negative and positive controls respectively. Dilutions are prepared as either duplicates or single wells depending on the number of samples to be tested and the amount of material available for testing. All steps prior to incubation were carried out with chilled buffers and on ice. Finally, the suspension was mixed with a wide-bore tip, and the plate was covered and incubated at 37 °C for the indicated time. After incubation, the cells were centrifuged for 5 min at 500 rcf, and 150 µL of the supernatant was transferred into a new 96-well clear-bottom plate. Absorbance was measured at 541 nm, and the resulting raw hemolysis figures were normalized to a matching set of RBCs incubated in the presence of 1% Triton X-100 (100% hemolysis control). The known RBC lytic peptide melittin was used as an internal standard in all assays performed. The background absorbance is subtracted from all samples, treating each pH grouping separately. The % hemolysis is calculated for each sample at varied concentrations as a % of the Triton X-100 sample (100% hemolysis), standard curves plotted, and the EC 50 values calculated using ADA. Unless indicated, all peptides were tested a minimum of three determinations at each pH, and the activity is reported as the mean. Standard deviations were determined for the compounds with larger n values, to provide some guidance regarding the variability of the assay.

3.3. Circular Dichroism Spectra

CD spectra were collected using a VPR706 spectropolarimiter (Jasco, Easton, MD, USA). The following instrument parameters were used:

Band width	1 nm
Response	2 sec
Sensitivity	High
Measurement range	300–200 nm
Data pitch	1 nm
Scanning speed	50 nm/min
Accumulation	1 or 3 scans as noted
Cell Length	0.1 cm
Temperature	Ambient

Peptides were dissolved in a minimum of TFE and were diluted into the appropriate buffer (pH 7.4 = PBS; pH 5.5 = MES) to give a final concentration of 25 µM. Runs are the average of three scans. Samples were prepared by mixing peptide stock solution and buffer directly in a 0.1 cm × 1 cm, 0.5 mL quartz cuvette. Cuvette was cleaned with an aspirating washer with dd-water and methanol until dry.

4. Conclusions

In summary, a systematic analysis of the sequence of the chimeric INF7-Tat peptide has demonstrated a clear SAR for lytic activity and pH selectivity. This SAR appears to be quite unique to the chimeric nature of these peptides and is disparate from previously observed SAR for the individual peptides. The observed lytic potency and selectivity has been shown to be optimizable by manipulating the pKa of the peptide sidechains to refine the point at which the peptides change secondary structure from a random coil to an alpha-helix. Simultaneously, enhancing/maximizing the overall amphiphilic nature of the peptide helix through targeted modifications of the appropriate lipophilic and charged polar residues also appears to be a key contributor to lytic potency. Several modified peptides were shown to have greatly enhanced lytic potency at late endosomal pH of 5.5 while also possessing much enhanced selectivity versus lysis at physiological pH. This study represents one of the first reports of a highly systematic, position-by-position SAR-based approach to the design and optimization of novel membrane active peptides. Our study clearly demonstrates that direct manipulation of the charge, lipophilicity, and overall amphiphilicity of helical, membrane active peptides can be used in a systematic manner to optimize their potency and pH selectivity. This general set of criteria can be useful to systematically optimize other classes of membrane active peptides such as antimicrobial peptides, CPPs, and various other endosomal escape peptides. Our data suggest that using a systematic, position-by-position optimization strategy for membrane active peptides may lead to significant improvements in activity, while also helping to develop novel chemical space that otherwise would remain largely unexplored. Based on the encouraging results of this preliminary effort, we are continuing to develop novel peptides that may be useful for delivery by enhancing endosomal escape. We are extending these design principles to the investigation of next generation peptides with novel charge distributions and enhanced endosomal escape properties that are membrane active but not membrane disruptive, and as such are less likely to cause safety issues than these highly lytic first-generation analogs. We will report on our continued efforts in due course.

Author Contributions: Conceptualization, T.J.T; D.M.T.; experimental procedures, T.J.T.; B.A.; A.O.; A.M.; W.P.; data analysis, A.M.; A.O., D.J.M.; W.P.; T.J.T.; Investigation, D.M.T.; T.J.T.; Methodology, B.A.; A.B.; A.M.; D.J.M.; W.P.; T.J.T.; D.M.T.; Validation, B.A.; D.J.M.; A.M.; W.P; writing-original draft preparation—T.J.T.; writing—review and editing, A.M.; D.J.M.; T.J.T.; D.M.T.; supervision—T.J.T.; D.M.T.

Funding: This work received no external funding.

Acknowledgments: The authors would like to acknowledge Tomi Sawyer for helpful discussions. The authors also acknowledge Biopeptek LLC for the prompt and high-quality preparation of many of the peptides described in this manuscript.

Conflicts of Interest: The authors declare no conflict of interest.

References and Notes

1. Fire, A.; Xu, S.; Montgomery, M.K.; Kostas, S.A.; Driver, S.E.; Mello, C.C. Potent and specific genetic interference by double-stranded RNA in Caenorhabditis elegans. *Nature* **1998**, *391*, 806–811. [CrossRef] [PubMed]
2. Stanton, M.G.; Colletti, S.L. Medicinal Chemistry of siRNA Delivery. *J. Med. Chem.* **2010**, *53*, 7887–7901. [CrossRef]
3. EErazo-Oliveras, A.; Muthukrishnan, N.; Baker, R.; Wang, T.Y.; Pellois, J.P. Improving the endosomal escape of cell-penetrating peptides and their cargos. *Pharmaceuticals* **2012**, *5*, 1177–1209. [CrossRef]
4. Endoh, T.; Ohtsuki, T. Cellular siRNA delivery using cell-penetrating peptides modified for endosomal escape. *Adv. Drug Del. Rev.* **2009**, *61*, 704–709. [CrossRef]

5. Weise, K.; Reed, J. Fusion peptides and transmembrane domains of fusion proteins are characterized by different but specific structural properties. *Chembiochem* **2008**, *9*, 934–943. [CrossRef]
6. Lundberg, P.; El-Andaloussi, S.; Sutlu, T.; Johansson, H.; Langel, U. Delivery of short interfering RNA using endosomolytic cell-penetrating peptides. *FASEB J.* **2007**, *21*, 2664–2671. [CrossRef]
7. Avci, F.G.; Akbulut, B.S.; Ozkirimli, E. Membrane active peptides and their biophysical characterization. *Biomolecules* **2018**, *8*, 77. [CrossRef]
8. Liu, Q.; Zhao, H.; Jiang, Y.; Tian, Y.; Wang, D.; Lao, Y.; Xu, N.; Li, Z. Development of a lytic peptide derived from BH3-only proteins. *Cell Death Discov.* **2016**, *2*, 16008. [CrossRef] [PubMed]
9. Epand, R.M. Fusion peptides and the mechanism of viral fusion. *Biochim. Biophys. Acta* **2003**, *1614*, 116–121. [CrossRef]
10. Wimley, W.C. Describing the mechanism of antimicrobial peptide action with the interfacial activity model. *ACS Chem. Bio.* **2010**, *5*, 905–917. [CrossRef]
11. Dufourc, E.J.; Buchoux, S.; Toupé, J.; Sani, M.A.; Jean-François, F.; Khemtémourian, L.; Grélard, A.; Loudet-Courrèges, C.; Laguerre, M.; Elezgaray, J.; et al. Membrane interacting peptides: from killers to helpers. *Curr. Prot. Pept. Sci.* **2012**, *13*, 620–631. [CrossRef]
12. Tamm, L.K.; Han, X. Viral Fusion Peptides: A tool set to disrupt and connect biological membranes. *Biosci. Rep.* **2000**, *20*, 501–518. [CrossRef] [PubMed]
13. Guidotti, G.; Brambilla, L.; Rossi, D. Cell-penetrating peptides: from basic research to clinics. *Trends Pharmacol. Sci.* **2017**, *38*, 406–424. [CrossRef] [PubMed]
14. Sugita, T.; Yoshikawa, T.; Mukai, Y.; Yamanda, N.; Imai, S.; Nagano, K.; Yoshida, Y.; Shibata, H.; Yoshiaok, Y.; Nakagawa, S.; et al. Improved cytosolic translocation and tumor-killing activity of Tat-shepherdin conjugates mediated by co-treatment with Tat-fused endosome-disruptive HA2 peptide. *Biochem. Biophys. Res. Comm.* **2007**, *363*, 1027–1032. [CrossRef] [PubMed]
15. Lee, Y.; Jophnson, G.; Pellois, J.P. Modeling of the Endosomolytic Activity of HA2-TAT Peptides with Red Blood Cells and Ghosts. *Biochemistry* **2012**, *49*, 7854–7866. [CrossRef] [PubMed]
16. Angeles-Boza, A.M.; Erazo-Oliveras, A.; Lee, Y.J.; Pellois, J.P. Generation of Endosomolytic Reagents by Branching of Cell-Penetrating Peptides: Tools for the Delivery of Bioactive Compounds to Live Cells in Cis or Trans. *Bioconj. Chem.* **2010**, *21*, 2164–2167. [CrossRef]
17. Lee, Y.; Johnson, G.; Peltier, G.C.; Pellois, J.P. A HA2-Fusion tag limits the endosomal release of its protein cargo despite causing endosomal lysis. *Biochim. Biophys. Acta* **2011**, *1810*, 752–758. [CrossRef]
18. Liou, J.; Liu, B.R.; Martin, A.L.; Huang, Y.; Chiang, H.-J.; Lee, H.-J. Protein transduction in human cells is enhanced by cell-penetrating peptides fused with an endosomolytic HA2 sequence. *Peptides* **2012**, *37*, 273–284. [CrossRef]
19. Ye, S.-F.; Tian, M.; Wang, T.-X.; Ren, L.; Wang, D.; Shen, L.-H.; Shang, T. Synergistic effects of cell-penetrating peptide Tat and fusogenic peptide HA2-enhanced cellular internalization and gene transduction of organosilica nanoparticles. *Nanomed. Nanotech Bio. Med.* **2012**, *8*, 833–841. [CrossRef]
20. Oliverira, S.; van Rooy, I.; Kranenburg, O.; Storm, G.; Schiffelers, R.M. Fusogenic peptides enhance endosomal escape improving siRNA-induced silencing of oncogenes. *Int. J. Pharm.* **2007**, *331*, 211–214. [CrossRef]
21. Thomas J. Tucker, Merck Research Laboratories, West Point, PA, USA. There are different Tat sequences that have been used in the literature for delivery; we chose the YG-Tat (YGRKKRRQRR) sequence for this particular study as unpublished internal data showed that this sequence exhibited the most consistent CPP behavior in multiple cell lines, and also in general showed very good physical properties and behavior, 2016.
22. Miletti, F. Cell-penetrating peptides: classes, origin, and current landscape. *Drug Disc. Today* **2012**, *17*, 850–860. [CrossRef]
23. Mechtler, K.; Wagner, E. Gene transfer mediated by influenza virus peptides: the role of peptide sequences. *New J. Chem.* **1997**, *21*, 105–111.
24. Sung, M.S.; Mun, J.Y.; Kwon, O.; Oh, D.B. Efficient myogenic differentiation of human adipose-derived stem cells by the transduction of engineered MyoD protein. *Biochem. Biophys. Res. Comm.* **2013**, *437*, 156–161. [CrossRef] [PubMed]
25. Lin, N.; Zheng, W.; Li, L.; Liu, H.; Wang, T.; Wang, P.; Ma, X. A novel system enhancing the endosomal escapes of peptides promotes Bak BH3 peptide inducing apoptosis in lung cancer A549 cells. *Targ. Oncol.* **2014**, *9*, 163–170. [CrossRef]

26. Garcia-Sosa, A.T.; Tulp, I.; Langel, K.; Langel, U. Peptide-ligand binding modeling of siRNA with cell penetrating peptides. *Biomed. Res. Int.* **2014**, *2014*, 257040. [CrossRef] [PubMed]
27. Friemann, K.; Arukuusk, P.; Kurrikoff, K.; Ferreira Vasconcelos, L.D.; Veiman, K.-L.; Uusna, J.; Margus, H.; Garcia-Sosa, A.T.; Pooga, M.; Langel, U. Optimization of in vivo delivery with NickFect peptide vectors. *J. Cont. Rel.* **2016**, *241*, 135–143. [CrossRef] [PubMed]
28. Durell, R.D.; Martin, I.; Ruysschaert, J.-M.; Shai, Y.; Blumenthal, R. What studies of fusion peptides tell us about viral envelope glycoprotein-mediated membrane fusion. *Mol. Memb. Biol.* **1997**, *14*, 97–112. [CrossRef]
29. Cross, K.J.; Wharton, S.A.; Skehel, J.J.; Wiley, D.C.; Steinhauser, D.A. Studies on influenza haemagglutinin fusion peptide mutants generated by reverse genetics. *EMBO J.* **2001**, *20*, 4432–4442. [CrossRef]
30. Han, X.; Bushweller, J.H.; Cafiso, D.S.; Tamm, L.K. Membrane structure and fusion-triggering conformational change of the fusion domain from influenza hemagglutinin. *Nat. Struct. Bio.* **2001**, *8*, 715–720. [CrossRef]
31. Lorieau, J.L.; Louis, J.M.; Bax, A. The complete influenza hemagglutinin fusion domain adopts a tight helical hairpin arrangement at the lipid:water interface. *Proc. Natl. Acad. Sci.* **2010**, *107*, 11341–11346. [CrossRef]
32. Lorieau, J.L.; Louis, J.M.; Bax, A. Helical Hairpin Structure of Influenza Hemagglutinin Fusion Peptide Stabilized by Charge–Dipole Interactions between the N-Terminal Amino Group and the Second Helix. *J. Am. Chem. Soc.* **2011**, *133*, 2824–2827. [CrossRef] [PubMed]
33. Midoux, P.; Kichler, A.; Boutin, V.; Maurizot, J.-C.; Monsigny, M. Membrane Permeabilization and Efficient Gene Transfer by a Peptide Containing Several Histidines. *Bioconj. Chem.* **1998**, *9*, 260–267. [CrossRef]
34. Schafmeister, C.E.; Po, J.; Verdine, G.L. An All-Hydrocarbon Cross-Linking System for Enhancing the Helicity and Metabolic Stability of Peptides. *J. Am. Chem. Soc.* **2000**, *122*, 5891–5892. [CrossRef]
35. Kutchukian, P.S.; Yang, J.S.; Verdine, G.L.; Shakhnovich, E.I. An all-atom model for stabilization of α-helical structure in peptides by hydrocarbon staples. *J. Am. Chem. Soc.* **2009**, *131*, 4622–4627. [CrossRef] [PubMed]
36. Kim, Y.-W.; Grossmann, T.N.; Verdine, G.L. Synthesis of all-hydrocarbon stapled α-helical peptides by ring-closing olefin metathesis. *Nat. Protoc.* **2011**, *6*, 761–771. [CrossRef] [PubMed]
37. Martin, I.; Teixido, M.; Giralt, E. Design, synthesis and characterization of a new anionic cell-penetrating peptide: SAP(E). *ChemBioChem* **2011**, *12*, 896–903. [CrossRef] [PubMed]
38. Sitaram, N. Antimicrobial peptides with unusual amino acid compositions and unusual structures. *Curr. Med. Chem.* **2006**, *13*, 679–696. [CrossRef]
39. Harris, F.; Dennison, S.R.; Phoenix, D.A. Anionic antimicrobial peptides from eukaryotic organisms and their mechanisms of action. *Curr. Chem. Bio.* **2011**, *5*, 142–153. [CrossRef]
40. Henry, S.M.; El-Sayed, M.E.; Pirie, C.M.; Hoffman, A.S.; Stayton, P.S. pH-responsive poly (styrene-alt-maleic anhydride) alkylamide copolymers for intracellular drug delivery. *Biomacromolecules* **2006**, *7*, 2407–2414. [CrossRef]

Sample Availability: Not Available.

molecules

MDPI

Article

Incorporation of Putative Helix-Breaking Amino Acids in the Design of Novel Stapled Peptides: Exploring Biophysical and Cellular Permeability Properties

Anthony W. Partridge [1,*], Hung Yi Kristal Kaan [1], Yu-Chi Juang [1], Ahmad Sadruddin [1], Shuhui Lim [1], Christopher J. Brown [2], Simon Ng [2], Dawn Thean [2], Fernando Ferrer [2], Charles Johannes [3], Tsz Ying Yuen [3], Srinivasaraghavan Kannan [4], Pietro Aronica [4], Yaw Sing Tan [4], Mohan R. Pradhan [4], Chandra S. Verma [4], Jerome Hochman [5], Shiying Chen [6], Hui Wan [6], Sookhee Ha [6], Brad Sherborne [6], David P. Lane [2] and Tomi K. Sawyer [7,*]

1 MSD International, 8 Biomedical Grove, #04-01/05 Neuros Building, Singapore 138665, Singapore; kristal.kaan@merck.com (H.Y.K.K.); angela.juang@merck.com (Y.-C.J.); ahmad.sadruddin@merck.com (A.S.); shuhui.lim@merck.com (S.L.)
2 p53Lab, Agency for Science, Technology and Research (A*STAR), 8A Biomedical Grove, #06-04/05 Neuros/Immunos, Singapore 138648, Singapore; CJBrown@p53lab.a-star.edu.sg (C.J.B.); simon.ng@merck.com (S.N.); dthean@p53Lab.a-star.edu.sg (D.T.); fjferrer@p53Lab.a-star.edu.sg (F.F.); dplane@p53Lab.a-star.edu.sg (D.P.L.)
3 Institute of Chemical and Engineering Sciences (ICES), Agency for Science, Technology and Research (A*STAR), 8 Biomedical Grove, #07, Neuros Building, Singapore 138665, Singapore; charles_johannes@p53lab.a-star.edu.sg (C.J.); yuenty@ices.a-star.edu.sg (T.Y.Y.)
4 Bioinformatics Institute (BII), Agency for Science, Technology and Research (A*STAR), 30 Biopolis Street, #07-01 Matrix, Singapore 138671, Singapore; raghavk@bii.a-star.edu.sg (S.K.); pietroa@bii.a-star.edu.sg (P.A.); tanys@bii.a-star.edu.sg (Y.S.T.); mohanrp@bii.a-star.edu.sg (M.R.P.); chandra@bii.a-star.edu.sg (C.S.V.)
5 Merck & Co., Inc., West Point, PA 19486, USA; jerome_hochman@merck.com
6 Merck & Co., Inc., Kenilworth, NJ 07033, USA; shiying.chen@merck.com (S.C.); hui.wan@merck.com (H.W.); sookhee_ha@merck.com (S.H.); tomi.sawyer@merck.com (B.S.)
7 Merck & Co., Inc., Boston, MA 02115, USA
* Correspondence: anthony_partridge@merck.com (A.W.P.); sawyerkrt@aol.com (T.K.S.)

Academic Editor: Derek J. McPhee
Received: 22 May 2019; Accepted: 16 June 2019; Published: 20 June 2019

check for updates

Abstract: Stapled α-helical peptides represent an emerging superclass of macrocyclic molecules with drug-like properties, including high-affinity target binding, protease resistance, and membrane permeability. As a model system for probing the chemical space available for optimizing these properties, we focused on dual Mdm2/MdmX antagonist stapled peptides related to the p53 N-terminus. Specifically, we first generated a library of ATSP-7041 (Chang et al., 2013) analogs iteratively modified by L-Ala and D-amino acids. Single L-Ala substitutions beyond the Mdm2/(X) binding interfacial residues (i.e., Phe^3, Trp^7, and Cba^{10}) had minimal effects on target binding, α-helical content, and cellular activity. Similar binding affinities and cellular activities were noted at non-interfacial positions when the template residues were substituted with their D-amino acid counterparts, despite the fact that D-amino acid residues typically 'break' right-handed α-helices. D-amino acid substitutions at the interfacial residues Phe^3 and Cba^{10} resulted in the expected decreases in binding affinity and cellular activity. Surprisingly, substitution at the remaining interfacial position with its D-amino acid equivalent (i.e., Trp^7 to D-Trp^7) was fully tolerated, both in terms of its binding affinity and cellular activity. An X-ray structure of the D-Trp^7-modified peptide was determined and revealed that the indole side chain was able to interact optimally with its Mdm2 binding site by a slight global re-orientation of the stapled peptide. To further investigate the comparative effects of D-amino acid substitutions we used linear analogs of

ATSP-7041, where we replaced the stapling amino acids by Aib (i.e., *R8*[4] to Aib[4] and *S5*[11] to Aib[11]) to retain the helix-inducing properties of α-methylation. The resultant analog sequence Ac–Leu–Thr–Phe–Aib–Glu–Tyr–Trp–Gln–Leu–Cba–Aib–Ser–Ala–Ala–NH_2 exhibited high-affinity target binding (Mdm2 K_d = 43 nM) and significant α-helicity in circular dichroism studies. Relative to this linear ATSP-7041 analog, several D-amino acid substitutions at Mdm2(X) non-binding residues (e.g., D-Glu[5], D-Gln[8], and D-Leu[9]) demonstrated decreased binding and α-helicity. Importantly, circular dichroism (CD) spectroscopy showed that although helicity was indeed disrupted by D-amino acids in linear versions of our template sequence, stapled molecules tolerated these residues well. Further studies on stapled peptides incorporating N-methylated amino acids, L-Pro, or Gly substitutions showed that despite some positional dependence, these helix-breaking residues were also generally tolerated in terms of secondary structure, binding affinity, and cellular activity. Overall, macrocyclization by hydrocarbon stapling appears to overcome the destabilization of α-helicity by helix breaking residues and, in the specific case of D-Trp[7]-modification, a highly potent ATSP-7041 analog (Mdm2 K_d = 30 nM; cellular EC_{50} = 600 nM) was identified. Our findings provide incentive for future studies to expand the chemical diversity of macrocyclic α-helical peptides (e.g., D-amino acid modifications) to explore their biophysical properties and cellular permeability. Indeed, using the library of 50 peptides generated in this study, a good correlation between cellular permeability and lipophilicity was observed.

Keywords: peptide permeability; stapled peptide; macrocyclic peptide; D-amino acid; helix-breaker

1. Introduction

Intracellular protein–protein interactions (PPIs) represent a plethora of potential drug targets across therapeutic classes. However, the discovery of disease-modifying molecules against PPI targets has proceeded slowly due to the limitations of traditional therapeutic strategies [1]. In particular, the large and flat surfaces of PPIs pose challenges for small molecules (<500 daltons) as potent inhibitors [1]. Monoclonal antibodies represent the other major class of therapeutics and are highly effective at inhibiting PPIs, however, methods for efficient intracellular delivery of such molecules have not yet been realized [2]. Peptides also have the capacity to compete with PPIs but generally have poor proteolytic stability and limited membrane permeability, which greatly hinder their therapeutic application to intracellular targets [3]. However, the macrocyclization of peptides has been shown to address both of these liabilities [4]. Most prominently, hydrocarbon stapling of helical peptides has emerged as a potential therapeutic approach with ALRN-6924—a first-generation molecule, currently undergoing clinical trials [5]. Hydrocarbon stapling generally involves covalently linking two α-methyl, olefin-containing amino acids on the same helical face (typically either at i to i +4 or i to i +7 positions) via ring closing metathesis [6–8]. Such hydrocarbon stapling (or other macrocyclization chemistries) has been reported to confer drug-like properties, including stabilization of the peptide into an α-helical conformation, increased target binding affinity, enhanced proteolytic stability and/or improved membrane permeability [4].

Although there have been several examples of stapled peptides with activity in cellular systems, most peptides reported thus far have marginal cellular permeability, as evidenced by the large disparity between their target binding biochemical and target-dependent cellular functional potencies. Therefore, a deeper understanding of the design rules governing stapled peptide cellular permeability would greatly enable their development as potential clinical candidates. Exploration of the peptide permeability determinants may be facilitated by expanded chemical diversity. Here, we show that α-helical stapled peptides unexpectedly tolerate residues that are generally considered α-helix breakers within the context of linear sequences. To study this, we used ATSP-7041 analogs [9]—stapled peptides with sequences related to the p53 N-terminus [10], those discovered by phage display (pDI [11] and pMI [12]), and with similarity to the literature staple peptides SAH-8 [13] and M06 [14]. Stapled peptide analogs harboring helix-breakers, such as D-amino acids, Pro, Gly, and N-methylated amino acids, generally retained their α-helical structure, binding affinity for Mdm2, and cellular functional activity (See Figure 1A,B for the sequence and structure of peptide templates used in this study). Overall, our work shows for the first time a compelling structural and chirality tolerance of macrocyclic α-helical peptides and provides impetus for future exploration of their biophysical and cellular permeability properties.

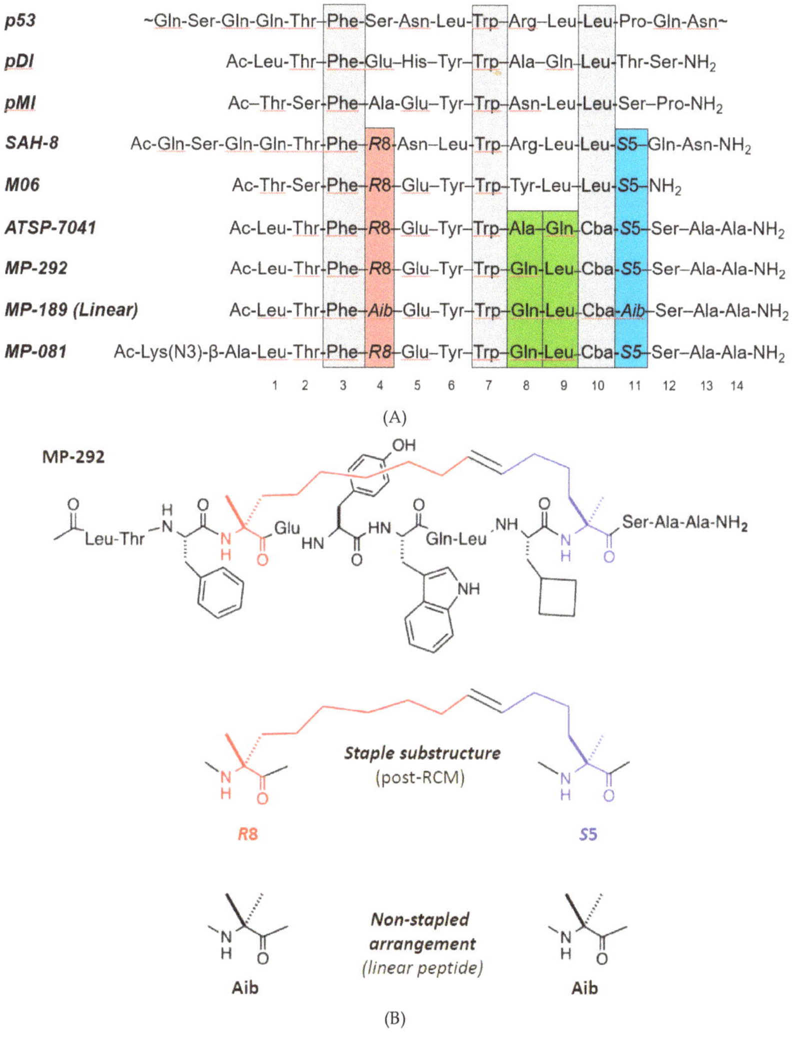

Figure 1. Template sequences used in this study and comparison to related literature peptides. (**A**) Sequences of p53; phage display peptides pDI and pMI; literature stapled peptides SAH-8, M06, and ATSP-7041; and ATSP-7041 variants used as template sequences in this work, MP-292, MP-189, and MP-018. (**B**) Chemical structure of MP-292, as well as the substructure of the stapling amino acids (*R*8 and *S*5) and Aib.

2. Methods

2.1. Peptide Synthesis

Peptides were synthesized using Rink Amide MBHA resin and Fmoc-protected amino acids, coupled sequentially with DIC/HOBt activating agents. Double coupling reactions were performed on the first amino acid and also at the stapling positions. At these latter positions, the activating reagents were switched to DIEA/HATU for better coupling efficiencies. Ring closing metathesis reactions were performed by first washing the resin three times with DCM, followed by the addition of the first-generation Grubbs Catalyst (20 mol % in DCM and allowed to react for 2 h; all steps with Grubbs Catalyst were performed in the dark). The RCM (ring closing metathesis) reaction was repeated to ensure a complete reaction. After the RCM was complete, a test cleavage was performed to ensure adequate yield. Peptides were cleaved and then purified as a mixture of cis-trans isomers by RP-HPLC.

2.2. Protein Production

For use in the peptide binding assay, a human Mdm2 1–125 sequence was cloned into a pNIC-GST vector. The TEV (tobacco etch virus) cleavage site was changed from ENLYFQS to ENLYFQG to give a fusion protein with the following sequence:

MSDKIIHSPILGYWKIKGLVQPTRLLLEYLEEKYEEHLYERDEGDKWRNKKFELGLEFPNLPYYI
DGDVKLTQSMAIIRYIADKHNMLGGCPKERAEISMLEGAVLDIRYGVSRIAYSKDFETLKVDFLSK
LPEMLKMFEDRLCHKTYLNGDHVTHPDFMLYDALDVVLYMDPMCLDAFPKLVCFKKRIEAIPQI
DKYLKSSKYIAWPLQGWQATFGGGDHPPKLEVLFQGHMHHHHHHSSGVDLGTENLYFQGMCN
TNMSVPTDGAVTTSQIPASEQETLVRPKPLLLKLLKSVGAQKDTYTMKEVLFYLGQYIMTKRLY
DEKQQHIVYCSNDLLGDLFGVPSFSVKEHRKIYTMIYRNLVVVNQQESSDSGTSVSEN-.

The corresponding plasmid was transformed into BL21 (DE3) Rosetta T1R *Escherichia coli* cells and grown under kanamycin selection. Bottles of 750 mL Terrific Broth, supplemented with appropriate antibiotics and 100 μL of antifoam 204 (Sigma-Aldrich, St. Louis, MO, USA, were inoculated with 20 mL seed cultures grown overnight. The cultures were incubated at 37 °C in the LEX system (Harbinger Biotech, Toronto, Canada) with aeration and agitation through the bubbling of filtered air through the cultures. The LEX system temperature was reduced to 18 °C when culture OD600 reached 2, and the cultures were induced after 60 min with 0.5 mM IPTG. Protein expression was allowed to continue overnight. Cells were harvested by centrifugation at 4000× *g*, at 15 °C for 10 min. The supernatants were discarded and the cell pellets were resuspended in a lysis buffer (1.5 mL per gram of cell pellet). The cell suspensions were stored at −80 °C before purification work.

The re-suspended cell pellet suspensions were thawed and sonicated (Sonics Vibra-Cell, Newtown, CO, USA) at 70% amplitude, 3 s on/off for 3 min, on ice. The lysate was clarified by centrifugation at 47,000× *g*, 4 °C for 25 min. The supernatants were filtered through 1.2 μm syringe filters and loaded onto the AKTA Xpress system (GE Healthcare, Fairfield, CO, USA). The purification regime is briefly described as follows. The lysates were loaded onto a 1 mL Ni-NTA Superflow column (Qiagen, Valencia, CA, USA) that had been equilibrated with 10 column volumes of wash 1 buffer. Overall buffer conditions were as follows: Immobilized metal affinity chromatography (IMAC) wash 1 buffer—20 mM HEPES ((4-(2-hydroxyethyl)-1-piperazineethanesulfonic acid), 500 mM NaCl, 10 mM Imidazole, 10% (*v*/*v*) glycerol, 0.5 mM TCEP (Tris(2-carboxyethyl)phosphine), pH 7.5; IMAC wash 2 buffer—20 mM HEPES, 500 mM NaCl, 25 mM Imidazole, 10% (*v*/*v*) glycerol, 0.5 mM TCEP, pH 7.5; IMAC Elution buffer—20 mM HEPES, 500 mM NaCl, 500 mM Imidazole, 10% (*v*/*v*) glycerol, 0.5 mM TCEP, pH 7.5. The sample was loaded until air was detected by the air sensor, 0.8 mL/min. The column was then washed with wash 1 buffer for 20 column volumes, followed by 20 column volumes of wash 2 buffer. The protein was eluted with five column volumes of elution buffer. The eluted proteins were collected and stored in sample loops on the system and then injected into gel filtration (GF) columns. Elution peaks were collected in 2 mL fractions and analyzed on SDS-PAGE gels. The entire purification was performed at 4 °C. Relevant peaks were pooled, TCEP was added to a total concentration of 2 mM. The protein sample was concentrated in Vivaspin 20 filter concentrators (VivaScience, Littleton, MA, USA) at 15 °C to approximately 15 mg/mL. (<18 kDa—5 K MWCO, 19–49 kDa—10 K MWCO, >50 kDa—30 K MWCO). The final protein concentration was assessed by measuring absorbance at 280 nm on Nanodrop ND-1000 (Thermo Fisher, Waltham, MA, USA). The final protein purity was assessed on SDS-PAGE gel. The final protein batch was then aliquoted into smaller fractions, frozen in liquid nitrogen and stored at −80 °C.

For x-ray crystallography, Mdm2 (6–125) was cloned as a GST-fusion protein using the pGEX-6P-1 GST expression vector (GE Healthcare). The GST-fused Mdm2 (6–125) construct was then transformed into *Escherichia coli* BL21(DE3) pLysS (Thermo Fisher, Waltham, MA, USA) competent cells. Cells were grown in Luria-Bertani (LB) medium at 37 °C and induced at OD600 nm of 0.6 with 0.5 mM Isopropyl β- D -1-thiogalactopyranoside (IPTG) at 16 °C. After overnight induction, the cells were harvested by centrifugation, resuspended in binding buffer (50 mM Tris-HCl pH 8.0, 150 mM NaCl), and lysed by sonication. After centrifugation for 60 min at 19,000× *g* at 4 °C, the cell lysate was then applied to a 5 mL GSTrap FF column (GE Healthcare) pre-equilibrated in wash buffer (50 mM Tris-HCl pH 8.0, 150 mM NaCl, 1 mM DTT). The GST-fused Mdm2 (6–125) was then cleaved on-column by PreScission protease (GE Healthcare) overnight at 4 °C and eluted off the column with wash buffer. The protein sample was then dialyzed into a buffer A solution (20 mM Bis-Tris, pH 6.5, 1 mM DTT) using HiPrep 26/10 Desalting column, and loaded onto a cation-exchange Resource S 1 mL column (GE Healthcare), pre-equilibrated in buffer A. The column was then washed in six column volumes of buffer A and the bound protein was eluted with a linear gradient in buffer comprising 1 M NaCl, 20 mM Bis-Tris pH 6.5, and 1 mM DTT over 30 column volumes. Protein purity as assessed by SDS-PAGE was ~95%, and the proteins were concentrated using Amicon-Ultra (3 kDa MWCO) concentrator (Millipore, Burlington, MA, USA). Protein concentration was determined using 280 nm absorbance measurements.

2.3. Crystallization and Data Collection

Mdm2 (6-125) was concentrated to 3.5 mg/mL and then incubated with the stapled peptide at a 1:3 molar ratio of protein to peptide at 4 °C overnight. The lyophilized stapled peptide (MP-594) was first dissolved in dimethyl sulfoxide (DMSO) to make a 100 mM stock solution before being directly added to the protein solutions. The sample was clarified by centrifugation before crystallization trials at 16 °C using the sitting drop vapor diffusion method. Crystals of Mdm2 (6–125) in complex with MP-594 were obtained by mixing the protein–peptide complex with the reservoir solution in a ratio of 1:1, with the reservoir solution containing 2.4 M di-sodium malonate. Mdm2/MP-594 complex crystals were frozen in an equivalent mother liquor solution containing 15% (*v*/*v*) glycerol and then flash frozen in liquid nitrogen. X-ray diffraction was collected at the Australian synchrotron (Aus.). See Table S1 for data collection statistics.

2.4. X-ray Structure and Refinement

X-ray datasets were processed and scaled with the XDS1 and CCP42 packages [15,16]. The structures were solved by molecular replacement with the program PHASER3, using the human Mdm2 (6-125) structure from the PDB:4UMN (chain A) as a search model [17]. The starting model was built and refined by iterative cycles of manual and automatic building with Coot4 and restrained refinement with Refmac5 [18,19]. The geometric restraints for the non-natural amino acids constituting the hydrocarbon staple and the covalent bond linking their respective side chains together, to form the macrocyclic linkage constraining the stapled peptide, were defined and generated using JLigand6 [20]. The final model was validated using RAMPAGE7 [21] and the MOLPROBITY8 [21] webserver. Structural overlays and analysis was performed using PYMOL software (Schrödinger, New York, NY, USA). See Table S1 for data collection and refinement statistics. The Mdm2: MP-594 complex structure was deposited in the PDB with the accession code 6AAW.

2.5. Mdm2 Binding Assay

Purified Mdm2 (1–125) protein was titrated against 50 nM carboxyfluorescein (FAM)—labeled 12/1 peptide13 (FAM-RFMDYWEGL-NH2). Dissociation constants for titration of Mdm2 against the FAM-labeled 12/1 peptide were determined by fitting the experimental data to a 1:1 binding model equation, shown below:

$$r = r_0 + (r_b - r_0) \times \frac{(K_d + [L]_t + [P]_t) - \sqrt{(K_d + [L]_t + [P]_t)^2 - 4[L]_t[P]_t}}{2[L]_t} \quad (1)$$

where $[P]$ is the protein concentration (Mdm2), $[L]$ is the labeled peptide concentration, r is the anisotropy measured, r_0 is the anisotropy of the free peptide, r_b is the anisotropy of the Mdm2–FAM-labeled peptide complex, K_d is the dissociation constant, $[L]_t$ is the total FAM-labeled peptide concentration, and $[P]_t$ is the total Mdm2 concentration. The determined apparent K_d value of FAM-labeled 12/1 peptide (13.0 nM) was used to determine the apparent K_d values of the respective competing ligands in subsequent competition assays in fluorescence anisotropy experiments. Titrations were carried out with the concentration of Mdm2 held constant at 250 nM and the labeled peptide at 50 nM. The competing molecules were then titrated against the complex of the FAM-labeled peptide and protein. Apparent K_d values were determined by fitting the experimental data to the equations shown below:

$$\begin{gathered} r = r_0 + (r_b - r_0) \times \frac{2\sqrt{(d^2-3e)}\cos(\theta/3)-9}{3K_{d1}+2\sqrt{(d^2-3e)}\cos(\theta/3)-d} \\ d = K_{d1} + K_{d2} + [L]_{st} + [L]_t - [P]_t \\ e = ([L]_t - [P]_t)K_{d1} + ([L]_{st} - [P]_t)K_{d2} + K_{d1}K_{d2} \\ f = -K_{d1}K_{d2}[P]_t \\ \theta = ar\cos\left[\frac{-2d^3+9de-27f}{2\sqrt{(d^2-3e)^3}}\right] \end{gathered} \quad (2)$$

where $[L]_{st}$ and $[L]_t$ denote labeled ligand and total unlabeled ligand input concentrations, respectively. K_{d2} is the dissociation constant of the interaction between the unlabeled ligand and the protein. In all competition experiments, it was assumed that $[P]_t > [L]_{st}$, otherwise considerable amounts of free labeled ligand would always be present and would interfere with measurements. K_{d1} is the apparent K_d for the labeled peptide used and was experimentally determined as described in the previous paragraph. The FAM-labeled peptide was dissolved in dimethyl sulfoxide (DMSO) at 1 mM and diluted into the experimental buffer. Readings were carried out with an Envision Multilabel Reader (PerkinElmer). Experiments were carried out in PBS (2.7 mM KCl, 137mM NaCl, 10 mM Na2HPO4, and 2 mM KH2PO4 (pH 7.4)) and 0.1% Tween 20 buffer. All titrations were carried out in triplicate. Curve-fitting was carried out using Prism 4.0 (GraphPad). To validate the fitting of a 1:1 binding model, we carefully ensured that the anisotropy value at the beginning of the direct titrations between Mdm2 and the FAM-labeled peptide did not differ significantly from the anisotropy value observed for the free fluorescently-labeled peptide. Negative control titrations of the ligands under investigation were also carried out with the fluorescently labeled peptide (in the absence of Mdm2) to ensure no interactions were occurring between the ligands and the FAM-labeled peptide. In addition, we ensured that the final baseline in the competitive titrations did not fall below the anisotropy value for the free FAM-labeled peptide, which would otherwise indicate an unintended interaction between the ligand and the FAM-labeled peptide to be displaced from the Mdm2 binding site.

2.6. p53 Beta-Lactamase Reporter Gene Cellular Functional Assay

HCT116 cells were stably transfected with a p53 responsive β-lactamase reporter and were seeded into a 384-well plate at a density of 8000 cells per well. Cells were maintained in McCoy's 5A Medium with 10% fetal bovine serum (FBS), Blasticidin, and Penicillin/Streptomycin. The cells were incubated overnight, followed by removal of cell growth media and replacement with Opti-MEM either containing 0% FBS or 10% FBS. Peptides were then dispensed to each well using a liquid handler, ECHO 555, and incubated for 4 or 16 h. The final working concentration of DMSO was 0.5%. β-lactamase activity was detected using the ToxBLAzer Dual Screen (Invitrogen), as per the manufacturer's instructions. Measurements were made using the Envision multiplate reader (Perkin–Elmer). Maximum p53 activity was defined as the amount of β-lactamase activity induced by 50 μM azide-ATSP-7041. This was determined as the highest amount of p53 activity induced by azide-ATSP-7041 from titrations on HCT116 cells.

2.7. *Lactate Dehydrogenase (LDH) Release Assay*

HCT116 cells were seeded into a 384-well plate at a density of 8000 cells per well. Cells were maintained in McCoy's 5A Medium with 10% fetal bovine serum (FBS), Blasticidin, and Penicillin/Streptomycin. The cells were incubated overnight, followed by the removal of cell media and the addition of Opti-MEM Medium without FBS. Cells were then treated with peptides for 4 or 16 h in Opti-MEM, either in 10% FBS or in serum free conditions. The final concentration of DMSO was 0.5%. Lactate dehydrogenase release was detected using the CytoTox-ONE Homogenous Membrane Integrity Assay Kit (Promega), as per the manufacturer's instructions. Measurements were carried out using the Tecan plate reader. Maximum LDH release was defined as the amount of LDH released as induced by the lytic peptide (iDNA79) and used to normalize the results.

2.8. *Tetracycline Beta-Lactamase Reporter Gene Cellular Assay (Counterscreen)*

This assay was based on Jump-In™ T-REx™ CHO-K1 BLA cells containing a stably integrated β-lactamase under the control of an inducible cytomegalovirus (CMV) promoter. Cells were seeded into a 384-well plate at a density of 4000 cells per well. Cells were maintained in Dulbecco's Minimal Eagle Medium (DMEM) with 10% fetal bovine serum (FBS), Blasticidin, and Penicillin/Streptomycin. The cells were incubated for 24 h, followed by cell media removal and replacement with Opti-MEM, either containing 10% FBS or 0% FBS. Peptides were then dispensed to each well using a liquid handler, ECHO 555 and incubated for 4 or 16 h. The final working concentration of DMSO was 0.5%. β-lactamase activity was detected using the ToxBLAzer Dual Screen (Invitrogen), as per the manufacturer's instructions. Measurements were carried out using the Envision multiplate reader (Perkin–Elmer). Counterscreen activity was defined as the amount of β-lactamase activity induced by tetracycline.

2.9. *Isothermal Titration Calorimetry (ITC)*

Overnight dialysis of protein and peptides were carried out in buffer containing 1× phosphate-buffered saline (PBS) pH 7.2, 3% DMSO, and 0.001% Tween-20. Approximately 100–200 μM of peptide was titrated into 20 μM of purified recombinant human Mdm2 protein (amino acids 1–125), over 40 injections of 1 μL each. Reverse ITC (200 μM of Mdm2 protein titrated into 20 μM of peptide) was carried out for peptides that are insoluble at high concentrations. All experiments were performed in duplicates using the MicroCal PEAQ-ITC Automated system. Data analysis was carried out using the MicroCal PEAQ-ITC Analysis Software.

2.10. *Circular Dichroism (CD)*

A total of 5 μL of the 10 mM stock peptide was mixed with 45 μL of 100% methanol, and dried for 2 h in the SpeedVac concentrator (Thermo Scientific). The dried peptide was reconstituted in a buffer (1 mM Hepes pH 7.4 and 5% methanol) to a concentration of 1 mM. The peptide sample was placed in a quartz cuvette with a path length of 0.2 cm. The peptide concentration was determined by the absorbance of the peptide at 280 nM. The CD spectrum was recorded from 300 to 190 nm using the Chirascan-plus qCD machine (Applied Photophysics, Surrey, UK), at 25 °C. All experiments were done in duplicates. The CD spectrum was converted to mean residue ellipticity, before deconvolution and estimation of the secondary structure components of the peptide using the CDNN software (distributed by Applied Photophysics).

2.11. Surface Plasmon Resonance (SPR)

SPR experiments were performed with Biacore T100 (GE Healthcare) at 25 °C. The site-specific mono-biotinylated Mdm2 was prepared by sortase-mediated ligation. The SPR buffer consisted of 50 mM Tris pH 7.4, 150 mM NaCl, 1 mM DTT, 0.05% Tween 20, and 3% DMSO. The CM5 chip was first conditioned with 100 mM HCl, followed by 0.1% SDS, 50 mM NaOH, and then water, all performed twice with 6 sec injection at a flow rate of 100 µL/min. With the flow rate set to 10 µL/min, streptavidin (S4762, Sigma-Aldrich) was immobilized on the conditioned chip through amine coupling, as described in the Biacore manual. Excess protein was removed by 30 s injection of the wash solution (50 mM NaOH + 1 M NaCl) at least eight times. The immobilized level was ~3000 RU. The biotinylated Mdm2 was captured by streptavidin, up to a level of ~400 RU. A flow cell consisting of only streptavidin was used as the reference surface. Using a flow rate of 30 µL/min, peptides dissolved in the SPR buffer were injected for 180 s. The dissociation was monitored for 300 s. For each peptide concentration, the peptide injection was followed by a similar injection of SPR buffer to allow the surface to be fully regenerated (though not completely for peptides with an extremely slow off-rate). After the run, responses from the target protein surface were transformed by: (i) correcting with the DMSO calibration curve, (ii) subtracting the responses obtained from the reference surface, and (iii) subtracting the responses of the buffer injections from those of peptide injections. The last step is known as double referencing, which corrects the systematic artefacts. The resulting responses were subjected to kinetic analysis by global fitting with a 1:1 binding model to obtain the *KD*, k_a (M-1 s-1), and k_d (s-1). Binding responses that did not have enough curvature during the association and dissociation were subjected to steady-state analysis, and the *KD* was obtained by fitting a plot of response at equilibrium against the concentration.

2.12. Computational Chemistry and Molecular Dynamics (MD) Studies

The crystal structure of the stapled peptide ATSP-7041 co-crystalized with the N-terminal domain of MdmX (PDB ID 4N5T) [9] was used to generate a model of ATSP-7041 bound to the N-terminal domain of Mdm2; the sequence identity between Mdm2 and MdmX was ~53% in their N-terminal domains. Following the mutation of Ala^8-Gln^9 to Gln^8-Leu^9, the stapled peptide analog (MP-292) and its complex with Mdm2 were used for generating all the systems explored in this study and for the MD simulations. The Xleap module of the program AMBER16 [22] was used to prepare the systems and the N- and C- termini of the peptide and Mdm2 were acetylated and amidated respectively. The parameters for the staple linkers were taken from our previous study [23]. All the simulation systems were prepared and simulated using protocols, as previously described [23]. MD simulations were carried out in triplicate for 250 ns each, using the pemed.cuda module from the AMBER 16 package in combination with the ff14SB force field [24]. To enhance the conformational sampling, each of these peptides was subjected to biasing potential replica exchange MD (BP-REMD) simulations [25] using eight replicas for 50 ns. Simulation trajectories were visualized using the program VMD [26] and images were generated using the program Pymol [27].

2.13. Whole Cell Homogenate Stability

Peptides at a concentration of 1 µM were incubated at 37 °C with HCT116 whole cell homogenates prepared from 1 million lysed cells/mL. The reaction was stopped at 0, 1, 2, 4, and 22 h with an organic solvent followed by centrifugation. The resulting supernatant was injected into LC/MS for detection of the tested peptide. The remaining percentage of each compound was normalized to the 0 h amount and reported. As a positive control, we used the ONEG peptide with the sequence PLGRPQLRRGQF [28].

2.14. Stapled Peptide Lipophilicity Analysis and Correlation with Cellular/Target Ratios

To explore the correlation between the stapled peptide lipophilicity and cellular permeability, two methods were adapted from the literature: HPLC-LogD [29] and ALogP [30,31]. As related to macrocyclic peptides, such experimental and predictive lipophilicity may be understood in terms of cellular uptake mechanisms ranging from passive permeability [32] to active transport (e.g., endocytosis and/or translocation) [33,34]. The correlation of HPLC-LogD and ALogP data to cellular potency normalized to target binding affinity (cellular EC_{50}/Mdm2 K_d) was then determined to explore whether lipophilicity may be a contributing factor to cellular permeability for the stapled peptides tested here.

2.15. Statistics

Experimental data was collected in at least triplicate and coefficients of variations (% CV) were all <30%. Binding and cellular potency values are reported as geometric means, whereas circular dichroism spectroscopy values are reported as arithmetic means.

3. Results and Discussion

3.1. MP-292 is a High Affinity Mdm2 Binder with On-Target Cellular Activity

To explore the effects of various residue types on stapled peptide secondary structure, binding affinity, and cellular activity, we selected MP-292, an analog of ATSP-7041 but with a substitution of the Ala^8-Gln^9 residues with Gln^8-Leu^9 (Figure 1A). To ensure stoichiometric binding, as well as on-target cellular activity [35], we applied a combination of competitive fluorescence polarization (FP), surface plasmon resonance (SPR), and isothermal titration calorimetry (ITC). Specific and high-affinity binding of MP-292 for Mdm2 was demonstrated through the ability of unlabeled peptides to compete for the fluorescent tracer by FP, canonical saturable SPR sensorgrams [36,37], and 1:1 stoichiometric binding by ITC (Figure 2A). In our cell-based p53 reporter assay, we determined this peptide to have a sub-micromolar EC_{50} in 0% serum (0.5 μM, Figure 2B) and with slightly weaker potencies in 2% and 10% serum (0.7 μM and 4.2 μM, respectively, data not shown). Critically, on-target cellular activity of this molecule was demonstrated, as MP-292 was inactive in our cellular counterscreen and was not able to compromise the plasma membrane, as it was inactive in our LDH release assay (Figure 2B). Indeed, all the stapled p53 peptides investigated here had EC_{50} values >50 μM in both the counterscreen and LDH assays (data not shown).

3.2. Ala Scanning of Stapled Peptide Analogs of MP-292 Confirms Key Residues for Target Binding

As a first step to explore the tolerance of MP-292 to structural substitutions, we performed Ala scanning substitution across the sequence, except for the $R8^4$ and $S5^{11}$ residues that were critical to the macrocyclization. In agreement with previously reported studies [5,9–11], Ala substitution at Phe^3, Trp^7, and Cba^{10} decreased Mdm2 binding affinity by approximately 10- to 100-fold, as measured by competitive fluorescence polarization (Table 1A) and surface plasmon resonance (Table S2). Lowered Mdm2 binding affinity was reflected by corresponding losses in cellular potency (Table 1A and Figure 3A). In contrast, Ala substitutions at other residues of MP-292 were well-tolerated, with minimal changes to Mdm2 binding affinities (Table 1A). These results were expected based on prior biophysical studies [5,9–11] and an X-ray co-crystal structure of the progenitor peptide ATSP-7041 bound to the MdmX protein [9]. Computational modeling of MP-292 with Mdm2 was consistent with Phe3, Trp7, and Cba10 as the most critical residues for molecular interactions with the target (Figure 3B, see Supplementary Section S1 for a discussion of homology model details). For the substitutions at non-interfacial residues, CD spectroscopy rationalized the lack of affinity changes, since the Ala substitutions showed minimal effects on α-helicity in free solution (Table 1A). Specifically, we determined an average value of approximately 40% α-helicity (ranging from 27.6 to 53.3%) for this stapled peptide series. These α-helicity values were consistent between runs and with distinct methods of sample preparation and concentration determination (data not shown). Computational modeling and MD simulations of the unbound peptides in solution also predicted a moderate level of helicity without any dramatic fluctuations in secondary structures (Figure S1). Further simulations predicted increased α-helicity (>85%) of all the stapled peptides in their Mdm2 bound state (Figure S1).

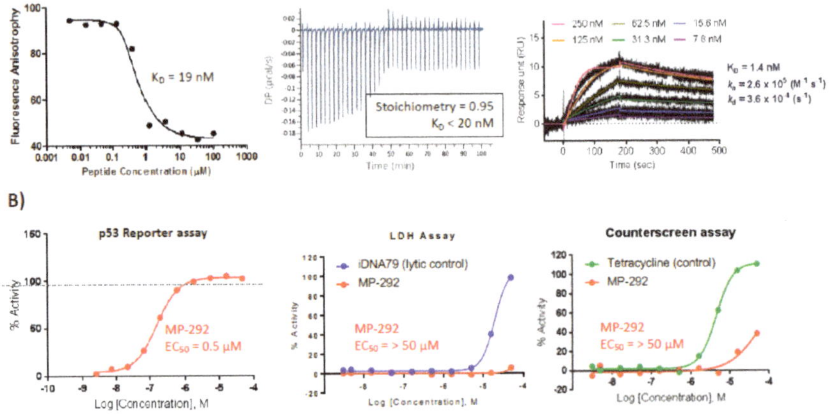

Figure 2. MP-292 is a bona fide Mdm2 binder with on-target cellular activity. (**A**) MP-292 binds to recombinant Mdm2 in a host of biophysical assays, including competitive fluorescence polarization (left panel), isothermal titration calorimetry (middle panel), and surface plasmon resonance (right panel). (**B**) MP-292 shows cellular activity in a β-lactamase-based p53 reporter assay (left panel) but not in counterscreen assays, such as those probing for disruption in membrane integrity (lactate dehydrogenase release, middle panel), nor a β-lactamase based reporter-assay driven from a tetracycline-dependent promoter (p53 independent, right panel).

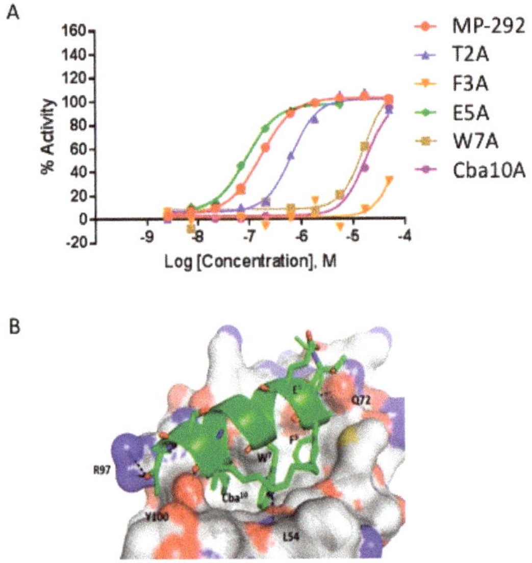

Figure 3. (**A**) Select dose response curves of MP-292 analogs containing Ala substations in the p53 reporter assay. (**B**) Model of MP-292 in complex with Mdm2. Mdm2 is shown as surface (Grey color) and the bound peptide (Green color) is shown as a cartoon. Peptide residues, staple linker, and interacting residues from Mdm2 are shown as lines, with Mdm2/MP-292 hydrogen bond interactions shown as dashed lines (black).

Table 1. Sequence, helicity, cellular activity (EC50), and Mdm2 binding (Kd) of MP-292 and derivatives. Ratio refers to the fold-shift between the binding affinity and cellular activity. Section A) Alanine scan of MP-292 highlights F3, W7 and Cba10 as key residues for Mdm2 binding and cellular activity. Section B) D-amino acid scan of MP-292 shows that most variants maintain Mdm2 binding and cellular activity. Section C) D-amino acids substitutions to MP-189, a linear equivalent of stapled peptide MP-292, disrupt secondary structure and binding to Mdm2.

Table section	Peptide	N-term	1	2	3	4	5	6	7	8	9	10	11	C-term	Helicity (%)	Cellular (µM)	Mdm2 (nM)	Ratio
A	MP-292	Ac-	L	T	F	R8	E	Y	W	Q	L	Cba	S5	-SAA-amide	32.8	0.54	18.6	29
	L1A	Ac-	A	T	F	R8	E	Y	W	Q	L	Cba	S5	-SAA-amide	53.3	0.50	17.6	28
	T2A	Ac-	L	A	F	R8	E	Y	W	Q	L	Cba	S5	-SAA-amide	36.2	1.0	21.3	47
	F3A	Ac-	L	T	A	R8	E	Y	W	Q	L	Cba	S5	-SAA-amide	48.4	37	3600	10
	E5A	Ac-	L	T	F	R8	A	Y	W	Q	L	Cba	S5	-SAA-amide	27.6	0.18	29.8	6
	Y6A	Ac-	L	T	F	R8	E	A	W	Q	L	Cba	S5	-SAA-amide	50.3	0.55	38.9	14
	W7A	Ac-	L	T	F	R8	E	Y	A	Q	L	Cba	S5	-SAA-amide	ND	8.8	5093	2
	Q8A	Ac-	L	T	F	R8	E	Y	W	A	L	Cba	S5	-SAA-amide	33.4	0.10	26.5	4
	L9A	Ac-	L	T	F	R8	E	Y	W	Q	A	Cba	S5	-SAA-amide	48.7	0.16	12.0	13
	Cba10A	Ac-	L	T	F	R8	E	Y	W	Q	L	A	S5	-SAA-amide	ND	11	176	61
	S12A	Ac-	L	T	F	R8	E	Y	W	Q	L	Cba	S5	-AAA-amide	36.5	0.35	20.4	17
B	L1(D-Leu)	Ac-	D-Leu	T	F	R8	E	Y	W	Q	L	Cba	S5	-SAA-amide	44.1	0.6	31	18
	T2(D-Thr)	Ac-	L	D-Thr	F	R8	E	Y	W	Q	L	Cba	S5	-SAA-amide	40.7	3.4	136	25
	F3(D-Phe)	Ac-	L	T	D-Phe	R8	E	Y	W	Q	L	Cba	S5	-SAA-amide	51.8	>50	6485	>8
	E5(D-Glu)	Ac-	L	T	F	R8	D-Glu	Y	W	Q	L	Cba	S5	-SAA-amide	38.2	1.0	32	30
	Y6 (D-Tyr)	Ac-	L	T	F	R8	E	D-Tyr	W	Q	L	Cba	S5	-SAA-amide	43.2	3.2	286	11
	W6(D-Trp) (MP-384)	Ac-	L	T	F	R8	E	Y	D-Trp	Q	L	Cba	S5	-SAA-amide	41.0	0.6	30	20
	Q8(D-Gln)	Ac-	L	T	F	R8	E	Y	W	D-Gln	L	Cba	S5	-SAA-amide	27.1	2.1	22	95
	L9(D-Leu)	Ac-	L	T	F	R8	E	Y	W	Q	D-Leu	Cba	S5	-SAA-amide	39.0	1.1	30	37
	Cba10(D-Cba)	Ac-	L	T	F	R8	E	Y	W	Q	L	D-Cba	S5	-SAA-amide	ND	8.1	1650	5
	S12(D-Ser)	Ac-	L	T	F	R8	E	Y	W	Q	L	Cba	S5	-(D-Ser)-AA-amide	41.2	1.2	8.6	140
	A13(D-Ala)	Ac-	L	T	F	R8	E	Y	W	Q	L	Cba	S5	-S-(D-Ala)-A-amide	41.8	0.6	17	35
	A14(D-Ala)	Ac-	L	T	F	R8	E	Y	W	Q	L	Cba	S5	-SA-(D-Ala)-amide	34.6	0.5	18	28
C	Linear Parent (MP-189)	Ac-	L	T	F	Aib	E	Y	W	Q	L	Cba	Aib	-SAA-amide	35.3	33.5	43.1	777
	Linear L1(D-Leu)	Ac-	D-Leu	T	F	Aib	E	Y	W	Q	L	Cba	Aib	-SAA-amide	37.2	>50	277	>180
	Linear E5(D-Glu)	Ac-	L	T	F	Aib	D-Glu	Y	W	Q	L	Cba	Aib	-SAA-amide	21.4	>50	135	>370
	Linear Q8(D-Gln)	Ac-	L	T	F	Aib	E	Y	W	D-Gln	L	Cba	Aib	-SAA-amide	21.8	>50	119	>370
	Linear L9(D-Leu)	Ac-	L	T	F	Aib	E	Y	W	Q	D-Leu	Cba	Aib	-SAA-amide	19.7	>50	88	>568

3.3. α-Helicity, Target Binding, and Cellular Activity Were Generally Unaffected by D-Amino Acid Substitutions into MP-292

Considering the helix-inducing propensity of alanine, it was not surprising that Ala substitution at non-interfacial positions of MP-292 had relatively minimal effects on binding affinities and cellular activities. To explore whether more drastic substitutions may be tolerated, we performed a D-amino acid scan of MP-292 (except for the $R8^4$ and $S5^{11}$ residues). As predicted, both D-Phe^3 and D-Cba^{10} substitutions resulted in stapled peptide analogs exhibiting significantly decreased Mdm2 binding affinities (Table 1B), details of the specific mechanisms for affinity loss were studied by MD simulations and are detailed in the Supplementary Information, Section S2. Unexpectedly, substitution of Trp^7 by D-Trp^7 gave an Mdm2 binding affinity and cellular activity similar to that of MP-292 (Table 1B); a result that was explained by biophysical (CD), computational modeling, and X-ray crystallography studies (vide infra). For the non-interfacial residues, D-amino acid substitutions were well-tolerated with respect to Mdm2 binding affinities or cellular activities (Table 1B). A comparative analysis of the α-helical content of the D-amino acid scan peptides with the aforementioned Ala-scan peptides by CD spectroscopy corroborated such biochemical and cellular data. Specifically, it was determined that the α-helical properties of the D-amino acid scan series of MP-292 analogs were similar to those of the Ala-scan peptides (Table 1 and Figures S1 and S2).

3.4. D-Amino Acid Scanning of Linear Peptides Results in Decreased α-Helicity, Target Binding, and Cellular Activity

To ascertain if the retention of α-helicity for the D-amino acid peptides was a consequence of conformational stabilization by the $R8^4$-to-$S5^{11}$ hydrocarbon stapling, we designed a series of linear peptides containing Aib^4 and Aib^{11} substitutions to impart α-helical inducing properties, albeit without the benefit of macrocyclization. With the exception of the D-Leu^1 substituted analog, the linear peptides containing D-amino acid replacements (e.g., D-Glu^5, D-Gln^8, and D-Leu^9) showed a dramatic loss in α-helical properties, as evidenced by less intense spectra and decrease of the minima at 222 nm (Figure 4), a hallmark of the α-helical conformation. Remarkably, despite the low helical content of the D-amino acid modified linear peptides, as determined by CD analysis, they exhibited relatively potent Mdm2 binding affinities (Table 1C), in line with a previous report, where binding was retained in a linear Mdm2-binding peptide (pMI) with D-amino acid substitutions at the C-terminus [38]. Importantly, and in contrast to the stapled peptide series, the linear peptide analogs possessed marginal, if any, cellular activity (Table 1C), a phenomenon likely due to a combination of compromised intracellular stability (vide infra) and cell permeability.

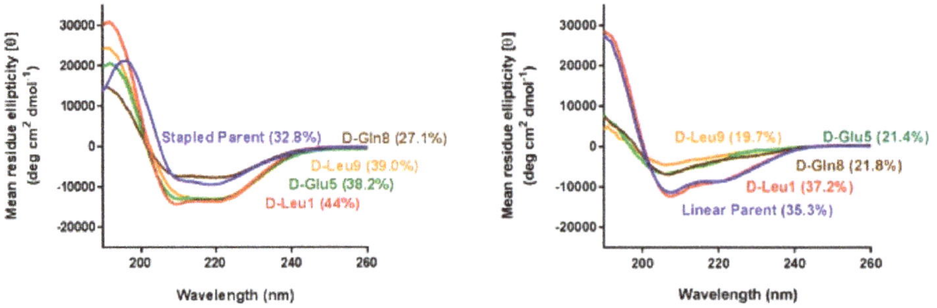

Figure 4. Circular dichroism spectra of stapled peptides bearing D-amino acid substitutions (left panel) and their corresponding linear counterparts (right panel). The table gives the sequences of the parent peptides.

3.5. D-Trp^7 Modified Stapled Peptide: Computational Modeling and X-Ray Crystallographic Studies with Mdm2

We next sought to understand why D-Trp^7 substitution at a critical interfacial position for Mdm2 molecular recognition did not abrogate binding. MD simulations showed that the D-Trp^7 side chain undergoes a re-orientation to adopt a conformation that is highly similar to that adopted by the L-Trp^7 sidechain in MP-292 (Figure S3, Movies 1,2), and allowed for the retention of critical hydrogen bonds. Given that the D-Trp^7 sidechain projects off the helical backbone with a significantly different spatial vector, compensating changes were requisite to enable the peptide analog to bind Mdm2 in a productive manner. Specifically, a combination of changes to the Phe^3 and Cba^{10} sidechain torsion angles and a cooperative shift in α-helical register was predicted to occur to allow the Phe^3, D-Trp^7, and Cba^{10} sidechains to bind effectively. This would also preserve a hydrogen bond between the D-Trp^7 indole nitrogen and the backbone carbonyl oxygen of Leu54. The rationale provided by such computational simulations was confirmed by solving the co-crystal structure of the D-Trp^7-modified stapled peptide MP-594 in complex with Mdm2 (6–125). The structure revealed a single complex in the asymmetric unit of the crystal. The p53 peptide binding groove in the Mdm2 complex was occupied by a single molecule of MP-594, wherein electron density in the 2Fo-Fc was observed for the entirety of the stapled peptide, interacting with the target protein by burying the residues Phe^3, D-Trp^7, and Cba^{10} into the same hydrophobic cleft where Nutlin and p53-derived peptides are known to interact (Figure 5A,B). The D-Trp^7-substituted stapled peptide aligns itself along the p53 peptide binding site in the same orientation as other stapled peptides co-crystallized with Mdm2, including M06 (PDB: 4UMN) and SAH-8 (PDB: 3V3B) (Figure 5C,D). Interestingly, when the Mdm2:MP-594 complex is overlaid with the Mdm2:M06 complex (Figure 5E), the D-Trp^7 sidechain is observed to occupy the same volume of space as the Trp in M06 without perturbing the spatial positions of the other critical side chains in relation to each other (Figure 5E) or the overall α-helical fold of the constrained peptide (Figure 5E). In addition, MP-594 maintained the same hydrogen bond formed as that which exists between the Trp of M06 and the carbonyl backbone group found on Leu^{54} of Mdm2. However, there were changes in the global conformation of MP-594 in relation to M06, whereby it translated further across the Mdm2 binding groove, resulting in a major change in the position of the Cα carbon backbone (Figure 5C,E). A similar displacement was observed in relation to the SAH-8 peptide (Figure 5D). These changes enable the side chain interactions of the critical residues to be maintained especially in relation to the D-Trp^7 of MP-594, where the re-orientation of the Cα allows the indole side chain to optimally pack with Mdm2. Interestingly, overlay of MP-594 with the pMI (N8A) linear peptide (PDB: 3LNZ) showed an even greater change in the bound conformation of the peptide, where a longitudinal translation down the pocket can be seen in combination with a movement across the binding groove on Mdm2 (Figure 5F). This result demonstrates the cumulative effects that hydrocarbon stapling of the linear peptide and introduction of the D-Trp^7 have on the conformation of the bound peptide. In the complex, the interaction of the hydrocarbon staple with the surface of Mdm2 and the accommodation of D-Trp^7 in the target binding pocket causes the dramatic re-orientation of MP-594 with respect to pMI.

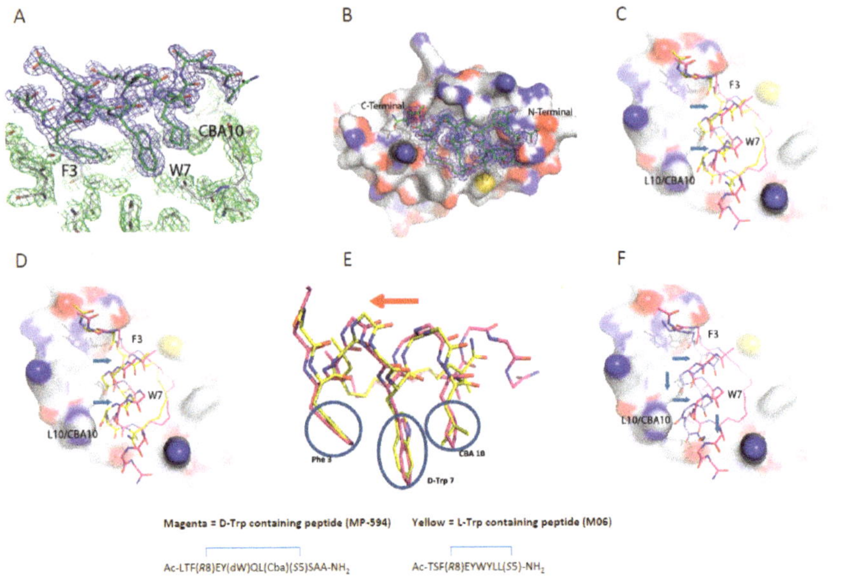

Figure 5. (**A**) The three critical residues (F3, D-Trp^7, and Cba^{10}) responsible for the interaction of the peptide with Mdm2 project into a hydrophobic groove on the surface of Mdm2. 2Fo-Fc map for ATSP-7041 variant with a W^7 to D-Trp substitution (MP-594) peptide is shown in blue and the 2Fo-Fc map for Mdm2 is shown in green (1.5σ). (**B**) Surface representation of Human Mdm2 (6–125) in complex with MP-594. The 2Fo-Fc electron density map for MP-594 is shown in blue mesh (1.5σ). (**C**) Alignment of MP-594 (magenta) with the M06 stapled peptide (chain C from PDB ID: 4UMN, yellow) (**D**) and the SAH-8 stapled peptide (chain B from PDB ID: 3V3B, cyan), both respectively in complex with Mdm2, highlighting the translation (blue arrows) of MP-594 across the peptide binding groove. (**E**) Overlay of MP-594 and M06, demonstrating that the D-Trp^7 sidechain of MP-594 occupies the same volume of space as the Trp^7 in M06 without perturbing the spatial positions of the other critical side chains in relation to each other or the overall α-helical fold of the constrained peptide. Only a global shift in register of the whole peptide occurs to maintain these critical interactions in their optimal positions with Mdm2. (**F**) Alignment of MP-594 (magenta) with the linear pMI N8A peptide (chain B from PDB ID: 3LNZ, blue), both in complex with Mdm2, where gross differences can be observed between both molecules in terms of displacement along and across the Mdm2 binding pocket (blue arrows).

3.6. Cell Homogenate Proteolytic Stability of D-Amino Acid Modified Stapled Versus Linear Peptides

Amongst the known benefits of incorporating D-amino acids in peptides is their capacity to confer resistance to proteolytic degradation. To explore whether such a benefit was realized in the context of the D-amino acid modified peptides investigated in this study, we subjected a subset of both linear and stapled analogs of MP-292 to stability analysis in whole-cell homogenates (Figure 6). As expected, MP-292 showed minimal degradation over 22 h despite being exposed to a multitude of cellular proteases. Thus, in the context of MP-292, further proteolytic stabilization through D-amino acid substitution was not requisite, and similar stability profiles were found for those D-amino acid modified analogs studied. In sharp contrast, the linear peptides were all significantly less stable than their stapled counterparts. However, the Aib^4 and Aib^{11} modified linear peptide MP-189 and D-amino acid modified analogs thereof displayed moderate stabilities (Figure 6). Interestingly, the D-Glu^5 modified linear peptide analog showed decreased stability, perhaps a result of locally perturbed secondary structure. Indeed, replica exchange simulations suggested that D-Glu^5 modification may compromise secondary structural stability, predicted as a result of H-bonding between the sidechains of Glu^5 and Thr^2.

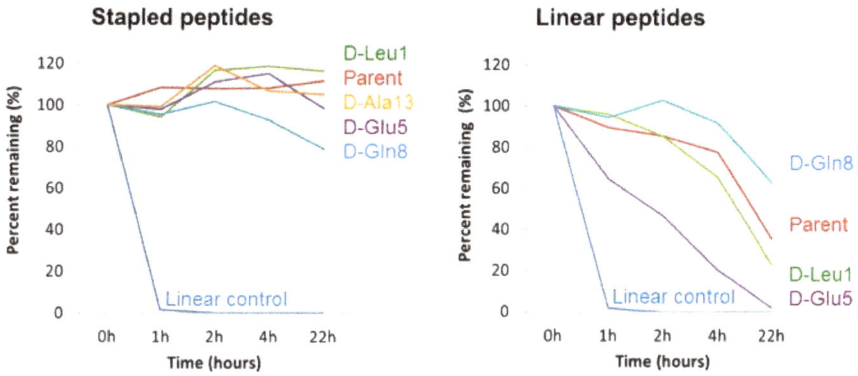

Figure 6. Stability of stapled and linear peptides in whole cell homogenate. Parent sequences correspond to MP-292 (left panel) and MP-189 (right panel). The linear control peptide is ONEG [38].

3.7. Aib, N-Me-Amino Acid, Pro, and Gly Substitutions Had Minimal Effects on a-Helicity, Target Binding, and Cellular Activity

To further explore the effects of helix-inducing or helix-disrupting amino acid substitutions, a series of stapled peptide analogs of MP-082—an N-terminal Lys(N3)-modified ATSP-7041 analog—were evaluated (Table 2). This series included Aib, L-Pro, Gly, and N-methylated amino acid modification at varying positions. Although D-amino acid scanning studies showed a tolerance for α-helicity within the stapled peptide analog of MP-292, it was anticipated that Aib (helix-inducing) versus N-methylated amino acid, Pro, or Gly (helix-disrupting) modifications would exemplify significant differences in α-helicity, as determined by CD studies. However, such modifications did not result in a significant change in α-helicity relative to the parent sequence MP-081 (Table 2). Furthermore, several analogs in this series of peptides exemplified relatively potent Mdm2 binding affinities (i.e., K_d < 100 nM), except for Aib^2 (K_d = 1,706 nM), N-Me-Thr^2 (K_d = 351 nM), N-Me-Ala^8 (K_d = 671 nM), Aib^8 (K_d = 119.4 nM) and N-Me-Gln^9 (K_d = 211 nM) substitutions. CD studies and MD simulations of this series of MP-081 analogs showed that they exhibited good α-helicity (e.g., >30% by CD). An explanation for the significantly decreased Mdm2 binding affinity of N-Me-Thr^2 or Aib^2-substituted MP-081 may be that it effected a local perturbation manifested in a loss of a critical H-bond between the backbone NH of Phe^3 of MP-081 and the sidechain amide moiety of Mdm2 residue Gln72 (Figure S4). Substitutions that disrupt contiguous helix-stabilizing intramolecular H-bonds involving the backbone amides at positions 8 and 9 of MP-081 (i.e., Ala^8 to N-Me-Ala^8, Gln^9 to N-Me-Gln^9 or Pro^9) decreased α-helicity to <30%, as measured by CD studies (Table 2). MD simulations predicted that N-methylation of Ala^8 and Gln^9 would disrupt α-helicity in both free and bound states (see further discussion with Figure S5). Both N-Me-Ala^8 and N-Me-Gln^9 substitutions abolished cellular activity (EC_{50} > 50 μM, Table 2). In contrast, Gln^9 to Pro^9 substitution with MP-081 maintained α-helicity (27.4%) and showed about three-fold lower Mdm2 binding affinity and six-fold decreased cellular potency (Table 2). Surprisingly, Gly substitutions at various positions were tolerated, with each of the MP-081 analogs tested showing α-helicities, Mdm2 binding affinities, and cellular activities similar to the parent sequence (a minor exception was the Glu^5 to Gly^5 substituted analog, which was determined to have 28.6% helicity). Noteworthy was the triple Gly-modified (i.e., $Gly^{1,5,8}$-substituted) MP-081 analog (Table 2), which showed moderately reduced α-helicity (20.4%), retained high binding affinity to Mdm2 (Kd 49.8 nM,), and only three-fold lower cellular activity. Single Gly substitutions for Leu^1, Glu^5, Gln^9, and Ser^{12} showed similar α-helicities and Mdm2 binding affinities relative to the parent sequence MP-081 (Table 2; see further molecular modeling discussion with Figure S6). Lastly, this series of Gly-substituted stapled peptides showed similar cellular potencies (ranging from 263.5–1697 nM), although the Gly^1 analog and the triple $Gly^{1,5,8}$ analog were approximately three-fold less potent than MP-081.

Table 2. Sequence, helicity, cellular activity (EC50), and Mdm2 binding (Kd) of MP-081 and derivatives. A variety of putative helix inducers and helix-breakers are accommodated in the context of stapled peptide MP-081 with most variants maintaining helical structure, Mdm2 binding and cellular activity. Ratio refers to the fold-shift between the binding affinity and cellular activity.

Peptide	N-term	1	2	3	4	5	6	7	8	9	10	11	C-term	Helicity (%)	Cellular (μM)	Mdm2 (nM)	Ratio
MP-081	Ac-K(N3)-(βA)-	L	T	F	R8	E	Y	W	A	Q	Cba	S5	-SAA-amide	49.6	0.42	19.0	22
L1(Aib)	Ac-K(N3)-(βA)-	Aib	T	F	R8	E	Y	W	A	Q	Cba	S5	-SAA-amide	42.7	0.49	29.5	17
T2(Aib)	Ac-K(N3)-(βA)-	L	Aib	F	R8	E	Y	W	A	Q	Cba	S5	-SAA-amide	38.3	2.9	1706	2
A8(Aib)	Ac-K(N3)-(βA)-	L	T	F	R8	E	Y	W	Aib	Q	Cba	S5	-SAA-amide	37.5	1.5	119.4	12
Q9(Aib)	Ac-K(N3)-(βA)-	L	T	F	R8	E	Y	W	A	Aib	Cba	S5	-SAA-amide	28	0.25	33.1	8
S12(Aib)	Ac-K(N3)-(βA)-	L	T	F	R8	E	Y	W	A	Q	Cba	S5	-(Aib)-AA-amide	37.3	0.25	24.4	10
A13(Aib)	Ac-K(N3)-(βA)-	L	T	F	R8	E	Y	W	A	Q	Cba	S5	-A-(Aib)-A-amide	34.4	0.59	25.7	23
L1(N-methyl L-Leu)	Ac-K(N3)-(βA)-	NMe-L	T	F	R8	E	Y	W	A	Q	Cba	S5	-SAA-amide	32.6	0.46	23.5	20
L1(N-methyl L-Ala)	Ac-K(N3)-(βA)-	NMe-A	T	F	R8	E	Y	W	A	Q	Cba	S5	-SAA-amide	47.2	1.49	15.4	97
T2(N-methyl L-Thr)	Ac-K(N3)-(βA)-	L	NMe-T	F	R8	E	Y	W	A	Q	Cba	S5	-SAA-amide	38.2	7.7	352.2	22
A8(N-methyl L-Ala)	Ac-K(N3)-(βA)-	L	T	F	R8	E	Y	W	NMe-A	Q	Cba	S5	-SAA-amide	16.9	>50	671.3	>75
Q9(N-methyl L-Gln)	Ac-K(N3)-(βA)-	L	T	F	R8	E	Y	W	A	NMe-Q	Cba	S5	-SAA-amide	20.2	>50	211.2	>237
A13(N-methyl L-Ala)	Ac-K(N3)-(βA)-	L	T	F	R8	E	Y	W	A	Q	Cba	S5	-S-(Nme-A)-A-amide	38.6	1.6	10.0	158
A14(N-methyl L-Ala)	Ac-K(N3)-(βA)-	L	T	F	R8	E	Y	W	A	Q	Cba	S5	-SA-(Nme-A)-amide	47.5	0.71	5.9	120
L1P	Ac-K(N3)-(βA)-	P	T	F	R8	E	Y	W	A	Q	Cba	S5	-SAA-amide	41.6	0.75	21.9	34
Q9P	Ac-K(N3)-(βA)-	L	T	F	R8	E	Y	W	A	P	Cba	S5	-SAA-amide	27.4	3.1	77.1	41
S12P	Ac-K(N3)-(βA)-	L	T	F	R8	E	Y	W	A	Q	Cba	S5	-PAA-amide	30.8	3.7	45.7	80
L1G	Ac-K(N3)-(βA)-	G	T	F	R8	E	Y	W	A	Q	Cba	S5	-SAA-amide	44.6	1.6	22.1	73
E5G	Ac-K(N3)-(βA)-	L	T	F	R8	G	Y	W	A	Q	Cba	S5	-SAA-amide	28.6	0.26	61.8	4
Q9G	Ac-K(N3)-(βA)-	L	T	F	R8	E	Y	W	A	G	Cba	S5	-SAA-amide	38.8	0.68	42.0	16
S12G	Ac-K(N3)-(βA)-	L	T	F	R8	E	Y	W	A	Q	Cba	S5	-GAA-amide	46.5	0.65	18.9	34
L1G, E5G, A8G	Ac-K(N3)-(βA)-	G	T	F	R8	G	Y	W	G	Q	Cba	S5	-SAA-amide	20.4	1.7	49.8	34

3.8. Membrane Permeability Correlates with Peptide Lipophilicity

Having amassed a sizable library of ATSP-7041 analogs (50 molecules), we looked for trends that might aid in the design of cellularly active stapled peptides. As an estimate for membrane permeability, we normalized peptide cellular potencies by their target-binding affinities (ratios listed in Tables 1 and 2). A visual inspection of these values revealed several instances where substitutions that increased lipophilicity correlated with a decreased cellular/binding ratio compared to its corresponding parent peptide, MP-292 or MP-081 (e.g., E5A, Q8A, and S12 in Table 1; T2(Aib), E5G, Q9G in Table 2). To probe this relationship more formally, we plotted the cellular/biochemical ratios against both experimentally derived lipophilicity (HPLC-logD) and calculated lipophilicity (AlogP) and found a reasonable linear relationship (Figure 7A, $R^2 = 0.46$ for HPLC-LogD and $R^2 = 0.52$ for ALogP). Thus, lipophilicity, at least for this family of peptides, appears to be a primary driver of cellular uptake. It was noted that cell/target ratios in the range of 1000 to 1 are interpreted to represent low to high cellular permeabilities (assuming similar stabilities toward intracellular proteases and cell uptake mechanisms). It was further surmised that stapled peptides having greater lipophilicities (e.g., HPLC-LogD or ALogP values >3) were aligned with superior cell/target ratios (1–10 range). As shown in Figure 7B, the hydrophobic residues of ATSP-7041 are also engaged in target binding, whereas the hydrophilic residues are exposed to solvent. Therefore, the amphipathic properties of this series of stapled peptides translates in terms of both membrane partitioning and target binding to achieve cellular potency.

3.9. Conclusions: A Macrocyclic α-Helical Peptide Model System to Explore Biophysical and Cellular Permeability Properties

To establish ATSP-7041 analogs as a compelling model system to study stapled peptide biophysical properties, cellular activities, and membrane permeability, we focused on MP-292 as a prototypic example. Indeed, this molecule proved to be ideal as a library template, as it showed: (i) 1:1 stoichiometric binding to Mdm2; (ii) sub-μM potency in our cellular assay (p53 reporter assay); (iii) an absence of activity in our cellular counterscreen (p53-independent reporter assay); (iv) an absence of activity in a cell membrane disruption assay (LDH release); and (v) highly proteolytically stable in a cell homogenate assay. As exemplified above by both Ala-scanning and D-amino acid scanning analysis of MP-292, as well as Aib, N-methylated amino acid, L-Pro, and Gly substitutions of MP-081, there are compelling future opportunities to further explore the biophysical and cellular permeability properties of this macrocyclic α-helical peptide model system. We have shown that (within the framework of a stapled α-helical peptide) it is possible to incorporate D-amino acids as well as other classic helix-breakers, such as N-methylated amino acids, L-Pro, and Gly, to expand chemical space without abolishing α-helical conformational properties. Indeed, a surprising result uncovered here was the ability of MP-594 (the D-Trp^7-modified stapled peptide analog) to maintain binding and cellular activity despite the change in stereochemistry at a key binding position—a result explained by modeling and a high-resolution X-ray crystal structure. Furthermore, the comparative analysis of the $Aib^{4,11}$-substituted MP-292 analogs with respect to α-helicity, Mdm2 binding affinity, cellular activity, and proteolytic stability provide insight to understand the unique biophysical and cellular permeability properties of the benchmark stapled peptide ATSP-7041. Lastly, the lipophilic properties of this series of stapled peptides were investigated in terms of determining their experimental and computational partition coefficients (HPLC-LogD and ALogP, respectively). A good correlation between these partition coefficients and the cell/target ratios was observed. The importance of lipophilicity and permeability has been noted in other studies [32–34]. Together, these studies and ours suggest that simply increasing lipophilic character while maintaining strong a binding affinity may enhance peptide permeability and cellular activity. Since a prerequisite for cellular permeability is partitioning of the peptide into an apolar membrane, it is reasonable to assume that a more lipophilic peptide may achieve enhanced partitioning. However, surpassing what may be defined as a peptide-dependent threshold, LogD will likely result in undesired physicochemical properties, such as poor solubility, aggregation, and/or nonspecific binding. Special attention should be given to the judicious regiospecific placement of amino acids to achieve an optimal balance of hydrophobic and hydrophilic surface topology. Interestingly, upon examination of the MdmX:ATSP-7041 co-crystal structure, an amphipathic distribution of hydrophobic amino acids is seen. In particular, a hydrophobic face composed of the hydrocarbon staple moiety and target binding residues (Phe^{3}, Trp^{7}, and Cba^{10}) is balanced by an opposing hydrophilic face (Thr^{2}, Glu^{5}, Gln^{9}, and Ser^{12}). We speculate that this spatial configuration may contribute to favorable aqueous-phase properties, membrane permeability, and ultimately to the sub-μM cellular activity determined for this molecule. Future work will focus more deeply on the cell uptake and intracellular exposure analysis, as well as further exploration of the relationship of lipophilicity to cellular permeability through the expanded chemical diversity of this macrocyclic α-helical peptide model system.

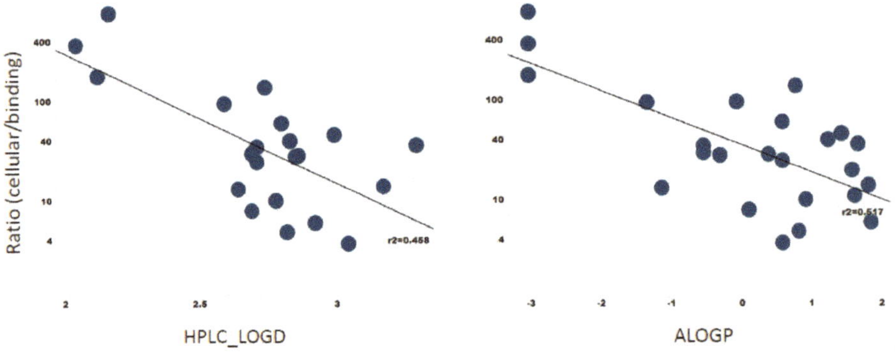

(A)

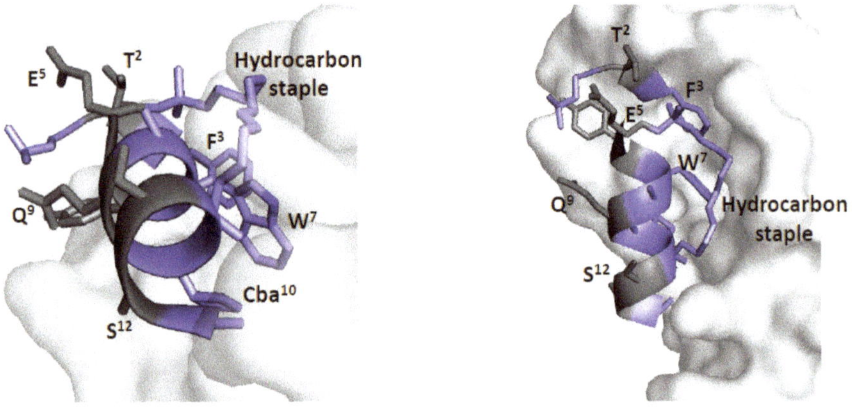

(B)

Figure 7. (**A**) Correlations between cellular/biochemical ratios (see Tables 1 and 2) and lipophilicity determinations; HPLC-LogD (Left panel) and ALogP (Right panel). (**B**) α-Helical structure of ATSP-7041 showing it amphipathicity in terms of hydrophobic surface in blue (F^{3}, W^{7}, Cba^{10}, hydrocarbon staple) that is interacting with Mdm2, whereas the hydrophilic surface in gray (T^{2}, E^{5}, Q^{9}, S^{12}) is exposed to the solvent. The X-ray crystal structure of ATSP-7041 complexed with Mdmx (PDB code, 4N5T) was used for this analysis.

Supplementary Materials: The Supplementary Materials are available online.

Author Contributions: Conceptualization, A.W.P., C.J., C.S.V., D.P.L. and T.K.S.; Data curation, H.Y.K.K., Y.-C.J., A.S., S.L., S.N., D.T., T.Y.Y., S.K., P.A., Y.S.T., M.R.P., S.C., H.W. and S.H.; Formal analysis, K.K., Y.-C.J., A.S., S.N., D.T., T.Y.Y., S.K., P.A., Y.S.T., M.R.P., S.C., H.W., S.H. and B.S.; Funding acquisition, S.L.; Investigation, A.W.P., C.J.B., F.F., C.J., C.S.V. and J.H.; Methodology, A.W.P., H.Y.K.K., Y.-C.J., A.S., S.L., C.J.B., S.N., D.T., F.F., C.J., T.Y.Y., S.K., P.A., Y.S.T., M.R.P., C.S.V., J.H., S.C., H.W., S.H. and B.S.; Project administration, A.W.P., C.J.B., C.J., C.S.V., D.P.L. and T.K.S.; Supervision, A.W.P., C.J.B., C.J., C.S.V., J.H., B.S. and D.P.L.; Writing—original draft, A.W.P. and T.K.S.; Writing—review & editing, C.J., C.S.V., J.H., B.S. and D.P.L.

Funding: This work was supported by a collaborative grant from MSD to A*STAR (p53lab, ICES, and BII) and an Industry Alignment Pre-Positioning Grant (Peptide Engineering Program) to A*STAR (p53lab, ICES, and BII).

Conflicts of Interest: The authors declare no conflict of interest.

References

1. Arkin, M.R.; Tang, Y.; Wells, J.A. Small-molecule inhibitors of protein-protein interactions: Progressing toward the reality. *Chem. Biol.* **2014**, *21*, 1102–1114. [CrossRef] [PubMed]
2. Sousa, F.; Castro, P.; Fonte, P.; Kennedy, P.J.; Neves-Petersen, M.T.; Sarmento, B. Nanoparticles for the delivery of therapeutic antibodies: Dogma or promising strategy? *Expert Opin. Drug Deliv.* **2017**, *14*, 1163–1176. [CrossRef] [PubMed]
3. Vlieghe, P.; Lisowski, V.; Martinez, J.; Khrestchatisky, M. Synthetic therapeutic peptides: Science and market. *Drug Discov. Today* **2010**, *15*, 40–56. [CrossRef] [PubMed]
4. Sawyer, T.K.; Partridge, A.W.; Kaan, H.Y.K.; Juang, Y.C.; Lim, S.; Johannes, C.; Yuen, Y.T.; Verma, C.; Kannan, S.; Aronica, P.; et al. Macrocyclic alpha helical peptide therapeutic modality: A perspective of learnings and challenges. *Bioorg. Med. Chem.* **2018**, *26*, 2807–2815. [CrossRef] [PubMed]
5. Carvajal, L.A.; Neriah, D.B.; Senecal, A.; Benard, L.; Thiruthuvanathan, V.; Yatsenko, T.; Narayanagari, S.R.; Wheat, J.C.; Todorova, T.I.; Mitchell, K.; et al. Dual inhibition of MDMX and MDM2 as a therapeutic strategy in leukemia. *Sci. Transl. Med.* **2018**, *10*, eaao3003. [CrossRef] [PubMed]
6. Schafmeister, C.E.; Po, J.; Verdine, G.L. An All-Hydrocarbon Cross-Linking System for Enhancing the Helicity and Metabolic Stability of Peptides. *J. Am. Chem. Soc.* **2000**, *122*, 5891–5892. [CrossRef]
7. Blackwell, H.E.; Sadowsky, J.D.; Howard, R.J.; Sampson, J.N.; Chao, J.A.; Steinmetz, W.E.; O'Leary, D.J.; Grubbs, R.H. Ring-closing metathesis of olefinic peptides: Design, synthesis, and structural characterization of macrocyclic helical peptides. *J. Org. Chem.* **2001**, *66*, 5291–5302. [CrossRef] [PubMed]
8. Blackwell, H.E.; Grubbs, R.H. Highly Efficient Synthesis of Covalently Cross-Linked Peptide Helices by Ring-Closing Metathesis. *Angew. Chem. Int. Ed. Engl.* **1998**, *37*, 3281–3284. [CrossRef]
9. Chang, Y.S.; Graves, B.; Guerlavais, V.; Tovar, C.; Packman, K.; To, K.H.; Olson, K.A.; Kesavan, K.; Gangurde, P.; Mukherjee, A.; et al. Stapled alpha-helical peptide drug development: A potent dual inhibitor of MDM2 and MDMX for p53-dependent cancer therapy. *Proc. Natl. Acad. Sci. USA* **2013**, *110*, E3445–E3454. [CrossRef]
10. Bernal, F.; Tyler, A.F.; Korsmeyer, S.J.; Walensky, L.D.; Verdine, G.L. Reactivation of the p53 tumor suppressor pathway by a stapled p53 peptide. *J. Am. Chem. Soc.* **2007**, *129*, 2456–2457. [CrossRef]
11. Hu, B.; Gilkes, D.M.; Chen, J. Efficient p53 activation and apoptosis by simultaneous disruption of binding to MDM2 and MDMX. *Cancer Res.* **2007**, *67*, 8810–8817. [CrossRef] [PubMed]
12. Pazgier, M.; Liu, M.; Zou, G.; Yuan, W.; Li, C.; Li, C.; Li, J.; Monbo, J.; Zella, D.; Tarasov, S.G.; et al. Structural basis for high-affinity peptide inhibition of p53 interactions with MDM2 and MDMX. *Proc. Natl. Acad. Sci. USA* **2009**, *106*, 4665–4670. [CrossRef] [PubMed]
13. Bernal, F.; Wade, M.; Godes, M.; Davis, T.N.; Whitehead, D.G.; Kung, A.L.; Wahl, G.M.; Walensky, L.D. A stapled p53 helix overcomes HDMX-mediated suppression of p53. *Cancer Cell* **2010**, *18*, 411–422.
14. Brown, C.J.; Quah, S.T.; Jong, J.; Goh, A.M.; Chiam, P.C.; Khoo, K.H.; Choong, M.L.; Lee, M.A.; Yurlova, L.; Zolghadr, K.; et al. Stapled Peptides with Improved Potency and Specificity That Activate p53. *ACS Chem. Biol.* **2013**, *8*, 506–512. [CrossRef] [PubMed]
15. Kabsch, W. XDS. *Acta Crystallogr. Sect. D Biol. Crystallogr.* **2010**, *66*, 125–132. [CrossRef] [PubMed]
16. Winn, M.D.; Ballard, C.C.; Cowtan, K.D.; Dodson, E.J.; Emsley, P.; Evans, P.R.; Keegan, R.M.; Krissinel, E.B.; Leslie, A.G.W.; McCoy, A.; et al. Overview of the CCP4 suite and current developments. *Acta Crystallogr. Sect. D Biol. Crystallogr.* **2011**, *67*, 235–242. [CrossRef] [PubMed]

17. McCoy, A.J.; Grosse-Kunstleve, R.W.; Adams, P.D.; Winn, M.D.; Storoni, L.C.; Read, R.J. Phaser crystallographic software. *J. Appl. Crystallogr.* **2007**, *40*, 658–674. [CrossRef] [PubMed]
18. Moriarty, N.A.-O.; Liebschner, D.; Klei, H.E.; Echols, N.; Afonine, P.V.; Headd, J.J.; Poon, B.K.; Adams, P.D. Interactive comparison and remediation of collections of macromolecular structures. *Protein Sci.* **2018**, *27*, 182–194. [CrossRef]
19. Murshudov, G.N.; Vagin, A.A.; Dodson, E.J. Refinement of macromolecular structures by the maximum-likelihood method. *Acta Crystallogr. Sect. D Biol. Crystallogr.* **1997**, *53*, 240–255. [CrossRef] [PubMed]
20. Lebedev, A.A.; Young, P.; Isupov, M.N.; Isupov, M.N.; Moroz, O.V.; Murshudov, G.N. JLigand: A graphical tool for the CCP4 template-restraint library. *Acta Crystallogr. Sect. D Biol. Crystallogr.* **2012**, *D64*, 431–440. [CrossRef]
21. Prisant, M.G.; Richardson, J.S.; Richardson, D.C. Structure validation by Calpha geometry: Phi,psi and Cbeta deviation. *Proteins* **2003**, *50*, 437–450.
22. Pearlman, D.A.; Case, D.A.; Caldwell, J.W.; Ross, W.S.; Cheatham, T.E.; DeBolt, S.; Ferguson, D.; George, S.; Kollman, P. AMBER, a package of computer programs for applying molecular mechanics, normal mode analysis, molecular dynamics and free energy calculations to simulate the structural and energetic properties of molecules. *Comput. Phys. Commun.* **1995**, *91*, 1–41. [CrossRef]
23. Tan, Y.S.; Reeks, J.; Brown, C.J.; Thean, D.; Ferrer Gago, F.J.; Yuen, T.Y.; Goh, E.T.L.; Lee, X.E.C.; Jennings, C.E.; Joseph, T.L.; et al. Benzene Probes in Molecular Dynamics Simulations Reveal Novel Binding Sites for Ligand Design. *J. Phys. Chem. Lett.* **2016**, *7*, 3452–3457. [CrossRef] [PubMed]
24. Maier, J.A.; Martinez, C.; Kasavajhala, K.; Wickstrom, L.; Hauser, K.E.; Simmerling, C. ff14SB: Improving the Accuracy of Protein Side Chain and Backbone Parameters from ff99SB. *J. Chem. Theory Comput.* **2015**, *11*, 3696–3713. [CrossRef] [PubMed]
25. Ostermeir, K.; Zacharias, M. Hamiltonian replica-exchange simulations with adaptive biasing of peptide backbone and side chain dihedral angles. *J. Comput. Chem.* **2014**, *35*, 150–158. [CrossRef] [PubMed]
26. Humphrey, W.; Dalke, A.; Schulten, K. VMD: Visual molecular dynamics. *J. Mol. Graph.* **1996**, *14*, 33–38. [CrossRef]
27. Delano, W.L. The PyMOL Molecular Graphics System. Available online: https://www.researchgate.net/publication/225159692_The_PyMOL_Molecular_Graphics_System_2002_DeLano_Scientific_Palo_Alto_CA_USA_httpwwwpymolorg (accessed on 17 June 2019).
28. Cruz, J.; Mihailescu, M.; Wiedman, G.; Herman, K.; Searson, P.C.; Searson, P.C.; Wimley, W.C.; Hristova, K. A membrane-translocating peptide penetrates into bilayers without significant bilayer perturbations. *Biophys. J.* **2013**, *104*, 2419–2428. [CrossRef]
29. Valko, K.; Bevan, C.; Reynolds, D. Chromatographic Hydrophobicity Index by Fast-Gradient RP-HPLC: A High-Throughput Alternative to log P/log D. *Analy. Chem.* **1997**, *69*, 2022–2029. [CrossRef] [PubMed]
30. Ghose, A.K.; Viswanadhan, V.N.; Wendoloski, J.J. Prediction of Hydrophobic (Lipophilic) Properties of Small Organic Molecules Using Fragmental Methods: An Analysis of ALOGP and CLOGP Methods. *J. Phys. Chem. A* **1998**, *102*, 3762–3772. [CrossRef]
31. Ghose, A.K.; Crippen, G.M. Atomic physicochemical parameters for three-dimensional-structure-directed quantitative structure-activity relationships. 2. Modeling dispersive and hydrophobic interactions. *J. Chem. Inform. Comput. Sci.* **1987**, *27*, 21–35. [CrossRef]
32. Furukawa, A.; Townsend, C.E.; Schwochert, J.; Pye, C.R.; Bednarek, M.A.; Lokey, R.S. Passive Membrane Permeability in Cyclic Peptomer Scaffolds Is Robust to Extensive Variation in Side Chain Functionality and Backbone Geometry. *J. Med. Chem.* **2016**, *59*, 9503–9512. [CrossRef]
33. Bird, G.H.; Mazzola, E.; Opoku-Nsiah, K.; Lammert, M.A.; Godes, M.; Neuberg, D.S.; Walensky, L.D. Biophysical determinants for cellular uptake of hydrocarbon-stapled peptide helices. *Nat. Chem. Biol.* **2016**, *12*, 845. [CrossRef] [PubMed]
34. Sakagami, K.; Masuda, T.; Kawano, K.; Futaki, S. Importance of Net Hydrophobicity in the Cellular Uptake of All-Hydrocarbon Stapled Peptides. *Mol. Pharm.* **2018**, *15*, 1332–1340. [CrossRef] [PubMed]
35. Ng, S.; Juang, Y.C.; Kaan, H.Y.K.; Sadruddinb, A.; Yuen, T.Z.; Ferrer, F.J.; Lee, X.C.; Xi, L.; Johannes, C.W.; Brown, C.J.; et al. De-risking drug discovery of intracellular targeting macrocyclic peptides: Screening strategies to eliminate false-positive hits. *BioRxiv* **2019**, 636563.

36. Rich, R.L.; Myszka, D.G. Survey of the 2009 commercial optical biosensor literature. *J. Mol. Recognit.* **2011**, *24*, 892–914. [CrossRef] [PubMed]
37. Myszka, D.G. Survey of the 1998 optical biosensor literature. *J. Mol. Recognit.* **1999**, *12*, 390–408. [CrossRef]
38. Li, X.; Liu, C.; Chen, S.; Hu, H.; Su, J.; Zou, Y. d-Amino acid mutation of PMI as potent dual peptide inhibitors of p53-MDM2/MDMX interactions. *Bioorg. Med. Chem. Lett.* **2017**, *27*, 4678–4681. [CrossRef] [PubMed]

Sample Availability: Samples of the compounds used in this study may be available from the authors pending sufficient stocks and execution of material transfer agreements.

molecules

MDPI

Article

LIR Motif-Containing Hyperdisulfide β-Ginkgotide is Cytoprotective, Adaptogenic, and Scaffold-Ready

Bamaprasad Dutta †, Jiayi Huang †, Janet To and James P. Tam *

School of Biological Sciences, Nanyang Technological University, 60 Nanyang Drive, Singapore 637551, Singapore

* Correspondence: jptam@ntu.edu.sg; Tel.: +65-6316-2833

† These authors contributed equally to this work.

Academic Editor: Henry Mosberg, Tomi Sawyer, Carrie Haskell-Luevano and Stefania Galdiero

check for updates

Received: 27 May 2019; Accepted: 28 June 2019; Published: 30 June 2019

Abstract: Grafting a bioactive peptide onto a disulfide-rich scaffold is a promising approach to improve its structure and metabolic stability. The ginkgo plant-derived β-ginkgotide β-gB1 is a highly unusual molecule: Small, hyperdisulfide, and found only in selected ancient plants. It also contains a conserved 16-amino-acid core with three interlocking disulfides, as well as a six-amino-acid inter-cysteine loop 2 suitable for grafting peptide epitopes. However, very little is known about this recently-discovered family of molecules. Here, we report the biophysical and functional characterizations of the β-ginkgotide β-gB1 from *G. biloba*. A circular dichroism spectroscopy analysis at 90 °C and proteolytic treatments of β-gB1 supported that it is hyperstable. Data mining revealed that the β-gB1 loop 2 contains the canonical LC3 interacting region (LIR) motif crucial for selective autophagy. Cell-based assays and pull-down experiments showed that β-gB1 is an adaptogen, able to maintain cellular homeostasis through induced autophagosomes formation and to protect cells by targeting intracellular proteins from stress-mediated damage against hypoxia and the hypoxia-reoxygenation of induced cell death. This is the first report of an LIR-containing peptide natural product. Together, our results suggest that the plant-derived β-ginkgotide is cytoprotective, capable of targeting intracellular proteins, and holds promise as a hyperdisulfide scaffold for engineering peptidyl therapeutics with enhanced structural and metabolic stability.

Keywords: adaptogenic; autophagy; β-ginkgotide; cytoprotective; cysteine-rich peptides; disulfide-rich scaffold; hyperdisulfide; hypoxia; LIR motif; ginkgo nuts

---

1. Introduction

Bioactive peptides, particularly peptide hormones that are small in size and flexible in structure, are useful drug leads. They have the advantages of being amenable to chemical synthesis, multiple derivatizations, combinatorial chemistries, and structure-activity relationship studies. However, they suffer the limitations of receptor selectivity, short serum half-life, and poor oral bioavailability [1,2].

For five decades, Hruby and his co-workers have addressed these limitations using a multi-disciplinary approach, combining structure analysis, pharmacology, and chemistry to achieve the desired bioactivity and receptor selectivity of peptide hormones such as α-, β- and γ-melanotropins, neuropeptides, and opioid peptides. In chemistry, they championed the use of structure-restricting tools through various combinations of backbone or side chain-side chain cyclization. For conformation-restricting tools, they pioneered peptidomimetics and conformationally-hindered amino acids. Their collective works have strongly impacted the design of peptidyl drugs and approaches to medicinal chemistry [1,3–6].

Nature also provides peptide natural products with various schemes of constraints to enhance their structure and metabolic stability. These schemes, especially features that provide exceptional stability against proteolysis, can be found in two rapidly expanding and highly diverse superfamilies of natural products: The ribosomally synthesized and post-translationally modified peptides (RiPPs) [7] and the cysteine-rich peptides (CRPs) [8,9].

RiPPs are richly represented by the microbial-derived peptides such as microcins, lanthipeptides, and lasso peptides [10]. CRPs are found in both plants and animals. In animals, they are well represented by the ion-channel modulating venom-peptide toxins, which are found in cone snails, insects, and snakes [11,12]. In plants, CRPs are often found as host-defense molecules against environmental stress, pests, and pathogen attacks [8,13].

Over the past 20 years, our laboratory has been interested in the discovery of novel CRPs from medicinal plants—particularly those CRPs with a high potential for oral activity [14–21]. To meet this goal, we have focused our efforts on disulfide-rich or cystine-dense plant peptides containing three or more disulfide bonds with a molecular size of <6 kDa. Such disulfide-rich peptides would have a high structural and metabolic stability because of multiple cross-braces by disulfides. In addition, such peptides would contain, on average, a cysteine in every four or five amino acids in their sequence or about 18–25% cysteine per molecule. Because of their structure and metabolic stability, disulfide-rich peptides have been used successfully as scaffolds to graft bioactive peptides [22–24].

Recently, we discovered hyperdisulfide peptides from medicinal plants. These peptides contain a cysteine in every three amino acids or about 30% cysteine per molecule. However, plant-derived hyperdisulfide peptides have not been explored as a scaffold for drug design. Their exceptional compact structure suggests that these hyperdisulfide peptides could also be a hyperstable scaffold for engineering peptides to enhance their metabolic stability while retaining their bioactivity.

Ginkgo biloba, commonly known as ginkgo or maidenhair tree, is one of the most ancient tree species. Both the leaves and nuts have been used in traditional medicines [22]. Recently, we have identified two CRP families in *G. biloba* nuts, α- and β-ginkgotides [18,19]. The α-ginkgotides are disulfide-rich and belong to the 8C-hevein-like peptide family. In contrast, the β-ginkgotides are hyperdisulfide peptides which contain a conserved six-cysteine core with a highly clustered cysteine spacing and a motif of C–CC–C–CC, an arrangement that has not been reported in cysteine-rich peptides. Furthermore, we found that the α-ginkgotides display anti-fungal activity, but the bioactivity of β-ginkgotides remains unexplored.

Here, we report the biophysical and functional characterizations of the hyperdisulfide-constrained the β-ginkgotide β-gB1 from *G. biloba*. We found that β-ginkgotide is highly resistant to heat and proteolytic degradation, suggesting it is a suitable scaffold for grafting peptide epitopes. Bioinformatics data-mining revealed that β-gB1 contains the canonical LIR (LC3 interacting region) motif. Functionally, we showed that the β-ginkgotide β-gB1 displays cytoprotective and adaptogenic properties to modulate cellular homeostasis and survivability against hypoxia-induced stress.

2. Results

2.1. *β-Ginkgotide: Synthesis and Biophysical Characterization*

2.1.1. Chemical Synthesis and Oxidative Folding of β-Ginkgotide

We prepared three forms of β-ginkgotide β-gB1: The folded form, the *S*-reduced form where all six cysteine residues remained as free sulfhydryls, and the *S*-alkylated form in which the *S*-reduced β-gB1 was *S*-alkylated with iodoacetamide (Scheme 1, legend). A synthetic β-ginkgotide β-gB1 was obtained from GL Biochem (Shanghai, China) by a stepwise solid phase peptide synthesis using Fmoc (*N*-(9-fuorenyl)methoxycarbonyl) chemistry. However, the acidolytic cleavage, HPLC purification, and oxidative folding were performed in our laboratory. The oxidative folding was performed according to the conditions previously reported using a mixture of reduced and oxidized glutathione together with dimethyl sulfoxide in a 75% yield before purification. The mass spectrometry (MS) spectra and HPLC chromatogram of the folded β-gB1 are shown in Supplementary Figure S1. A co-elution test and 2D NMR comparison in our previous study showed that under this folding condition, the folded β-gB1 shared the same peptide fold as the native β-gB1 extracted from *G. biloba* [19].

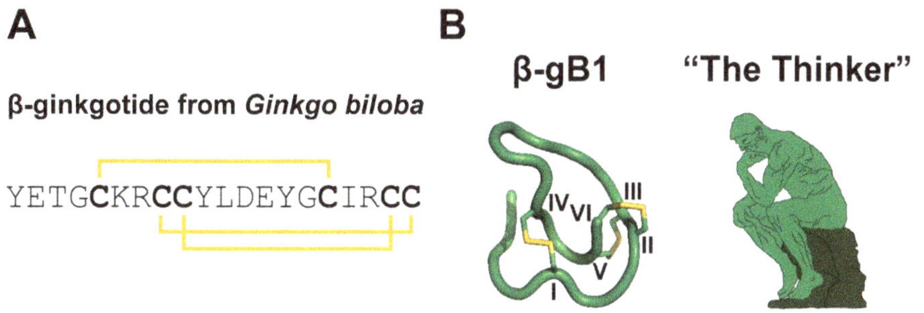

Scheme 1. β-ginkgotide, β-gB1 from *Ginkgo biloba*. (**A**) Primary sequence and disulfide connectivities (Cys I-IV, Cys II-VI, and Cys III-V) of β-gB1. (**B**) Cartoon representation of the NMR structure of synthetic β-gB1 (PDB: 5XIV) resembles the Rodin sculpture "The Thinker (Le Penseur)." The central loop 2 (between Cys III and Cys IV, the vicinal cysteine is counted as one cysteine) containing the peptide epitope YLDEYG forms the head and the back of "The Thinker." Two additional forms of the β-ginkgotide β-gB1 (not shown in the scheme) are: The *S*-reduced form where all six cysteines remained as free sulfhydryls, and the *S*-alkylated form in which the reduced β-gB1 was *S*-alkylated with iodoacetamide.

2.1.2. β-Ginkgotide Secondary Structure and Stability

The secondary structure and thermal stability of the synthetic β-gB1 were assessed using circular dichroism (CD) spectroscopy. The far-UV CD data of β-gB1 were acquired at 20 °C, and secondary structure composition was predicted using the CDSSTR algorithm [23] with a normalized root mean square deviation (RMSD) value of 0.021. The CD spectroscopy spectra agreed with the predicted secondary structure of folded β-gB1, which consists 28% strands, 16% turns, 1% helices, and 55% unordered structures (Figure 1A). The spectrum is in strike contrast with that of the *S*-reduced β-gB1, which is devoid of a secondary structure (Figure 1A). Heating the folded β-gB1 peptide up to 90 °C did not alter its CD spectrum (Figure 1B), thus indicating that this hyperdisulfide peptide is highly resistant to thermal denaturation, which is consistent with our previous observations [19].

To assess the proteolytic stability of β-gB1, it was treated with trypsin or pepsin for 6 h. Figure 1C reveals that about 90% of the β-gB1 remained intact after a six hour trypsin or pepsin treatment. In contrast, the *S*-alkylated β-gB1 was completely degraded after a five minute treatment with trypsin at 37 °C. Similarly, the *S*-alkylated β-gB1 was degraded completely by pepsin within 30 min. Our results suggest that the presence of multiple disulfide bonds is essential for the stability of β-gB1 against proteolytic degradation. This result is also consistent with our previous observations that the hyper-constrained β-gB1 is hyperstable [19]. Prolonging the proteolytic treatment does not change the trend of degradation. This is in agreement with other plant CRPs that contain a compact structure, whose proteolytic stability was examined up to six hours treatment [14,17,18,24].

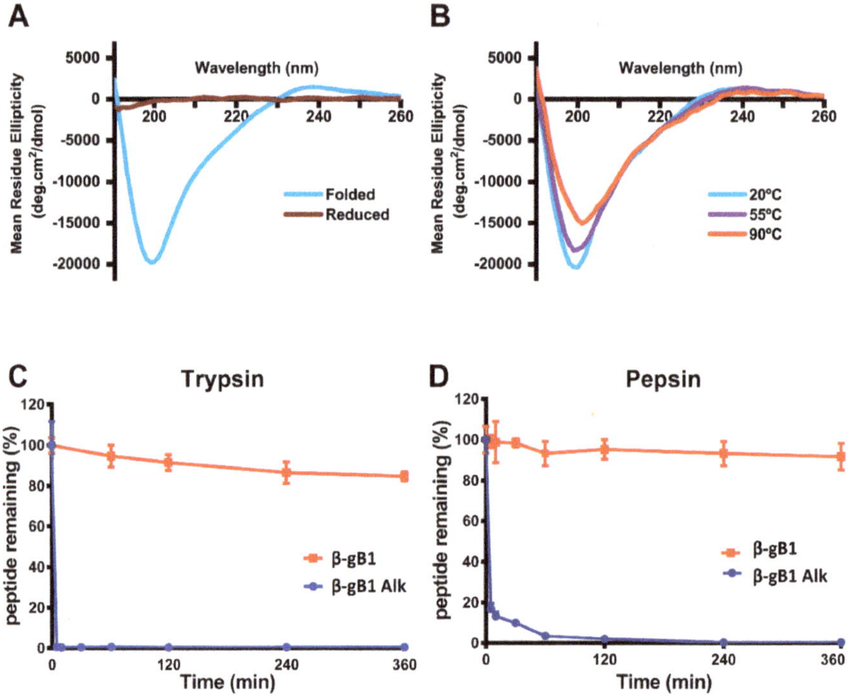

Figure 1. Comparison of the stability of the folded β-gB1 and *S*-reduced and *S*-alkylated forms. (**A**) Far-UV CD spectra of folded and *S*-reduced β-gB1 peptides at 20 °C. (**B**) Far-UV CD spectra of the folded β-gB1 peptide at 20, 55 and 90 °C. Proteolytic stability of β-gB1 against (**C**) trypsin and (**D**) pepsin for six hours in the buffer (pH 7.8) at 37 °C. The *S*-alkylated β-gB1 (β-gB1 Alk) was used as a control.

2.2. Intrinsic Functions of β-Ginkgotide

2.2.1. β-Ginkgotide Contains the LIR Motif and Induces Autophagosomes Formation

We performed a motif search of β-gB1 using the eukaryotic linear motif (ELM) resource and found that the hexapeptide sequence DEYGCI in the loop 2 of β-gB1 (Scheme 1) matches the canonical LC3-interacting region (LIR) motif [25]. The LIR-containing proteins regulate autophagosome formation by interacting with the protein Atg8 (autophagy-related gene, Atg) family through their LIR sequences [26]. Based on this data mining information, we examined β-gB1 in autophagy using the neuronal-like SH-SY5Y cells. The SH-SY5Y cells were cultured with or without β-gB1. The autophagy markers, Beclin-1 (BECN1), LC3B-I, and LC3B-II, were identified and quantified by western blot analysis. Beclin-1 plays an important role in regulating both autophagy and cell death [27], whereas LC3B is an important component of the autophagy pathway and the most widely used marker for autophagosomes. Two of the processed LC3B protein are LC3B-I and LC3B-II. LC3B-I is a truncated LC3B. In contrast, LC3B-II is a truncated and lipidated version of LC3B-I [28,29]. Importantly, LC3B-II is centrally involved in the events of autophagosome membrane expansion and fusion.

Figure 2A,B shows the expression of all three autophagy markers by western blot analysis. The β-gB1 treatment did not alter the expression of the LC3B-I isoform. In contrast, the β-gB1-treated cells increased the expression of the LC3B-II isoform by 2.8-fold. Figure 2C shows that the LC3B-II/LC3B-I ratio increased about 3-fold upon β-gB1 treatment compared to the control. In addition, the β-gB1-treated cells increased the BECN1 expression by 1.5-fold (Figure 2A,B). The elevated expression of both the LC3B-II isoform and BECN1 suggest that β-gB1 induced autophagosomes formation in SH-SY5Y cells. To show that β-gB1 was not involved in apoptosis, the SH-SY5Y cells were treated with β-gB1. Our results showed that the expression of caspase-3 and caspase-9, two enzymes that are critical to the apoptotic pathway, remained unchanged in the treated cells (Figure 2D,E), suggesting that no β-gB1-induced apoptosis occurs.

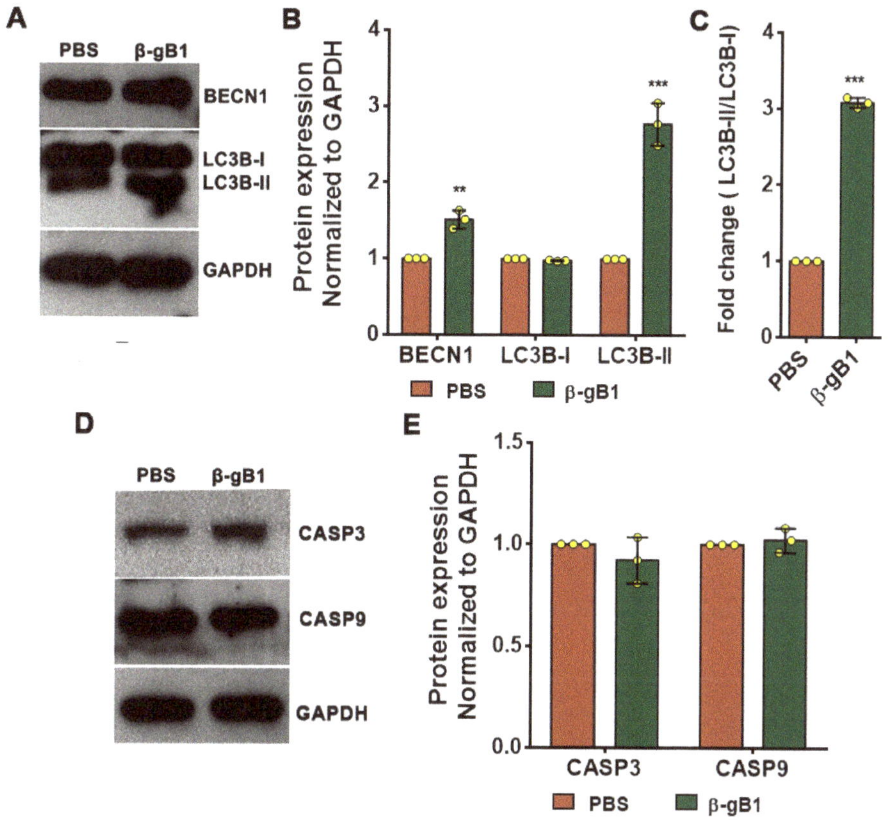

Figure 2. β-ginkgotide-induced autophagy. **A**. Western blot of BECN1, LC3B-I, and LC3B-II in β-gB1-treated and untreated cells. **B**. Expression of BECN1, LC3B-I, and LC3B-II compared with the control. **C**. Ratio of LC3B-II/ LC3B-I upon β-gB1 treatment. **D**. Western blot of caspases CASP3 and CASP9 in β-gB1-treated and untreated cells. **E**. Expression of caspases CASP3 and CASP9 I compared with the control. Quantification was based on western blot band intensity, and data are shown as mean values. Statistical significance was calculated from biological triplicates (** $p < 0.005$ and *** $p < 0.0005$).

2.2.2. β-Ginkgotide Protects Hypoxia-Induced Cell Death

Autophagy is an integrated stress response that clears the subcellular damages. Previous studies have shown that such damages can be induced by hypoxia and hypoxia-reoxygenation stress. Clearing subcellular damages would increase survivability [30–32]. In traditional medicine, *G. biloba* is used as an herbal remedy for acute ischemic stroke and post-stroke recovery [33–35]. To examine the effects of β-gB1 in hypoxia stress, we used cardio-myoblast H9c2 and SH-SY5Y cells. Cells were cultured with or without β-gB1 and incubated in a hypoxic environment for 48 h before the assessment of cell survival by the MTT assay. Figure 3A shows that 10 μM of β-gB1 increases H9c2 survivability by 37%. A comparable cytoprotective effect was also observed in SH-SY5Y cells. Importantly, when the concentration of β-gB1 was reduced tenfold from 10 to 1 μM, a 22–24% increase of survivability was still observed in H9c2 and SH-SY5Y cells (Figure 3A–D). In contrast, no cytoprotective effect was observed in cells treated with a control peptide, the linear S-alkylated β-gB1 (Figure 3C,D), suggesting that the folded form of β-gB1 is important for the cytoprotective activity. No change in cell viability was observed during a normal oxygenated environment (normoxia) in both β-gB1 and S-alkylated β-gB1–treated H9c2 and SH-SY5Y cells (Figure 4C,D), suggesting that β-gB1 or its S-alkylated form has no effect on cell proliferation and cell death. Collectively, these results confirm the cytoprotective effects are exerted by the folded hyperdisulfide form but not the S-alkylated form of β-gB1.

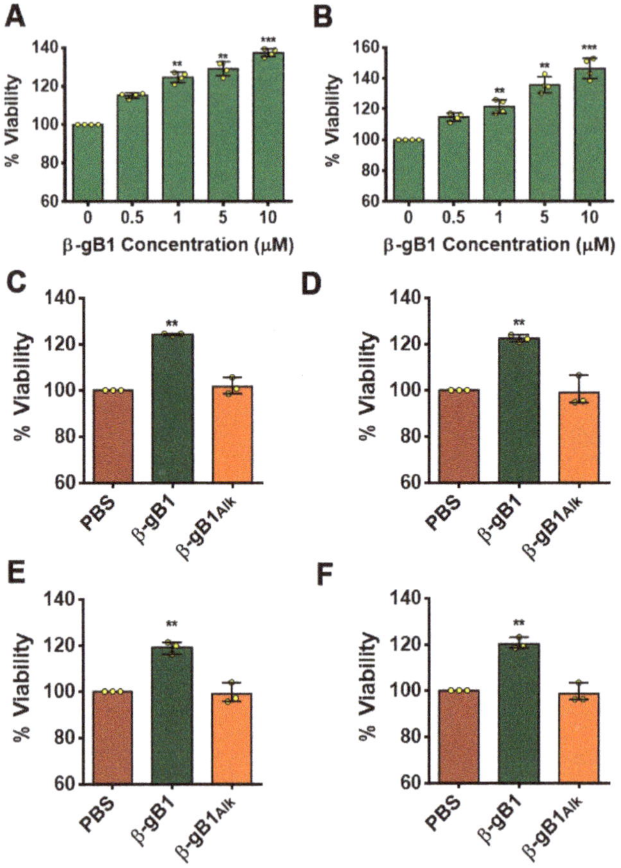

Figure 3. Effect of β-ginkgotide against hypoxia and hypoxia-reoxygenation-induced cell death. Cells were cultured with β-gB1/S-alkylated β-gB1 (β-gB1$_{Alk}$, see Scheme 1 legend) under hypoxia/hypoxia-reoxygenation condition for 48h, and viability was measured by an MTT assay. PBS was used as a vehicle control. Dose-response of β-gB1 upon cell survivability of H9c2 (**A**) and SH-SY5Y (**B**) cells under a hypoxic environment. Relative survival of H9c2 (**C**) and SH-SY5Y (**D**) cells upon 1μM β-gB1 treatment during 48h hypoxia. Relative survivals of H9c2 (**E**) and SH-SY5Y (**F**) cells upon 1μM β-gB1 treatment during hypoxia-reoxygenation stress. Viabilities are expressed as mean values, and statistical significance was calculated from three independent experimental replicates. ** p <0.005 and *** $p < 0.0005$.

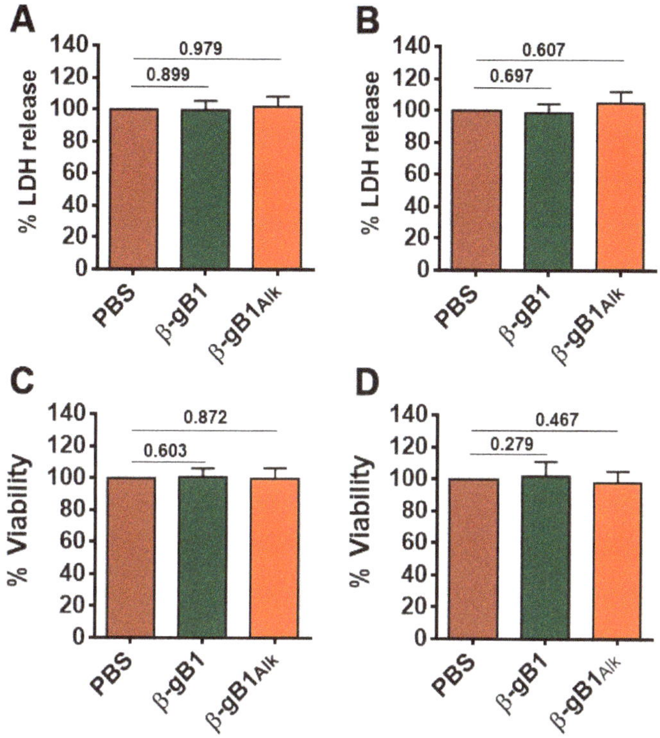

Figure 4. Effect of β-ginkgotide in cell growth and death. The cytotoxicity and plasma membrane-damaging effect was measured by a lactate dehydrogenase (LDH) release assay. Cells were cultured and with or without 10μM of β-gB1/*S*-alkylated β-gB1 (β-gB1$_{Alk}$) for 48 h, and an LDH release was measured by an LDH assay kit. PBS was used as a vehicle control. The Y-axis represents the % LDH release by H9c2 (**A**) and SH-SY5Y (**B**) cells compared to their vehicle control counterpart. Statistical significance was determined from experimental triplicates. Cells were cultured with or without 10μM of β-gB1 and *S*-alkylated β-gB1 (β-gB1$_{Alk}$) for 48 h, and viability was measured by an MTT assay. The relative viability of H9c2 (**C**) and SH-SY5Y (**D**) cells are expressed as mean values, and statistical significance was calculated from independent experimental triplicates.

2.2.3. β-Ginkgotide Protects Cells from Hypoxia-Reoxygenation Injury

The cytoprotective effect of β-ginkgotides against hypoxic stress led us to examine the effect of β-gB1 under hypoxia-reoxygenation stress. Cells were cultured with or without β-gB1 and its *S*-alkylated β-gB1, first under the hypoxic condition for 24 h and then at a normal oxygen environment for another 24 h. The cell viability under hypoxia-reoxygenation condition was assessed by the MTT assay. Upon β-gB1 treatment, cell survivability was increased by 24% and 19% in H9c2 and SH-SY5Y cells, respectively (Figure 3E,F). In contrast, the *S*-alkylated β-gB1 did not produce any cytoprotective effect against hypoxia-reoxygenation injury (Figure 3E,F). Again, our results confirm the importance of the folded structure of β-gB1 against hypoxia-reoxygenation injury.

2.2.4. β-Ginkgotide in Cytotoxicity

Previously, we showed that β-gB1 does not exhibit an antimicrobial effect against *Escherichia coli*, *Candida albicans*, and *Candida tropicalis* at concentrations up to 100 μM. In addition, β-gB1 is non-toxic to Vero and BHK (baby hamster kidney) cell lines based on an MTT assay [19]. To show that β-gB1 is membrane-permeable to target intracellular proteins that induce autophagy formation and cytoprotective against hypoxia, we used a lactate dehydrogenase (LDH) release assay to test the non-toxic effect of β-gB1 in H9c2 and SH-SY5Y cells. LDH is a cytoplasmic enzyme which is rapidly released into the cell culture medium upon plasma membrane damage and is widely used as a marker for cytotoxicity. Thus, an LDH-release assay measures the level of plasma membrane damage to a cell population. Indeed, an LDH-release assay showed that 10 μM of β-gB1 or the *S*-alkylated β-gB1 treatment produced no significant cytotoxicity or cell-membrane damaging effects on both cell lines (Figure 4A,B). An MTT-based cell proliferation assay showed that treatment of 10 μM of β-gB1 or *S*-alkylated β-gB1 has no significant effect on the growth or death of H9c2 and SH-SY5Y cells (Figure 4C,D). Together, our experimental data suggest that both the linear *S*-alkylated and folded forms of β-gB1 have no cytotoxic effect on our tested cell lines in the 10 μM dose range.

3. Discussion

This report describes, for the first time, that the hyperdisulfide peptide, the β-ginkgotide β-gB1 derived from the ginkgo plant, is cytoprotective against hypoxia stress. It also acts as an adaptogen because it induces autophagy, an adaptive process that maintains cellular homeostasis and promotes cell survival. Overall, our findings suggest that the observed cytoprotective and adaptogenic effects of β-ginkgotide agree with the ethnomedicinal uses of ginkgo for treating ischemic stroke, post-stroke recovery cognitive disorders, and Alzheimer's disease [22–24]. The following discussion further amplifies the significance and salient features of this highly unusual molecule.

Autophagy, a degradation process for macromolecules and organelles, maintains homeostasis in cells and tissues. Historically, autophagy has been viewed solely as a degradation process to replenish the nutrition and energy of cells during starvation. However, recent research has described various forms of selective autophagy which have relevance to the treatment of various pathological conditions which include cancer, neurodegenerative diseases, muscular dystrophy, ageing, and innate immunity [36].

A major driving force for this change of view is the discovery of specific autophagy receptors that sequester cargo into forming autophagosomes (phagophores) [26]. In turn, these double-membraned phagophores merge with lysosomes for degradation. The key to this selectivity is the LC3-interacting region (LIR) motif, which guards and locks the targeting of autophagy receptors to LC3 or other ATG8 family proteins anchored in the phagophore membrane. LIR-containing proteins include a complex array of receptors, proteins associated with basal autophagy apparatus, vesicles formation and their transporters, GTPase activating proteins, and specific signaling proteins [26].

The LIR-containing proteins which interact with ATG8 contain a consensus sequence **W/F/Y**-X-X-**L/I/V**, a sequence motif with two essential hydrophobic amino acids (in bold) separated by two amino acids [37]. This LIR motif is often preceded by two acidic amino acid residues to form a six-amino-acid recognition sequence that fits tightly into the basic and hydrophobic pocket on ATG8, the LIR-docking site (LDS). Thus, the six-amino-acid LIR is the minimal required sequence to interact with the Atg proteins. The loop 2 sequences of β-gB1 and β-gB1-like peptides from different ancient plants are highly conserved. In particular, some contain the consensus LIR motif DEYGCI (Scheme 2), suggesting that they could play a role in autophagy [38].

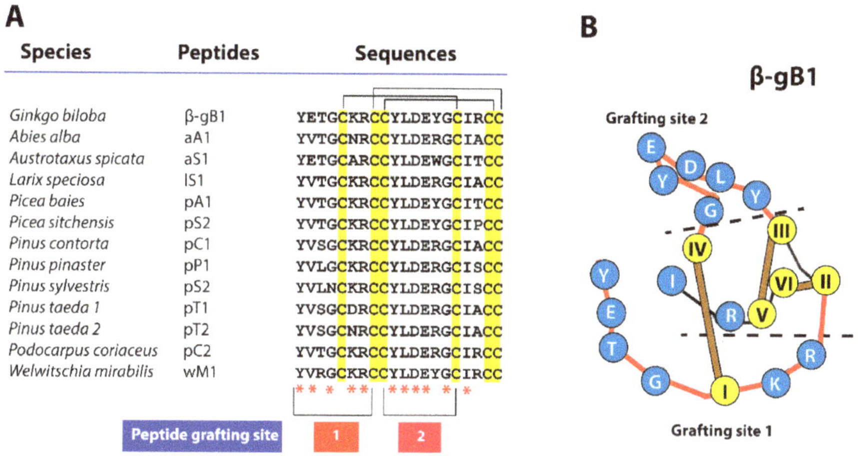

Scheme 2. Sequences and the suitable grafting sites of β-ginkgotide and β-ginkgotide-like peptides. (**A**) Sequence comparison between the β-ginkgotide β-gb1 and twelve selected β-ginkgotide-like peptides with highly conserved sequences. The two suitable grafting sites, 1 and 2, are indicated. (**B**) The schematic representation of the grafting sites 1 and 2 are colored in red. * Represents highly and absolutely conserved residues.

The conversion of the LC3-I isoform (soluble form of LC3) to the lipidated LC3-II isoform is an essential step of autophagosome formation [39,40]. The LC3-II isoform is stably associated with the autophagosome and is widely used as an essential indicator of autophagosome formation [40]. We show that the β-ginkgotide β-gB1 increases the expression of the lipidated LC3B-II isoform. The autophagosome will fuse with an available lysosome as a special waste management and disposal process for degradation of the toxic protein aggregates, implicated in the neurodegenerative diseases [36,39]. In addition, we showed that BECN1 expression, a key pathogenic factor for the pathogenesis of neurodegenerative diseases including Alzheimer's disease, is elevated, and the overexpression of BECN1 has been found to reduce disease pathogenesis through the autophagy-mediated clearance of the toxic amyloid precursor [33].

As a part of the integrated stress response to maintain cellular homeostasis which increases cellular survivability, autophagy involves the clearing of the subcellular damages induced by environmental stress, including hypoxia and hypoxia-reoxygenation stress [40–42]. Thus, the autophagy-inducing property of β-gB1 could be beneficial for minimizing the pathogenic effects of different environmental stresses including hypoxia. Resected circulation reduces the oxygenation levels in tissues, a condition which is commonly known as hypoxia [19]. The restoration of circulation after hypoxia results in hypoxia-reoxygenation stress, resulting in the alternation of several important pathways including ion channels, reactive oxygen species, inflammation, and endothelial dysfunction, followed by apoptosis-induced cell death and tissue damage [30,31,43]. Those two adverse physical factors are the key mediators for the pathogenesis of diseases including ischemic heart diseases, stroke, and cancer [30–32,43–47]. Thus far, the limited knowledge and availability of the therapeutics has complicated the treatment against hypoxia-induced pathogenesis. In this regard, our results are promising in showing the adaptogenic and cytoprotective effects of the β-ginkgotide β-gB1, effects which could minimize hypoxia- and hypoxia-reoxygenation-induced pathogenesis and increase cell survivability in cardiomyocyte and neuronal cells.

The interactions of β-gB1 with the intracellular protein targets in autophagy and hypoxia pathways suggest that it is membrane permeable. These data, coupled with our results, show that the cell membranes are not damaged based on an LDH release assay. In addition, we previously showed that β-gB1 is not a membranolytic antimicrobial [19]. Furthermore, our data have shown that the linear *S*-alkylated form of β-gB1 is not cytoprotective or adaptogenic, strongly suggesting that the folded and structurally compact β-gB1 is necessary for membrane permeability to interact with its intracellular targets.

A distinguishing feature of the β-ginkgotide β-gB1 is its high amount of cysteine residues. The intercysteinyl distance of the hyperdisulfide β-gB1 is relatively small, with 16 residues between the first and six cysteine residues, accounting for 38% of cysteine. In contrast, the average cysteine content of most plant six-cysteine-containing CRPs contain 17–27% of cysteine [19].

Scheme 2 compares the sequences of β-ginkgotide with 12 β-ginkgotide-like peptides, and it shows that they are highly conserved with 80% sequence identity. Two suitable epitope grafting sites can be envisioned. Site 1 is the *N*-terminus, whereas site 2 is the longer and highly conserved loop 2 with six amino acids. If necessary, the four residues of the amino terminus of site 1 can be combine with site 2 for grafting even longer peptides.

Table 1 compares the cysteine frameworks of the β-gB1 with three hyperdisulfide peptides from the conotoxin family, the scratch peptide, BtIIIA, and Mr3e (ConoServer, the database of conotoxins (http://www.conoserver.org)). From the standpoint of grafting a peptide epitope, β-gB1 would be the most suitable. First, it contains the longest interdisulfide loop among the selected hyperdisulfide peptides, loop 2 with six amino acids, which is highly amenable for grafting peptides. In contrast, the other three hyperdisulfide peptides listed in Table 1 contain less than four amino acids in their intercysteinyl loops. Secondly, the intrinsic property of β-gB1 is cytoprotective, which makes it more desirable than a toxin derived from the conotoxin family. Thirdly, β-gB1 is membrane permeable and could target intracellular proteins. Overall, our results suggest that the β-ginkgotide β-gB1 is a novel hyperdisulfide scaffold that is suitable for grafting bioactive peptides to improve their structures and metabolic stability.

Table 1. Comparison of β-gB1 with three hyperdisulfide conotoxin peptides.

Peptides	Cysteine motif [1]	No. of aa [2]	Cys (%) [3]
Scratch peptide	$C^{I}C^{II}\bullet\bullet C^{III}\bullet\bullet C^{IV}\bullet\bullet C^{V}C^{VI}$	12	50
BtIIIA	$C^{I}C^{II}\bullet\bullet\bullet C^{III}\bullet\bullet C^{IV}\bullet\bullet C^{V}C^{VI}$	13	46
Mr3e	$XC^{I}C^{II}\bullet\bullet\bullet\bullet C^{III}\bullet\bullet\bullet C^{IV}\bullet C^{V}C^{VI}X$	14	43
β-gB1	$X_4CI\bullet\bullet C^{II}C^{III}\bullet\bullet\bullet\bullet\bullet\bullet C^{IV}\bullet\bullet C^{V}C^{VI}$	16	38

[1] The red dots represent the amino acids in the longest intercysteinyl loop suitable for grafting peptide epitopes. [2] Number of amino acids (aa) within Cys I and Cys VI; [3] Cys (%) = (number of Cys/total number of amino acids between Cys I and Cys VI) × 100.

4. Materials and Methods

4.1. Reagents

All reagents were purchased from Sigma-Aldrich unless otherwise indicated (Sigma-Aldrich, Madison, WI, USA). Antibodies against GAPDH (6C5) (sc-32233) were from Santa Cruz Biotechnology, Santa Cruz, CA, and the Anti-LC3B (L7543) antibody was purchased from Sigma-Aldrich, WI. Beclin-1 (D40C5) (3495), Caspase-3 (9662), and Caspase-9 (9502) antibodies were procured from Cell Signaling Technology, Danvers, MA. Clarity Max™ Western ECL blotting substrates (1705062) were purchased from Bio-Rad Laboratories, Segrate, Italy.

4.2. Synthesis and Oxidative Folding of β-Ginkgotide β-gB1

A synthetic β-ginkgotide β-gB1 was obtained from GL Biochem (Shanghai, China) by solid phase peptide synthesis using Fmoc (*N*-(9-fluorenyl) methoxycarbonyl) chemistry and purified by C_{18}-reversed-phase HPLC to 85% purity. The oxidative folding was performed and modified as previous report [19]. Briefly, the oxidative folding was initiated by adding 1 mg of synthetic, reduced β-gB1 to 1 mL of a 0.1 M ammonium bicarbonate buffer (pH 8.5) containing 20 mM of reduced glutathione, 4 mM of oxidized glutathione and 10% (*v*/*v*) dimethyl sulfoxide (DMSO). After a 2-h incubation, the reaction was quenched 0.1% trifluoroacetic acid solution and purified by C_{18}-reversed-phase HPLC.

4.3. Circular Dichroism Spectroscopy

Far-UV CD spectra were recorded for the synthetic and folded β-ginkgotide β-gB1 (42 μM) in a sodium phosphate buffer (pH 7.5) on a Chirascan™ CD spectrometer (Applied Photophysics, Leatherhead, UK) equipped with a temperature controller. Spectra were acquired between 190 and 260 nm from 20 to 90 °C using a 1 mm path-length quartz cuvette, a 1 nm spectral bandwidth, and a 1 nm step size. CD spectroscopy data were analyzed for secondary structure content using CDSSTR [23]. CD data were expressed as mean residue ellipticity (in deg $cm^2 dmol^{-1}$).

4.4. Enzymatic Stability

The folded β-gB1 (28 μg) was added to 100 μL of a 0.1 M ammonium bicarbonate buffer (pH 7.8) containing 800 U/mL of trypsin or 4 mg/mL of pepsin and incubated at 37 °C for 6 h. At each time-point (0, 1, 2, 4, and 6 h), 20 μL of the treated sample was aliquoted and quenched by adding 5 μL of 1 M hydrochloric acid or 0.8 μL of 1 M sodium hydroxide. The reduced β-gB1 was alkylated with iodoacetamide (*S*-alkylated β-gB1) and used as a control in this study. The reaction mixture was analyzed by MALDI-TOF MS and C_{18}-reversed-phase HPLC to determine its stability.

4.5. Cell Culture

Rat cardio-myoblast cells (H9c2) and mouse neuron-like SH-SY5Y cells were purchased from ATCC and maintained in DMEM (Dulbecco's modified eagle medium) medium supplemented with 10% fetal bovine serum (FBS), 10,000 U/mL of penicillin, and 10,000 μg/mL of streptomycin at 37 °C, 5% CO_2.

4.6. Hypoxia and Hypoxia-Reoxygenation Model

Cells were seeded in a cell culture medium with/without β-gB1 and incubated at 37 °C, 5% CO_2 overnight. The next day, the cells were locked inside a BD GasPak EZ anaerobe pouch system (BD Diagnostics, MD) and incubated at 37 °C for the next 48 h for the hypoxia condition. In addition, the cells were cultured under a normal oxygenated environment for the normoxic control. In hypoxia-reoxygenation experiments, the cells were incubated for 24 h in hypoxic conditions before being incubated for another 24 h under normoxia.

4.7. MTT Assay

Cells were cultured in DMEM with or without β-gB1/*S*-alkylated β-gB1 (β-gB1$_{Alk}$) for 48 h under normoxia, hypoxia, and hypoxia-reoxygenation conditions. Phosphate-buffered saline (PBS) was used as a vehicle control. After 48 h, MTT (3-(4,5-dimethylthiazol-2-yl)-2,5-diphenyltetrazolium bromide) reagent was added with a final concentration of 0.5 mg/mL, and it was incubated at 37 °C for 2 h. The culture medium was then aspirated, and purple formazan crystals were dissolved in DMSO for colorimetric quantification at 570 nm using a microplate reader with a reference wavelength of 630 nm. Experiments were performed in triplicates, and statistical calculations and bar graphs were done using GraphPad Prism software (GraphPad Prism version 6.01, La Jolla, California, USA). Data are presented as means ± SD, and multiple comparisons were performed by one-way ANOVA. *P*-values of less than 0.05 were considered significant.

4.8. LDH Assay

An LDH release assay was performed using the CytoSelect™ LDH cytotoxicity assay kit (CBA-241, Cell Biolabs, Inc., San Diego, CA, USA). In brief, cells were cultured in DMEM with or without 10 μM of β-gB1 and *S*-alkylated β-gB1 (β-gB1$_{Alk}$) for 48 h at 37 °C and 5% CO_2. PBS was used for the vehicle control experiment. The culture medium was transferred and mixed with the LDH assay reagent in a ratio of 9:1. The reaction mixture was incubated at 37 °C for 2 h, and colorimetric quantification was performed using a 450 nm wavelength. The assay was performed in experimental triplicates, and statistical calculations and bar graphs were done using GraphPad Prism software (Version 6.01). Data are presented as means ± SD, and multiple comparisons were performed by one-way ANOVA. *P*-values pf less than 0.05 were considered significant.

4.9. Western Blot Analysis

A 25 μg equivalent quantity of each protein samples were resolved on a 10% and 15% SDS-PAGE gel accordingly and transferred onto a nitrocellulose membrane. Immunoblotting was performed using anti-protein antibodies against glyceraldehyde 3-phosphate dehydrogenase (GAPDH) (1:5000), LC3B (1:1500), Beclin-1 (1:1500), Caspase-3 (1:1500), and Caspase-9 (1:1500). Blots were developed with Clarity Max Western ECL blotting substrates. Protein bands were quantitated densitometrically using ImageJ software (ImageJ15.0b, Wayen Rasband, NIH, Bethesda, Maryland, USA), expressed relative to GAPDH, and normalized to the vehicle control cells. Statistical calculations and bar graphs were done using GraphPad Prism software (Version 6.01), and three individual experimental data sets were used for the calculation. Data are presented as means ± SD and compared by the Holm–Sidak multiple *t*-tests method. P-values pf less than 0.05 were considered significant.

4.10. Bioinformatics Analysis

A short linear motifs (SLiMs) search was performed using the online bioinformatics tool the eukaryotic linear motif (ELM) resource (http://elm.eu.org) [25]. The sequences of β-ginkgotide-like peptides were obtained from the GenBank database as previously described [19].

Supplementary Materials: The following are available online, Figure S1: Mass spectrometry and HPLC Spectrum of folded β-gB1.

Author Contributions: J.P.T., B.D., J.Y.H., and J.T. conceived and designed the experiments. J.P.T., B.D., J.Y.H., and J.T. performed the experiments, analyzed the data, and wrote the manuscript. J.P.T. revised the manuscript. All authors read and approved the final version of the manuscript.

Funding: This work was supported by a Nanyang Technological University internal funding–Synzymes and Natural Products Center (SYNC) and the AcRF Tier 3 funding (MOE2016-T3-1-003).

Conflicts of Interest: The authors declare no conflict of interest.

References

1. Hruby, V.J. Designing peptide receptor agonists and antagonists. *Nat. Rev. Drug Discov.* **2002**, *1*, 847–858. [CrossRef] [PubMed]
2. Craik, D.J.; Fairlie, D.P.; Liras, S.; Price, D. The future of peptide-based drugs. *Chem. Biol. Drug Des.* **2013**, *81*, 136–147. [CrossRef] [PubMed]
3. Haskell-Luevano, C.; Shenderovich, M.D.; Sharma, S.D.; Nikiforovich, G.V.; Hadley, M.E.; Hruby, V.J. Design, synthesis, biology, and conformations of bicyclic alpha-melanotropin analogues. *J. Med. Chem.* **1995**, *38*, 1736–1750. [CrossRef] [PubMed]
4. Sawyer, T.K.; Hruby, V.J.; Darman, P.S.; Hadley, M.E. [half-Cys4,half-Cys10]-alpha-Melanocyte-stimulating hormone: A cyclic alpha-melanotropin exhibiting superagonist biological activity. *Proc. Natl. Acad. Sci. USA* **1982**, *79*, 1751–1755. [CrossRef]
5. Cai, M.; Hruby, V.J. Design of cyclized selective melanotropins. *Biopolymers* **2016**, *106*, 876–883. [CrossRef] [PubMed]
6. Chang, Y.S.; Graves, B.; Guerlavais, V.; Tovar, C.; Packman, K.; To, K.-H.; Olson, K.A.; Kesavan, K.; Gangurde, P.; Mukherjee, A.; et al. Stapled α–helical peptide drug development: A potent dual inhibitor of MDM2 and MDMX for p53-dependent cancer therapy. *Proc. Natl. Acad. Sci. USA* **2013**, *110*, E3445–E3454. [CrossRef] [PubMed]

7. Arnison, P.G.; Bibb, M.J.; Bierbaum, G.; Bowers, A.A.; Bugni, T.S.; Bulaj, G.; Camarero, J.A.; Campopiano, D.J.; Challis, G.L.; Clardy, J.; et al. Ribosomally synthesized and post-translationally modified peptide natural products: Overview and recommendations for a universal nomenclature. *Nat. Prod. Rep.* **2013**, *30*, 108–160. [CrossRef] [PubMed]
8. Tam, J.P.; Wang, S.; Wong, K.H.; Tan, W.L. Antimicrobial Peptides from Plants. *Pharmaceuticals* **2015**, *8*, 711–757. [CrossRef] [PubMed]
9. Jennings, C.; West, J.; Waine, C.; Craik, D.; Anderson, M. Biosynthesis and insecticidal properties of plant cyclotides: The cyclic knotted proteins from *Oldenlandia affinis*. *Proc. Natl. Acad. Sci. USA* **2001**, *98*, 10614–10619. [CrossRef]
10. Hetrick, K.J.; van der Donk, W.A. Ribosomally synthesized and post-translationally modified peptide natural product discovery in the genomic era. *Curr. Opin. Chem. Biol.* **2017**, *38*, 36–44. [CrossRef]
11. Olivera, B.; Gray, W.; Zeikus, R.; McIntosh, J.; Varga, J.; Rivier, J.; de Santos, V.; Cruz, L. Peptide neurotoxins from fish-hunting cone snails. *Science* **1985**, *230*, 1338–1343. [CrossRef] [PubMed]
12. Goudet, C.; Chi, C.-W.; Tytgat, J. An overview of toxins and genes from the venom of the Asian scorpion Buthus martensi Karsch. *Toxicon* **2002**, *40*, 1239–1258. [CrossRef]
13. Shafee, T.M.A.; Lay, F.T.; Phan, T.K.; Anderson, M.A.; Hulett, M.D. Convergent evolution of defensin sequence, structure and function. *Cell. Mol. Life Sci.* **2017**, *74*, 663–682. [CrossRef] [PubMed]
14. Kini, S.G.; Wong, K.H.; Tan, W.L.; Xiao, T.; Tam, J.P. Morintides: Cargo-free chitin-binding peptides from Moringa oleifera. *BMC Plant. Biol.* **2017**, *17*, 68. [CrossRef] [PubMed]
15. Kumari, G.; Serra, A.; Shin, J.; Nguyen, P.Q.; Sze, S.K.; Yoon, H.S.; Tam, J.P. Cysteine-Rich Peptide Family with Unusual Disulfide Connectivity from Jasminum sambac. *J. Nat. Prod.* **2015**, *78*, 2791–2799. [CrossRef] [PubMed]
16. Nguyen, G.K.; Zhang, S.; Nguyen, N.T.; Nguyen, P.Q.; Chiu, M.S.; Hardjojo, A.; Tam, J.P. Discovery and characterization of novel cyclotides originated from chimeric precursors consisting of albumin-1 chain a and cyclotide domains in the Fabaceae family. *J. Biol. Chem.* **2011**, *286*, 24275–24287. [CrossRef] [PubMed]
17. Nguyen, P.Q.; Luu, T.T.; Bai, Y.; Nguyen, G.K.; Pervushin, K.; Tam, J.P. Allotides: Proline-Rich Cystine Knot α-Amylase Inhibitors from Allamanda cathartica. *J. Nat. Prod.* **2015**, *78*, 695–704. [CrossRef] [PubMed]
18. Wong, K.H.; Tan, W.L.; Serra, A.; Xiao, T.; Sze, S.K.; Yang, D.; Tam, J.P. Ginkgotides: Proline-Rich Hevein-Like Peptides from Gymnosperm Ginkgo biloba. *Front. Plant Sci.* **2016**, *7*, 1639. [CrossRef]
19. Wong, K.H.; Tan, W.L.; Xiao, T.; Tam, J.P. beta-Ginkgotides: Hyperdisulfide-constrained peptides from Ginkgo biloba. *Sci. Rep.* **2017**, *7*, 6140. [CrossRef]
20. Huang, J.; Wong, K.H.; Tay, S.V.; Serra, A.; Sze, S.K.; Tam, J.P. Astratides: Insulin-Modulating, Insecticidal, and Antifungal Cysteine-Rich Peptides from Astragalus membranaceus. *J. Nat. Prod.* **2019**, *82*, 194–204. [CrossRef]
21. Shen, Y.; Xu, L.; Huang, J.; Serra, A.; Yang, H.; Tam, J.P. Potentides: Novel Cysteine-Rich Peptides with Unusual Disulfide Connectivity from Potentilla anserina. *ChemBioChem* **2019**. [CrossRef] [PubMed]
22. Mahady, G.B. Ginkgo biloba: A review of quality, safety, and efficacy. *Nutr. Clin. Care* **2001**, *4*, 140–147. [CrossRef]
23. Whitmore, L.; Wallace, B.A. DICHROWEB, an online server for protein secondary structure analyses from circular dichroism spectroscopic data. *Nucleic Acids Res.* **2004**, *32*, W668–W673. [CrossRef] [PubMed]
24. Tam, J.P.; Nguyen, G.K.T.; Loo, S.; Wang, S.; Yang, D.; Kam, A. Ginsentides: Cysteine and Glycine-rich Peptides from the Ginseng Family with Unusual Disulfide Connectivity. *Sci. Rep.* **2018**, *8*, 16201. [CrossRef] [PubMed]
25. Gouw, M.; Michael, S.; Samano-Sanchez, H.; Kumar, M.; Zeke, A.; Lang, B.; Bely, B.; Chemes, L.B.; Davey, N.E.; Deng, Z.; et al. The eukaryotic linear motif resource - 2018 update. *Nucleic. Acids Res.* **2018**, *46*, D428–D434. [CrossRef] [PubMed]
26. Birgisdottir, A.B.; Lamark, T.; Johansen, T. The LIR motif - crucial for selective autophagy. *J. Cell Sci.* **2013**, *126*, 3237–3247. [CrossRef]
27. Kang, R.; Zeh, H.J.; Lotze, M.T.; Tang, D. The Beclin 1 network regulates autophagy and apoptosis. *Cell Death Differ.* **2011**, *18*, 571–580. [CrossRef]

28. Kirisako, T.; Ichimura, Y.; Okada, H.; Kabeya, Y.; Mizushima, N.; Yoshimori, T.; Ohsumi, M.; Takao, T.; Noda, T.; Ohsumi, Y. The reversible modification regulates the membrane-binding state of Apg8/Aut7 essential for autophagy and the cytoplasm to vacuole targeting pathway. *J. Cell Biol.* **2000**, *151*, 263–276. [CrossRef]
29. Weidberg, H.; Shpilka, T.; Shvets, E.; Abada, A.; Shimron, F.; Elazar, Z. LC3 and GATE-16 N termini mediate membrane fusion processes required for autophagosome biogenesis. *Dev. Cell* **2011**, *20*, 444–454. [CrossRef]
30. Turer, A.T.; Hill, J.A. Pathogenesis of myocardial ischemia-reperfusion injury and rationale for therapy. *Am. J. Cardiol.* **2010**, *106*, 360–368. [CrossRef]
31. Li, X.; Arslan, F.; Ren, Y.; Adav, S.S.; Poh, K.K.; Sorokin, V.; Lee, C.N.; de Kleijn, D.; Lim, S.K.; Sze, S.K. Metabolic adaptation to a disruption in oxygen supply during myocardial ischemia and reperfusion is underpinned by temporal and quantitative changes in the cardiac proteome. *J. Proteome Res.* **2012**, *11*, 2331–2346. [CrossRef] [PubMed]
32. Semenza, G.L.; Agani, F.; Feldser, D.; Lyer, N.; Kotch, L.; Laughner, E.; Yu, A. Hypoxia, HIF-1, and the Pathophysiologi of Common Human Diseases. In *Oxygen Sensing: Molecule to Man*; Lahiri, S., Prabhakar, N.R., Forster, R.E., Eds.; Springer US: Boston, MA, USA, 2002; pp. 123–130.
33. Aziz, T.A.; Hussain, S.A.; Mahwi, T.O.; Ahmed, Z.A. Efficacy and safety of Ginkgo biloba extract as an "add-on" treatment to metformin for patients with metabolic syndrome: A pilot clinical study. *Ther. Clin. Risk Manag.* **2018**, *14*, 1219–1226. [CrossRef] [PubMed]
34. Canevelli, M.; Adali, N.; Kelaiditi, E.; Cantet, C.; Ousset, P.J.; Cesari, M. Effects of Gingko biloba supplementation in Alzheimer's disease patients receiving cholinesterase inhibitors: Data from the ICTUS study. *Phytomedicine* **2014**, *21*, 888–892. [CrossRef] [PubMed]
35. Zeng, X.; Liu, M.; Yang, Y.; Li, Y.; Asplund, K. Ginkgo biloba for acute ischaemic stroke. *Cochrane Database Syst. Rev.* **2005**. [CrossRef] [PubMed]
36. Guo, F.; Liu, X.; Cai, H.; Le, W. Autophagy in neurodegenerative diseases: Pathogenesis and therapy. *Brain Pathol.* **2018**, *28*, 3–13. [CrossRef] [PubMed]
37. Jacomin, A.-C.; Samavedam, S.; Promponas, V.; Nezis, I.P. iLIR database: A web resource for LIR motif-containing proteins in eukaryotes. *Autophagy* **2016**, *12*, 1945–1953. [CrossRef] [PubMed]
38. Jing, K.; Lim, K. Why is autophagy important in human diseases? *Exp Mol Med* **2012**, *44*, 69–72. [CrossRef] [PubMed]
39. Nixon, R.A. The role of autophagy in neurodegenerative disease. *Nat. Med.* **2013**, *19*, 983–997. [CrossRef]
40. Kroemer, G.; Marino, G.; Levine, B. Autophagy and the integrated stress response. *Mol. Cell* **2010**, *40*, 280–293. [CrossRef]
41. Ryter, S.W.; Cloonan, S.M.; Choi, A.M. Autophagy: A critical regulator of cellular metabolism and homeostasis. *Mol. Cells* **2013**, *36*, 7–16. [CrossRef]
42. Youle, R.J.; Narendra, D.P. Mechanisms of mitophagy. *Nat. Rev. Mol.* **2010**, *12*, 9. [CrossRef] [PubMed]
43. Li, C.; Jackson, R.M. Reactive species mechanisms of cellular hypoxia-reoxygenation injury. *Am. J. Physiol. Cell Physiol.* **2002**, *282*, C227–C241. [CrossRef] [PubMed]
44. Abe, H.; Semba, H.; Takeda, N. The Roles of Hypoxia Signaling in the Pathogenesis of Cardiovascular Diseases. *J. Atheroscler Thromb* **2017**, *24*, 88–894. [CrossRef] [PubMed]
45. Merelli, A.; Rodriguez, J.C.G.; Folch, J.; Regueiro, M.R.; Camins, A.; Lazarowski, A. Understanding the Role of Hypoxia Inducible Factor During Neurodegeneration for New Therapeutics Opportunities. *Curr. Neuropharmacol.* **2018**, *16*, 1484–1498. [CrossRef] [PubMed]
46. Navarrete-Opazo, A.; Mitchell, G.S. Therapeutic potential of intermittent hypoxia: A matter of dose. *Am. J. Physiol Regul Integr Comp. Physiol* **2014**, *307*, R1181–R1197. [CrossRef] [PubMed]
47. Gallart-Palau, X.; Serra, A.; Hase, Y.; Tan, C.F.; Chen, C.P.; Kalaria, R.N.; Sze, S.K. Brain-derived and circulating vesicle profiles indicate neurovascular unit dysfunction in early Alzheimer's disease. *Brain Pathol.* **2019**. [CrossRef] [PubMed]

molecules

MDPI

Article

A Structure—Activity Relationship Study of Bis-Benzamides as Inhibitors of Androgen Receptor—Coactivator Interaction

Tae-Kyung Lee [1], Preethi Ravindranathan [2], Rajni Sonavane [2], Ganesh V. Raj [2] and Jung-Mo Ahn [1,*]

1 Department of Chemistry and Biochemistry, University of Texas at Dallas, Richardson, TX 75080, USA
2 Departments of Urology and Pharmacology, University of Texas Southwestern Medical Center at Dallas, Dallas, TX 75390, USA
* Correspondence: jungmo.ahn@utdallas.edu; Tel.: +1-972-883-2917

Academic Editors: Henry Mosberg, Tomi Sawyer and Carrie Haskell-Luevano
Received: 13 June 2019; Accepted: 30 July 2019; Published: 31 July 2019

check for updates

Abstract: The interaction between androgen receptor (AR) and coactivator proteins plays a critical role in AR-mediated prostate cancer (PCa) cell growth, thus its inhibition is emerging as a promising strategy for PCa treatment. To develop potent inhibitors of the AR–coactivator interaction, we have designed and synthesized a series of bis-benzamides by modifying functional groups at the N/C-terminus and side chains. A structure–activity relationship study showed that the nitro group at the N-terminus of the bis-benzamide is essential for its biological activity while the C-terminus can have either a methyl ester or a primary carboxamide. Surveying the side chains with various alkyl groups led to the identification of a potent compound **14d** that exhibited antiproliferative activity (IC_{50} value of 16 nM) on PCa cells. In addition, biochemical studies showed that **14d** exerts its anticancer activity by inhibiting the AR–PELP1 interaction and AR transactivation.

Keywords: α-helix mimetics; bis-benzamide scaffold; protein–protein interaction; prostate cancer; androgen receptor; coactivator PELP1

1. Introduction

Prostate cancer (PCa) is one of the leading causes of cancer death worldwide, accounting for an estimated 1.28 million new cases and 358,000 deaths in 2018 [1]. Initiation and progression of PCa are dependent on the androgen receptor (AR)-mediated signaling pathway triggered by androgens [2]. Upon androgen binding, AR undergoes a conformational change in the ligand-binding domain (LBD) to form a hydrophobic cleft, termed activation function-2 (AF-2), that is recognized by AR coactivator proteins. AR subsequently translocates to the nucleus and activates transcription of the AR related genes leading to cell proliferation [3].

Various strategies have been developed to deprive androgens or block their effects. Surgical or chemical castration suppresses PCa growth by lowering circulating androgen levels. Chemical castration is achieved by blocking testicular and adrenal androgen synthesis with luteinizing hormone-releasing hormone (LH-RH) analogues [4]. Alternatively, antiandrogens have been developed to inhibit AR activities by competitively blocking androgens from binding to AR LBD [3]. Although antiandrogens are initially effective to suppress tumor growth, PCa ultimately turns into an incurable androgen-resistant state [5]. The transition to androgen-resistant state frequently involves AR mutations, overexpression of AR and its splice variants, increased production of intratumoral androgens, upregulation of AR coactivators and so on [5,6].

AR coactivators enhance the transcriptional activity of AR via multiple mechanisms including stabilization/cellular trafficking of AR, chromatin remodeling, and recruitment of general transcription factors [7]. Many coactivators interact with AR through an α-helical LXXLL motif in which L is a leucine and X is any amino acid. The side chains of three leucines at the i, $i + 3$, and $i + 4$ positions in the LXXLL motif fit in the hydrophobic pocket at the AF-2 domain of AR [8]. The interaction between the LXXLL motif and the AF-2 domain results in the AR-mediated gene transcription [8], thus the LXXLL motif is a high potential target to suppress PCa growth and overcome drug resistance in PCa [9,10]. As a coactivator, proline-, glutamic acid-, and leucine-rich protein 1 (PELP1) enhances the function of nuclear receptors like AR by coupling them with various signaling factors including transcriptional, chromatin, cytoskeleton, and cell cycle regulators. PELP1 is often found to be overexpressed in several cancers including PCa, and its dysregulation contributes to therapy resistance [11,12].

Short peptide segments encompassing the LXXLL motif can block interactions between the LXXLL motif and the AF-2 domain [13]. However, their therapeutic use is compromised by the intrinsic properties of peptides, such as rapid metabolic degradation, low bioavailability, and poor cell permeability [14]. To overcome these drawbacks, we previously developed oligo-benzamide-based α-helix mimetics that can place its substituents in the same spatial arrangement found in an α-helix, thereby reproducing the structure and function of the helix [15]. Nonpeptidic α-helix mimetics offer advantages of proteolytic stability and cell permeability over natural peptide segments [16]. Previously, we designed a bis-benzamide **D2** with two isobutyl groups based on the canonical LXXLL motif [10]. It disrupts AR–PELP1 interaction in PCa cells, and inhibits transcription and proliferation, suggesting the utility of the bis-benzamide as a therapeutic candidate in PCa treatment [10].

We herein report a structure–activity relationship study of the bis-benzamide and its analogs as potent inhibitors of the AR–coactivator interaction. Cell-based assays identified potent compounds with higher antiproliferative activity compared to **D2** in PCa cells. Further biochemical experiments demonstrated that these compounds were able to disrupt the AR–coactivator interaction and inhibit AR transactivation.

2. Results

For the structure–activity relationship study, we focused on three positions in the structure of the bis-benzamide **D2**: the N-terminal nitro group, the C-terminal methyl ester, and two isobutyl substituents at the O-alkylated side chains (Figure 1). To explore the effects of N-terminal substituents, a series of bis-benzamides with different substituents were prepared starting from **D2** that was synthesized by making an amide bond between 3-isobutoxy-4-nitrobenzoyl chloride **1b** and methyl 4-amino-3-isobutoxybenzoate **2** (Scheme 1a) [10]. The nitro group was reduced with tin (II) chloride to make the corresponding amine **4**. Coupling of the aromatic **4** with acyl chlorides produced compounds (**5a** and **5b**) containing N-acylamido groups. Compound **5c** containing a carboxylic acid was obtained by reacting the amine **4** with succinic anhydride. Coupling Boc-Gly to the amine **4** and removing the Boc protecting group from the resulting compound **5d** gave amine-containing compound **5e**. Compound **3** with no substituent at the N-terminus was synthesized from 3-isobutoxybenzoyl chloride **1b** (Scheme 1a).

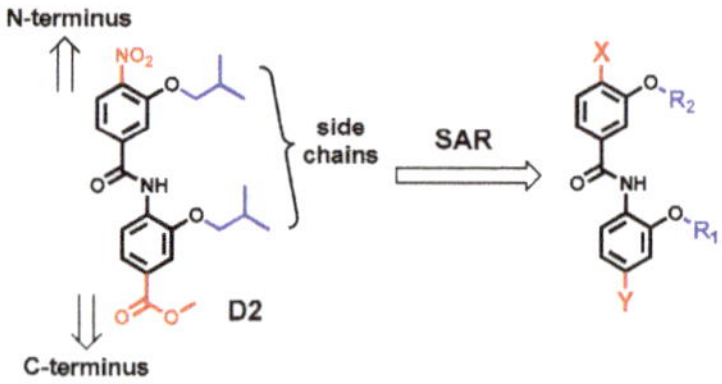

Figure 1. The structure of **D2** and the structure-activity relationship study at the N/C-terminus (X and Y) and side chains (R_1 and R_2).

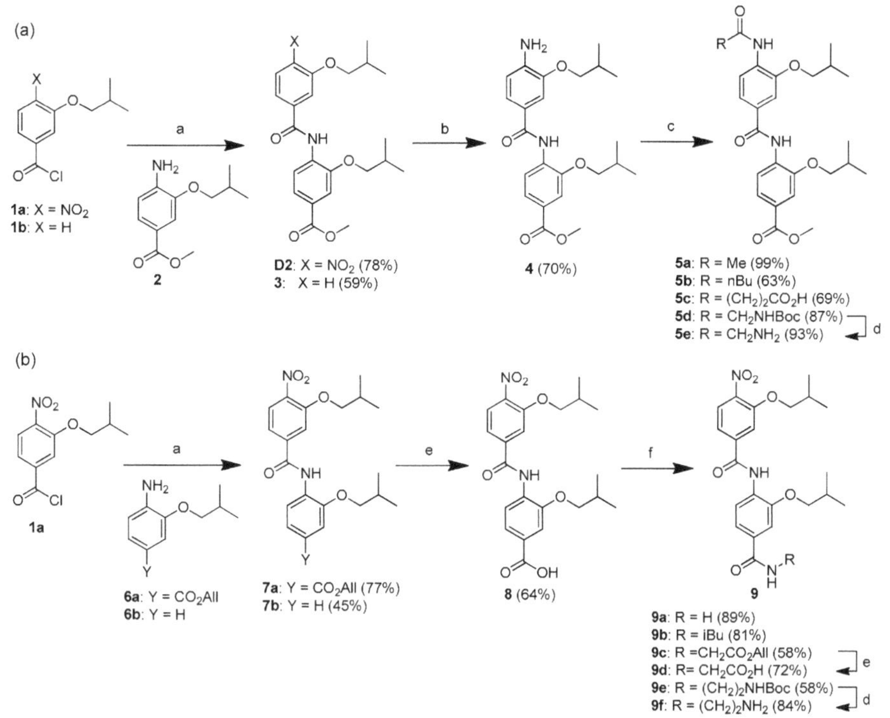

Scheme 1. Synthesis of bis-benzamide **D2** analogs. Reagents and conditions: (**a**) DIEA, DCM, rt, 12 h; (**b**) $SnCl_2$, DMF, rt, 12 h; (**c**) RCOCl, DIEA, DCM, rt, 12 h for **5a** and **5b**, $(RCO)_2O$, DCM, rt, 12 h for **5c** and **5d**; (**d**) TFA, rt, 1 h; (**e**) $Pd(PPh_3)_4$, $PhSiH_3$, THF, rt, 1 h; (**f**) RNH_2, PyBOP, DIEA, DMF, rt, 24 h.

We next synthesized bis-benzamides with different substituents at the C-terminus. These compounds were prepared from compound **7a** [10] (Scheme 1b). The allyl ester of compound **7a** was removed with $Pd(PPh_3)_4$ affording the carboxylic acid **8** [17]. Treatment of **8** with ammonium chloride [18] and isobutylamine in the presence of PyBOP provided the primary carboxamide **9a** and the N-isobutyl amide **9b**, respectively. Another carboxylic acid-containing compound **9d** was also obtained by introducing a glycine as a spacer at the C-terminus. The carboxylic acid **8** was reacted with glycine allyl ester to yield compound **9c**, of which the allyl group was removed with $Pd(PPh_3)_4$ giving compound **9d**. An amino group (**9f**) was introduced by coupling compound **8** with N-Boc-protected ethylenediamine and removing the Boc group from compound **9e**. Compound **7b** with no substituent at the C-terminus was obtained from 2-isobutoxyaniline **6b** (Scheme 1b).

These bis-benzamides were examined for their antiproliferative activity on LNCaP cells by MTT assays which quantify cell viability by measuring the activity of mitochondrial enzymes in live cells that reduce MTT (Table 1). Elimination of the N-terminal nitro group (**3**) or its replacement with either an amino (**4**) or N-acylamido group (**5a** or **5b**) led to a significant reduction in the inhibitory activity compared to **D2**. Introducing polar substituents at the N-terminus, such as a carboxylic acid (**5c**) or an aliphatic amine (**5e**) also resulted in complete loss of activity. These data suggest that the nitro group is critical for the biological activity of **D2**.

Among the substituents at the C-terminus, the carboxylic acid **8** was found to be moderately potent (IC_{50} = 90 nM) while the primary carboxamide **9a** (IC_{50} = 57 nM) showed improvement from the carboxylic acid **8**. In fact, it is comparable to **D2** (IC_{50} = 40 nM). However, other C-terminal amide derivatives containing isobutyl (**9b**), carboxylic acid (**9d**), or aliphatic amine (**9f**) did not show any activity (Table 1). The primary carboxamide **9a** appears to be a promising lead since carboxamides tends to have favorable properties, such as superior proteolytic stability [19] and aqueous solubility [20] when compared with methyl esters.

Table 1. Antiproliferative activity of bis-benzamides [a].

Compound	IC_{50} (nM)	Compound	IC_{50} (nM)
3	n.d. [b]	**8**	90
4	n.d. [b]	**9a**	57
5a	n.d. [b]	**9b**	n.d. [b]
5b	n.d. [b]	**9d**	n.d. [b]
5c	n.d. [b]	**9f**	n.d. [b]
5e	n.d. [b]	**D2**	40
7b	n.d. [b]		

[a] MTT assay on LNCaP cells. [b] Not determined due to weak or no inhibition.

Next, we examined the effect of the side chains of the bis-benzamide **9a** by constructing and evaluating a small library of bis-benzamides. Since the side chains of the LXXLL motifs make a hydrophobic surface to interact with the AF-2 domain of the AR [8], we focused on hydrophobic groups as substitutions. Larger hydrocarbon chains compared to the isobutyl group of the leucine residues of the LXXLL motifs may cause steric clash in the AF-2 domain. Indeed, compounds containing isopentyl or benzyl groups at the side chains were found to be inactive in the MTT assay (data not shown). Therefore, five alkyl groups of identical or a smaller size than the original isobutyl moiety, such as n-propyl, isopropyl, n-butyl, isobutyl, and sec-butyl groups, were selected to generate a 24-member bis-benzamide library, from which a compound containing two isobutyl groups (**9a**) is excluded (Scheme 2).

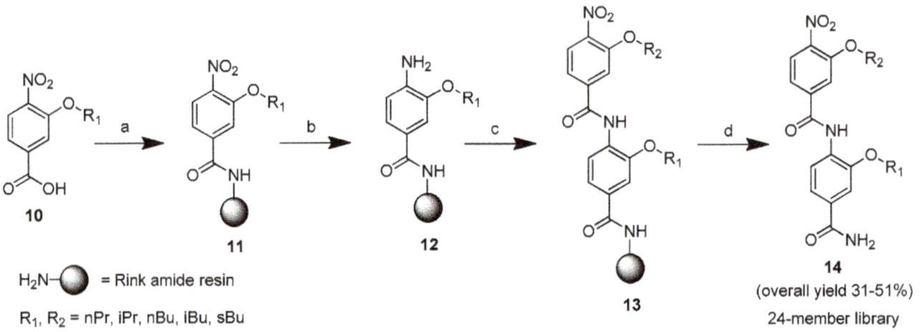

Scheme 2. Synthesis of a bis-benzamide library **14**. Reagents and conditions: (**a**) Rink amide resin, PyBOP, DIEA, DMF, rt, 24 h; (**b**) $SnCl_2$, THF/HCl/AcOH, rt, 24 h; (**c**) **10**, HATU, DIEA, DMF, rt, 24 h; (**d**) TFA, rt, 1 h.

The library synthesis commenced with the loading of 3-alkoxy-4-nitrobenzoic acids **10** onto Rink amide resin (Scheme 2). The nitro group of **11** was then reduced with tin (II) chloride under acidic conditions. The resulting amines **12** was reacted with 3-alkoxy-4-nitrobenzoic acids **10** using HATU to form a resin-bound bis-benzamides **13**. After cleavage with TFA, 24-membered bis-benzamide library **14** was prepared in high purity (92%–99%) [21].

The bis-benzamide library **14** was screened to evaluate their antiproliferative activity at 200 nM by MTT assays (Figure 2). Using a cutoff at 80% inhibition, 13 compounds were selected for follow-up studies. Dose-response experiments were carried out for the selected compounds, and their activities are summarized in Table 2. Among them, **14d** and **14s** were found to be highly potent with the IC_{50} values of 16 and 24 nM, respectively (Figure 3). Additionally, compound **14d** exhibits approximately 6-fold increase in inhibitory activity compared to compound **9a** (IC_{50} = 90 nM) and 2.5-fold increase to the original compound **D2** (IC_{50} = 40 nM).

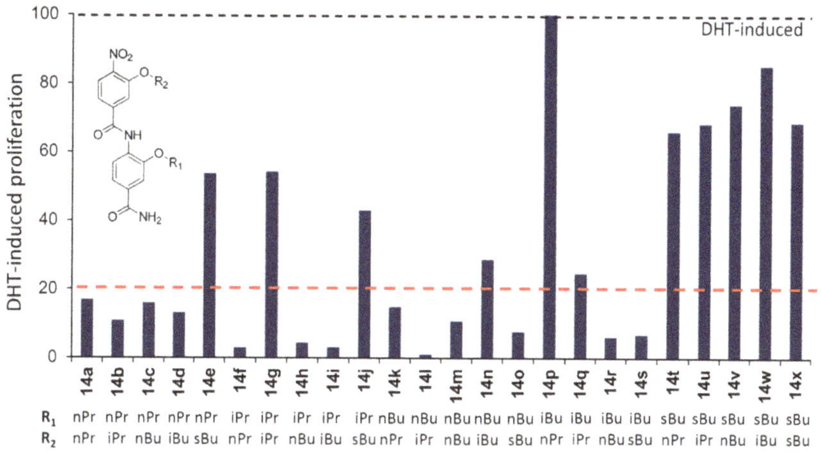

Figure 2. Antiproliferative activity of the bis-benzamide library **14** at 200 nM on LNCaP cells by MTT assay.

Table 2. Antiproliferative activity of bis-benzamides **14** [a].

Compound	IC_{50} (nM)	Compound	IC_{50} (nM)
14a	120	**14k**	76
14b	97	**14l**	66
14c	50	**14m**	51
14d	16	**14o**	57
14f	70	**14r**	44
14h	74	**14s**	24
14i	81		

[a] MTT assay on LNCaP cells.

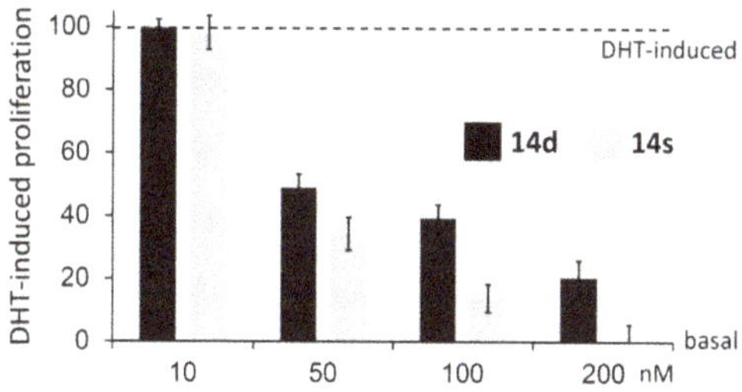

Figure 3. Dose-response experiments of bis-benzamides **14d** and **14s** for the growth inhibition of LNCaP cells by MTT assay.

Compounds **14f**, **14h**, **14i**, and **14l** showed the highest efficacy resulting in complete inhibition at 200 nM (Figure 2), however their IC_{50} values range from 66 to 81 nM (Table 2). On the other hand, compounds such as **14c**, **14m**, **14o**, and **14r** exhibited the inhibitory activity with the IC_{50} values of 44–57 nM. Compounds **14d**, **14s**, and **14o** demonstrated that the order of substituents at the side chains seems to be important to achieve high inhibitory activity, as observed in total loss of inhibition of PCa proliferation when the order of substituents is reversed (e.g., **14p**, **14w**, and **14v**) (Figure 2). These results suggest that the interaction of the bis-benzamides on the AF-2 domain of AR is specific, and topology of the side chain groups is critical for high affinity. However, isopropyl and n-butyl groups (**14h** and **14l**) are interchangeable without a considerable loss in potency (Table 2).

To determine if **14d** and **14s** can block the AR–coactivator interaction, we carried out co-immunoprecipitation (co-IP) experiments of AR and PELP1 on LNCaP cells (Figure 4a). Treatment of LNCaP cells with **14d** blocked 5α-dihydrotestosterone (DHT)-induced AR–PELP1 complex formation, resulting in complete inhibition at a concentration of 100 nM. Compound **14s** also inhibited the protein complex formation, but with slightly less efficiency.

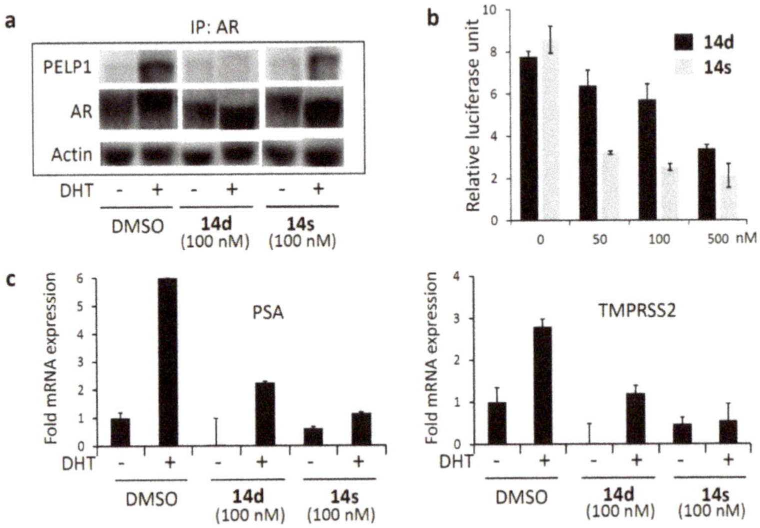

Figure 4. Inhibition of androgen receptor (AR)–coactivator interaction and AR-mediated transcriptional activity by compounds **14d** and **14s**. (**a**) The effects of **14d** and **14s** on the interaction of AR with PELP1 on LNCaP cells. (**b**) The effects of **14d** and **14s** on ARE-luciferase activity on LNCaP cells. (**c**) The effects of **14d** and **14s** on the expression levels of AR target genes, prostate specific antigen (PSA) and TMPRSS2, in LNCaP cells.

After AR associates with coactivators, the complex subsequently enhances transcription of AR target genes [3]. Thus, the effects of **14d** and **14s** on AR transactivation were assessed by luciferase activity on LNCaP cells transfected with ARE-luciferase reporter gene (Figure 4b). Compounds **14d** and **14s** significantly attenuated DHT-induced transcriptional activity with their IC_{50} values in the nanomolar range. Expression of well-known AR target genes such as prostate specific antigen (PSA) and transmembrane protease serine 2 (TMPRSS2) was also measured by quantitative reverse transcription PCR (qRT-PCR). Compound **14s** significantly reduced the expression of PSA and TMPRSS2 mRNA (5.2- and 5.0-fold, respectively) in the presence of DHT. Similarly, compound **14d** decreased PSA and TMPRSS2 mRNA levels by 2.7- and 2.3-fold, respectively (Figure 4c). These results indicate that blockage of the AR–coactivator interaction and AR transactivation accounts for the antiproliferative activities of compounds **14d** and **14s**.

We next examined the specificity of compounds **14d** and **14s** for the cell growth inhibition. Compounds **14d** and **14s** have little effect on the transcription of AR target genes in the absence of DHT (Figure 4c). In addition, cell proliferation was unaffected by **14d** and **14s** in the absence of DHT (Supplementary Materials Figure S1a), suggesting compounds **14d** and **14s** are dependent on androgen for their inhibitory activity. The specificity of compounds **14d** and **14s** for the cell growth inhibition was also tested using AR-negative PC3 prostate cancer cells. While **14d** and **14s** were effective in inhibiting AR-positive LNCaP cells (Figure 3), they had no effect on the growth of PC3 cells, confirming that the antiproliferative properties are specific to AR-dependent PCa cells (Supplementary Materials Figure S1b).

To investigate the binding mode of compound **14d** to the AF-2 domain of AR, molecular docking studies were carried out by using AutoDock Vina (version 1.1.2, The Scripps Research Institute, La Jolla, CA, USA) [22]. Docking calculations were performed five times with random seed numbers, and 20 conformers from each docking were collected. The resulting 100 conformers of **14d** were clustered by using clustering of conformer's script in Maestro (version 9.1, Schrödinger, LLC, New York, NY, USA, 2010) (see Supplementary Materials Tables S1 and S2 for the mean binding energy value, the number of conformers, and the lowest energy binding mode of each cluster). The docked conformations were further minimized in the MacroModel suite of Maestro (OPLS-2005 force filed).

Representative binding modes of **14d** and **D2** are shown in Figure 5. Like **D2** and the LXXLL motifs, compound **14d** interacts with the AF-2 domain by projecting its side chains (e.g., n-propyl and isobutyl groups) into the pockets designated for the leucine residues at the *i* and *i* + 4 positions of the LXXLL motif (Figure 5). However, compounds **14d** and **D2** show subtle differences in the binding mode. Compound **14d** appears to make hydrogen bonds to Lys720, whereas **D2** makes a hydrogen bond to Arg726 (Figure 5b,c). In particular, whereas the methyl ester moiety of **D2** is exposed to solvent (Figure 5c), the primary carboxamide of **14d** is buried inside the cavity near the pocket (Figure 5b). This additional interaction may explain the stronger affinity of **14d** to AR and the increased cell growth inhibition activity of **14d** compared to **D2**.

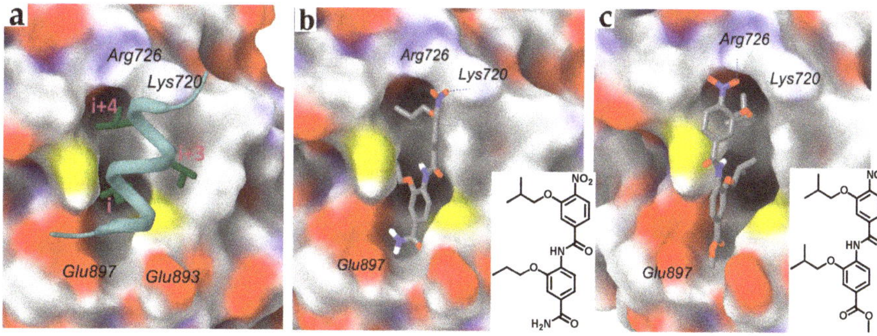

Figure 5. Molecular docking studies of **14d** on the AF-2 domain of AR. (**a**) Crystal structure (PDB code 1T63) of the LXXLL motif bound on the AF-2 domain. (**b**) Predicted binding mode of **14d**. (**c**) Predicted binding mode of **D2**.

3. Discussion

The interaction between AR–coactivators presents a viable and orthogonal target for overcoming PCa resistance to current antiandrogens. Several synthetic molecules targeting the interaction have been reported based on scaffolds like pyrimidines [23], dihydroperimidine [24], and diarylhydrazides [25]. However, these molecules showed only weak inhibition even at micromolar levels. Thus, there is a continuing need to develop novel and potent inhibitors.

We previously developed a nonpeptidic oligo-benzamide scaffold mimicking the structure and function of α-helical segments [15]. Designed to mimic the LXXLL motif, a bis-benzamide **D2** effectively inhibited the PCa cell growth by blocking the AR–coactivator interaction and AR-mediated gene transcription. This bis-benzamide scaffold is particularly attractive as a therapeutic candidate because of its favorable properties including metabolic stability, cell permeability, and bioavailability [10].

In this study, we performed a structure-activity relationship study of the bis-benzamide to identify structural requirements and to improve anticancer activity. N-terminal functionality had a dramatic effect on antiproliferative activity on LNCaP cells. A nitro group of **D2** was found to be critical for the inhibitory activity, whereas compounds possessing either no substituent (**3**) or an amine (**4**) were inefficient to inhibit the PCa cell growth. N-acylamido derivatives containing methyl (**5a**), n-butyl (**5b**), a carboxylic acid (**5c**) or an aliphatic amine (**5e**) also failed to show any activity (Table 1).

On the other hand, substitution at the C-terminus is more tolerable than at the N-terminus. A carboxylic acid (**8**) and a primary carboxamide (**9a**) at the C-terminus retained inhibitory activity, whereas compounds possessing no substituent (**7b**) or other N-alkyl amides (**9b**, **9d**, and **9f**) were found to be inactive (Table 1). Carboxamides are often preferred over methyl esters when considering proteolytic stability [19] and aqueous solubility [20]. Furthermore, the carboxamide at the C-terminus allowed us to use solid-phase synthetic techniques for the construction of a small library of bis-benzamides [26].

We next investigated the effects of the side chains of compound **9a** on the inhibitory activity. Since substituents larger than isobutyl groups or aromatic groups showed no significant inhibitory activity (data not shown), five alkyl chains (n-propyl, isopropyl, n-butyl, isobutyl, and sec-butyl groups) were selected as side chains, and a small bis-benzamide library was constructed by combination of different side chain groups. Single-dose screening and follow-up dose-response experiments identified that compounds **14d** and **14s** are the most potent with their IC_{50} values of 16 and 24 nM, respectively, showing significant improvement over **D2** and **9a** (Figure 2 and Table 2). It is noteworthy that the n-propyl group of **14d** at R_1 position and sec-butyl group of **14s** at R_2 position have higher activity than isobutyl groups at the corresponding positions.

As shown previously, **D2** exerts its anti-proliferative effect by inhibiting the AR–coactivator interaction and AR transactivation [10]. We examined whether **14d** and **14s** have a mechanism of action similar to that of **D2**. Co-IP experiments showed that **14d** was able to block the AR interaction with PELP1 in the presence of DHT at a dose of 100 nM (Figure 4a). In AR luciferase and qRT-PCR assays, **14d** and **14s** were also effective in inhibiting DHT-induced AR transactivation in the nanomolar range (Figure 4b). Importantly, the compounds were found to depend on androgen and AR for the inhibitory activity as shown by gene expression assays in the absence of DHT (Figure 4c) and cell viability assays using AR-negative PC3 cells (Supplementary Materials Figure S1).

On the other hand, compound **14s** had similar effects on AR transactivation compared to **14d**, but only weakly inhibited the recruitment of PELP1 to AR (Figure 4a). Since a number of coactivators including steroid receptor coactivators (SRCs) also possess the LXXLL motif for their interactions with AR and enhance the transcriptional activity of AR [8], compound **14s** may block such coactivators in addition to PELP1 to display its inhibitory activity on AR transactivation.

4. Materials and Methods

All chemical reagents and solvents were obtained from commercial sources and used without additional purification. Thin-layer chromatography (TLC) was performed on silica gel plates (250 μm, Sorbent Technologies, Atlanta, GA, USA) and the plates were visualized under UV at 254 nm. Standard grade silica gel (230–400 mesh, Sorbent Technologies, Atlanta, GA, USA) was used for flash column chromatography. ^1H and ^{13}C nuclear magnetic resonance (NMR) spectra were recorded on a Bruker Avance III HD 600 MHz NMR or JEOL Model DELTA-270 (270 MHz) NMR spectrometer. Chemical shifts are reported in parts per million (δ) from an internal standard of residual DMSO-d_6 (2.50 or 39.5 ppm) or $CDCl_3$ (7.27 or 77.2 ppm). Data are reported as follows: chemical shift (δ), multiplicity (s, singlet; d, doublet; dd, doublet of doublet; t, triplet; dt, doublet of triplet, q, quartet; sep, septet; br s, broad singlet; m, multiplet), coupling constant (J) in Hertz (Hz), integration. High resolution mass spectrometry (HRMS) data were obtained on an Applied Biosystem 4000 Q TRAP® LC/MS/MS system using electrospray ionization (ESI). Low-resolution mass spectra (LRMS) were recorded on a Shimadzu AXIMA Confidence MALDI-TOF mass spectrometer (nitrogen UV laser, 50 Hz, 337 nm) by using α-cyano-4-hydroxycinnamic acid (CHCA) as a matrix. Melting points were determined with a Mel-Temp® capillary apparatus (Cole-Parmer, Staffordshire, UK) and are uncorrected. High performance liquid chromatography (HPLC) analyses were carried out on Agilent 1100 series HPLC system (Foster City, CA) equipped with a diode-array UV detector and a C18-bounded HPLC column (Vydac 218TP104, 4.6 × 250 mm, 10 μm) by using a 40 min-gradient elution from 10% to 90% acetonitrile in water (0.1% TFA) and a flow rate of 1.0 mL/min. Eluents were monitored at 280 nm. Solid-phase reactions were carried out in 12 mL polypropylene cartridges with 20 μ PE frit (Applied Separations, Allentown, PA) and a labquake tube shaker (Fisher Scientific, Pittsburgh, PA) was used for mixing.

4.1. Synthesis of Bis-Benzamides

Methyl 3-isobutoxy-4-[(3-isobutoxybenzoyl)amino]benzoate (**3**): Oxalyl chloride (0.26 mL, 3.0 mmol) was slowly added to a solution of 3-isobutoxybenzoic acid (300 mg, 1.5 mmol) in DCM (20 mL). The resulting mixture was stirred at room temperature for 2 h. The solvent and excess oxalyl chloride were then removed under reduced pressure, and the residue was dissolved in DCM (5 mL). The resulting solution was then slowly added to a solution of methyl 4-amino-3-isobutoxybenzoate (226 mg, 1.0 mmol) and DIEA (0.52 mL, 3.0 mmol) in DCM (20 mL). After stirring at room temperature for 12 h, the resulting solution was concentrated under reduced pressure, and diluted with EtOAc (20 mL) and 1N HCl (20 mL). The layers were separated, and the aqueous layer was extracted with EtOAc (20 mL). The organic layers were combined, washed with saturated $NaHCO_3$ and brine, dried over anhydrous sodium sulfate, and concentrated under reduced pressure. The resulting solid was washed with EtOAc and dried in vacuo to afford the compound **3** as a white solid (240 mg, 59%). ^{1}H NMR (DMSO-d_6, 600 MHz): δ 9.44 (br s, 1 H), 8.12 (d, J = 8.3 Hz, 1 H), 7.63 (dd, J = 8.3, 1.7 Hz, 1 H), 7.56 (d, J = 1.7 Hz, 1 H), 7.49 (d, J = 7.7 Hz, 1 H), 7.46 (d, J = 7.7 Hz, 1 H), 7.45 (d, J = 7.7 Hz, 1 H), 7.19–7.17 (m, 1 H), 3.92 (d, J = 6.2 Hz, 2 H), 3.86 (s, 3 H), 3.83 (d, J = 6.6 Hz, 2 H), 2.14–2.01 (m, 2 H), 1.02 (d, J = 6.6 Hz, 6 H), 1.00 (d, J = 6.7 Hz, 6 H). ^{13}C NMR (DMSO-d_6, 150 MHz): δ 165.8, 164.6, 158.9, 149.5, 135.7, 131.8, 129.9, 125.9, 122.0, 121.9, 119.4, 118.5, 112.8, 112.0, 74.5, 73.9, 52.1, 27.8, 27.7, 18.99, 18.97. MALDI-TOF (m/z): [M+H]$^+$ calcd for $C_{23}H_{30}NO_5$: 400.21, found 400.81.

Methyl 4-[(4-amino-3-isobutoxybenzoyl)amino]-3-isobutoxybenzoate (**4**): *The title compound was synthesized* as previously described [10].

Methyl 4-[(4-acetamido-3-isobutoxybenzoyl)amino]-3-isobutoxybenzoate (**5a**): Acetyl chloride (0.015 mL, 0.21 mmol) was slowly added to a solution of compound **4** (60 mg, 0.14 mmol) and DIEA (0.097 mL, 0.56 mmol) in EtOAc (10 mL). After stirring at room temperature for 6 h, the resulting solution was concentrated under reduced pressure, and diluted with EtOAc (20 mL) and 1N HCl (10 mL). The layers were separated, and the aqueous layer was extracted with EtOAc (20 mL). The organic layers were combined, washed with saturated $NaHCO_3$ and brine, dried over anhydrous sodium sulfate, and concentrated under reduced pressure. The crude product was purified by flash column chromatography (hexanes/DCM 1:1) to afford the compound **5a** as a light yellow solid (63 mg, 99%). Rf = 0.16 (hexanes/EtOAc 4:1). ^{1}H NMR (DMSO-d_6, 600 MHz): δ 9.37 (br s, 1 H), 9.10 (br s, 1 H), 8.15 (d, J = 8.4 Hz, 1 H), 8.12 (d, J = 8.3 Hz, 1 H), 7.63 (dd, J = 8.3, 1.5 Hz, 1 H), 7.56 (d, J = 1.5 Hz, 1 H), 7.54 (d, J = 1.5 Hz, 1 H), 7.51 (dd, J = 8.3, 1.5 Hz, 1 H), 3.92 (d, J = 6.6 Hz, 2 H), 3.89 (d, J = 6.6 Hz, 2 H), 3.86 (s, 3 H), 2.19–2.11 (m, 2 H), 2.15 (s, 3 H), 1.03 (d, J = 7.0 Hz, 12 H). ^{13}C NMR (DMSO-d_6, 150 MHz): δ 168.8, 165.8, 164.2, 149.3, 148.4, 131.9, 131.1, 129.5, 125.6, 122.1, 121.6, 121.1, 119.8, 112.0, 110.8, 74.8, −74.6, 52.1, 27.8, 27.5, 24.0, 19.10, 19.05. MALDI-TOF (m/z): [M + Na]$^+$ calcd for $C_{25}H_{32}N_2NaO_6$: 479.52, found 479.79.

Methyl 3-isobutoxy-4-[[3-isobutoxy-4-(pentanoylamino)benzoyl]amino]benzoate (**5b**): The title compound was prepared following the same procedure as for compound **5a**, using compound **4** (250 mg, 0.60 mmol) and valeroyl chloride (0.15 mL, 1.21 mmol). The crude product was purified by flash column chromatography (hexanes/EtOAc 2:1) to afford the compound **5b** as a white solid (189 mg, 63%). Rf = 0.49 (hexanes/EtOAc 2:1). ^{1}H NMR (DMSO-d_6, 600 MHz): δ 9.37 (br s, 1 H), 9.02 (br s, 1 H), 8.15 (d, J = 8.4 Hz, 1 H), 8.08 (d, J = 8.4 Hz, 1 H), 7.64 (dd, J = 8.3, 1.7 Hz, 1 H), 7.56 (d, J = 1.8 Hz, 1 H), 7.54 (d, J = 1.8 Hz, 1 H), 7.51 (dd, J = 8.4, 1.8 Hz, 1 H), 3.92 (d, J = 6.2 Hz, 2 H), 3.89 (d, J = 6.6 Hz, 2 H), 3.86 (s, 3 H), 2.44 (t, J = 7.3 Hz, 2 H), 2.17–2.09 (m, 2 H), 1.61–1.56 (m, 2 H), 1.37–1.31 (m, 2 H), 1.03 (d, J = 6.6 Hz, 12 H), 0.90 (t, J = 7.3 Hz, 3 H). ^{13}C NMR (DMSO-d_6, 150 MHz): δ 171.6, 165.8, 164.2, 149.3, 148.6, 131.9, 131.0, 129.6, 125.6, 122.1, 121.5, 121.3, 119.8, 111.9, 110.7, 74.7, 74.5, 52.1, 36.0, 27.8, 27.6, 27.3, 21.7, 19.1, 13.7. MALDI-TOF (m/z): [M + H]$^+$ calcd for $C_{28}H_{39}N_2O_6$: 499.28, found 499.82.

4-[2-Isobutoxy-4-[(2-isobutoxy-4-methoxycarbonylphenyl)carbamoyl]anilino]-4-oxobutanoic acid (**5c**): Succinic anhydride (3.4 g, 33.8 mmol) was added to a solution of compound **4** (2.8 g, 6.8 mmol) in DCM (300 mL). After stirring at room temperature for 12 h, the resulting precipitate was collected by vacuum filtration, washed with DCM, and dried in vacuo to afford compound **5c** as a white solid (2.4 g, 69%). ^{1}H NMR (DMSO-d_6, 600 MHz): δ 12.14 (br s, 1 H), 9.37 (br s, 1 H), 9.12 (br s, 1 H), 8.15 (d, J = 8.1 Hz, 1 H), 8.13 (d, J = 7.4 Hz, 1 H), 7.63 (dd, J = 8.3, 1.7 Hz, 1 H), 7.56 (d, J = 1.7 Hz, 1 H), 7.54 (d, J = 1.7 Hz, 1 H), 7.51 (dd, J = 8.3, 1.7 Hz, 1 H), 3.92 (d, J = 6.2 Hz, 2 H), 3.89 (d, J = 6.6 Hz, 2 H), 3.86 (s, 3 H), 2.69 (t, J = 6.7 Hz, 2 H), 2.53 (t, J = 6.7 Hz, 2 H), 2.19–2.10 (m, 2 H), 1.04 (d, J = 6.7 Hz, 6 H), 1.03 (d, J = 6.7 Hz, 6 H). ^{13}C NMR (DMSO-d_6, 150 MHz): δ 173.8, 170.6, 165.8, 164.2, 149.2, 148.3, 131.9, 131.1, 129.4, 125.6, 122.1, 121.5, 120.7, 119.9, 111.9, 110.7, 74.8, 74.5, 52.1, 31.3, 28.9, 27.8, 27.6, 19.12, 19.05. MALDI-TOF (*m*/*z*): [M + H]$^+$ calcd for $C_{27}H_{35}N_2O_8$: 515.24, found 515.69.

[2-[2-Isobutoxy-4-[(2-isobutoxy-4-methoxycarbonylphenyl)carbamoyl]anilino]-2-oxoethyl]ammonium trifluoroacetate (**5e**): Compound **5d** was synthesized as previously described [10]. Then, compound **5d** (1.8 g, 3.2 mmol) was dissolved in 50% TFA in DCM (40 mL) and the mixture was stirred at room temperature for 1 h. The reaction mixture was concentrated under reduced pressure. The product was precipitated by adding cold diethyl ether, washed with diethyl ether, and dried in vacuo. The TFA salt of compound **5e** was obtained as a white solid (1.7 g, 93%). ^{1}H NMR (DMSO-d_6, 600 MHz): δ 9.73 (br s, 1 H), 9.43 (br s, 1 H), 8.15 (d, J = 8.1 Hz, 1 H), 8.13 (d, J = 8.4 Hz, 1 H), 8.00 (br s, 3 H), 7.64 (dd, J = 8.4, 1.5 Hz, 1 H), 7.60 (d, J = 1.5 Hz, 1 H), 7.57–7.56 (m, 2 H), 3.92 (d, J = 5.5 Hz, 4 H), 3.91 (s, 2 H), 3.86 (s, 3 H), 1.04 (d, J = 5.8 Hz, 6 H), 1.03 (d, J = 6.2 Hz, 6 H). ^{13}C NMR (DMSO-d_6, 150 MHz): δ 165.8, 164.2, 158.4, 158.2, 149.4, 148.7, 131.9, 130.4, 129.9, 125.8, 122.1, 121.8, 121.3, 120.0, 112.0, 111.0, 75.0, 74.6, 52.1, 41.4, 27.8, 27.5, 19.13, 19.06. MALDI-TOF (*m*/*z*): [M + H]$^+$ calcd for $C_{25}H_{34}N_3O_6$: 472.24, found 472.67.

3-Isobutoxy-N-(2-isobutoxyphenyl)-4-nitrobenzamide (**7b**): The title compound was prepared following the same procedure as for compound **3**, using 3-isobutoxy-4-nitrobenzoic acid (431 mg, 0.18 mmol) and 2-isobutoxyaniline (**6b**) (200 mg, 1.2 mmol). Recrystallization from EtOAc/hexanes afforded compound **7b** as a light yellow solid (210 mg, 45%). ^{1}H NMR (DMSO-d_6, 600 MHz): δ 9.70 (br s, 1 H), 8.01 (d, J = 8.1 Hz, 1 H), 7.80 (s, 1 H), 7.66 (d, J = 8.1 Hz, 1 H), 7.60 (d, J = 8.4 Hz, 1 H), 7.23–7.20 (m, 1 H), 7.10–7.09 (m, 1 H), 6.99–6.97 (m, 1 H), 4.02 (d, J = 6.2 Hz, 2 H), 3.80 (d, J = 6.2 Hz, 2 H), 2.10–2.00 (m, 2 H), 0.99 (d, J = 6.6 Hz, 6 H), 0.97 (d, J = 6.6 Hz, 6 H). ^{13}C NMR (DMSO-d_6, 150 MHz): δ 163.2, 151.5, 150.9, 140.8, 139.5, 126.4, 126.2, 125.0, 124.9, 120.0, 119.3, 113.6, 112.4, 75.1, 75.0, 74.1, 27.7, 27.5, 18.9, 18.6. MALDI-TOF (*m*/*z*): [M + H]$^+$ calcd for $C_{21}H_{27}N_2O_5$: 387.19, found 387.67.

3-Isobutoxy-4-[(3-isobutoxy-4-nitrobenzoyl)amino]benzoic acid (**8**): Compound **7a** was synthesized as previously described [10]. Then, $Pd(PPh_3)_4$ (198 mg, 0.17 mmol) and $PhSiH_3$ (0.43 mL, 3.4 mmol) were added to a solution of compound **7a** (800 mg, 1.7 mmol) in DCM (30 mL). After stirring at room temperature for 1 h, the reaction mixture was concentrated under reduced pressure. The product was precipitated by adding diethyl ether, washed with diethyl ether, and dried in vacuo. Compound **8** was obtained as a white solid (465 mg, 64%), m.p. 242–245 °C. ^{1}H NMR (DMSO-d_6, 600 MHz): δ 12.98 (br s, 1 H), 9.78 (br s, 1 H), 8.03 (d, J = 8.4 Hz, 1 H), 7.96 (d, J = 8.4 Hz, 1 H), 7.80 (d, J = 1.4 Hz, 1 H), 7.62–7.60 (m, 2 H), 7.57 (d, J = 1.5 Hz, 1 H), 4.03 (d, J = 6.2 Hz, 2 H), 3.89 (d, J = 6.6 Hz, 2 H), 2.11–2.05 (m, 2 H), 1.005 (d, J = 6.4 Hz, 6 H), 0.995 (d, J = 6.3 Hz, 6 H). ^{13}C NMR (DMSO-d_6, 150 MHz): δ 167.4, 164.0, 151.6, 150.8, 141.7, 139.8, 131.3, 128.6, 125.6, 123.6, 122.4, 120.0, 114.3, 113.0, 75.8, 75.0, 40.2, 28.3, 28.1, 19.5, 19.2. MALDI-TOF (*m*/*z*): [M + Na]$^+$ calcd for $C_{22}H_{26}N_2NaO_7$: 453.16, found 453.67.

3-Isobutoxy-4-[(3-isobutoxy-4-nitrobenzoyl)amino]benzamide (**9a**): DIEA (0.16 mL, 0.92 mmol) was added to a solution of compound **8** (200 mg, 0.46 mmol) and PyBOP (263 mg, 0.51 mmol) in DMF (10 mL). After stirring at room temperature for 1 h, ammonium chloride (246 mg, 4.6 mmol) and additional DIEA (0.80 mL, 4.6 mmol) were added. The resulting mixture was stirred at room temperature for 12 h and diluted with EtOAc (50 mL) and 1N HCl (30 mL). The layers were separated, and the aqueous layer was extracted with EtOAc (30 mL). The organic layers were combined, washed with saturated

$NaHCO_3$, and concentrated under reduced pressure. The resulting solid was washed with EtOAc and dried in vacuo to afford the compound **9a** as a white solid (175 mg, 89%), m.p. 249–251 °C. ^{1}H NMR (DMSO-d_6, 270 MHz): δ 9.76 (br s, 1 H), 8.02 (d, J = 8.4 Hz, 1 H), 8.00 (br s, 1 H), 7.84 (d, J = 8.2 Hz, 1 H), 7.79 (d, J = 1.2 Hz, 1 H), 7.60 (dd, J = 8.4, 1.2 Hz, 1 H), 7.57 (d, J = 1.5 Hz, 1 H), 7.53 (dd, J = 8.2, 1.5 Hz, 1 H), 7.37 (br s, 1 H), 4.02 (d, J = 6.7 Hz, 2 H), 3.87 (d, J = 6.4 Hz, 2 H), 2.12–2.00 (m, 2 H), 0.994 (d, J = 6.7 Hz, 6 H), 0.992 (d, J = 6.7 Hz, 6 H). ^{13}C NMR (DMSO-d_6, 150 MHz): δ 167.2, 163.5, 151.0, 150.6, 141.1, 139.4, 131.9, 129.2, 125.1, 123.5, 119.8, 119.5, 113.8, 111.4, 75.3, 74.5, 27.8, 27.6, 19.1, 18.7. MALDI-TOF (*m/z*): $[M + Na]^+$ calcd for $C_{22}H_{27}N_3NaO_6$: 452.18, found 452.54.

3-Isobutoxy-4-[(3-isobutoxy-4-nitrobenzoyl)amino]-N-isobutylbenzamide (**9b**): DIEA (0.084 mL 0.48 mmol) was added to a mixture of compound **8** (50 mg, 0.12 mmol) and PyBOP (73 mg, 0.14 mmol) in DMF (5 mL), followed by isobutylamine (0.024 mL, 0.24 mmol). After stirring at room temperature for 12 h, the resulting solution was diluted with EtOAc (20 mL) and 1N HCl (20 mL). The layers were separated, and the aqueous layer was extracted with EtOAc (20 mL). The organic layers were combined, washed with saturated $NaHCO_3$ and brine, dried over anhydrous sodium sulfate, and concentrated under reduced pressure. The crude product was purified by flash column chromatography (hexanes/EtOAc 1:1) to afford the compound **9b** as a light yellow solid (47 mg, 81%). Rf = 0.41 (hexanes/EtOAc 1:1). ^{1}H NMR (DMSO-d_6, 600 MHz): δ 9.77 (br s, 1 H), 8.47 (d, J = 5.7 Hz, 1 H), 8.02 (d, J = 8.2 Hz, 1 H), 7.84 (d, J = 8.2 Hz, 1 H), 7.80 (br s, 1 H), 7.61 (dd, J = 8.2, 1.4 Hz, 1 H), 7.54 (br s, 1 H), 7.51 (d, J = 8.2 Hz, 1 H), 4.03 (d, J = 6.2 Hz, 2 H), 3.88 (d, J = 6.2 Hz, 2 H), 3.09 (t, J = 6.4 Hz, 2 H), 2.11–2.04 (m, 2 H), 1.90–1.82 (m, 1 H), 1.00 (d, J = 5.7 Hz, 6 H), 0.996 (d, J = 5.7 Hz, 6 H), 0.90 (d, J = 6.6 Hz, 6 H). ^{13}C NMR (DMSO-d_6, 150 MHz): δ 165.5, 163.4, 151.0, 150.7, 141.1, 139.4, 132.4, 128.9, 125.1, 123.7, 119.5, 119.4, 113.8, 111.1, 75.2, 74.5, 46.8, 28.1, 27.8, 27.6, 20.2, 19.1, 18.7. MALDI-TOF (*m/z*): $[M + H]^+$ calcd for $C_{26}H_{36}N_3O_6$: 486.26, found 486.76.

2-[[3-Isobutoxy-4-[(3-isobutoxy-4-nitrobenzoyl)amino]benzoyl]amino]acetic acid (**9d**): DIEA (0.35 mL, 2.0 mmol) was added to a solution of compound **8** (430 mg, 1.0 mmol) and PyBOP (624 mg, 1.2 mmol) in DMF (20 mL). After stirring at room temperature for 1 h, glycine allyl ester trifluoroacetate (344 mg, 1.5 mmol) and additional DIEA (0.35 mL, 2.0 mmol) were added. The resulting mixture was stirred at room temperature for 12 h and diluted with EtOAc (50 mL) and 1N HCl (30 mL). The layers were separated, and the aqueous layer was extracted with EtOAc (20 mL). The organic layers were combined, washed with saturated $NaHCO_3$ and brine, dried over anhydrous sodium sulfate, and concentrated under reduced pressure. Recrystallization from EtOAc/hexanes afforded compound **9c** as a white solid (308 mg, 58%). Then, $Pd(PPh_3)_4$ (54 mg, 0.047 mmol) and $PhSiH_3$ (0.12mL, 0.94 mmol) were added to a solution of compound **9c** (250 mg, 0.47 mmol) in THF (20 mL). After stirring at room temperature for 1 h, the reaction mixture was concentrated under reduced pressure. The product was precipitated by adding diethyl ether, washed with diethyl ether, and dried in vacuo. Compound **9d** was obtained as a white solid (165 mg, 72%). ^{1}H NMR (DMSO-d_6, 600 MHz): δ 12.6 (br s, 1 H), 9.79 (br s, 1 H), 8.86 (t, J = 5.7 Hz, 1 H), 8.02 (d, J = 8.4 Hz, 1 H), 7.88 (d, J = 8.1 Hz, 1 H), 7.81 (br s, 1 H), 7.62 (d, J = 8.4 Hz, 1 H), 7.58 (br s, 1 H), 7.54 (d, J = 8.2 Hz, 1 H), 4.03 (d, J = 6.6 Hz, 2 H), 3.94 (d, J = 5.9 Hz, 2 H), 3.89 (d, J = 6.2 Hz, 2 H), 2.12–2.05 (m, 2 H), 1.01 (d, J = 6.6 Hz, 6 H), 1.00 (d, J = 6.7 Hz, 6 H). ^{13}C NMR (DMSO-d_6, 150 MHz): δ 171.4, 165.8, 163.5, 151.1, 150.7, 141.1, 139.4, 131.4, 129.4, 125.1, 123.6, 119.7, 119.5, 113.8, 111.1, 75.3, 74.6, 41.3, 27.8, 27.7, 19.1, 18.7. MALDI-TOF (*m/z*): $[M + Na]^+$ calcd for $C_{24}H_{29}N_3NaO_8$: 510.19, found 510.68.

2-[[3-Isobutoxy-4-[(3-isobutoxy-4-nitrobenzoyl)amino]benzoyl]amino]ethylammonium trifluoroacetate (**9f**): The title compound was synthesized as previously described [10].

4.2. Synthesis of Bis-Benzamides Library 14

These compounds were synthesized as previously described [21]. We briefly describe their syntheses. Fmoc-Rink amide MBHA resin (0.50 mmol/g, 300 mg, 0.15 mmol) was swollen in DMF for 2 h and washed with DMF (×3). The Fmoc protecting group was removed by treating with piperidine

(20% in DMF, 5 × 30 min), and washed with DMF (×3). Then, 3-alkoxy-4-nitrobenzoic acid **10** was introduced by using a preactivated ester which was prepared by mixing 3-alkoxy-4-nitrobenzoic acid **10** (4.0 equiv.), PyBOP (4.0 equiv), and DIEA (4.0 equiv) in DMF (8 mL) for 5 min. The solution was added to the resin and shaken at room temperature for 24 h. The resin was then filtered and washed with DMF (×3) affording compound **11**. The nitro group of the compound **11** was swollen in AcOH (50% in H_2O)/HCl (0.5 N in H_2O)/THF (1:1:6, 8 mL) for 20 min and treated with $SnCl_2{\cdot}2H_2O$ (5.0 equiv.). The reaction mixture was shaken at room temperature for 24 h. The resin was filtered, and washed with HCl (0.5 N in H_2O)/DMF (1:6) (×3), H_2O/DMF (1:6) (×3) and DMF (×3) affording compound **12**. Then 3-alkoxy-4-nitrobenzoic acid **10** was introduced by using a preactivated HOAt ester which was prepared by mixing 3-alkoxy-4-nitrobenzoic acid **10** (4.0 equiv.), HATU (4.0 equiv), and DIEA (4.0 equiv) in DMF (8 mL) for 1 h. The solution was added to the resin and shaken at room temperature for 24 h. The resin was then filtered and washed with DMF (×3) affording the resin-bound bis-benzamide **13**. The bis-benzamide **13** was washed with DCM (×3) and dried in vacuo. The dried resin was treated with a cleavage mixture of TFA/H_2O (95:5, 6 mL) for 90 min. The TFA solution was then filtered, and the resin was washed with TFA (2 mL). The combined TFA solution was concentrated to a volume of approximately 0.5 mL with a gentle stream of nitrogen. The product was precipitated by adding cold diethyl ether, washed with diethyl ether, and dried in vacuo affording compound **14**.

4-[(4-Nitro-3-propoxybenzoyl)amino]-3-propoxybenzamide (**14a**): Light yellow solid, 22 mg, 47% overall yield, 95% purity by HPLC. ^{1}H NMR (DMSO-d_6, 270 MHz): δ 9.76 (br s, 1 H), 8.01 (d, J = 8.4 Hz, 1 H), 7.99 (br s, 1 H), 7.85 (d, J = 8.2 Hz, 1 H), 7.80 (d, J = 1.4 Hz, 1 H), 7.61 (dd, J = 8.4, 1.5 Hz, 1 H), 7.58 (d, J = 1.6 Hz, 1 H), 7.53 (dd, J = 8.0, 1.6 Hz, 1 H), 7.37 (br s, 1 H), 4.22 (t, J = 6.4 Hz, 2 H), 4.05 (t, J = 6.4 Hz, 2 H), 1.82–1.73 (m, 4 H), 0.988 (t, J = 7.2 Hz, 3 H), 0.986 (t, J = 7.2 Hz, 3 H). ^{13}C NMR (DMSO-d_6, 150 MHz): δ 167.2, 163.5, 151.0, 150.4, 141.2, 139.4, 131.8, 129.2, 125.0, 123.4, 119.7, 119.5, 114.0, 111.4, 70.8, 69.9, 22.0, 21.8, 10.4, 10.2. MALDI-TOF (*m*/*z*): [M + Na]$^+$ calcd for $C_{20}H_{23}N_3NaO_6$: 424.15, found 424.87.

4-[(3-Isopropoxy-4-nitrobenzoyl)amino]-3-propoxybenzamide (**14b**): Light yellow solid, 22 mg, 37% overall yield, 97% purity by HPLC. ^{1}H NMR (DMSO-d_6, 270 MHz): δ 9.74 (br s, 1 H), 7.99 (br s, 1 H), 7.97 (d, J = 8.4 Hz, 1 H), 7.86 (d, J = 8.2 Hz, 1 H), 7.85 (br s, 1 H), 7.81 (d, J = 8.3, 1 H), 7.57 (br s, 1 H), 7.53 (d, J = 8.4, 1 H), 7.37 (br s, 1 H), 4.94 (sep, J = 6.2, 1 H), 4.05 (t, J = 6.3 Hz, 2 H), 1.82–1.71 (m, 2 H), 1.33 (d, J = 6.2, 6 H), 0.99 (t, J = 7.3 Hz, 3 H). ^{13}C NMR (DMSO-d_6, 150 MHz): δ 167.2, 163.6, 150.4, 149.7, 142.3, 139.2, 131.7, 129.2, 124.9, 123.3, 119.7, 119.6, 115.1, 111.4, 72.5, 69.9, 22.0, 21.6, 10.4. MALDI-TOF (*m*/*z*): [M + Na]$^+$ calcd for $C_{20}H_{23}N_3NaO_6$: 424.15, found 424.97.

4-[(3-Butoxy-4-nitrobenzoyl)amino]-3-propoxybenzamide (**14c**): Light yellow solid, 30 mg, 48% overall yield based on the loading of Fmoc-Rink amide resin, 95% purity by HPLC, m.p. 247–248 °C. ^{1}H NMR (DMSO-d_6, 270 MHz): δ 9.76 (br s, 1 H), 8.00 (d, J = 8.2 Hz, 1 H), 7.99 (br s, 1 H), 7.85 (d, J = 8.2 Hz, 1 H), 7.81 (d, J = 1.5 Hz, 1 H), 7.60 (dd, J = 8.4, 1.5 Hz, 1 H), 7.58 (d, J = 1.7 Hz, 1 H), 7.53 (dd, J = 8.2, 1.7 Hz, 1 H), 7.37 (br s, 1 H), 4.26 (t, J = 6.3 Hz, 2 H), 4.05 (t, J = 6.3 Hz, 2 H), 1.85–1.69 (m, 4 H), 1.51–1.38 (m, 2 H), 0.99 (t, J = 7.4 Hz, 3 H), 0.94 (t, J = 7.7 Hz, 3 H). ^{13}C NMR (DMSO-d_6, 68 MHz): δ 167.8, 164.1, 151.5, 150.9, 141.8, 140.0, 132.3, 129.8, 125.6, 123.9, 120.3, 120.0, 114.5, 112.0, 70.5, 70.0, 30.9, 22.6, 19.1, 14.1, 11.0. HRMS-ESI (*m*/*z*): [M + H]$^+$ calcd for $C_{21}H_{26}N_3O_6$: 416.1822, found 416.1815.

4-[(3-Isobutoxy-4-nitrobenzoyl)amino]-3-propoxybenzamide (**14d**): Light yellow solid, 32 mg, 51% overall yield based on the loading of Fmoc-Rink amide resin, 93% purity by HPLC, m.p. 255–257 °C. ^{1}H NMR (DMSO-d_6, 270 MHz): δ 9.76 (br s, 1 H), 8.02 (d, J = 8.2 Hz, 1 H), 7.99 (br s, 1 H), 7.86 (d, J = 8.2 Hz, 1 H), 7.79 (d, J = 1.6 Hz, 1 H), 7.61 (dd, J = 8.3, 1.6 Hz, 1 H), 7.58 (d, J = 1.7 Hz, 1 H), 7.53 (dd, J = 8.2, 1.7 Hz, 1 H), 7.37 (br s, 1 H), 4.05 (t, J = 6.4 Hz, 2 H), 4.03 (d, J = 6.5 Hz, 2 H), 2.12–2.02 (m, 1 H), 1.85–1.72 (m, 2 H), 0.994 (t, J = 7.2 Hz, 3 H), 0.992 (d, J = 6.7 Hz, 6 H). ^{13}C NMR (DMSO-d_6, 68 MHz): δ 167.8, 164.1, 151.6, 151.0, 141.7, 140.0, 132.3, 129.8, 125.6, 123.9, 120.3, 120.1, 114.5, 112.0, 75.8, 70.5, 28.2, 22.6, 19.3, 11.2. HRMS-ESI (*m*/*z*): [M + H]$^+$ calcd for $C_{21}H_{26}N_3O_6$: 416.1816, found 416.1822.

3-Isopropoxy-4-[(4-nitro-3-propoxy-benzoyl)amino]benzamide (**14f**): Light yellow solid, 24 mg, 40% overall yield, 95% purity by HPLC. ^{1}H NMR (DMSO-d_6, 270 MHz): δ 9.66 (br s, 1 H), 8.01(d, J = 8.4 Hz, 1 H), 7.98 (br s, 1 H), 7.91 (d, J = 8.2 Hz, 1 H), 7.78 (d, J = 1.4 Hz, 1 H), 7.60 (dd, J = 8.2, 1.4 Hz, 1 H), 7.58 (d, J = 1.5 Hz, 1 H), 7.52 (dd, J = 8.4, 1.6 Hz, 1 H), 7.37 (br s, 1 H), 4.70 (sep, J = 6.2 Hz, 1 H), 4.23 (t, J = 6.4 Hz, 2 H), 1.83–1.71 (m, 2 H), 1.32 (d, J = 5.7 Hz, 6 H), 0.99 (t, J = 7.4 Hz, 3 H). ^{13}C NMR (DMSO-d_6, 150 MHz): δ 167.2, 163.6, 151.0, 148.9, 141.2, 139.5, 131.5, 130.2, 125.1, 123.1, 119.9, 119.4, 114.1, 113.1, 71.2, 70.8, 21.8, 21.7, 10.2. MALDI-TOF (*m*/*z*): [M + Na]$^+$ calcd for $C_{20}H_{23}N_3NaO_6$: 424.15, found 424.62.

4-[(3-Butoxy-4-nitrobenzoyl)amino]-3-isopropoxybenzamide (**14h**): Light yellow solid, 28 mg, 45% overall yield based on the loading of Fmoc-Rink amide resin, 96% purity by HPLC, m.p. 213–214 °C. ^{1}H NMR (DMSO-d_6, 270 MHz): δ 9.65 (br s, 1 H), 8.01 (d, J = 8.4 Hz, 1 H), 7.99 (br s, 1 H), 7.92 (d, J = 8.4 Hz, 1 H), 7.79 (br s, 1 H), 7.59 (d, J = 8.3 Hz, 1 H), 7.58 (br s, 1 H), 7.52 (d, J = 8.4 Hz, 1 H), 7.37 (br s, 1 H), 4.70 (sep, J = 5.9 Hz, 1 H), 4.27 (t, J = 6.4 Hz, 2 H), 1.79–1.68 (m, 2 H), 1.51–1.37 (m, 2 H), 1.32 (d, J = 5.9 Hz, 6 H), 0.93 (t, J = 7.4 Hz, 3 H). ^{13}C NMR (DMSO-d_6, 150 MHz): δ 167.2, 163.5, 150.9, 148.9, 141.2, 139.4, 131.5, 130.2, 125.0, 122.9, 119.9, 119.4, 114.0, 113.0, 71.2, 69.1, 30.3, 21.8, 18.5, 13.5. MALDI-TOF (*m*/*z*): [M + Na]$^+$ calcd for $C_{21}H_{25}N_3NaO_6$: 438.16, found 438.51.

4-[(3-Isobutoxy-4-nitrobenzoyl)amino]-3-isopropoxybenzamide (**14i**): Light yellow solid, 31 mg, 48% overall yield, 93% purity by HPLC. ^{1}H NMR (DMSO-d_6, 270 MHz): δ 9.66 (br s, 1 H), 8.02 (d, J = 8.4 Hz, 1 H), 7.99 (br s, 1 H), 7.92 (d, J = 8.2 Hz, 1 H), 7.77 (br s, 1 H), 7.59 (d, J = 8.3 Hz, 1 H), 7.58 (br s, 1 H), 7.52 (d, J = 8.4 Hz, 1 H), 7.36 (br s, 1 H), 4.70 (sep, J = 5.9 Hz, 1 H), 4.04 (d, J = 6.4 Hz, 2 H), 2.11–2.02 (m, 1 H), 1.32 (d, J = 5.7 Hz, 6 H), 0.99 (d, J = 6.7 Hz, 6 H). ^{13}C NMR (DMSO-d_6, 150 MHz): δ 167.2, 163.5, 151.0, 148.9, 141.1, 139.5, 131.5, 130.2, 125.1, 123.0, 119.9, 119.4, 114.0, 113.0, 75.2, 71.2, 27.6, 21.8, 18.7. MALDI-TOF (*m*/*z*): [M + Na]$^+$ calcd for $C_{21}H_{25}N_3NaO_6$: 438.16, found 438.95.

3-Butoxy-4-[(4-nitro-3-propoxybenzoyl)amino]benzamide (**14k**): Light yellow solid, 23 mg, 37% overall yield, >99% purity by HPLC. ^{1}H NMR (DMSO-d_6, 270 MHz): δ 9.75 (br s, 1 H), 8.01 (d, J = 8.4 Hz, 1 H), 7.99 (br s, 1 H), 7.85 (d, J = 8.2 Hz, 1 H), 7.80 (d, J = 1.2 Hz, 1 H), 7.60 (dd, J = 8.4, 1.4 Hz, 1 H), 7.58 (d, J = 1.4 Hz, 1 H), 7.52 (dd, J = 8.4, 1.5 Hz, 1 H), 7.37 (br s, 1 H), 4.22 (t, J = 6.4 Hz, 2 H), 4.09 (t, J = 6.4 Hz, 2 H), 1.84–1.70 (m, 4 H), 1.52–1.38 (m, 2 H), 0.99 (t, J = 7.4 Hz, 3 H), 0.91 (t, J = 7.4 Hz, 3 H). ^{13}C NMR (DMSO-d_6, 150 MHz): δ 167.2, 163.5, 150.9, 150.4, 141.2, 139.4, 131.8, 129.2, 125.0, 123.3, 119.8, 119.5, 114.0, 111.4, 70.8, 68.1, 30.7, 21.8, 18.7, 13.7, 10.2. MALDI-TOF (*m*/*z*): [M + Na]$^+$ calcd for $C_{21}H_{25}N_3NaO_6$: 438.16, found 438.75.

3-Butoxy-4-[(3-isopropoxy-4-nitrobenzoyl)amino]benzamide (**14l**): Light yellow solid, 25 mg, 40% overall yield based on the loading of Fmoc-Rink amide resin, >99% purity by HPLC, m.p. 233–235 °C. ^{1}H NMR (DMSO-d_6, 270 MHz): δ 9.73 (br s, 1 H), 7.99 (br s, 1 H), 7.97 (d, J = 8.4 Hz, 1 H), 7.86 (d, J = 8.2 Hz, 1 H), 7.81 (d, J = 1.2 Hz, 1 H), 7.59 (dd, J = 8.2, 1.2 Hz, 1 H), 7.58 (d, J = 1.4 Hz, 1 H), 7.52 (dd, J = 8.3, 1.4 Hz, 1 H), 7.37 (br s, 1 H), 4.94 (sep, J = 5.9 Hz, 1 H), 4.09 (t, J = 6.2 Hz, 2 H), 1.80–1.70 (m, 2 H), 1.52–1.38 (m, 2 H), 1.33 (d, J = 6.2 Hz, 6 H), 0.91 (t, J = 7.4 Hz, 3 H). ^{13}C NMR (DMSO-d_6, 150 MHz): δ 167.2, 163.5, 150.4, 149.7, 142.3, 139.2, 131.7, 129.2, 124.9, 123.3, 119.7, 119.6, 115.1, 111.4, 72.5, 68.2, 30.7, 21.5, 18.7, 13.7. MALDI-TOF (*m*/*z*): [M + H]$^+$ calcd for $C_{21}H_{26}N_3O_6$: 416.18, found 416.56.

3-Butoxy-4-[(3-butoxy-4-nitrobenzoyl)amino]benzamide (**14m**): Light yellow solid, 20 mg, 31% overall yield based on the loading of Fmoc-Rink amide resin, 92% purity by HPLC, m.p. 249–251 °C. ^{1}H NMR (DMSO-d_6, 270 MHz): δ 9.74 (br s, 1 H), 8.00 (d, J = 8.4 Hz, 1 H), 7.99 (br s, 1 H), 7.86 (d, J = 8.4 Hz, 1 H), 7.80 (d, J = 1.2 Hz, 1 H), 7.60 (dd, J = 8.4, 1.4 Hz, 1 H), 7.58 (br s, 1 H), 7.52 (dd, J = 8.3, 1.4 Hz, 1 H), 7.37 (br s, 1 H), 4.26 (t, J = 6.2 Hz, 2 H), 4.09 (t, J = 6.2 Hz, 2 H), 1.80–1.69 (m, 4 H), 1.52–1.37 (m, 4 H), 0.94 (t, J = 7.2 Hz, 3 H), 0.91 (t, J = 7.3 Hz, 3 H). ^{13}C NMR (DMSO-d_6, 68 MHz): δ 167.8, 164.1, 151.5, 151.0, 141.8, 140.0, 132.3, 129.8, 125.6, 123.9, 120.3, 120.1, 114.5, 112.0, 69.7, 68.7, 31.2, 30.9, 19.3, 19.1, 14.3, 14.1. MALDI-TOF (*m*/*z*): [M + Na]$^+$ calcd for $C_{22}H_{27}N_3NaO_6$: 452.18, found 452.56.

3-Butoxy-4-[(3-sec-butoxy-4-nitrobenzoyl)amino]benzamide (**14o**): Light yellow solid, 20 mg, 31% overall yield based on the loading of Fmoc-Rink amide resin, 94% purity by HPLC, m.p. 218–220 °C. ^{1}H NMR (DMSO-d_6, 270 MHz): δ 9.73 (br s, 1 H), 7.99 (br s, 1 H), 7.97 (d, J = 8.4 Hz, 1 H), 7.87 (d, J = 8.2 Hz, 1 H), 7.80 (d, J = 1.2 Hz, 1 H), 7.580 (d, J = 1.4 Hz, 1 H), 7.578 (dd, J = 8.2, 1.5 Hz, 1 H), 7.52 (dd, J = 8.3, 1.6 Hz, 1 H), 7.37 (br s, 1 H), 4.81–4.70 (m, 1 H), 4.09 (d, J = 6.4 Hz, 2 H), 1.80–1.63 (m, 4 H), 1.52–1.38 (m, 2 H), 1.30 (d, J = 5.9 Hz, 3 H), 0.93 (t, J = 7.4 Hz, 3 H), 0.90 (t, J = 7.4 Hz, 3 H). ^{13}C NMR (DMSO-d_6, 150 MHz): δ 167.2, 163.6, 150.4, 150.0, 142.2, 139.2, 131.7, 129.2, 124.9, 123.3, 119.8, 119.5, 114.8, 111.4, 77.0, 68.2, 30.7, 28.4, 18.7, 18.7, 13.7, 9.2. MALDI-TOF (m/z): [M + Na]$^+$ calcd for $C_{22}H_{27}N_3NaO_6$: 452.18, found 452.60.

4-[(3-Butoxy-4-nitrobenzoyl)amino]-3-isobutoxybenzamide (**14r**): Light yellow solid, 20 mg, 31% overall yield based on the loading of Fmoc-Rink amide resin, 92% purity by HPLC, m.p. 239–240 °C. ^{1}H NMR (DMSO-d_6, 270 MHz): δ 9.76 (br s, 1 H), 8.01 (d, J = 8.2 Hz, 1 H), 7.99 (br s, 1 H), 7.83 (d, J = 8.4 Hz, 1 H)), 7.81 (br s, 1 H), 7.60 (dd, J = 8.3, 1.4 Hz, 1 H), 7.57 (br s, 1 H), 7.52 (dd, J = 8.2, 1.5 Hz, 1 H), 7.37 (br s, 1 H), 4.25 (t, J = 6.2 Hz, 2 H), 3.87 (d, J = 6.4 Hz, 2 H), 2.14–2.00 (m, 1 H), 1.79–1.68 (m, 2 H), 1.51–1.40 (m, 2 H), 0.99 (d, J = 6.7 Hz, 6 H), 0.93 (t, J = 7.4 Hz, 3 H). ^{13}C NMR (DMSO-d_6, 68 MHz): δ 167.8, 164.1, 151.5, 151.2, 141.8, 140.0, 132.5, 129.7, 125.6, 124.1, 120.3, 120.1, 114.5, 112.0, 75.1, 69.7. 30.9, 28.4, 19.6, 19.1, 14.1. HRMS-ESI (m/z): [M + Na]$^+$ calcd for $C_{22}H_{27}N_3NaO_6$: 452.1798, found 452.1792.

4-[(3-sec-Butoxy-4-nitrobenzoyl)amino]-3-isobutoxybenzamide (**14s**): Light yellow solid, 26 mg, 40% overall yield based on the loading of Fmoc-Rink amide resin, >99% purity by HPLC, m.p. 216–218 °C. ^{1}H NMR (DMSO-d_6, 270 MHz): δ 9.75 (br s, 1 H), 7.99 (br s, 1 H), 7.97 (d, J = 8.4 Hz, 1 H), 7.83 (d, J = 8.2 Hz, 1 H), 7.81 (br s, 1 H), 7.59 (d, J = 8.2 Hz, 1 H), 7.59 (br s, 1 H), 7.53 (d, J = 8.4 Hz, 1 H), 7.37 (br s, 1 H), 4.78–4.71 (m, 1 H), 3.86 (d, J = 6.4 Hz, 2 H), 2.11–2.02 (m, 1 H), 1.73–1.62 (m, 2 H), 1.29 (d, J = 6.2 Hz, 3 H), 0.98 (d, J = 6.7 Hz, 6 H), 0.93 (t, J = 7.4 Hz, 3 H). ^{13}C NMR (DMSO-d_6, 68 MHz): δ 167.8, 164.1, 151.3, 150.6, 142.8, 139.8, 132.5, 129.8, 125.5, 124.3, 120.3, 120.0, 115.3, 112.0, 77.6, 75.1, 29.0, 28.4, 19.6, 19.3, 9.8. HRMS-ESI (m/z): [M + Na]$^+$ calcd for $C_{22}H_{27}N_3NaO_6$: 452.1798, found 452.1798.

4.3. Proliferation Assays

LNCaP cells were obtained from the American Type Culture Collection (ATCC, Manassas, VA) and maintained in T medium (Invitrogen, Carlsbad, CA, USA) supplemented with 5% fetal bovine serum (FBS). All growth media were supplemented with penicillin (100 IU/mL) and streptomycin (100 µg/mL). For androgen deprivation, LNCaP cells were plated (2–10 × 10^3 per well) in 96-well plates and washed with PBS. The growth medium then changed to phenol-red-free RPMI 1640 with 1%–5% charcoal-stripped fetal bovine serum (CSF) for 48 h. The cells were pretreated with DMSO (vehicle control), or compounds (inhibitors) for 2 h. Media containing ethanol (vehicle control) or DHT was then added to a final concentration of 10 nM and cells cultured for another 72 h. Cell proliferation was measured using the MTT colorimetric assay (Roche Diagnostics, Indianapolis, IN). All experiments were performed in triplicate and the average of experiments displayed.

4.4. Western Blot and Immunoprecipitation Analyses

After treatments as indicated, total cellular protein was extracted and Western blotting and/or immunoprecipitation analyses using Protein G Dynabeads (Invitrogen) were performed as previously described [27].

4.5. Luciferase Assays

Cells were transfected as indicated with Lipofectamine Plus (Invitrogen), then equally divided into 24-well plates and allowed to attach. The culture medium was replaced after 24 h with androgen deprivation medium containing DHT or vehicle control for 48 h. All experiments were performed in triplicate. Luciferase activity was measured using the Dual Luciferase assay system (Promega,

Madison, WI, USA) and normalized to sample protein concentration. Results are presented as fold change over untreated cells.

4.6. *Quantitative Real-Time Reverse Transcription Polymerase Chain Reaction (qRT-PCR)*

Total cellular RNA was extracted with the RNeasy mini kit according to the manufacturer's instructions (Qiagen, Valencia, CA, USA). Complementary DNA (cDNA) was then synthesized from 1 μg RNA using the cDNA synthesis kit (Bio-Rad, Hercules, CA, USA). PCR was performed as previously described [10].

4.7. *Molecular Docking Study*

AutoDock Tools 1.5.6 (ADT; The Scripps Research Institute, La Jolla, CA, USA) was used to create input PDBQT files of a receptor and a ligand. The input file of AR was prepared using the published coordinates (PDB 1T63). Water molecules were removed from the protein structure and hydrogens were added. All other atom values were generated automatically by ADT. The docking area was assigned visually around the peptide ligand. The grid box was centered to cover the AF-2 domain of the AR and to accommodate ligand to move freely. The grid box was set to 22 Å × 22 Å × 22 Å, and the x,y,z coordinates of the center of the grid box were set to $x = -37.7$, $y = 25.1$, and $z = 20.1$, respectively. The input files of compound **14d** and **D2** were created from its energy-minimized conformation using ADT. Docking calculations were performed with AutoDock Vina 1.1.2 [22]. A search exhaustiveness of 16 was used and all other parameters were left as default values. The docked conformations were minimized in the MacroModel suite of Maestro (OPLS-2005 force filed, version 9.1, Schrödinger, LLC, New York, NY, USA, 2010). The predicted binding modes were visualized using Maestro.

5. Conclusions

In this study, we examined the effects of functional group modifications at the N/C-terminus and the side chains of bis-benzamide **D2**, which were previously found to be effective at inhibiting cell growth of prostate cancer cells (LNCaP). The nitro group at the N-terminus of **D2** appears to be critical for its biological activity. At the C-terminus, a primary carboxamide showed potent growth inhibition as comparable to the methyl ester of **D2**. To survey the optimal substituents at the side chains, we constructed a small bis-benzamide library containing various alkyl groups which differ in substitution pattern and the length of carbon chain. The bis-benzamide library was examined for the antiproliferative activity and identified compound **14d** as the most potent inhibitor with an IC_{50} value of 16 nM. Compound **14d** was found to exert anticancer activity by disrupting the AR–PELP1 interaction and AR transactivation. This study suggests that the bis-benzamide structure is an effective scaffold for producing a chemical library and identifying potent inhibitors of the AR–coactivator interaction.

Supplementary Materials: The following are available online: Synthesis of compounds **1b**, **6b**, and **10** (Scheme S1), Dependence of compounds **14d** and **14s** on AR-signaling (Figure S1), Clusters of docked poses of compound **14d** on the AF-2 domain of AR (Table S1), Clusters of docked poses of compound **D2** on the AF-2 domain of AR (Table S2), ^{1}H and ^{13}C NMR spectra of all products, HPLC chromatograms of bis-benzamide library **14**.

Author Contributions: Conceptualization, T.-K.L., G.V.R., and J.-M.A.; Methodology, T.-K.L., P.R., and R.S.; Software, T.-K.L.; Writing—Original Draft Preparation, T.-K.L.; Writing—Review and Editing, T.-K.L., P.R., G.V.R., and J.-M.A.; Funding Acquisition, G.V.R. and J.-M.A.

Funding: This research was funded in part by Welch Foundation [AT-1595, J.-M.A.], Department of Defense Prostate Cancer Research Program [W81XWH-12-1-0288, G.V.R.], and Cancer Prevention and Research Institute of Texas [RP120717-P4, J.-M.A.].

Acknowledgments: We appreciate Kara Kassees for her generous help in editing the manuscript.

Conflicts of Interest: The authors declare no conflict of interest.

Abbreviations

CAN	acetonitrile
ADT	androgen deprivation therapy
AF-2	activation function-2
AR	androgen receptor
ARE	androgen response element
Boc	*tert*-butoxycarbonyl
$CDCl_3$	deuterated chloroform
CHC	α-cyano-4-hydroxycinnamic acid
DIEA	N,N-diisopropylethylamine
DMF	N,N-dimethylformamide
DCM	dichloromethane
DHT	5α-dihydrotestosterone
DMSO-d_6	deuterated dimethyl sulfoxide
EtOAc	ethyl acetate
ESI	electrospray ionization
Fmoc	9-fluorenylmethoxycarbonyl
HATU	2-(7-aza-1H-benzotriazol-1-yl)-1,1,3,3-tetramethyluronium hexafluorophosphate
HOAt	1-hydroxy-7-azabenzotriazole
HPLC	high performance liquid chromatography
IC_{50}	half-maximal inhibitory concentration
HRMS	high resolution mass spectrometry
LBD	ligand-binding domain
LNCaP	lymph node carcinoma of the prostate
MALDI-TOF MS	matrix-assisted laser desorption/ionization time-of flight mass spectrometry
MTT	3-(4,5-dimethylthiazol-2-yl)-2,5-diphenyltetrazolium bromide
NMR	nuclear magnetic resonance
PCa	prostate cancer
PELP1	proline-, glutamic acid-and leucine-rich-protein-1
PyBOP	(benzotriazol-1-yloxy)tripyrrolidinophosphonium hexafluorophosphate
TFA	trifluoroacetic acid
THF	tetrahydrofuran
TLC	thin-layer chromatography

References

1. Bray, F.; Ferlay, J.; Soerjomataram, I.; Siegel, R.L.; Torre, L.A.; Jemal, A. Global cancer statistics 2018: GLOBOCAN estimates of incidence and mortality worldwide for 36 cancers in 185 countries. *CA Cancer J. Clin.* **2018**, *68*, 394–424. [CrossRef] [PubMed]
2. Zhou, Y.; Bolton, E.C.; Jones, J.O. Androgens and androgen receptor signaling in prostate tumorigenesis. *J. Mol. Endocrinol.* **2015**, *54*, R15–R29. [CrossRef] [PubMed]
3. Tan, M.H.E.; Li, J.; Xu, H.E.; Melcher, K.; Yong, E.-L. Androgen receptor: Structure, role in prostate cancer and drug discovery. *Acta Pharmacol. Sin.* **2014**, *36*, 3–23. [CrossRef] [PubMed]
4. Helsen, C.; Van den Broeck, T.; Voet, A.; Prekovic, S.; Poppel, H.V.; Joniau, S.; Claessens, F. Androgen receptor antagonists for prostate cancer therapy. *Endocr. Relat. Cancer* **2014**, *21*, T105–TK118. [CrossRef] [PubMed]
5. Watson, P.A.; Arora, V.K.; Sawyers, C.L. Emerging mechanisms of resistance to androgen receptor inhibitors in prostate cancer. *Nat. Rev. Cancer* **2015**, *15*, 701–711. [CrossRef] [PubMed]
6. Tsao, C.-K.; Galsky, M.D.; Small, A.C.; Yee, T.; Oh, W.K. Targeting the androgen receptor signalling axis in castration-resistant prostate cancer (CRPC). *BJU Int.* **2012**, *110*, 1580–1588. [CrossRef]
7. Culig, Z. Androgen receptor coactivators in regulation of growth and differentiation in prostate cancer. *J. Cell. Physiol.* **2016**, *231*, 270–274. [CrossRef]
8. Estébanez-Perpiñá, E.; Moore, J.M.R.; Mar, E.; Delgado-Rodrigues, E.; Nguyen, P.; Baxter, J.D.; Buehrer, B.M.; Webb, P.; Fletterick, R.J.; Guy, R.K. The molecular mechanisms of coactivator utilization in ligand-dependent transactivation by the androgen receptor. *J. Biol. Chem.* **2005**, *280*, 8060–8068. [CrossRef]

9. Chang, C.Y.; McDonnell, D.P. Androgen receptor–cofactor interactions as targets for new drug discovery. *Trends Pharmacol. Sci.* **2005**, *26*, 225–228. [CrossRef]
10. Ravindranathan, P.; Lee, T.-K.; Yang, L.; Centenera, M.M.; Butler, L.; Tilley, W.D.; Hsieh, J.-T.; Ahn, J.-M.; Raj, G.V. Peptidomimetic targeting of critical androgen receptor–coregulator interactions in prostate cancer. *Nat. Commun.* **2013**, *4*, 1923. [CrossRef]
11. Ravindranathan, P.; Lange, C.A.; Raj, G.V. Minireview: Deciphering the cellular functions of PELP1. *Mol. Endocrinol.* **2015**, *29*, 1222–1229. [CrossRef] [PubMed]
12. Sareddy, G.R.; Vadlamudi, R.K. PELP1: Structure, biological function and clinical significance. *Gene* **2016**, *585*, 128–134. [CrossRef] [PubMed]
13. Zhou, X.E.; Suino-Powell, K.M.; Li, J.; He, Y.; Mackeigan, J.P.; Melcher, K.; Yong, E.-L.; Xu, H.E. Identification of SRC3/AIB1 as a preferred coactivator for hormone-activated androgen receptor. *J. Biol. Chem.* **2010**, *285*, 9161–9171. [CrossRef] [PubMed]
14. Sood, A.; Panchagnula, R. Peroral route: An opportunity for rrotein and peptide drug delivery. *Chem. Rev.* **2001**, *101*, 3275–3304. [CrossRef] [PubMed]
15. Ahn, J.-M.; Han, S.-Y. Facile synthesis of benzamides to mimic an α-helix. *Tetrahedron Lett.* **2007**, *48*, 3543–3547. [CrossRef]
16. Henchey, L.K.; Jochim, A.L.; Arora, P.S. Contemporary strategies for the stabilization of peptides in the alpha-helical conformation. *Curr. Opin. Chem. Biol.* **2008**, *12*, 692–697. [CrossRef]
17. Ahn, J.-M.; Gitu, P.M.; Medeiros, M.; Swift, J.R.; Trivedi, D.; Hruby, V.J. A new approach to search for the bioactive conformation of glucagon: Positional cyclization scanning. *J. Med. Chem.* **2001**, *44*, 3109–3116. [CrossRef]
18. Wang, W.; McMurray, J.S. A selective method for the preparation of primary amides: Synthesis of Fmoc-l-4-carboxamidophenylalanine and other compounds. *Tetrahedron Lett.* **1999**, *40*, 2501–2504. [CrossRef]
19. Breitenlechner, C.B.; Wegge, T.; Berillon, L.; Graul, K.; Marzenell, K.; Friebe, W.-G.; Thomas, U.; Schumacher, R.; Huber, R.; Engh, R.A.; et al. Structure-based optimization of novel azepane derivatives as PKB Inhibitors. *J. Med. Chem.* **2004**, *47*, 1375–1390. [CrossRef]
20. Yalkowsky, S.H.; He, Y.; Jain, P. The aqueous solubilities of benzamide and methyl benzoate have been reported to be 0.110 and 0.031 mol/L, respectively. In *Handbook of Aqueous Solubility Data*, 2nd ed.; Yalkowsky, S.H., He, Y., Jain, P., Eds.; CRC Press: Boca Raton, FL, USA, 2010; pp. 385–479. ISBN 9781439802465.
21. Raj, G.V.; Sareddy, G.R.; Ma, S.; Lee, T.-K.; Viswanadhapalli, S.; Li, R.; Liu, X.; Murakami, S.; Chen, C.-C.; Lee, W.-R.; et al. Estrogen receptor coregulator binding modulators (ERXs) effectively target estrogen receptor positive human breast cancers. *ELife* **2017**, *6*, e26857. [CrossRef]
22. Trott, O.; Olson, A.J. AutoDock Vina: Improving the speed and accuracy of docking with a new scoring function, efficient optimization, and multithreading. *J. Comput. Chem.* **2010**, *31*, 455–461. [CrossRef] [PubMed]
23. Gunther, J.R.; Parent, A.A.; Katzenellenbogen, J.A. Alternative inhibition of androgen receptor signaling: Peptidomimetic pyrimidines as direct androgen receptor/coactivator disruptors. *ACS Chem. Biol.* **2009**, *4*, 435–440. [CrossRef] [PubMed]
24. Axerio-Cilies, P.; Lack, N.A.; Nayana, M.R.S.; Chan, K.H.; Yeung, A.; Leblanc, E.; Guns, E.S.T.; Rennie, P.S.; Cherkasov, A. Inhibitors of androgen receptor activation function-2 (AF2) site identified through virtual screening. *J. Med. Chem.* **2011**, *54*, 6197–6205. [CrossRef] [PubMed]
25. Caboni, L.; Kinsella, G.K.; Blanco, F.; Fayne, D.; Jagoe, W.N.; Carr, M.; Williams, D.C.; Meegan, M.J.; Lloyd, D.G. "True" antiandrogens-selective non-ligand-binding pocket disruptors of androgen receptor-coactivator interactions: Novel tools for prostate cancer. *J. Med. Chem.* **2012**, *55*, 1635–1644. [CrossRef] [PubMed]
26. Lee, T.-K.; Ahn, J.-M. Solid-phase synthesis of tris-benzamides as α-helix mimetics. *ACS Comb. Sci.* **2011**, *13*, 107–111. [CrossRef] [PubMed]
27. Yang, L.; Ravindranathan, P.; Ramanan, M.; Kapur, P.; Hammes, S.R.; Hsieh, J.-T.; Raj, G.V. Central role for PELP1 in nonandrogenic activation of the androgen receptor in prostate cancer. *Mol. Endocrinol.* **2012**, *26*, 550–561. [CrossRef] [PubMed]

Sample Availability: Samples of the compounds are not available from the authors.

molecules

MDPI

Article

Replacement of L-Amino Acids by D-Amino Acids in the Antimicrobial Peptide Ranalexin and Its Consequences for Antimicrobial Activity and Biodistribution

Cornelius Domhan [1], Philipp Uhl [2], Christian Kleist [2], Stefan Zimmermann [3], Florian Umstätter [2], Karin Leotta [2], Walter Mier [2] and Michael Wink [1,*]

1 Institute of Pharmacy and Molecular Biotechnology, Heidelberg University, 69120 Heidelberg, Germany
2 Department of Nuclear Medicine, Heidelberg University Hospital, 69120 Heidelberg, Germany
3 Department of Infectious Diseases, Medical Microbiology and Hygiene, Heidelberg University Hospital, 69120 Heidelberg, Germany
* Correspondence: wink@uni-heidelberg.de; Tel.: +49-6221-544880; Fax: +49-6221-544884

Academic Editors: Henry Mosberg, Tomi Sawyer and Carrie Haskell-Luevano
Received: 1 August 2019; Accepted: 16 August 2019; Published: 17 August 2019

check for updates

Abstract: Infections caused by multidrug-resistant bacteria are a global emerging problem. New antibiotics that rely on innovative modes of action are urgently needed. Ranalexin is a potent antimicrobial peptide (AMP) produced in the skin of the American bullfrog *Rana catesbeiana*. Despite strong antimicrobial activity against Gram-positive bacteria, ranalexin shows disadvantages such as poor pharmacokinetics. To tackle these problems, a ranalexin derivative consisting exclusively of D-amino acids (named danalexin) was synthesized and compared to the original ranalexin for its antimicrobial potential and its biodistribution properties in a rat model. Danalexin showed improved biodistribution with an extended retention in the organisms of Wistar rats when compared to ranalexin. While ranalexin is rapidly cleared from the body, danalexin is retained primarily in the kidneys. Remarkably, both peptides showed strong antimicrobial activity against Gram-positive bacteria and Gram-negative bacteria of the genus *Acinetobacter* with minimum inhibitory concentrations (MICs) between 4 and 16 mg/L (1.9–7.6 μM). Moreover, both peptides showed lower antimicrobial activities with MICs ≥32 mg/L (≥15.2 μM) against further Gram-negative bacteria. The preservation of antimicrobial activity proves that the configuration of the amino acids does not affect the anticipated mechanism of action, namely pore formation.

Keywords: Ranalexin; peptide therapeutics; antibiotics; configuration; antimicrobial activity

---

1. Introduction

Bacteria that possess multidrug-resistance against common antibiotics are spreading worldwide [1]. Infections with bacteria cause increasing numbers of deaths and thus endanger the achievements of modern medicine [2]. To circumvent a return to a pre-antibiotic state, innovative antibiotics are urgently needed.

Antimicrobial peptides (AMPs) are highly effective, amphiphilic, cationic peptides produced by a wide variety of lifeforms [3]. Ranalexin is an AMP that is produced in the skin of the North American bullfrog *Rana catesbeiana* [4]. This peptide of 20-amino acid length has strong antimicrobial activity against Gram-positive bacteria, and its efficacy was previously shown in animal infection models [5]. So far, no host-defense peptide has been approved as an antibiotic drug [6]. Because of their amino acid backbone, AMPs possess intrinsic weaknesses such as a short plasma half-life and degradability by proteolytic enzymes [7,8].

Peptide bonds formed by D-amino acids are resistant to degradation by proteolytic enzymes [9]. A specific substitution of L-amino acids would impair the antimicrobial activity of an AMP [10]. Therefore, we substituted all L-amino acids of ranalexin with D-amino acids (hereinafter named danalexin). Danalexin and ranalexin were tested for their antimicrobial activity against a broad variety of bacteria, including multidrug-resistant pathogens. Further, the antimicrobial kinetics of both substances were investigated by time-kill curves. The biodistribution of danalexin in a rat model was investigated by scintigraphy and positron emission tomography (PET). For both in vivo imaging modalities, specially designed tracer peptides were required. For scintigraphy, an additional D-tyrosine was coupled to danalexin (D-Tyr-danalexin), whereas for PET imaging, the chelating moiety DOTA was covalently attached to danalexin (DOTA-D-Tyr-danalexin). Amino acid sequences of the synthesized peptides are shown in Table 1.

Table 1. Amino acid sequences of the synthesized peptides.

Peptide	Amino Acid Sequence																			
Ranalexin	F	L	G	G	L	I	K	I	V	P	A	M	I	C	A	V	T	K	K	C
Ranalexin-D-Tyr	F	L	G	G	L	I	K	I	V	P	A	M	I	C	A	V	*y*[1]	K	K	C
Danalexin	*f*	*l*	G	G	*l*	*i*	*k*	*i*	*v*	*p*	*a*	*m*	*i*	*c*	*a*	*v*	*t*	*k*	*k*	*c*
D-Tyr-danalexin	*Y*[1]	*l*	G	G	*l*	*i*	*k*	*i*	*v*	*p*	*a*	*m*	*i*	*c*	*a*	*v*	*t*	*k*	*k*	*c*
DOTA-D-Tyr-danalexin	*y*	*l*	G	G	*l*	*i*	*k*	*i*	*v*	*p*	*a*	*m*	*i*	*c*	*a*	*v*	*t*	*k*	*K*[2]	*c*

The amino acid sequences are shown in one-letter code. D-amino acids are printed in lowercase. Basic amino acids are highlighted in blue. Cysteines (yellow) are linked via disulfide bonds. [1] Position of the coupling with ^{125}iodine. [2] Position of the coupling with ^{68}Ga-DOTA.

We found that danalexin retains the spectrum of antibacterial efficacy of ranalexin. The antimicrobial time-kill kinetics of both substances were comparable. Furthermore, in vivo imaging of danalexin was found to be superior to that of ranalexin, because of accumulation and prolonged retention in the kidneys.

2. Results

2.1. Peptide Synthesis

Pure batches of the peptides were obtained by peptide synthesis. Their calculated molecular masses and the results of the HPLC-MS analyses are shown in Table 2, proving that the synthesis was correct.

Table 2. Mass spectrometric analyses by HPLC-MS. Calculated mass, observed mass and interpretation of the identity of the detected species.

Peptide	Calculated Mass [Da]	Observed Mass [Da]	Detected Species
Ranalexin	2103.1890	2104.1768	$[M + H]^+$
Ranalexin-D-Tyr	2165.0267	1083.6002	$[M + 2H]^{2+}$
Danalexin	2103.1890	2104.1047	$[M + H]^+$
D-Tyr-danalexin	2119.1839	2120.1700	$[M + H]^+$
DOTA-D-Tyr-danalexin	2506.0098	2506.1562	$[M]^+$

2.2. Antimicrobial Susceptibility of Clinical Isolates

The results of the antimicrobial susceptibility testing of clinical isolates from Heidelberg University Hospital are shown in Table 3. The results of the antimicrobial testing of the clinical isolate *Acinetobacter baumannii* SC322333 has been published before [11]. In *A. baumannii* SC411190, a $bla_{OXA\text{-}23}$ resistance gene was found, coding for a carbapenemase enzyme. *Enterococcus faecium* UL407074 contains a *vanA* resistance gene. *Klebsiella pneumoniae* BL809453 contains a bla_{KPC} resistance gene, coding for a KPC-2 (*K. pneumoniae* carbapenemase) enzyme. All three Gram-negative clinical isolates belong to the

4-MRGN (multidrug-resistant Gram-negative bacteria) group. The results substantiate that colistin often constitutes the last-line antibiotic against multidrug-resistant Gram-negative infections.

Table 3. Antibiograms of the clinical isolates.

	A. baumannii SC303336 4-MRGN	*A. baumannii* SC411190 4-MRGN, OXA-23	*E. faecium* UL407074 VanA	*K. pneumoniae* BL809453 4-MRGN, KPC
Amoxicillin/Clavulanic acid	nt	R	R	nt
Piperacillin	R	R	nt	R
Piperacillin/Tazobactam	R	R	nt	R
Cefuroxime	nt	nt	R	R
Imipenem	R	R	R	R
Meropenem	R	R	nt	R
Ciprofloxacin	R	R	R	R
Gentamicin	R	R	nt	I
Tobramycin	R	R	nt	R
Amikacin	R	R	nt	nt
Tigecycline	I	nt	S	S
Trimethoprim/Sulfamethoxazole	R	R	R	R
Vancomycin	nt	nt	R	nt
Teicoplanin	nt	nt	R	nt
Erythromycin	nt	nt	R	nt
Linezolid	nt	nt	S	nt
Colistin	S	S	nt	S

All isolates are multidrug-resistant (R-red). Only a few antibiotics remain active (S-green). *A. baumannii* SC303336, *A. baumannii* SC411190 and *K. pneumoniae* BL809543 belong to the 4-MRGN group. *E. faecium* UL407074 contains a vanA resistance gene. OXA-23 carbapenemases are produced by *A. baumannii* SC411190. *K. pneumoniae* produces a KPC-2 carbapenemase. I: intermediate (yellow), nt: not tested.

2.3. Antimicrobial Activity of Ranalexin and Danalexin

The results of antimicrobial testing are documented in Table 4. All experiments were performed in triplicates in three independent experiments. Ranalexin and danalexin showed a similar spectrum of antimicrobial activity. Both peptides have strong antimicrobial activity against Gram-positive bacteria and Gram-negative bacteria of the genus *Acinetobacter* with minimum inhibitory concentrations (MICs) in the range of 4–16 mg/L. Against other Gram-negative bacteria, only weak antimicrobial activity (32–>64 mg/L) could be observed. The activities of ranalexin and danalexin were comparable.

2.4. Time-Kill Curves

For the estimation of antimicrobial kinetics, time-kill curves of ranalexin and danalexin against the well examined Gram-positive bacterium *S. aureus* ATCC 25923 and the Gram-negative bacterium *E. coli* ATCC 25922 were performed ($n = 1$). Results are displayed in Figure 1. Ranalexin and danalexin showed fast, concentration-dependent time-kill kinetics. Between danalexin und ranalexin, no difference in antibacterial kinetics could be observed. At concentrations of 4× MIC, no living bacteria could be detected after 30 min of incubation. At concentrations of 1× MIC, no living bacteria could be detected after 4 h of incubation. Both substances were superior when compared to the established cephalosporin antibiotic cefuroxime, which needed concentration-dependent 8–12 h until no living bacteria could be detected. Cefuroxime was selected as a control compound because it is active against both strains tested.

Table 4. Minimum inhibitory concentrations (MICs) of ranalexin, danalexin and positive controls against a representative selection of bacteria. Both peptides have strong antimicrobial activity against Gram-positive bacteria and Gram-negative bacteria of the genus *Acinetobacter*. Against other Gram-negative bacteria, only weak antimicrobial activity could be shown.

Bacterium	MIC [mg/L] (μM) Ranalexin	Danalexin	Positive Control
Gram-positive bacteria			
Bacillus megaterium DSM 32	4 (1.9)	4 (1.9)	vancomycin 0.13
B. subtilis DSM 10	4 (1.9)	4 (1.9)	vancomycin 0.13
Clostridium pasterianum DSM 525	16 (7.6)	8 (3.8)	vancomycin 0.25
Corynebacterium spheniscorum DSM 44757	16 (7.6)	8 (3.8)	vancomycin 0.50
Enterococcus casseliflavus ATCC 700327 VanC [1]	8 (3.8)	8 (3.8)	vancomycin 8
E. faecalis ATCC 29212	16 (7.6)	16 (7.6)	vancomycin 1
E. faecium UL407074[2] VanA [3]	16 (7.6)	8 (3.8)	vancomycin 640
Staphylococcus aureus ATCC 25923	8 (3.8)	4 (1.9)	vancomycin 1
S. aureus NCTC 10442 MRSA [4]	8 (3.8)	8 (3.8)	vancomycin 1
S. epidermidis ATCC 14990	16 (7.6)	16 (7.6)	vancomycin 2
S. saprophyticus ATCC 15305	8 (3.8)	16 (7.6)	vancomycin 2
Gram-negative bacteria			
Acinetobacter baumannii SC303336[2] 4-MRGN [5]	4 (1.9)	4 (1.9)	colistin 0.25 [6]
A. baumannii SC322333[2] 4-MRGN [5]	8 (3.8)	16 (7.6)	colistin 1 [6]
A. baumannii SC411190[2] 4-MRGN [5]	4 (1.9)	8 (3.8)	colistin 0.25 [6]
Escherichia coli ATCC 25922	32 (15.2)	32 (15.2)	colistin 0.25 [6]
E. coli 0157:H7 ATCC 35150 EHEC [7]	32 (15.2)	32 (15.2)	colistin 0.50 [6]
Klebsiella pneumoniae ATCC 700603	>64 (>30.4)	>64 (>30.4)	colistin 1 [6]
K. pneumoniae BL809453 [2]	>64 (>30.4)	>64 (>30.4)	colistin 0.25 [6]
Pseudomonas aeruginosa ATCC 27853	64 (30.4)	64 (30.4)	colistin 0.25 [6]
P. fluorescens DSM 50090	>64 (>30.4)	>64 (>30.4)	doxycycline 0.50
Yersinia mollaretii DSM 18520	>64 (>30.4)	>64 (>30.4)	colistin 0.25 [6]

[1] *Enterococcus casseliflavus* ATCC 700327 possesses a natural low-level resistance against vancomycin, [2] Clinical isolate of Heidelberg University Hospital, [3] *E. faecium* UL407074 possesses a high-level resistance against vancomycin of the type vanA, [4] Methicillin-resistant *Staphylococcus aureus*, [5] Multidrug-resistant Gram-negative bacteria against four different groups of antibiotics, [6] The MICs of colistin are lower than expected, due to the use of non-absorbent material [12], [7] Enterohemorrhagic *Escherichia coli*.

2.5. Scintigraphy

To gain insight into the in vivo behavior of the AMPs, scintigraphic images of ^{125}I-labeled D-Tyr-danalexin and ranalexin-D-Tyr were obtained after intravenous injection into the tail vein of a Wistar rat. Scintigraphy images of ranalexin-D-Tyr are shown in Figure 2. The images clearly indicate that ranalexin-D-Tyr is predominantly detected in the kidneys. Additionally, smaller amounts of ranalexin-D-Tyr are found in the liver. The excretion occurs rapidly via the urine. Three hours post injection, the vast majority of the substance is already excreted. Minor amounts can be found in the kidneys and in the gut.

D-Tyr-danalexin shows a superior biodistribution because of prolonged renal retention when compared to ranalexin, so it might be applied for the treatment of renal infections (Figure 3). The peptide is mainly distributed in the kidneys and accumulates there for a minimum of 5 h. Even 24 h post injection, D-Tyr-danalexin can be found in the kidneys. Small amounts are distributed in the liver. The excretion takes place via the urine.

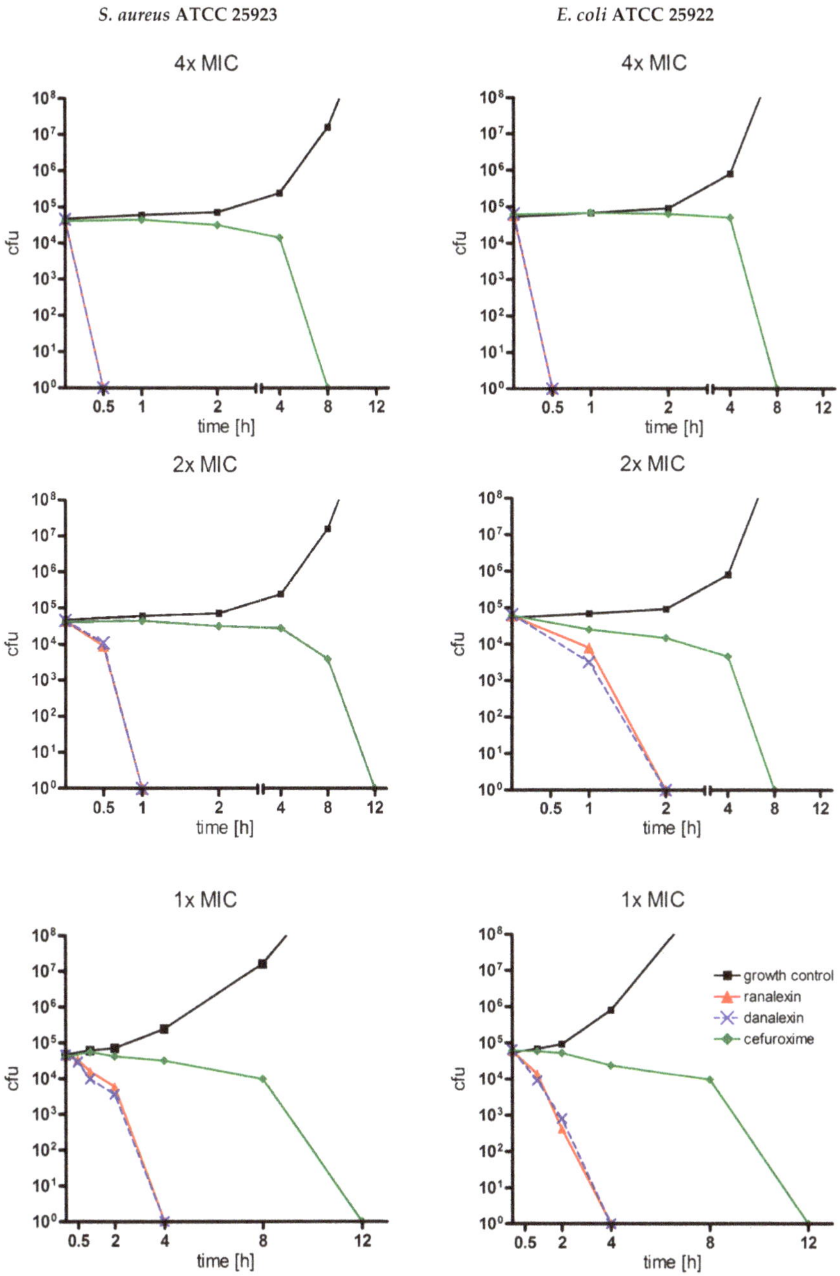

Figure 1. Time-kill curves of ranalexin and danalexin (n = 1). Time-kill curves were determined at 1×, 2× and 4× MIC against *E. coli* ATCC 25922 and *S. aureus* ATCC 25923. Ranalexin (red) and danalexin (blue) showed a fast, concentration-dependent mode of action. Both substances were more bactericidal compared to cefuroxime (green).

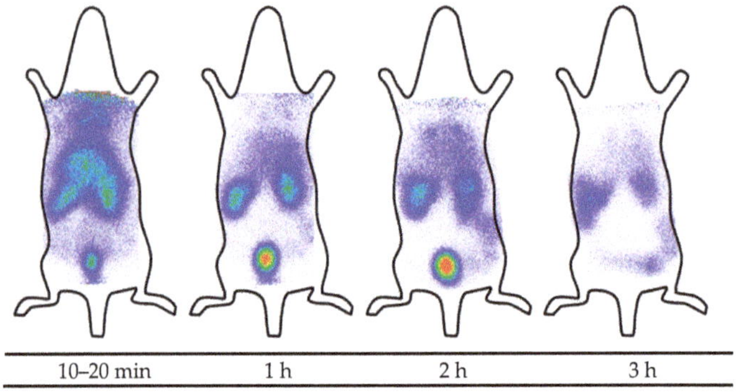

Figure 2. Scintigraphic imaging of ranalexin-D-Tyr in rats. Images were recorded 10–20 min, 1 h, 2 h and 3 h post injection into the tail vein of a Wistar rat. The peptide is excreted by the kidneys. At 1 h post injection, the majority of the substance is found in the bladder.

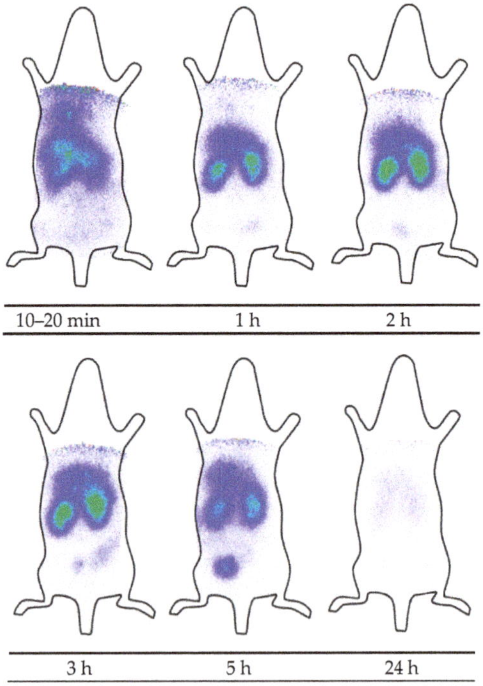

Figure 3. Scintigraphic images of D-Tyr-danalexin. Images were recorded 10–20 min, 1 h, 2 h, 3 h, 5 h and 24 h post injection into the tail vein of a Wistar rat. An accumulation of D-Tyr-danalexin in the kidneys is clearly visible. Even 24 h post injection, radioactivity is still visible in the kidneys.

2.6. Micro-PET Imaging

For higher resolution images, PET imaging of ^{68}Ga-labelled DOTA-D-Tyr-danalexin was performed. The images are shown in Figure 4. For comparison, the PET images of DOTA-ranalexin were published previously [11]. After injection into the tail vein of a Wistar rat, DOTA-D-Tyr-danalexin is distributed in the heart, liver and kidneys. At 20 min post injection, accumulation in the kidneys dominates. Even 3 h post injection, enhanced accumulation in the kidneys is visible. Excretion takes place via the urine. Standard uptake values (SUVs) are shown in Figure 5, substantiating the accumulation of DOTA-D-Tyr-danalexin in the kidneys.

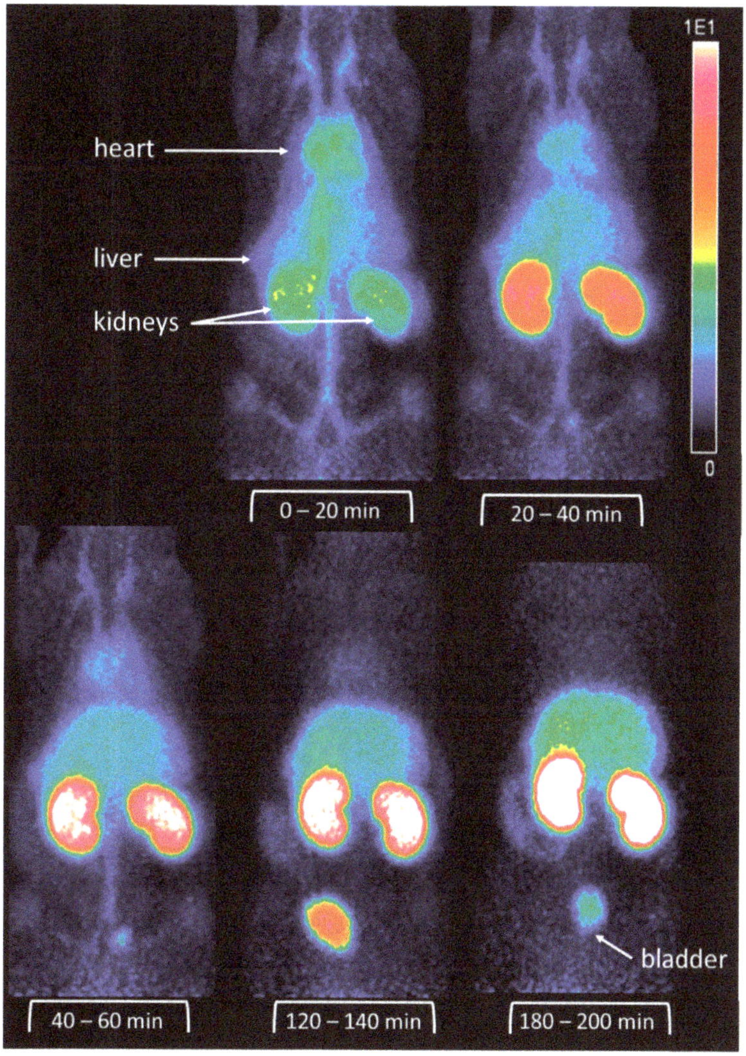

Figure 4. Positron emission tomography (PET) images of DOTA-D-Tyr-danalexin in a Wistar rat. After injection into the tail vein, distribution in the circulation (as reflected by the perfusion of the heart, kidneys, liver and the blood vessels) is visible. At 20 min after injection, an accumulation in the kidneys is clearly visible. This accumulation in the kidneys remains for at least 3 h. Smaller amounts of DOTA-D-Tyr-danalexin are taken up by the liver.

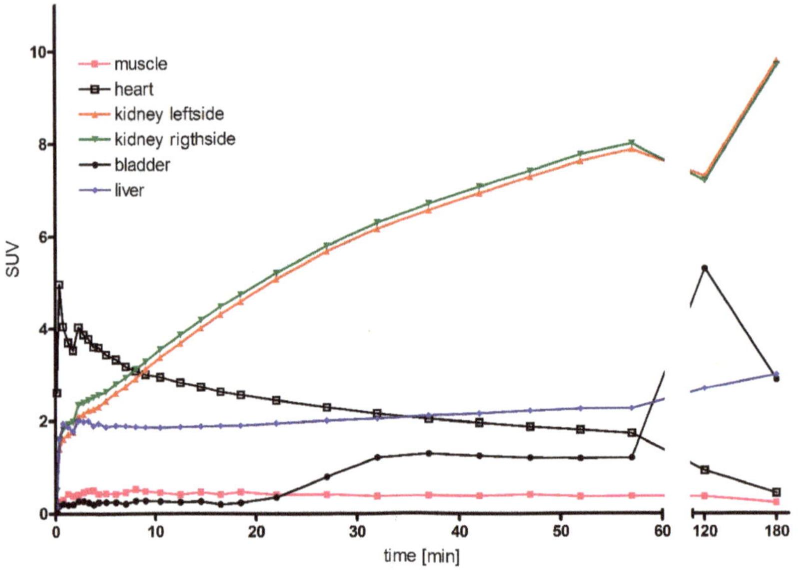

Figure 5. Standard uptake values (SUVs) of DOTA-D-Tyr-danalexin after injection into the tail vein of a Wistar rat. The SUV is used for the quantification of radioactivity in the individual organs. The accumulation of the substance in the kidneys is clearly visible. Smaller amounts are found in the liver. DOTA-D-Tyr-danalexin is excreted via the bladder.

3. Discussion

In this study, the influence of the substitution of proteinogenic amino acids on the antimicrobial activity and biodistribution of the AMP ranalexin was investigated. Solid phase peptide synthesis provided a suitable method for manufacturing peptides containing D-amino acids [13]. HPLC-MS analysis confirmed the purity of the obtained peptides. Ranalexin is an intensively investigated AMP, known for strong antimicrobial activity against Gram-positive bacteria with a rapid bactericidal mode of action [4,14]. The short plasma half-life in vivo is a general disadvantage of AMPs consisting of L-amino acids [8]. Truncated lipopeptide derivatives of ranalexin were found to overcome problems such as short plasma half-life and lack of activity against Gram-negative bacteria [11]. An all D-amino acid derivative was synthesized, because the substitution of only a few amino acids would change the secondary structure of the peptide, eventually leading to a loss of function [10,15]. In cases of AMPs with unspecific antibacterial modes of action, the substitution of all L-amino acids by D-amino acids might allow the retention of their antimicrobial activity [16]. A ranalexin derivative consisting exclusively of D-amino acids had previously been synthesized. Unfortunately, in this peptide, the L-isoleucine moieties had been substituted by D-leucine due to cost reasons [17]. In the peptide designed for this study, the original isoleucine was maintained—and thus incorporated as D-isoleucine—to prevent potential influences of a changed amino acid on the AMP conformation. Danalexin was found to retain the antimicrobial spectrum of ranalexin, including its activity against Gram-positive bacteria and, remarkably, Gram-negative bacteria of the genus *Acinetobacter*. This could be explained by the composition of the outer membranes of these bacteria, which contain higher amounts of carbohydrates and lower amounts of lipopolysaccharides when compared to other Gram-negative bacteria [18]. There were no or negligible differences in MICs between ranalexin and danalexin on the strains tested. This finding sustains the assumption of an unspecific membrane-targeted mode of action [16]. A specific mode of action would most probably be influenced by the conformation of the amino acids. For ranalexin, a rapid, bactericidal mode of action had already been shown [14]. The time-kill curves of ranalexin and danalexin revealed that both substances show similar fast antibacterial kinetics, which also underlines their unspecific mode of action. Compared to previously performed time-kill curves of ranalexin, herein minor differences occurred, because only one set of experiments was carried out due to the laborious and costly character of performing time-kill curves. Notably, both peptides showed superior antimicrobial kinetics when compared to the established bactericidal cefuroxime. Another important objective of this study was the investigation of the effect of the D-amino acids on the in vivo behavior of the modified AMP. Naturally occurring AMPs consisting of L-amino acids suffer from the disadvantage of a short plasma half-life and rapid renal clearance [8]. For ranalexin, a rapid renal clearance was shown before [11]. For non-proteinogenic amino acid-containing peptides such as polymyxins, an accumulation in the kidneys has previously been reported due to their stability against proteolytic degradation [19]. Both scintigraphy and micro-PET imaging revealed that the exchange with D-amino acids leads to a prolonged retention of the peptide danalexin (or its degradation products) in the kidneys.

4. Material and Methods

4.1. Peptide Synthesis

Peptides were manufactured by solid-phase peptide synthesis using the Fmoc strategy on an Applied Biosystems 433A synthesizer (Thermo Fisher Scientific, Darmstadt, Germany) [20]. For coupling of the chelator 1,4,7,10-tetraazacyclododecane-1,4,7,10-tetraacetic acid (DOTA), Fmoc-Lys(alloc) as C-terminal lysine was used [21]. Cleavage from the resin was achieved by trifluoroacetic acid (TFA, Biosolve, Valkenswaard, The Netherlands), as described previously by Brings et al. [21]. Disulfide bridges were formed by dropwise addition of 30 mg/mL iodine (Merck, Darmstadt, Germany) in acetic acid (Sigma-Aldrich, Steinheim, Germany). Excessive iodine was inactivated with ascorbic acid (Merck, Darmstadt, Germany). Purification of the peptides was achieved by preparative HPLC on a Gilson 321 high-performance liquid chromatography (HPLC) system with a Reprosil Gold 120 C18 4-µm 150 × 120 mm column (Dr. Maisch HPLC, Ammerbuch, Germany) [20]. The purity of the peptides was determined by HPLC-MS using an Exactive Orbitrap system (Thermo Fisher Scientific, Bremen, Germany) equipped with a C18 column (Hypersil Gold aQ, Thermo Fisher).

4.2. Antimicrobial Activity

Bacillus megaterium DSM 32, *Bacillus subtilis* DSM 10, *Clostridium pasterianum* DSM 525, *Corynebacterium spheniscorum* DSM 44757, *Pseudomonas fluorescens* DSM 50090 and Yersinia mollaretii DSM 18520 were purchased from the Leibniz Institute DSMZ (Deutsche Sammlung von Mikroorganismen und Zellkulturen - German Collection of Microorganisms and Cell Cultures, Braunschweig, Germany). Other bacteria were obtained from the Department of Medical Microbiology and Hygiene, Heidelberg University Hospital (Heidelberg, Germany). Minimum inhibitory concentrations (MICs) were determined by broth microdilution according to European Committee on Antimicrobial Susceptibility Testing (EUCAST) [22]. In detail, the protocol was described previously [11]. For *C. spheniscorum*, cation-adjusted Mueller–Hinton broth supplemented with 5% lysed horse blood was used. For *C. pasterianum*, supplemented Brucella Broth according to Clinical and Laboratory Standards Institute (CLSI) was used [23]. The anaerobic atmosphere for the incubation of *C. pasterianum* was generated with Anaerocult®C mini systems (Merck, Darmstadt, Germany). After 20 h of incubation at 35 +/− 1 °C, respectively, 30 +/− 1 °C for *B. subtilis*, *B. megaterium*, *P. fluorescens* and *Y. mollaretii*, MIC was determined as the lowest concentration without visible growth. For *C. spheniscorum* and *C. pasterianum*, 40 h of incubation was necessary to obtain significant growth. As positive controls, vancomycin (potency 994 µg/mg; Sigma-Aldrich, Steinheim, Germany), respectively, colistin (potency 753 µg/mg; Carl Roth, Karlsruhe) or doxycycline (potency 842 µg/mg; Sigma-Aldrich, Steinheim, Germany) were used. All experiments were performed in triplicates in three independent experiments. For automated antimicrobial susceptibility testing of the clinical isolates, a Vitek®-2 system (Biomerieux Deutschland,

Nürtingen, Germany) was used. Interpretation criteria for susceptibility and resistance were obtained from EUCAST. For the determination of resistance genes, PCR methods were employed [24,25].

4.3. Time-Kill Curves

Time-kill curves were performed according to the guideline of CLSI [26]. The detailed protocol has been described before [11]. Ranalexin, danalexin, cefuroxime (potency 88.6%) (Sigma-Aldrich, Steinheim, Germany) and physiological saline solution (growth control; Braun, Melsungen, Germany) were incubated with an adjusted inoculum (1×10^6 cfu/mL) of *Staphylococcus aureus* ATCC 25923 or *Escherichia coli* ATCC 25922. After 0, 0.5, 1, 2, 4, 8 and 12 h, aliquots of 1× MIC, 2× MIC and 4× MIC were withdrawn, serially diluted in saline (1:10) and spread onto agar plates (Columbia agar with 5% sheep blood, Biomerieux Deutschland, Nürtingen, Germany). After 24 h of incubation at 37 °C, colonies on the plates were counted.

4.4. Radioactive Labeling and In Vivo Imaging

Male Wistar rats with a weight of 200–250 g were purchased from Janvier Labs (Saint-Berthevin Cedex, France) and kept at the animal facility of the Department of Nuclear Medicine until use for scintigraphic/PET imaging and biodistribution studies. For the animal experiments, approval was obtained from the Animal Welfare Board of the governmental office (Karlsruhe, Germany) and the University of Heidelberg Committee for Ethics on Laboratory Animal Experimentation, and testing was performed in compliance with the following institutional guidelines: the German law for animal protection, the Directive 2010/63/EU of the European Union on the protection of animals used for scientific purposes and FELASA (Federation of European Laboratory Animal Science Associations, Ipswich, UK) guidelines and recommendations.

The peptides were radiolabeled by the use of ^{125}iodine (^{125}I, Hartmann Analytic, Braunschweig, Germany) for scintigraphy studies. For the labeling procedure, the chloramine T method was used as described before [27]. Purification was achieved by preparative HPLC containing a Chromolith performance RP-18e that was equipped with a gamma detector [20]. ^{68}Gallium (^{68}Ga) was eluted from an iThemba LABS ^{68}Ge/^{68}Ga generator (DSD Pharma, Purkersdorf, Austria). Complexation of ^{68}Ga with the chelator DOTA at pH 3.8 in acetate buffer and the subsequent purification of the labeled peptide were performed as previously described [20].

5. Conclusions

We were able to synthesize an all D-amino acid derivative of the AMP ranalexin with prolonged in vivo retention. Furthermore, the spectrum of antimicrobial activity and the antimicrobial kinetics remained constant upon exchange of the configuration of the amino acids. Therefore, the modification of AMPs with D-amino acids could be a step to overcome the disadvantages of natural AMPs such as proteolytic degradation and rapid excretion.

Author Contributions: Conceptualization, C.D., W.M. and M.W.; methodology, P.U., S.Z., F.U. and C.K.; formal analysis, C.D., P.U., W.M. and M.W.; investigation, C.D., P.U., C.K., F.U., K.L. and W.M.; resources, S.Z. and M.W.; data curation, C.D., P.U., C.K., F.U., K.L. and W.M.; writing—original draft preparation, C.D., P.U. and M.W.; writing—review and editing, C.D., P.U., C.K., S.Z., F.U., K.L., W.M. and M.W.

Funding: The authors received financial support from the Deutsche Forschungsgemeinschaft and Ruprecht-Karls-Universität Heidelberg within the funding program Open Access Publishing.

Conflicts of Interest: The authors declare no conflict of interest.

References

1. Ventola, C.L. The antibiotic resistance crisis: Part 1: Causes and threats. *Pharm. Therap.* **2015**, *40*, 277–283.
2. Santajit, S.; Indrawattana, N. Mechanisms of antimicrobial resistance in ESKAPE pathogens. *Biomed. Res. Int.* **2016**, *2016*, 2475067. [CrossRef] [PubMed]
3. Fox, J.L. Antimicrobial peptides stage a comeback. *Nat. Biotechnol.* **2013**, *31*, 379–382. [CrossRef] [PubMed]

4. Clark, D.P.; Durell, S.; Maloy, W.L.; Zasloff, M. Ranalexin. A novel antimicrobial peptide from bullfrog (*Rana catesbeiana*) skin, structurally related to the bacterial antibiotic, polymyxin. *J. Bio. Chem.* **1994**, *269*, 10849–10855.
5. Desbois, A.P.; Sattar, A.; Graham, S.; Warn, P.A.; Coote, P.J. MRSA decolonization of cotton rat nares by a combination treatment comprising lysostaphin and the antimicrobial peptide ranalexin. *J. Antimicrob. Chemother.* **2013**, *68*, 2569–2575. [CrossRef]
6. Kosikowska, P.; Lesner, A. Antimicrobial peptides (AMPs) as drug candidates: A patent review (2003–2015). *Expert. Opin. Ther. Pat.* **2016**, *26*, 689–702. [CrossRef] [PubMed]
7. Kang, H.K.; Kim, C.; Seo, C.H.; Park, Y. The therapeutic applications of antimicrobial peptides (AMPs): A patent review. *J. Microbiol.* **2017**, *55*, 1–12. [CrossRef]
8. Hancock, R.E.; Sahl, H.G. Antimicrobial and host-defense peptides as new anti-infective therapeutic strategies. *Nat. Biotechnol.* **2006**, *24*, 1551–1557. [CrossRef]
9. Hancock, R.E.; Chapple, D.S. Peptide antibiotics. *Antimicrob. Agents Chemother.* **1999**, *43*, 1317–1323. [CrossRef]
10. Wakabayashi, H.; Matsumoto, H.; Hashimoto, K.; Teraguchi, S.; Takase, M.; Hayasawa, H. *N*-Acylated and D enantiomer derivatives of a nonamer core peptide of lactoferricin B showing improved antimicrobial activity. *Antimicrob. Agents Chemother.* **1999**, *43*, 1267–1269. [CrossRef]
11. Domhan, C.; Uhl, P.; Meinhardt, A.; Zimmermann, S.; Kleist, C.; Lindner, T.; Leotta, K.; Mier, W.; Wink, M. A novel tool against multiresistant bacterial pathogens: Lipopeptide modification of the natural antimicrobial peptide ranalexin for enhanced antimicrobial activity and improved pharmacokinetics. *Int. J. Antimicrob. Agents* **2018**, *52*, 52–62. [CrossRef]
12. CLSI. M100-S24: Performance Standards for Antimicrobial Susceptibility Testing. Available online: https://clsi.org/media/2663/m100ed29_sample.pdf (accessed on 15 July 2019).
13. Zoller, F.; Schwaebel, T.; Markert, A.; Haberkorn, U.; Mier, W. Engineering and functionalization of the disulfide-constrained miniprotein min-23 as a scaffold for diagnostic application. *ChemMedChem* **2012**, *7*, 237–247. [CrossRef]
14. Aleinein, R.A.; Hamoud, R.; Schafer, H.; Wink, M. Molecular cloning and expression of ranalexin, a bioactive antimicrobial peptide from *Rana catesbeiana* in *Escherichia coli* and assessments of its biological activities. *Appl. Microbiol. Biotechnol.* **2013**, *97*, 3535–3543. [CrossRef]
15. Matsuzaki, K. Control of cell selectivity of antimicrobial peptides. *Biochim. Biophys. Acta* **2009**, *1788*, 1687–1692. [CrossRef]
16. Papo, N.; Shahar, M.; Eisenbach, L.; Shai, Y. A novel lytic peptide composed of DL-amino acids selectively kills cancer cells in culture and in mice. *J. Biol. Chem.* **2003**, *278*, 21018–21023. [CrossRef]
17. Zapotoczna, M.; Forde, E.; Hogan, S.; Humphreys, H.; O'Gara, J.P.; Fitzgerald-Hughes, D.; Devocelle, M.; O'Neill, E. Eradication of *Staphylococcus aureus* biofilm infections using synthetic antimicrobial peptides. *J. Infect. Dis.* **2017**, *215*, 975–983. [CrossRef]
18. Thorne, K.J.; Thornley, M.J.; Glauert, A.M. Chemical analysis of the outer membrane and other layers of the cell envelope of *Acinetobacter* sp. *J. Bacteriol.* **1973**, *116*, 410–417.
19. Jerala, R. Synthetic lipopeptides: A novel class of anti-infectives. *Expert. Opin. Investig. Drugs* **2007**, *16*, 1159–1169. [CrossRef]
20. Wischnjow, A.; Sarko, D.; Janzer, M.; Kaufman, C.; Beijer, B.; Brings, S.; Haberkorn, U.; Larbig, G.; Kubelbeck, A.; Mier, W. Renal targeting: Peptide-based drug delivery to proximal tubule cells. *Bioconjug. Chem.* **2016**, *27*, 1050–1057. [CrossRef]
21. Brings, S.; Fleming, T.; De Buhr, S.; Beijer, B.; Lindner, T.; Wischnjow, A.; Kender, Z.; Peters, V.; Kopf, S.; Haberkorn, U.; et al. A scavenger peptide prevents methylglyoxal induced pain in mice. *Biochim. Biophys. Acta* **2017**, *1863*, 654–662. [CrossRef]
22. EUCAST. Determination of minimum inhibitory concentrations (MICs) of antimicrobial agents by broth dilution. *Clin. Microbiol. Infect.* **2003**, ix–xv.
23. CLSI. M11-A6: Methods for susceptibility testing of anaerobic bacteria. Available online: https://infostore.saiglobal.com/en-au/Standards/CLSI-M11-A6-6ED-2004-357434_SAIG_CLSI_CLSI_814197/ (accessed on 15 July 2019).

24. Klein, S.; Zimmermann, S.; Kohler, C.; Mischnik, A.; Alle, W.; Bode, K.A. Integration of matrix-assisted laser desorption/ionization time-of-flight mass spectrometry in blood culture diagnostics: A fast and effective approach. *J. Med. Microbiol.* **2011**, *61*, 323–331. [CrossRef]
25. Hofko, M.; Mischnik, A.; Kaase, M.; Zimmermann, S.; Dalpke, A.H. Detection of carbapenemases by Real-Time PCR and melt curve analysis on the BD max system. *J. Clin. Microbiol.* **2014**, *52*, 1701–1704. [CrossRef]
26. NCCLS. M26: Methods for Determining Bactericidal Activity of Antimicrobial Agents. Available online: https://clsi.org/media/1462/m26a_sample.pdf (accessed on 15 July 2019).
27. Uhl, P.; Helm, F.; Hofhaus, G.; Brings, S.; Kaufman, C.; Leotta, K.; Urban, S.; Haberkorn, U.; Mier, W.; Fricker, G. A liposomal formulation for the oral application of the investigational hepatitis B drug Myrcludex B. *Eur. J. Pharm. Biopharm.* **2016**, *103*, 159–166. [CrossRef]

Sample Availability: Samples of the compounds tested in this study are available from the authors.

molecules

MDPI

Article

Development of *N*-Acetylated Dipalmitoyl-*S*-Glyceryl Cysteine Analogs as Efficient TLR2/TLR6 Agonists

Yang Zhou †, **Abid H. Banday** †, **Victor J. Hruby** and **Minying Cai** *

Department of Chemistry and Biochemistry, The University of Arizona, Tucson, AZ 85721, USA; yangzhou@email.arizona.edu (Y.Z.); abidrrl@gmail.com (A.H.B.); hruby@email.arizona.edu (V.J.H.)
* Correspondence: mcai@email.arizona.edu; Tel.: +1-520-621-8617
† These authors contributed equally.

Academic Editors: Henry Mosberg, Tomi Sawyer and Carrie Haskell-Luevano
Received: 28 August 2019; Accepted: 25 September 2019; Published: 27 September 2019

check for updates

Abstract: Cancer vaccine is a promising immunotherapeutic approach to train the immune system with vaccines to recognize and eliminate tumors. Adjuvants are compounds that are necessary in cancer vaccines to mimic an infection process and amplify immune responses. The Toll-like receptor 2 and 6 (TLR2/TLR6) agonist dipalmitoyl-*S*-glyceryl cysteine (Pam_2Cys) was demonstrated as an ideal candidate for synthetic vaccine adjuvants. However, the synthesis of Pam_2Cys requires expensive *N*-protected cysteine as a key reactant, which greatly limits its application as a synthetic vaccine adjuvant in large-scaled studies. Here, we report the development of N-acetylated Pam_2Cys analogs as TLR2/TLR6 agonists. Instead of *N*-protected cysteine, the synthesis utilizes *N*-acetylcysteine to bring down the synthetic costs. The *N*-acetylated Pam_2Cys analogs were demonstrated to activate TLR2/TLR6 in vitro. Moreover, molecular docking studies were performed to provide insights into the molecular mechanism of how N-acetylated Pam_2Cys analogs bind to TLR2/TLR6. Together, these results suggest *N*-acetylated Pam_2Cys analogs as inexpensive and promising synthetic vaccine adjuvants to accelerate the development of cancer vaccines in the future.

Keywords: cancer vaccine; synthetic vaccine; adjuvant; Toll-like receptor; Pam_2Cys; *N*-acetylated Pam_2Cys

1. Introduction

In the recent past, cellular immunotherapy has come up as one of the most suitable approaches for treating major diseases, such as infection and cancer, due to its high selectivity. The Chimeric Antigen Receptor T (CAR-T) therapy involves collecting T cells from patients and genetically modifying them to recognize specific antigens that are only expressed on tumor cells [1]. As immunotherapy approaches parallel to CAR-T therapy, cancer vaccines and synthetic vaccines utilize isolated or synthesized antigens to train the immune system to recognize tumors or pathogens [2]. The antigens used in cancer vaccines can be designed based on information collected from individual patients, thus opening up opportunities for personalized cancer treatment [3]. However, many isolated or synthetic antigens have poor immunogenicity on their own [4], and require adjuvants to help enhance the magnitude and quality of immune responses specific to various antigens [5].

Adjuvants include liposomes, lipopeptides, single stranded DNA etc., that mimic a natural infection to activate various immune components such as dendritic cells, macrophages and lymphocytes to produce desired immunological effects [6]. As a result, vaccine adjuvants can substantially reduce the number of requisite immunizations as well as the amount of antigen required [7]. The bacterial cell wall constituents Pam_2Cys and Pam_3Cys, together with the synthetic analogue Pam_2CSK_4 (Figure 1), have been shown as successful vaccine adjuvants due to their ability to activate Toll-like receptors (TLRs) [8–10]. Specifically, Pam_2Cys was shown to be recognized by the toll-like receptor 2

(TLR2) and Toll-like receptor 6 (TLR6) heterodimers [11]. These adjuvants can induce TLR activation, which further activates NF-kB pathway on both innate and adaptive immune system to induce cytokine production and enhance immune responses against synthetic antigens [12].

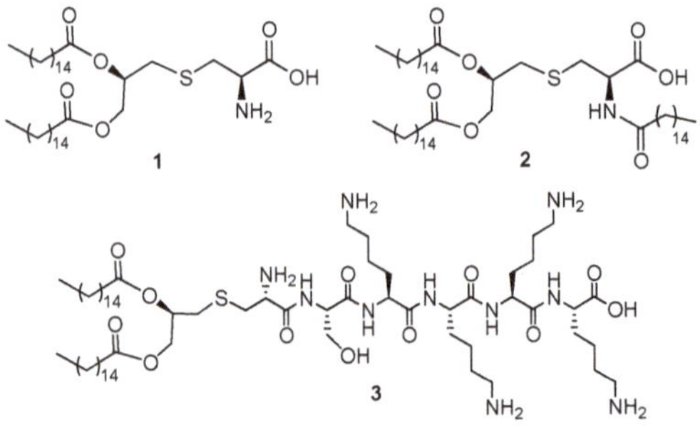

Figure 1. Structures of Pam_2Cys (**1**), Pam_3Cys (**2**) and Pam_2CysSK_4 (**3**).

Although the synthesis and many structural-activity relationship (SAR) studies of Pam_2Cys and its analogues have been described [13–17], efficient large-scale synthesis of Pam_2Cys analogues as synthetic vaccines adjuvants is still difficult due to its high cost. All previously reported synthetic methods involve costly synthetic strategies of orthogonal protection-deprotection techniques [13–15]. To ensure that the primary amine group on cysteine does not participate in any reactions during the synthesis, it has to be protected with either Boc [14,15] or Fmoc [13] protecting groups, which are cost inefficient for large scale synthesis. For the receptor-ligand interactions, an X-ray crystal structure of Pam_2Cys bound to TLR2/TLR6 dimer suggests that the primary amine of the Cys residue does not have a major contribution to the ligand-receptor interactions through any hydrogen bonding interactions [11]. In addition, introducing N-acetylation to Pam_2Cys analogs was shown to have minimal impact on the compound's ability to induce immune responses [18].

In this research, novel synthetic pathways were developed using the inexpensive reactant *N*-acetylcysteine to synthesize *N*-acetyl Pam_2Cys analogs, which can avoid orthogonal protection-deprotection steps and greatly reduce the costs for the synthesis of vaccine adjuvants. The ability of *N*-acetyl lipopeptides to activate TLR2/TLR6 signaling were examined in an NF-kB activation assay in comparison with the commercially available synthetic vaccine adjuvant candidate Pam_2CysSK_4 [8]. Molecular docking studies were performed to simulate the ligand-receptor interactions between *N*-acetyl Pam_2Cys and TLR2/TLR6. Our results confirmed that N-acetyl Pam_2Cys analogs can cause TLR2/TLR6 activation, and thus are promising candidates for cancer vaccine and synthetic vaccine adjuvants.

2. Results

2.1. Synthesis

Scheme 1 shows the novel synthetic design, which uses *N*-acetylcysteine instead of *N*-protected cysteine to avoid orthogonal protection-deprotection steps and lower synthetic costs. 1-hydroxyl and 2-hydroxyl groups on glycerol (**1**) were first protected by cyclohexanone (**2**) to form compound **3**. The hydroxyl group on compound **3** was charged by *p*-TsCl (**4**) to form compound **5**. The thiol group on N-acetylcysteine (**6**) reacts with compound **5**, yielding the thioether compound **7**. The two hydroxyl groups were first exposed by removing the protecting group with AcOH to yield compound **8**, and then coupled with fatty acids of different lengths to form the final products of **AHB 1–4** (Scheme 1, Table 1). The diastereomers were separated when they were first encountered in the synthesis i.e., from **6** to **7**. Product **7** used for further synthesis was diastereomerically pure. No further stereochemical complexity is observed thereafter. The AHB1-SK_4 was further synthesized using standard Fmoc solid-phase peptide synthesis (Table 1).

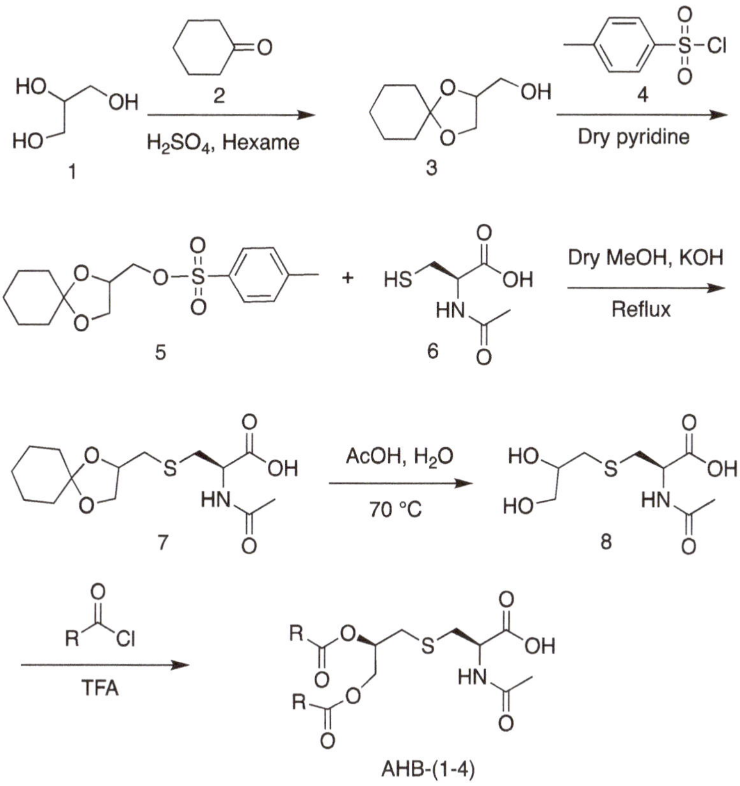

Scheme 1. Synthesis of *N*-acetyl diacyl-*S*-glyceryl cysteine analogs.

Table 1. Structures of various lapidated N-acetyl cysteine analogs analyzed for their TLR2/TLR6 agonist activity.

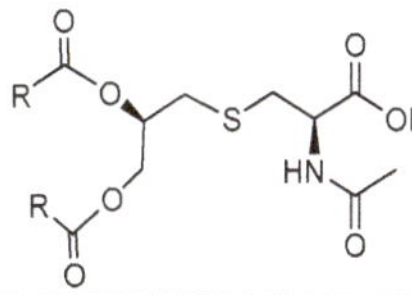

Entry	Nature of R	Nature of R′	Yield (%)
AHB1	CH_3-$(CH_2)_{16}$-	-H	87
AHB2	CH_3-$(CH_2)_{14}$-	-H	83
AHB3	CH_3-$(CH_2)_{12}$-	-H	78
AHB4	CH_3-$(CH_2)_{10}$-	-H	79
AHB1-SK_4	CH_3-$(CH_2)_{14}$-	-SK_4	54

2.2. *In Vitro TLR2/6 Activation*

It was previously reported that the acyl chain lengths of Pam_2Cys analogs can affect the TLR activation [15]. To optimize the ability of N-acetyl lipopeptides to activate TLR2/TLR6, different analogs with varying diacyl chain lengths (12, 14, 16 or 18 carbons, Table 1) were synthesized. To test their abilities to activate TLR2/TLR6, TLR2 and TLR6 as well as an ELAM-SEAP reporter gene were transfected into HEK293 cells. Cells were treated with indicated compounds at 1 μM for 6 h, and the TLR2/TLR6 activation was tested by an NF-kB based activation assay. Specifically, TLR activation leads to the activation of the transcription factor NF-kB, which is recognized by the ELAM promoter to initiate the transcription/translation of the SEAP reporter. The SEAP protein is then quantified due to its ability to catalyze the hydrolysis of *p*-Nitrophenyl phosphate producing a yellow end product. *N*-acetyl lipopeptide with 18 carbons in the acyl chain (AHB-1) was shown to have the highest level of TLR2 and TLR6 activation (Figure 2A). To compare *N*-acetyl lipopeptides with the commercially available standard compound Pam_2CSK_4 [8] in the ability to activate the TLR2/TLR6, AHB-1 was conjugated with the short peptide SKKKK. The ability of AHB-$1SK_4$ and Pam_2CSK_4 to activate TLR2/6 were tested in the NF-kB based activation assay. The results indicated that AHB-$1SK_4$ was able to achieve 67% of the TLR2/TLR6 activation comparing to Pam_2CysSK_4 at 1 μM concentration (Figure 2B), suggesting that AHB-1 analogs can be effectively used as vaccine adjuvants through activating TLR2/6.

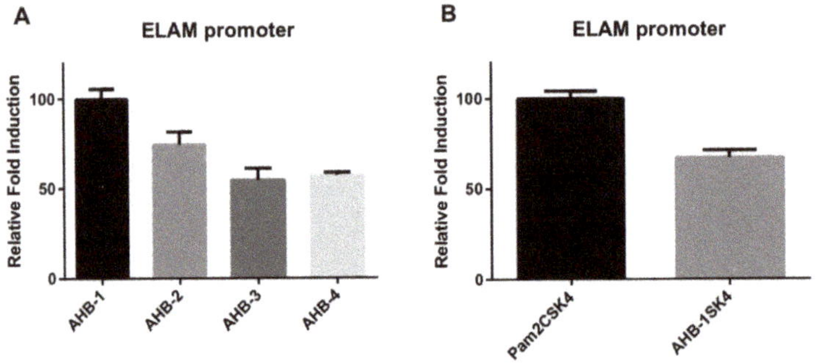

Figure 2. TLR2 and TLR6 activation by *N*-acetyl Pam_2Cys and analogues. HEK293 cells were transfected with plasmids encoding TLR2, TLR6 and the ELAM-SEAP reporter. After 24 h, cells were treated with 1 μM of indicated compounds for 6h. SEAP activities were measured by spectrophometer (OD_{412}). The data shown are representative of three independent experiments. (**A**) TLR2 and TLR6 activation studies using synthetic compounds AHBs; (**B**) Comparison of TLR2 and TLR6 activation via AHB-$1SK_4$ and Pam_2CysSK_4.

2.3. Docking Studies

To understand the effect of the *N*-acetyl group on lipopeptide binding to TLR2 and TLR6, in-silico molecular docking experiments were performed. The structure of Pam_2CysSK_4 bound to active TLR2 and TLR6 was previously determined [11] and was retrieved from Protein Data Bank (3A79). Since there are more than 50 rotatable bonds in Pam_2CysSK_4, which lead to inaccuracy in Glide flexible docking [19], the four lysine residues which do not interact with the receptor [20] were deleted and the diacyl chains were trimmed to six carbons to form the model structure of $Cap_2CysSer$ and N-acetyl $Cap_2CysSer$ molecules. The $Cap_2CysSer$ fits well into the binding pocket (Figure 3), with a Glide docking score of −8.149. With N-acetyl $Cap_2CysSer$, a docking score of −10.025 was achieved, suggesting that the extra *N*-acetyl group does not abolish the interactions between lipopeptides and TLR2/6. What is more interesting, is that comparing to the original position of Cap2CysS, the N-acetyl Cap_2CysS was found to be inserted deeper into the binding pocket (Figure 3). Our docking results suggest that the extra N-acetyl group can be tolerated during binding of N-acetyl Pam_2Cys analogs to TLR2/6.

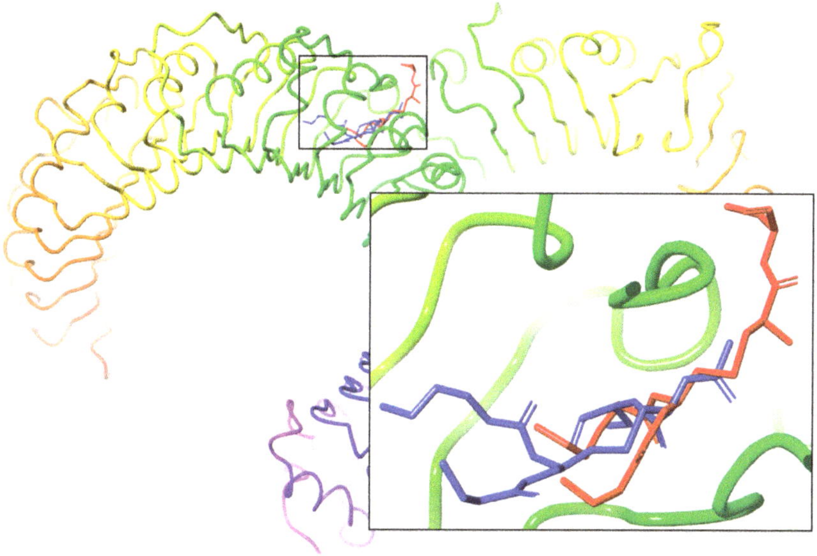

Figure 3. Comparison of the best flexible docking result (lowest docking score) of *N*-acetyl Cap2Cys (in blue) with the original conformation of the Cap2Cys (in red). Ligands are inserted into the binding pocket from up right to bottom left. The *N*-acetyl Cap2Cys is much more embedded into the binding pocket comparing to the position of Cap2Cys.

3. Discussion

Though Pam_2Cys analogs are widely considered as promising candidates for synthetic vaccine adjuvants [8], application in large scales can be limited by its relatively high synthetic costs. Here, we provide novel synthetic pathways to synthesize *N*-acetyl Pam_2Cys analogs with inexpensive materials and avoiding extra orthogonal protection-deprotection steps. Our bioassay results confirmed that the N-acetyl Pam_2Cys analogs can effectively activate TLR2/6, which is consistent with previous findings that an extra N-acetyl group did not produce any substantial difference in the ability of an Pam_2CSK_4 analog to induce CD80 expression [18]. Moreover, our docking results suggest that the extra N-acetyl group can be tolerated during ligand-receptor interactions. Given that the reported synthetic procedure of N-acetyl lipopeptides can effectively reduce the production cost, it is promising that N-acetyl lipopeptides will serve as adjuvants for synthetic vaccines in the future.

4. Materials and Methods

4.1. Synthesis of (1,4-Dioxa-spiro[4,5]dec-2-yl)-methanol (**3**)

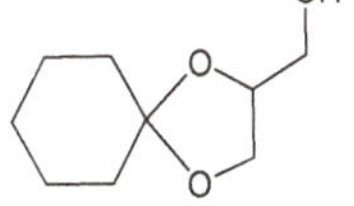

To a solution of glycerol 1 (5.0 g, 54.34 mmol) and cyclohexanone 2 (6.39 g, 65.16 mmol) in *n*-hexane (54.25 mL) was added conc. H_2SO_4 (3 mL) drop wise at 0 °C over a period of 15 min. The reaction mixture was slowly allowed to attain the room temperature and stirred for further 12 h. After completion of the reaction, as monitored by TLC, upper Hexane layer was separated. Then, powdered K_2CO_3 (1.41 g, 8.8 mmol) was charged for trapping the traces of acid that might be present in the organic layer. Finally, hexane layer was evaporated under vacuum to yield the crude product (10.0 g). The crude mixture was subjected to vacuum distillation to afford pure product 3 (8.41 g, 48.86 mmol, 89.9% yield) as a colorless syrupy liquid.

^{1}H-NMR ($CDCl_3$, 200 MHz): δ 1.41–1.64 (m,10 H), 3.55–3.61 (m, 1 H), 3.76–3.82 (m, 2 H), 3.99–4.07 (m, 1 H), 4.21–4.26 (m, 1 H). ESI-MS: 173 (M + H^+).

4.2. Synthesis of Toluene-4-sulfonic acid 1,4-dioxaspiro[4,5]dec-2-yl-methyl ester (**5**)

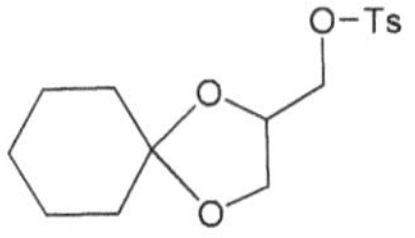

Compound **3** (8.41 g, 48.86 mmol) was dissolved in dry pyridine (35 mL) and immersed into an ice bath under nitrogen atmosphere. *p*-toluenesulfonyl chloride 4 (9.32 g, 48.0 mmol) was added slowly over a period of 20 min. to it and then the reaction mixture was slowly allowed to attain the room temperature and stirred for further 12 h. After completion of the reaction, as monitored by TLC, the reaction mixture was poured on to the crushed ice. The desired cyclohexanone protected glyceryl tosylate was obtained in its crude form after repeated extraction with water: EtOAc (4–25 mL). The crude product was purified using silica gel (100–200 mesh) chromatography to afford pure product 5as a colorless solid (10.95 g, 33.6 mmol, 70% yield).

^{1}H-NMR ($CDCl_3$, 200 MHz): δ 1.38–1.54 (m, 10 H), 2.46 (s, 3 H), 3.73–3.80 (m, 1 H), 3.92–4.12 (m, 3 H), 4.23–4.32 (m, 1 H), 7.37 (d, 2 H, J = 8.09 Hz), 7.81 (d, 2 H, J = 8.29 Hz). ESI-MS: 349 (M + Na^+).

4.3. Synthesis of 2-Acetyl amino-3-(1,4-dioxa-spiro[4,5]dec-2-ylmethyl sulfanyl)-propionic acid (**7**)

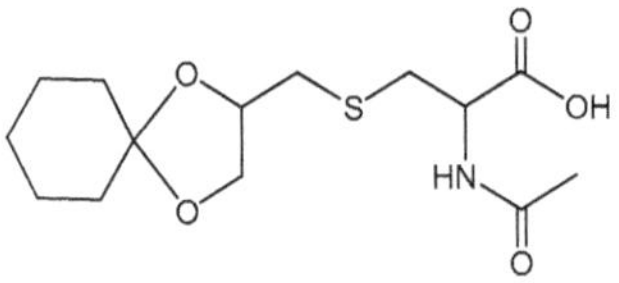

To the stirred suspension of N-acetyl cysteine 6 (5.47 g, 33.6 mmol) in methanolic KOH (2.81 g, 49.0 mmol in 40 mL methanol) solution, was added toluene-4-sulfonic acid 1,4-dioxa-spiro[4,5]dec-2-yl-methyl ester 5 (10.95 g, 33.6 mmol) under nitrogen at room temperature. Reaction mixture was heated at reflux for 8–10 h. After completion of the reaction, as monitored by TLC, reaction mixture was filtered off (potassium tosylate was precipitated during the course of reaction) and was acidified to 2 pH using 2 N HCl. Organic compound was extracted with DCM (3 × 100 mL) and Ethyl acetate (2 × 100 mL). The combined organic layers were dried over sodium sulphate and evaporated under vacuum to give the crude product which was purified on flash column chromatogram (silica gel as stationary phase, DCM: MeOH as mobile phase) to yield the product 7 in its pure form (8.2 g, 25.86 mmol, 77% yield).

^{1}H-NMR ($CDCl_3$, 200 MHz): δ 1.40–1.61 (m, 10 H), 2.05 (s, 3 H), 2.66–2.91 (m, 3 H), 3.29–3.31 (m, 1 H), 3.66–3.70 (m, 1 H), 4.03–4.11 (m, 1 H), 4.23–4.27 (m, 1 H), 4.59–4.63 (m, 1 H). ESI-MS: 340 (M + Na^+).

4.4. Synthesis of 2-Acetyl amino-3-(2,3-dihydroxy-propyl sulfanyl)-propionic acid (**8**)

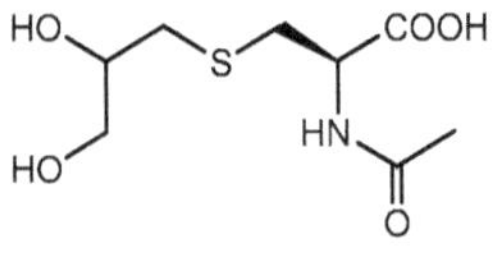

Compound 7 (8.2 g, 25.86 mmol) was dissolved in 75% aqueous acetic acid (20 mL) and heated to reflux for 3 h. After completion of the reaction, as monitored by TLC, the mixture was evaporated under vacuum to yield the crude product. The crude mass was purified through chromatography (Silica gel, 300–400 mesh) using chloroform: methanol gradient as the eluant to yield the pure compound 8 (5.80 g, 24.5 mmol, 94.6% yield).

^{1}H-NMR ($CDCl_3$, 200 MHz): δ 2.05 (s, 3 H), 2.68–2.93 (m, 3 H), 3.29–3.35 (m, 1 H), 3.68–3.76 (m, 1 H), 4.03–4.08 (m, 1 H), 4.27–4.30 (m, 1 H), 4.57–4.66 (m, 1 H). ESI-MS: 260 (M + Na^+).

4.5. Synthesis of N-Acetyl Pam2Cys and Analogs (**AHB-1–4**)

To the stirred solution of compound 8 (1 g, 4.20 mmol, 1 equation), in TFA (Trifluoroacetic acid) (30 mL) was added palmitoyl chloride (2.45 g, 8.40 mmol, 2 eq.) slowly under nitrogen at room temperature. Reaction mixture was stirred for 30 min. After the completion of the reaction, as monitored by TLC, reaction mixture was dried under vacuum to yield the crude product (3.5 g), which was purified by flash chromatography (silica gel, 200–400 mesh) using chloroform and methanol gradient as eluant to afford *N*-Acetyl Pam2Cys (AHB2) in its pure form (2.69 g, 3.77mmol, 89.8% yield). The assignment of NMR peaks is given as under for AHB1 as the assignment will be same for all other compounds and only the number of methylene protons in the fatty chain will change. (**AHB2–4** do not show carbon numbers.) C1–17 in both the fatty chains are the same, thus we have given the same number to all such carbons in both the chains. Their protons and carbons have exactly the same chemical shift values.

Hexadecanoic acid 2-(2-acetylamino-2-carboxy-ethylsulfanyl)-1-octadecanoyl-oxy methyl–ethyl ester (*N*-Acetyl Str2Cys) (AHB1):

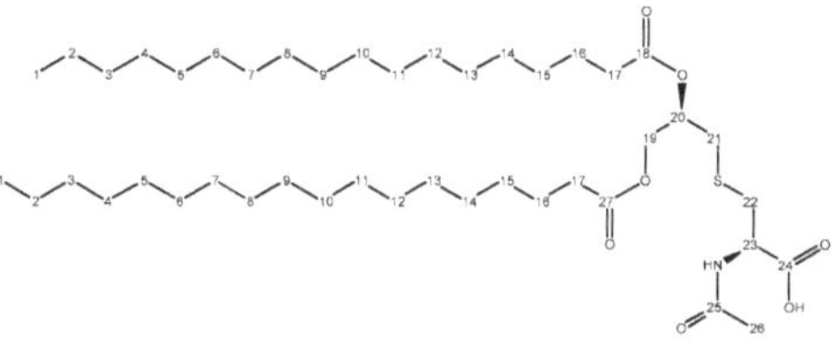

$[\alpha]_D^{25}$ −15.2 (c 0.10, CHCl3), 1H-NMR (CDCl3, 400 MHz): 0.87–0.90 (t, 6H) [6Hs on two C1], 1.24–1.45 (m, 56H) [Protons on C2–15], 1.58–1.63 (m, 4H) [Protons on C16], 2.12 (s, 3H) [Protons on C27], 2.30–2.36 (m, 4H) [Protons on C17], 2.75 (m, 2H) [Protons on C21], 3.06–3.15 (m, 2H) [Protons on C22], 4.12–4.17 (m, 1H) [Proton on C19], 4.34–4.40 (m, 1H) [Next Proton on C19], 4.82 (m, 1H) [Protons on C23], 5.18 (m, 1H) [Protons on C20], 6.86–6.92 (m, 1H) [-NH proton] (Total assigned protons 82, Carboxyl proton out of range). 13C-NMR (CDCl3, 400 MHz): 14.12 [C1], 22.68 [C2], 24.88 [C26], 29.36, 29.48, 29.61[C3-C16 and C22], 31.90 [C17], 52.18 [C21], 52.51 [C23], 63.72 [C19], 70.25 [C20], 171.74 [C18], 172.58 [C27], 173.52 [C25], 173.66 [C24]. IR (KBr, cm^{-1}): 3014, 2921, 2360, 1741, 1703, 1658, 1530, 1345, 1215, 1167, 964, 756. ESI-MS: 792 (M + Na+). Anal. Calcd. for C44H83NO7S, C, 68.61; H, 10.86; N, 1.82. Found C, 68.64; H, 10.83; N, 1.86.

Hexadecanoic acid 2-(2-acetylamino-2-carboxy-ethylsulfanyl)-1-hexadecanoyl-oxy methyl–ethyl ester (N-Acetyl Pam2Cys) (**AHB2**):

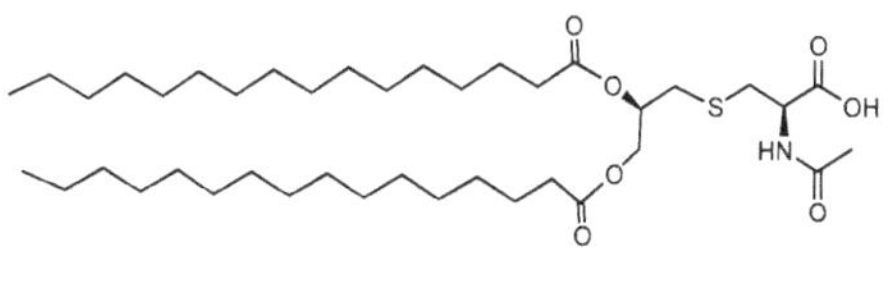

Specific rotation: $[\alpha]_D^{25}$ −21.2 (c 0.10, CHCl3), ^{1}H-NMR ($CDCl_3$, 400 MHz): δ 0.87–0.92 (m, 6H), 1.24–1.31 (m, 48H), 1.58–1.66 (m, 4H), 2.14 (s, 3H), 2.33–2.43 (m, 4H), 2.78 (d, 2H, *J* = 6.37 Hz), 3.10–3.17 (d, 2H, *J* = 54 Hz), 4.16–4.26 (m, 2H), 4.79 (m, 1H), 5.16 (m, 1H), 6.78–6.82 (m, 1H). ^{13}C-NMR ($CDCl_3$,

400 MHz): δ14.13, 22.70, 22.80, 24.71, 24.87, 29.12, 29.31, 29.38, 29.52, 29.71, 31.93, 32.93, 33.97, 34.11, 34.40, 52.04, 52.22, 63.72, 70.23, 70.27, 171.48, 172.99, 173.62, 173.69. IR (KBr, cm^{-1}): 3013, 2921, 2851, 2360, 1741, 1703, 1658, 1530, 1464, 1452, 1374, 1345, 1215, 1167, 964, 755. ESI-MS: 713 (M + H^+). Anal. Calcd. for $C_{40}H_{75}NO_7S$, C, 62.28; H, 10.59; N, 1.96. Found C, 62.31; H, 10.55; N, 1.93.

Hexadecanoic acid 2-(2-acetylamino-2-carboxy-ethylsulfanyl)-1-tetradecanoyl-oxy methyl–ethyl ester (*N*-Acetyl Myr2Cys) (**AHB3**):

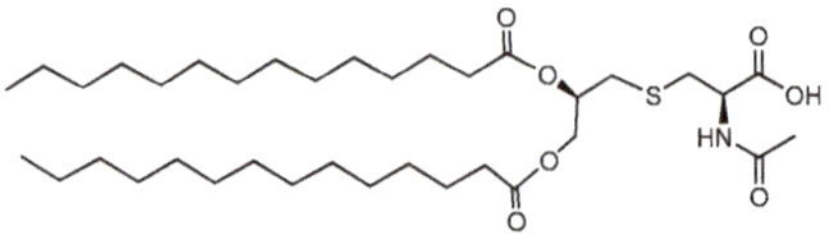

$[\alpha]_D^{25}$ −27.7 (c 0.10, $CHCl_3$), ^{1}H-NMR ($CDCl_3$, 400 MHz): δ 0.86–0.92 (t, 6H), 1.22–1.33 (m, 40H), 1.56–1.63 (m, 4H), 2.13 (s, 3H), 2.30–2.36 (m, 4H), 2.76 (m, 2H), 3.06–3.16 (m, 2H), 4.13–4.17 (m, 1H), 4.33–4.40 (m, 1H), 4.81 (m, 1H), 5.17 (m, 1H), 6.86–6.91 (m, 1H). ^{13}C-NMR ($CDCl_3$, 400 MHz): δ14.08, 22.66, 24.88, 29.36, 29.48, 29.61, 31.90, 52.18, 52.51, 63.72, 70.23, 70.27, 171.74, 172.52, 173.54, 173.67. IR (KBr, cm^{-1}): 3012, 2921, 2851, 2360, 1741, 1701, 1658, 1530, 1464, 1452, 1376, 1345, 1215, 1167, 964, 754. ESI-MS: 680 (M + Na^+), Anal. Calcd. for $C_{36}H_{67}NO_7S$, C, 65.71; H, 10.26; N, 2.13. Found C, 65.82; H, 10.28; N, 2.10.

Hexadecanoic acid 2-(2-acetylamino-2-carboxy-ethylsulfanyl)-1-dodecanoyl-oxy methyl ethyl ester (*N*-Acetyl Lau2Cys) (**AHB4**):

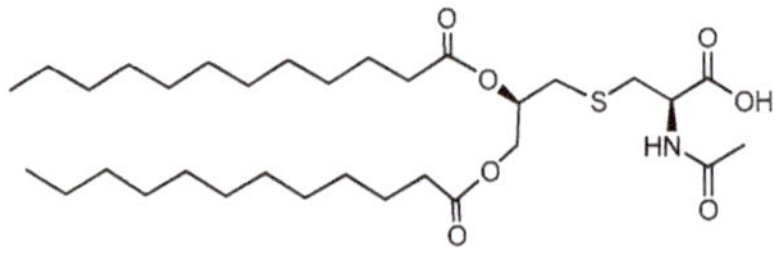

$[\alpha]_D^{25}$ −31.3 (c 0.10, $CHCl_3$), ^{1}H-NMR ($CDCl_3$, 400 MHz): δ 0.88–0.91 (t, 6H), 1.24–1.35 (m, 32H), 1.59–1.65 (m, 4H), 2.12 (s, 3H), 2.30–2.36 (m, 4H), 2.75 (m, 2H), 3.06–3.15 (m, 2H), 4.12–4.17 (m, 1H), 4.34–4.40 (m, 1H), 4.82 (m, 1H), 5.18 (m, 1H), 6.86–6.90 (m, 1H). ^{13}C-NMR ($CDCl_3$, 400 MHz): δ14.09, 22.68, 24.88, 29.36, 29.48, 29.61, 31.90, 52.18, 52.51, 63.72, 70.24, 70.27, 171.74, 172.58, 173.54, 173.68. IR (KBr, cm^{-1}): 3014, 2921, 2851, 2360, 1741, 1703, 1658, 1530, 1464, 1452, 1376, 1345, 1215, 1167, 964, 756. ESI-MS: 601 (M + H^+). Anal. Calcd. for $C_{32}H_{59}NO_7S$, C, 63.86; H, 9.88; N, 2.33. Found C, 63.85; H, 9.83; N, 2.37.

4.6. Cell Culture

HEK293 cells were grown in the MEM medium (Minimum Essential Medium) (Gaithersburg, MD, USA) with 1sodium pyruvate (Sigma-Aldrich, St. Louis, MO, USA), 10% fetal bovine serum (Sigma-Aldrich, MO, USA) and 1% Pen-Strep (Sigma-Aldrich, MO, USA) at 37 °C in 5% CO_2 incubator.

4.7. NF-kB Activation Assay

HEK293 cells (5 × 10^6) were transiently transfected with 5.7 μg of ELAM-SEAP reporter gene (Invivogen, San Diego, CA, USA) and 0.3 μg of TLR2/TLR6 expression vector (Invivogen, CA) using the FuGENE 6 transfection kit (Roche Diagnostics, Mannheim, Germany). The cells were seeded into 96-well plates 6 h after transfection. After 24 h, the cells were treated with lipopeptides (1 μM) and the medium was collected 6 h after stimulation. SEAP activity was measure using SEAP reporter assay kit (Invivogen, CA) and μQuant Microplate Reader (BioTek, Winooski, VT, USA) at OD_{412}.

4.8. Molecular Docking

The structure of the Pam_2CSK_4 bound to active TLR2 and TLR6 were retrieved from the 2.9Å crystal structure (PDB: 3A79) [20]. The TLR2/TLR6 structure was prepared by protein preparation wizards in Maestro with the force field of OPLS 2005. The ligand binding pocket was defined in the prepared receptor structure to generate a receptor grid by Glide receptor grid generation. The scaling factor was set to 1.0 and the partial charge cutoff was set to 0.25. The four lysine residues and 10 methylenes in each diacyl chain were deleted from the Pam_2CSK_4 structure to create the model of Cap_2CS molecule. An acetyl group was added to the amide group of cysteine to create the model for N-acetyl Cap_2CS. The structures of Cap_2CS and *N*-acetyl Cap_2CS were optimized using ligand preparation before docking. The ligand structures were docked into the receptor grid using Glide docking in flexible docking mode. The scaling factor was 0.8 and the partial charge cutoff was 0.15. The poses with the lowest docking score for each ligand were used for comparison. Poses were rejected if the Coulomb-vdW energy were greater than 0 kcal/mol. Extra precision (XP) was used in docking experiments.

Author Contributions: Conceptualization, A.H.B.; synthesis, A.H.B.; bioassays, Y.Z.; docking studies, Y.Z.; writing, Y.Z and A.H.B.; experimental design, writing and funding acquisition, M.C. and V.J.H.

Funding: This work was funded in part by the US Public Health Service, NIH NIDA, Grant RO1 DA 13449.

Acknowledgments: A.B. thanks UGC, India for the award of Raman postdoctoral fellowship under Singh–Obama 21st century knowledge initiative. The authors dedicate this paper to Victor J. Hruby in honor of his 80th birthday and would like to thank him for his extraordinary guidance.

Conflicts of Interest: The authors declare no conflict of interest.

References

1. Kingwell, K. CAR T therapies drive into new terrain. *Nat. Rev. Drug Discov.* **2017**, *16*, 301–304. [CrossRef] [PubMed]
2. Temizoz, B.; Kuroda, E.; Ishii, K.J. Vaccine adjuvants as potential cancer immunotherapeutics. *Int. Immunol.* **2016**, *28*, 329–338. [CrossRef] [PubMed]
3. Ott, P.A.; Hu, Z.; Keskin, D.B.; Shukla, S.A.; Sun, J.; Bozym, D.J.; Zhang, W.; Luoma, A.; Giobbie-Hurder, A.; Peter, L.; et al. An immunogenic personal neoantigen vaccine for patients with melanoma. *Nature* **2017**, *547*, 217–221. [CrossRef] [PubMed]
4. Skwarczynski, M.; Toth, I. Peptide-based synthetic vaccines. *Chem. Sci.* **2016**, *7*, 842–854. [CrossRef] [PubMed]
5. Leroux-Roels, G. Unmet needs in modern vaccinology: Adjuvants to improve the immune response. *Vaccine* **2010**, *28* (Suppl. 3), C25–C36. [CrossRef]
6. Gavin, A.L.; Hoebe, K.; Duong, B.; Ota, T.; Martin, C.; Beutler, B.; Nemazee, D. Adjuvant-enhanced antibody responses in the absence of toll-like receptor signaling. *Science* **2006**, *314*, 1936–1938. [CrossRef] [PubMed]
7. Schijns, V.E. Immunological concepts of vaccine adjuvant activity. *Curr. Opin. Immunol.* **2000**, *12*, 456–463. [CrossRef]
8. Jackson, D.C.; Lau, Y.F.; Le, T.; Suhrbier, A.; Deliyannis, G.; Cheers, C.; Smith, C.; Zeng, W.; Brown, L.E. A totally synthetic vaccine of generic structure that targets Toll-like receptor 2 on dendritic cells and promotes antibody or cytotoxic T cell responses. *Proc. Natl. Acad. Sci. USA* **2004**, *101*, 15440–15445. [CrossRef] [PubMed]
9. Aliprantis, A.O.; Yang, R.B.; Mark, M.R.; Suggett, S.; Devaux, B.; Radolf, J.D.; Klimpel, G.R.; Godowski, P.; Zychlinsky, A. Cell activation and apoptosis by bacterial lipoproteins through toll-like receptor-2. *Science* **1999**, *285*, 736–739. [CrossRef] [PubMed]
10. Moyle, P.M.; Toth, I. Self-adjuvanting lipopeptide vaccines. *Curr. Med. Chem.* **2008**, *15*, 506–516. [CrossRef] [PubMed]
11. Kang, J.Y.; Nan, X.; Jin, M.S.; Youn, S.J.; Ryu, Y.H.; Mah, S.; Han, S.H.; Lee, H.; Paik, S.G.; Lee, J.O. Recognition of lipopeptide patterns by Toll-like receptor 2-Toll-like receptor 6 heterodimer. *Immunity* **2009**, *31*, 873–884. [CrossRef] [PubMed]
12. Iwasaki, A.; Medzhitov, R. Toll-like receptor control of the adaptive immune responses. *Nat. Immunol.* **2004**, *5*, 987–995. [CrossRef] [PubMed]

13. Metzger, J.W.; Wiesmuller, K.H.; Jung, G. Synthesis of N alpha-Fmoc protected derivatives of S-(2,3-dihydroxypropyl)-cysteine and their application in peptide synthesis. *Int. J. Pept. Protein Res.* **1991**, *38*, 545–554. [CrossRef] [PubMed]
14. Wu, W.; Li, R.; Malladi, S.S.; Warshakoon, H.J.; Kimbrell, M.R.; Amolins, M.W.; Ukani, R.; Datta, A.; David, S.A. Structure-activity relationships in toll-like receptor-2 agonistic diacylthioglycerol lipopeptides. *J. Med. Chem.* **2010**, *53*, 3198–3213. [CrossRef] [PubMed]
15. Agnihotri, G.; Crall, B.M.; Lewis, T.C.; Day, T.P.; Balakrishna, R.; Warshakoon, H.J.; Malladi, S.S.; David, S.A. Structure-activity relationships in toll-like receptor 2-agonists leading to simplified monoacyl lipopeptides. *J. Med. Chem.* **2011**, *54*, 8148–8160. [CrossRef] [PubMed]
16. Zeng, W.; Eriksson, E.; Chua, B.; Grollo, L.; Jackson, D.C. Structural requirement for the agonist activity of the TLR2 ligand Pam2Cys. *Amino Acids* **2010**, *39*, 471–480. [CrossRef] [PubMed]
17. Azuma, M.; Sawahata, R.; Akao, Y.; Ebihara, T.; Yamazaki, S.; Matsumoto, M.; Hashimoto, M.; Fukase, K.; Fujimoto, Y.; Seya, T. The peptide sequence of diacyl lipopeptides determines dendritic cell TLR2-mediated NK activation. *PLoS ONE* **2010**, *5*. [CrossRef] [PubMed]
18. Wright, T.H.; Brooks, A.E.S.; Didsbury, A.J.; McIntosh, J.D.; Burkert, K.; Yeung, H.; Williams, G.M.; Dunbar, P.R.; Brimble, M.A. An Improved Method for the Synthesis of Lipopeptide TLR2-Agonists Using Click Chemistry. *Synlett* **2013**, *24*, 1835–1841. [CrossRef]
19. Friesner, R.A.; Banks, J.L.; Murphy, R.B.; Halgren, T.A.; Klicic, J.J.; Mainz, D.T.; Repasky, M.P.; Knoll, E.H.; Shelley, M.; Perry, J.K.; et al. Glide: A new approach for rapid, accurate docking and scoring. 1. Method and assessment of docking accuracy. *J. Med. Chem.* **2004**, *47*, 1739–1749. [CrossRef] [PubMed]
20. Jin, M.S.; Kim, S.E.; Heo, J.Y.; Lee, M.E.; Kim, H.M.; Paik, S.G.; Lee, H.; Lee, J.O. Crystal structure of the TLR1-TLR2 heterodimer induced by binding of a tri-acylated lipopeptide. *Cell* **2007**, *130*, 1071–1082. [CrossRef] [PubMed]

Sample Availability: Samples of the compounds are not available from the authors.

molecules

MDPI

Article

Application of *N*-Dodecyl L-Peptide to Enhance Serum Stability while Maintaining Inhibitory Effects on Myometrial Contractions Ex Vivo

Julien Poupart [1], Xin Hou [2], Sylvain Chemtob [2] and William D. Lubell [1,*]

1 Département de Chimie, Pavillon Roger Gaudry, Université de Montréal, CP 6128 and Succursale Centre-ville, Montréal, QC H3C 3J7, Canada; julien.poupart@umontreal.ca

2 Centre de recherches du Centre Hospitalier Universitaire Sainte-Justine, Montréal City, QC H3T 1C5, Canada; xin.hou82@gmail.com (X.H.); sylvain.chemtob@gmail.com (S.C.)

* Correspondence: william.lubell@umontreal.ca; Tel.: +1-514-343-7339

Academic Editors: Henry Mosberg, Tomi Sawyer and Carrie Haskell-Luevano
Received: 15 October 2019; Accepted: 7 November 2019; Published: 15 November 2019

check for updates

Abstract: *N*-Alkylation and *N*-acylation of the prostaglandin-$F_{2\alpha}$ allosteric modulator L-PDC31 were performed to install various alkyl, PEG and isoprenoid groups onto the L-enantiomer of the peptide. Among the different bio-conjugates studied, the *N*-dodecyl analog reduced prostaglandin-$F_{2\alpha}$-induced mouse myometrium contractions ex vivo. Furthermore, *N*-dodecyl-L-PDC31 exhibited improved stability in a mouse serum assay, likely due to protection from protease degradation by the lipid chain.

Keywords: bioconjugation; lipidation; prostaglandin $F_{2\alpha}$; preterm labor; myometrium contractions

1. Introduction

Preterm labor is a challenging contemporary target of modern medicinal chemistry. Preterm birth (PTB), defined as less than 37 weeks of gestational age, accounts for 5–13% of all births [1]. Responsible for an increased risk of neonatal and infantile mortality [2] PTB is associated with various other complications, including developmental disorders [3], vision and hearing impairments [4,5], and chronic metabolic conditions [6]. Since 2012, PTB has been the single most expensive medical urgency per patient in the United States [7], in part due to a lack of so-called tocolytic drugs that can effectively and safely delay delivery.

In less affluent countries, PTB is more problematic: >60% of PTBs occur in Africa and South-Asia. Ineffective healthcare to treat mother and child in less affluent countries is associated with a higher percentage of neonatal and infantile mortality: 90% for very preterm babies of <28 weeks. In developed countries, <10% of newborns suffering similar PTB conditions experience the same fate [7].

The currently available medications, including the oxytocin receptor antagonist Atosiban [8], calcium channel blockers [9], β_2 agonists [10], a myosin light chain inhibitor [11], and prostaglandin-endoperoxide synthase inhibitors [12], all rarely delay labor for >48 h [13,14] and many have risks of serious side effects for both mother and infant. New approaches exploring different pathways to tocolytic agents are essential for the development of more effective treatments with minimal side effects. For ideal distribution to third-world countries, such tocolytic agents would be produced cost-effectively.

The prostaglandin F2α receptor (FP) is a promising target for delaying labor because of its relevant involvement in parturition. At the beginning of labor and preterm labor, FP expression increases [15,16]. Moreover, FP-knockout mice do not go into labor, even when induced by oxytocin [17]. Targeting FP, the tocolytic prototype PDC31 is currently undergoing clinical trials [18,19]. In a phase Ib clinical trial of women with primary dysmenorrhea, PDC31 was demonstrated to be safe in reducing intrauterine pressure and pain associated with excessive uterine contractility [20].

The development of PDC31 originated from a library of sequences based on the second extracellular loop of FP. Short lead peptides were analyzed initially using *in vitro* and ex vivo analyses [19]. The lead peptide PDC113 (H-ile-leu-Gly-his-arg-asp-tyr-lys-OH, small letters refer to D amino acids) was identified as an active FP inhibitor [18]. Replacement of the arginine residue with citrulline yielded PDC31 (H-ile-leu-Gly-his-cit-asp-tyr-lys-OH, cit = D-citrulline), which exhibited notable efficacy (>85%) and potency (IC_{50} = 13 nM) [18]. Selectively modulating the downstream signaling of FP, the mechanism of action of PDC31 is suggested to involve allosteric inhibition at a site different from the "othosteric", native ligand-binding site [19,21].

The relatively high price of D-amino acid building blocks can influence the cost of production of PDC31, which is composed of seven of D-amino acids including D-citrulline. The L-amino acid version of PDC31 has been observed to exhibit some antagonist activity but failed to do so in a myometrial tissue-based assay, probably owing to the relatively low metabolic stability of linear L-peptides. To improve the metabolic stability of L-PDC31, the peptide *N*-terminal has now been modified with lipid chains. Previously, *N*-acetylation had abolished the activity of PDC113 analogs. Thus, instead of acylation, a strategy was pursued to maintain the basic nitrogen by alkylation with different hydrophobic moieties: linear hydrocarbons, PEG and farnesyl chains.

Polyethylene glycol grafts onto polyamide structures have demonstrated success for improving pharmacodynamic properties, particularly duration of action [22,23]. Protein PEGylation has enhanced water solubility, prolonged half-life, improved metabolic stability and diminished immunogenicity compared to the unmodified molecule. Polyethylene glycol chains are often employed as a distribution of related lengths grafted indiscriminately on various residues [24,25]. Successful examples on which polyethylene glycol grafts enhanced potency and duration of action of larger proteins include Pegasys© for hepatitis C [26] and Pegvisomant for the treatment of acromegaly (Somavert©) [27]. Moreover, modification of the glucagon-like peptide 1 (GLP-1)-based drug Liraglutide®, which features a C16 lipid chain responsible, in part, for its longer duration of action, by adding a PEG-like spacer gave Semaglutide®, which can be administered once weekly and is used in the treatment of type 2 diabetes and obesity [28,29]. Lipid attachment has also been used to improve metabolic stability and lipophilicity [30,31] to enhance the stability of larger peptides, as well as to improve their specificity and association with membranes [32]. Lipopeptide natural products, such as daptomycin and related antibiotics have exhibited promising activity against Gram-positive pathogens [33]. Lipid conjugation has also been applied to smaller peptides. For example, Hruby and co-workers have attached hexanoyl and decanoyl chains onto α-Melanocyte Stimulating Hormone (αMSH) [34] analogs to obtain equipotent conjugates with prolonged duration of action [31,35]. In contrast, longer chains (palmitic and myristic acids) resulted in less potent molecules, probably because of the increased lipophilicity [31,35]. Peptide-based vaccines have been created with lipid components that act as adjuvants [36]. Amphiphiles, peptides bearing both a hydrophobic lipid chain and a charged moiety have been showed to aggregate in liposomes that can act as carriers for targeted drug delivery [37,38]. The strategy called reversible aqueous lipidation (REAL) has been used to improve the bioavailability of prodrugs that release the active molecule in the organism and applied to facilitate oral delivery of small peptides [30]. Metabolic stability and membrane permeability were improved by acylation of small peptides with a palmitoyl chain that facilitated anchoring in membranes and may enhance peptide folding [39].

Prenylation is an important post-translational protein and peptide modification, which enhances typically cell membrane association [40–43]. Farnesyl transferase enzymes introduce farnesyl subunits that may serve to anchor the modified protein or peptide in the membrane. Disruption of prenylation has been suggested to play an important role in cancer because of the significance of membrane-associated proteins in the cellular life cycle [44]. Prenylation by prenyl transferases of small molecules, such as prenylflavonoids may also influence biological effects by favoring membrane association [45].

Seeking to improve the pharmacokinetic properties of L-PDC31, a variety of analogs were developed. Different *N*-alkyl terminal grafts were introduced by solid phase methods featuring reductive amination and sulfonamide alkylation. Among the analogs evaluated in a murine ex vivo myometrium contraction assay, the best was selected for study in a mouse serum stability test and in an in vivo PTB model.

2. Results

2.1. Chemistry

The influence of the different hydrophobic chains was initially evaluated by a computational model in which logP values were predicted using the HyperChem software [46,47] and compared with PDC-31 (Figure 1). Small PEG chains of 4 to 16 atoms had limited impact and lowered the logP of the peptide analogs. Alternatively, the addition of *n*-alkyl chains caused a notable increase with a nearly linear correlation in log P with increasing carbon length.

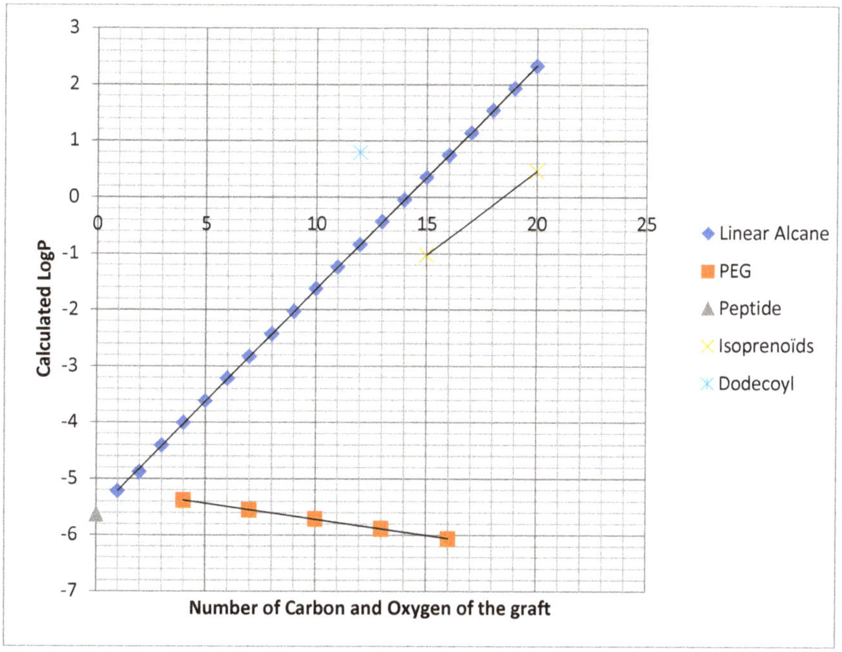

Figure 1. *c*LogP of L-PDC31 analogs relative to the number of heavy atoms present in their grafts.

The branched prenyl group increased logP with the effect appearing to be related to the longest linear chain. For example, the 15-carbon farnesyl chain produced a peptide derivative that was predicted to have a logP as that of the peptide possessing a linear 12-carbon alkyl chain. Similarly, the branched 20-carbon geranyl-geranyl group exhibited a logP lower than its 16-carbon linear alkyl chain equivalent.

Based on the above predictions, a set of analogs of the L-peptide variant of PDC31 were targeted possessing *N*-terminal chains consisting of 6-, 11-, 12-, 13- and 18-carbon linear alkyl, tetra-ethylene glycol [48] and farnesyl groups. In addition, *N*-dodeconyl-L-PDC31 (**8**) was synthesized as an acyl control using lauric acid.

Linear sequences of L- and D-PDC31 linked to 2-chlorotrityl resin (L- and D-**1**) were obtained by solid phase peptide synthesis using standard Fmoc/t-Bu protocols [49]. Peptide resin L-**1** was treated with the appropriate aldehyde **2** (Scheme 1). The imine resin was washed to remove excess aldehyde, and reductive amination was performed using sodium cyanoborohydride to provide secondary amine resin **3**. Removal of the protecting groups and resin cleavage were achieved using a cocktail of 95:2.5:2.5 TFA:TES:H_2O to provide *N*-alkyl- and *N*-PEG-grafted peptides **4**, which were purified by RP-HPLC (Table 1). Except for peptide **4e**, bearing the 18-carbon alkyl chain, peptides **4** were all soluble in water. Peptide **4f** required a small amount of DMSO to completely dissolve. An inseparable mixture of mono- and bis-*N*-alkyl peptides was isolated by HPLC from reaction with aldehyde of shorter chain length.

Farnesyl peptide **7** was synthesized by a route featuring sulfonylation followed by alkylation with farnesol under Mitsunobu conditions. Resin L-**1** was swollen in DMF and reacted with *ortho*-nitrobenzenesulfonyl (*o*NBS) chloride and di-*iso*-propylethylamine (Scheme 2). With the *o*NBS group installed, sulfonamide resin **5** was treated with di-*iso*-propyl azodicarboxylate (DIAD), triphenylphosphine and farnesol. *N*-Farnesyl peptide resin **6** was provided in 55% conversion as demonstrated by LC-MS analysis of material after resin cleavage [50–53]. The *o*NBS group was removed by treatment with thiophenol and DBU in DMF [52]. *N*-Farnesyl peptide resin **6** was cleaved with concomitant removal of the side chain protection using a cocktail of 95:2.5:2.5 TFA:TES:H_2O. Purification by RP-HPLC and freeze-drying of the collected fractions gave *N*-farnesyl peptide **7** as white powder, which was soluble in water (Table 1).

Finally, *N*-dodecoyl-L-PDC31 (**8**) was synthesized from resin L-**1** by coupling with lauric acid using HBTU and DIEA, resin cleavage and removal of side chain protection as described above. Purification by RP-HPLC gave **8** as white powder after freeze-drying (Table 1). The poor solubility of *N*-dodecoyl-L-PDC31 (**8**) necessitated dissolving in 0.1 N HCl and freeze-drying to give the hydrochloride salt as white powder that dissolved readily in water.

Among the peptides synthesized, only peptides **4f** and **8** displayed aqueous solubility issues, which were in agreement with their calculated >0 *c*LogP values (Figure 1). Increased lipophilic character may promote peptide aggregation and decrease solubility in aqueous solvent. The potential to aggregate may increase due to the amphiphilic character of the *N*-alkyl PDC-31 analogs which possess hydrophobic and charged residues respectively at the *N*- and *C*-terminals. For biological assays, solubility issues were surmounted by forming salts and using small amounts of DMSO. The influence of their amphiphilic character during purification by RP-HPLC and double alkylation from the reductive amination sequence may account for the lower isolated yields of peptides **4**, **7** and **8**.

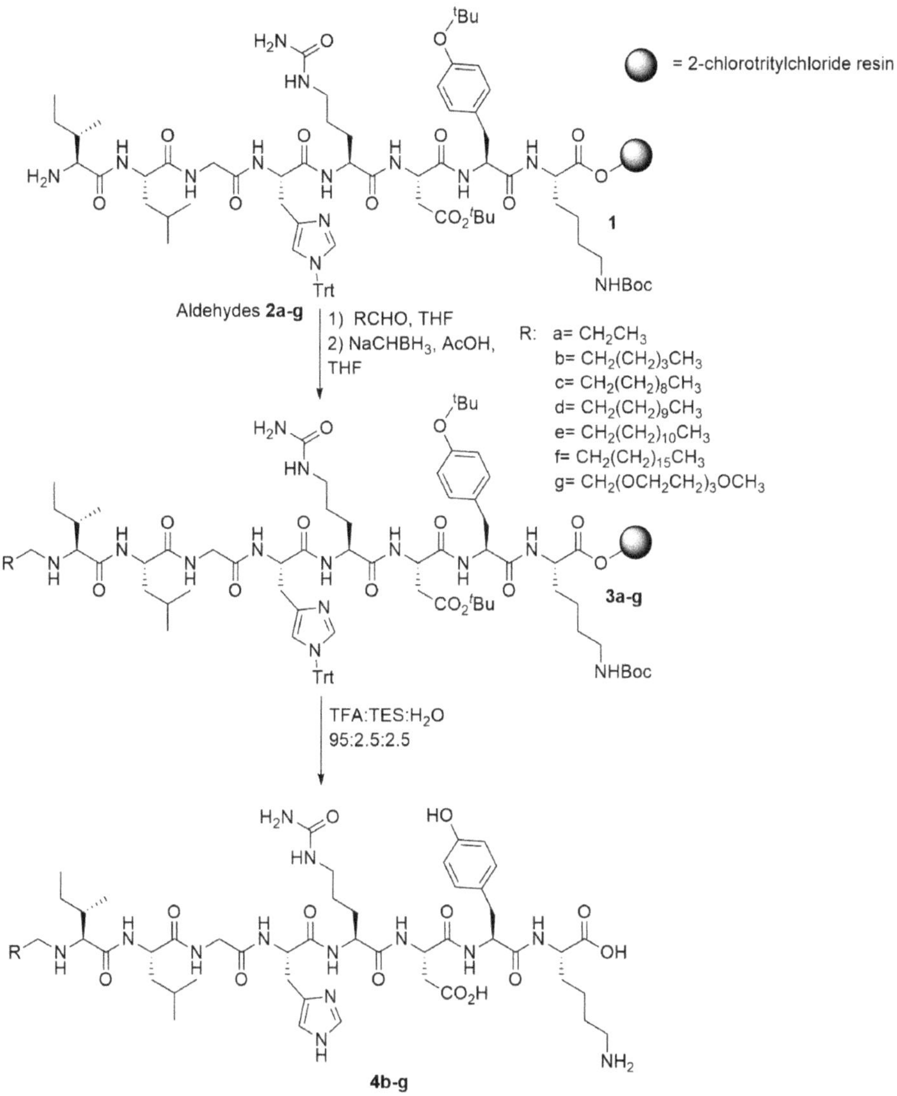

Scheme 1. Synthesis of peptides L–**4b**–**4g**.

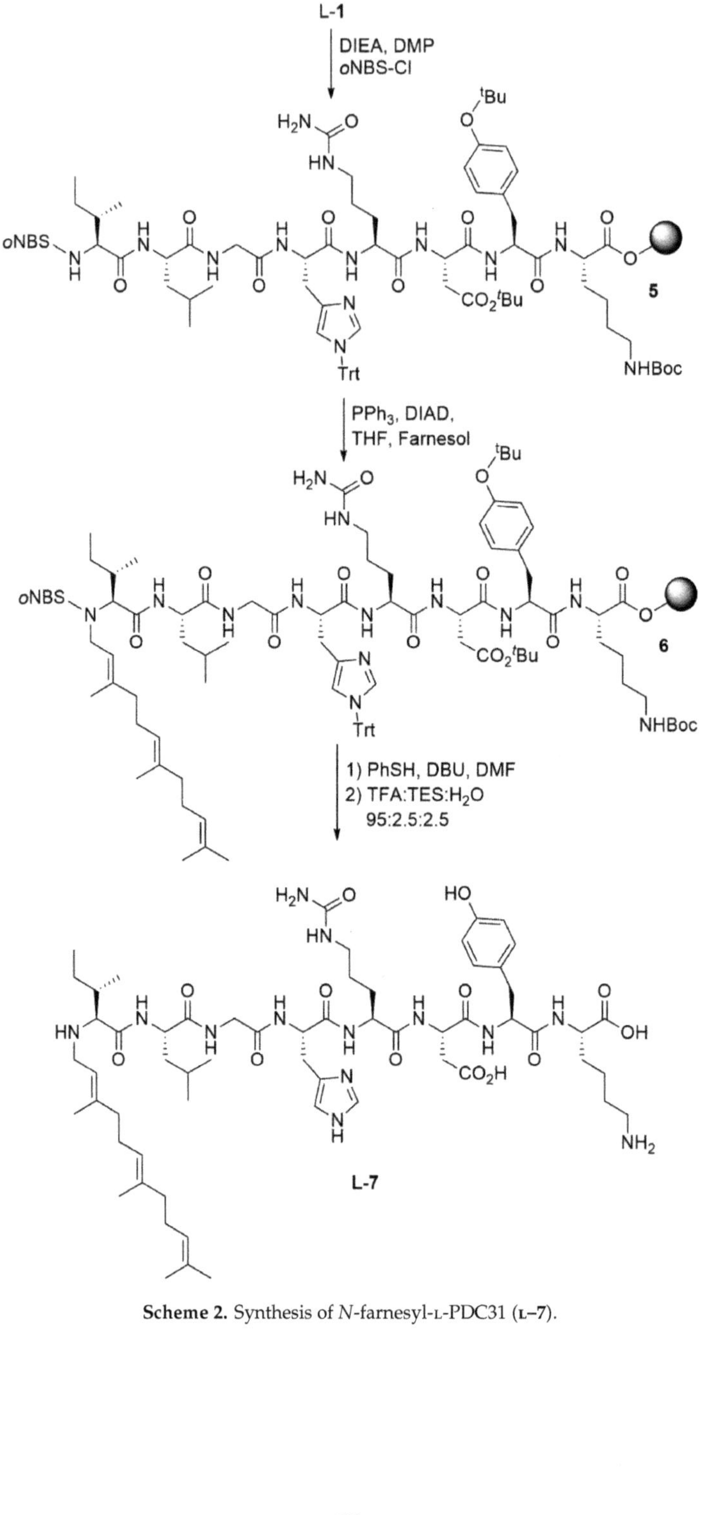

Scheme 2. Synthesis of *N*-farnesyl-L-PDC31 (L–7).

Table 1. Retention time, purity, exact mass and overall yield of peptides **4b–4g**, **7** and **8**.

Peptide	R-ILGHCitDYK R =	Retentin Time MeCN (min)	Retentin Time MeOH (min)	Purity (%)	[M + H]+ Calc.	[M + H]+ Found	TotalYield (%)
L-PDC31	H-	10.8 [a]	9.9 [b]	>97	1002.5367	1002.5366	7.7
4b	$H_3C(CH_2)_5$-	9.8 [a]	9.7 [b]	>92	1086.6306	1086.633	0.3
4c	$H_3C(CH_2)_{10}$-	11.1 [a]	11.9 [b]	>89	1158.7089	1158.7034	1.4
L-4d	$H_3C(CH_2)_{11}$-	12.6 [c]	13.4 [d]	>95	1170.7245	1170.7251	0.7
D -4d	$H_3C(CH_2)_{11}$-	13.0 [a]	13.1 [b]	>94	1170.7245	1170.7238	1.2
4e	$H_3C(CH_2)_{12}$-	13.9 [a]	14.2 [b]	>99	1184.7402	1084.7387	0.4
4f	$H_3C(CH_2)_{15}$-	15.0 [a]	15.1 [b]	>94	627.9128 ($[M + 2H]^{2+}$)	627.9105 ($[M + 2H]^{2+}$)	0.3
4g	$H_3C[O(CH_2)_2]_4$-	10.0 [a]	9.6 [b]	>86	1192.6572	1192.6605	2.9
7	Farnesyl-	10.0 [a]	13.3 [b]	>89	1206.7245	1206.7263	2.5
8	$H_3C(CH_2)_{10}CO$-	7.1[c]	10.2 [d]	>99	1184.7038	1184.7061	15.0

[a] Polar-RP, 5–50% MeCN with 0.1% formic acid (FA) in water (0.1% FA) over 20 min at 0.5 mL/min. [b] Polar-RP 30–90% MeOH (0.1% FA) in water (0.1% FA) over 20 min at 0.5mL/min. [c] C_{18}, 10–90% MeCN (0.1% FA) in water (0.1% FA) over 15 min at 0.5 mL/min. [d] C_{18}, 10–90% MeOH (0.1% FA) in water (0.1% FA) over 15 min at 0.5 mL/min.

2.2. Biology

All the peptides were initially tested in an ex vivo mouse myometrial tissue contraction assay. Contractile activity was measured on tissue that was harvested post-partum and treated with prostaglandin $F_{2\alpha}$ (PGF_{α}) alone (control) or in the presence of peptides L-**4b-4g**, L-**7**, and L-**8**. Among all the peptides tested, only *N*-dodecyl-L-PDC31 (L-**4d**) exhibited a significant reduction of contractions (Figure 2). Peptides D-**4d**, L-**4b** and L-**4f**, all exhibited trends suggesting protective effects against $PGF_{2\alpha}$-induced contractions. Mean tension induced by KCl (as a positive control) was not affected by L-**4d**.

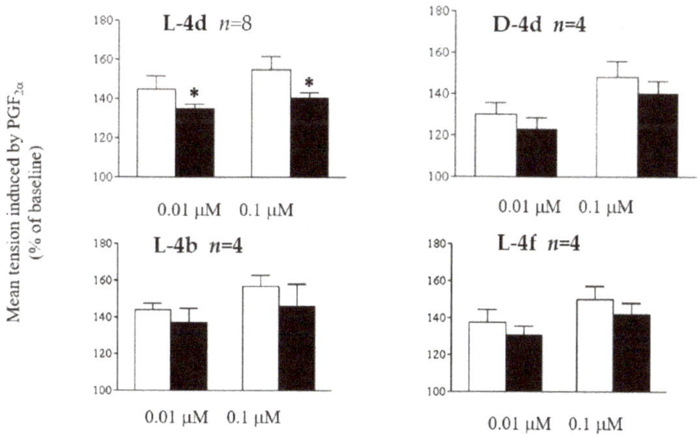

Figure 2. Mean tension induced by PGF_{α} on murine myometrial tissue alone (white bar) and in the presence of peptide at two different concentrations. * $p < 0.05$ compared with vehicle-treated.

Peptide L-**4d** was further examined for stability in serum and compared to L-PDC31. The two peptides were incubated at 37 °C in mouse plasma. Aliquots were removed at different time intervals and analyzed by mass spectrometry (MS/MS) to detect remaining amount of peptide (Figure 3). Although L-PDC31 was completely degraded within 5 minutes, the *N*-alkylated peptide L-**4d** exhibited a half-life of about 30 minutes and was still present after 2 hours of incubation. The *N*-dodecyl group substantially improved the stability of the peptide in plasma, likely by conferring resistance to proteolysis.

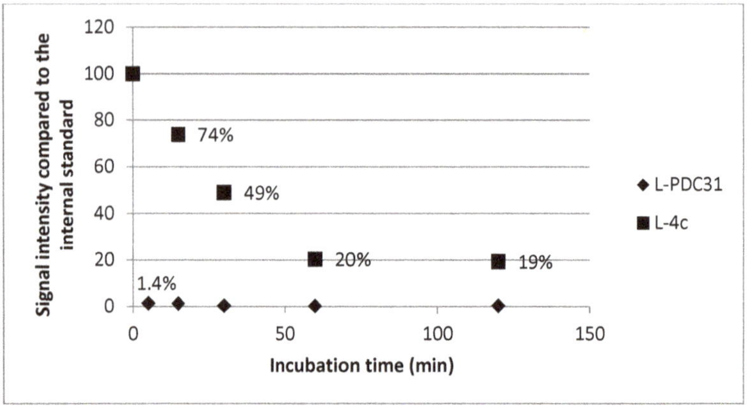

Figure 3. Intensity of MS signal of L-PDC31 and L-**4d** compared to the internal standard **L-4f** as a function of incubation time in mouse plasma.

The ability of peptide L-**4d** to delay labor in vivo was next tested in mice near term and treated with lipopolysaccharide (LPS) *Escherichia coli* endotoxin, as a pathogen associated molecular pattern, which is known to promote a general inflammatory state resulting in prostaglandin synthesis and induced premature delivery. Following LPS injection into mice (n = 4–5) at gestational day 16, all the animals tested delivered within 12–24 h. In contrast to PDC-31 and small molecule mimics, which have previously been shown to delay labor in the PTB model [54–56], L-**4d** was unable to exhibit a statistically significant reduction in the time of delivery (Figure 4).

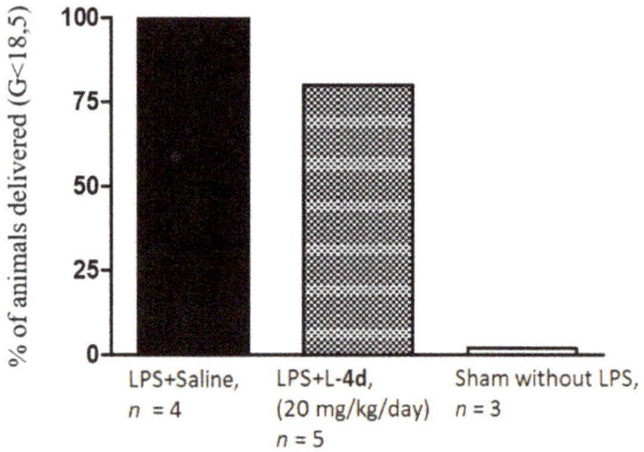

Figure 4. In LPS-induced mouse PTB assay, peptide L-**4d** exhibited no significant ability to delay labor.

3. Discussion

The D-peptide PDC-31 was previously shown to reduce both the strength and length of spontaneous and PGF2α-induced contractions in postpartum mice myometrium [18]. Examination of peptide conjugates L-**4b-g**, L-**7** and L-**8** for ability to inhibit PGF2α-induced contractions in the same assay demonstrated that *N*-dodecyl peptide L-**4d** was able to reduce uterine contractions induced by PGF2α in mice myometrial tissue [57]. Moreover, addition of the dodecyl chain enhanced plasma stability. In contrast, the parent L-peptide, L-PDC-31, did not show any inhibitory activity against PGF2α-induced contractions and was rapidly degraded in plasma. Myometrial tissue is rich in proteases [58], which may degrade and render the linear L-peptide inactive. The related *N*-hexanyl and *N*-octadecanyl peptides L-**4b** and L-**4f** exhibited trends in the myometrium contraction assay which may suggest an inhibitory potential, but the results were not statistically significant (Figure 2). Octadecanyl peptide **4f** was poorly soluble in water and needed slight amounts of DMSO to be tested, which, in turn, could explain the poor activity in the ex vivo assay. Neither PEGylated peptide L-**4g** nor *N*-farnesyl peptide L-**7** exhibited activity. Similarly, *N*-dodecanoyl peptide L-**8** and its HCl salt were both inactive. The latter result was consistent with the inactivity of *N*-acetyl-PDC31 [19] and highlighted the importance of a basic amine terminal for peptide activity.

In addition to *N*-alkylation rendering the L-peptide more stable to degradation in plasma, the lipid chain may compliment the hydrophobic (Ile-Leu-Gly) *N*-terminus to anchor the peptide in cell membranes and enhance activity and affinity for the membrane-bound receptor. To explore the latter hypothesis, the dodecyl chain was added onto PDC-31 to give D-**4d**. Although it exhibited a tendency similar to the activity of L-**4d**, D-**4d** affected myometrial contraction with a lower potency than the unmodified D-peptide, PDC-31 [18]. Thus, the alkyl chain appears to interfere with receptor binding [18] and likely exhibits its effect by enhancing resistance to proteolytic degradation.

Although activity was maintained and plasma stability was improved by the addition of a dodecyl chain to L-PDC-31, L-**4d** failed to prolong labor in vivo in the LPS-induced mouse model. The high lipophilicity of the dodecyl chain may inhibit delivery to the target receptor; instead, L-**4d** may be trapped in adipose tissue or cellular membranes, an effect that has been reported in other lipid-peptide conjugates [59].

4. Materials and Methods

4.1. General

Unless otherwise noted, synthetic grade reagents were obtained from commercial sources and used without further purification. Anhydrous solvents (THF, DMF and DCM) were obtained by passage through solvent filtration systems (GlassContour, Irvine, CA). Solution phase reactions were performed under argon atmosphere. Dodecanal and farnesol were purchased from commercial sources and used without further purification. Hexanal [60], undecanal [61], tridecanal [62], octadecanal [63], and 2,5,8,11-tetraoxatridecan-13-al [64] all were obtained by oxidation of the corresponding primary alcohol and exhibited characterization consistent with the published literature. Final purity assessments were made based on an analytical RP-HPLC-MS system from Agilent Technologies Inc. (Santa Clara, CA, USA) using the following columns and conditions: Phenomenex Synergi Polar-RP (Phenomenex, Torrance, CA, USA), 4,6 mm × 150 mm, 4 µm, UV detection (Agilent Technologies Inc., Santa Clara, CA, USA) at 250 nm or 280 nm, 5–50% MeCN with 0.1% formic acid (FA) in water (0.1% FA) over 20 min at 0.5 mL/min, or 30–90% MeOH (0.1% FA) in water (0.1% FA) over 20 min at 0.5 mL/min; Phenomenex C18 4.6 mm × 50 mm, 4 µM, UV detection at 280 nm, 10–90% MeCN (0.1% FA) in water (0.1% FA) over 15 min at 0.5 mL/min, or 10–90% MeOH (0.1% FA) in water (0.1% FA) over 15 min at 0.5 mL/min. Analytical RP-HPLC (Agilent Technologies Inc., Santa Clara, CA, USA) was performed on a Phenomenex SunFire C18 column, 2.1 × 50 mm, 3.5 um, with UV detection at 254 or 280 nm, using a gradient of 10–90% water (0.1% FA) in acetonitrile (0.1% FA) over 10 minutes at 0.35 mL/min. Accurate mass measurements were performed on a LC-MS-TOF instrument from Agilent Technologies Inc. (Santa Clara, CA, USA) using the positive electrospray mode for high resolution MS (HRMS) analysis, which was performed at the Centre regional de spectrométrie de masse de l'Université de Montréal (Montréal, PQ, Canada). Protonated ions $[M + H]^+$ were used for empirical formula confirmation.

4.2. Chemistry

4.2.1. Resin Loading and Capping

2-Chlorotrityl chloride resin (GLS Biochem, 1g, 0.8 mmol) swollen in DMF was treated with Fmoc-L-Lys(Boc)-OH (1.124 g, 2.4 mmol), HBTU (910 mg, 2.4 mmol) and diisopropyl ethylamine (835 µL, 4.8 mmol) in 10 mL of DMF. The reaction mixture was agitated on an orbital shaker for 3 h, the resin was filtered, and the coupling was repeated. The resin was filtered and washed with DMF (3 × 15 mL), isopropyl alcohol (3 × 15 mL) and DCM (3 × 15 mL). The resin was swollen in DMF (25 mL), treated with diisopropyl ethylamine (835 μL, 4.8 mmol) in 10 mL methanol, and agitated for 2 h. The resin was filtered, washed with DMF (3 × 15 mL), isopropyl alcohol (3 × 15 mL) and DCM (3 × 15 mL) and dried under vacuum. The efficiency of the coupling was determined after Fmoc removal and analysis of the dibenzofulvene adduct using UV analysis [65].

4.2.2. Automated Peptide Synthesis

Peptide synthesis was performed using a CEM Liberty microwave peptide synthesizer (CEM, Matthews, NC, USA), employing the following protected amino acids: Fmoc-Lys(Boc)-OH, Fmoc-Tyr(^{t}Bu)-OH, Fmoc-Asp(^{t}Bu)-OH, Fmoc-Cit-OH, Fmoc-His(Tr)-OH, Fmoc-Gly-OH, Fmoc-Leu-OH, and Fmoc-Ile-OH. The Fmoc group was removed by using two treatments with 20% piperidine in DMF with microwave irradiation at 75 °C (35W) at first for 30 sec, and then for 180 sec in the second treatment. After the resin was washed (4 × 25 mL DMF), couplings were performed in DMF with N^{α}-Fmoc amino acid (300 mol%, 0.2 M), HBTU (300 mol%, 0.5 M) and DIEA (600 mol%, 2 M). Typically, the N^{α}-Fmoc amino acid solution (30 mL, 6 mmol) was added to the resin, followed by the HBTU (12 mL, 6 mmol) and DIEA (6 mL, 12 mmol) solutions. For all the amino acids except histidine, the coupling cycle was performed with irradiation at 75 °C (25W) for 300 sec. In the case of histidine, the coupling cycle was performed without irradiation initially at 50 °C for 120 sec, followed by irradiation at 50 °C (25W) for 240 sec. The resin was washed (3 × 25 mL DMF) prior to each coupling step. All the residues were coupled using a single reaction cycle. Upon completion of the sequence, the resin was washed with 10 mL of DCM and transferred to the receiving flask using 3 × 10 mL volumes of DCM. The final Fmoc group removal was done manually by swelling the resin in a solution of 20% piperidine in DMF (25 mL) and agitating for 30 min. The resin was filtered and washed with DMF (3 × 25 mL), isopropanol (3 × 25 mL), dichloromethane (3 × 25 mL) and ethyl ether (1 × 30 mL), dried under vacuum and stored at −20 °C.

4.2.3. Peptide Cleavage and Purification

After removal of the terminal Fmoc group as described above, the resin was treated with a cleavage cocktail of TFA:TES:H_2O (95:2,5:2,5) for 2 h and filtered. The resin was washed once with TFA and once with DCM. The washing and filtrate were combined and evaporated to an oil, which was washed with cold ether and purified by RP-HPLC using a Synergi RP-Polar C18, 150 mm × 21.2 mm column, 10 mL/min flow rate, detection at 254 nm or 280 nm, and 5–90% MeCN (0.1% FA) in water (0.1% FA) as eluent over 40 min. Collected fractions were freeze-dried to afford pure peptides (Table 1).

H-Ile-Leu-Gly-His-Cit-Asp-Tyr-Lys-OH (L-**PDC31**): Resin L-**1** (221 mg, 0.07 mmol) was agitated with a mixture of 15 mL of TFA:TES:H_2O (95:2.5:2.5) for 2 h, filtered and washed with TFA (1 × 5 mL) and DCM (1 × 5 mL). The filtrate and washings were combined and evaporated to an oil, which was washed with cold ether and purified by RP-HPLC using 5–50% MeCN (0.1% FA) in H_2O (0.1% FA). Free-drying of the collected fractions gave L-**PDC31** as white solid (5 mg).

N-Hexanyl-Ile-Leu-Gly-His-Cit-Asp-Tyr-Lys-OH (L-**4b**): A dry sample of 912 mg (0.3 mmol) of Ile-Leu-Gly-His(Tr)-Cit-Asp(tBu)-Tyr(tBu)-Lys(Boc) resin L-**1** in a plastic syringe tube equipped with Teflon™ filter, stopcock and stopper was swollen in THF (15 mL) and treated with hexanal (613 mg, 6 mmol) agitated on an orbital shaker for 18 h at room temperature, filtered and washed with DMF (3 × 15 mL), dichloromethane (3 × 15 mL) and THF (1 × 20 mL). The resin was swollen in THF (15 mL), treated with sodium cyanoborohydride (150 mg, 2.4 mmol), agitated on an orbital shaker for 18 h, filtered and washed with DMF (3 × 15 mL), isopropanol (3 × 15 mL) and dichloromethane (3 × 15 mL). The resin was exposed to a mixture of TFA:TES:H_2O (95:2.5:2.5), stirred for 2 h, filtered and washed with TFA (1 × 5 mL) and DCM (1 × 5 mL). The filtrate and washing were combined, evaporated to a residue, which was washed with cold ether and purified by RP-HPLC using 5–50% MeCN (0.1%

FA)/H_2O (0.1% FA). Freeze drying of the collected fractions gave *n*-hexyl peptide L-**4b** as a white solid (1 mg).

N-Undecanyl-Ile-Leu-Gly-His-Cit-Asp-Tyr-Lys-OH (L-**4c**): The protocol for the synthesis of hexanyl peptide L-**4b** described above was adapted for undecanal. The obtained oil was purified by RP-HPLC using 5–50% MeCN (0.1% FA)/H_2O (0.1% FA). Freeze-drying of the collected fractions gave L-**4c** as white solid (8 mg).

N-Dodecyl-Ile-Leu-Gly-His-Cit-Asp-Tyr-Lys-OH (L-**4d**): The protocol for the synthesis of hexanyl peptide L-**4b** described above was adapted for dodecanal. The obtained oil was purified by RP-HPLC using 5–50% MeCN (0.1% FA)/H_2O (0.1% FA). Freeze-drying of the collected fractions gave L-**4d** as white solid (2 mg).

N-Dodecyl-D-Ile-D-Leu-Gly-D-His-D-Cit-D-Asp-D-Tyr- D-Lys-OH (D-**4d**): The protocol for the synthesis of hexanyl peptide L-**4b** described above was adapted for dodecanal on H- D -Ile- D -Leu-Gly- D -His(Tr)- D -Cit-D-Asp(tBu)-D-Tyr(tBu)- D -Lys(Boc) resin **D-1**. The oil was purified by RP-HPLC using 5–50% MeCN (0.1% FA)/H_2O (0.1% FA). Freeze-drying of the collected fractions provided D-**4d** as a white solid (4 mg).

N-Tridecanyl-Ile-Leu-Gly-His-Cit-Asp-Tyr-Lys-OH (L-**4e**): The protocol for the synthesis of hexanyl peptide L-**4b** described above was adapted for tridecanal. The oil was purified by RP-HPLC using 5–50% MeCN (0.1%FA)/H_2O (0.1% FA). Freeze-drying of the collected fractions gave octadecanyl peptide L-**4e** as white solid (3 mg).

N-Octadecanyl-Ile-Leu-Gly-His-Cit-Asp-Tyr-Lys-OH (L-**4f**): The protocol for the synthesis of hexanyl peptide L-**4b** described above was adapted for octadecanal. The oil was purified by RP-HPLC using 5–50% MeCN (0.1%FA)/H_2O (0.1% FA). Freeze-drying of the collected fractions gave octadecanyl peptide L -**4f** as white solid (1 mg).

N-2,7,8,11-tetraoxytetradecane-Ile-Leu-Gly-His-Cit-Asp-Tyr-Lys-OH (L-**4g**): The protocol for the synthesis of hexanyl peptide L-**4b** described above was adapted for 2,5,8,11-tetraoxatridecan-13-al. The resulting oil was purified by RP-HPLC (5–50% MeCN (0.1% FA)/H_2O + 0.1% FA). Freeze-drying of the collected fractions gave L-**4g** as white solid (10 mg).

N-o-Nitrophenylsulfonyl-Ile-Leu-Gly-His(Tr)-Cit-Asp(tBu)-Tyr(tBu)-Lys(Boc) Resin **5**: Resin L-**1** (917 mg, 0.3 mmol) was swollen in DMF, treated with diisopropyl ethylamine (0.742 µL, 1.68 mmol) and 2-nitrobenzenesulfonyl chloride (190 mg, 0.85 mmol) in 10 mL of DMF, agitated on an orbital shaker for 48 h at room temperature, filtered, and washed with DMF (3 × 15 mL), isopropyl alcohol (3 × 15 mL) and DCM (3 × 15 mL). An aliquot of resin was cleaved with 1 mL of a cocktail of TFA:TES:H_2O (95:2.5:2.5), filtered and evaporated to a residue that was examined by LC-MS analysis, which showed complete conversion [Rt = 4.33 min, C_{18}, 10–90% MeCN (0.1% FA) in water (0.1% FA) over 15 min at 0.5 mL/min.]; *m*/*z* = $[M]^+$ 1187.5. The resin was used in the next step without further treatment.

N-o-(NBS)-N-farnesyl-Ile-Leu-Gly-His(Tr)-Cit-Asp(tBu)-Tyr(tBu)-Lys(Boc) Resin **6**: The Mitsunobu reaction was performed using conditions previously reported. [53a] In brief, resin **5** (0.3 mmol) was swollen in THF, treated with triphenylphosphine (441 mg, 1.68 mmol) and diisopropyl azodicarboxylate (DIAD, 330 µL, 1.68 mmol) in 10 mL of THF, agitated for 10 min on an orbital shaker, treated with farnesol (420 µL, 1.68 mmol) and agitated at room temperature for 48 h. The resin was washed with DMF (3 × 15 mL), isopropanol (3 × 15 mL) and DCM (3 × 15 mL). An aliquot of resin was cleaved with 1 mL of a cocktail of TFA:TES:H_2O (95:2.5:2.5), filtered and evaporated to a residue, that was examined by LC-MS analysis, which showed 65% conversion [Rt = 5.68 min, C_{18}, 10–90% MeCN (0.1% FA) in water (0.1% FA) over 15 min at 0.5 mL/min]; *m*/*z* = $[M + 2H]^{2+}$ 696.5. The resin was used in the next step without further purification.

N-Farnesyl-Ile-Leu-Gly-His-Cit-Asp-Tyr-Lys-OH (L-**7**): Resin 6 was swollen in 15 mL of DMF, treated with thiophenol (300 μL, 2.93 mmol) and DBU (500 μL, 3.34 mmol), agitated on an orbital shaker for 6 h, filtered and washed with DMF (3 × 15 mL), isopropanol (3 × 15 mL) and DCM (3 × 15 mL). The resin was treated with 10 mL of a cocktail of TFA:TES:H_2O (95:2.5:2.5), agitated for 2 h, filtered, and washed with TFA (1 × 5 mL) and DCM (1 × 5 mL). The filtrate and washings were combined and evaporated to an oil, which was washed with cold ether and purified by RP-HPLC using 5–50% MeCN (0.1% FA)/H_2O (0.1% FA). Freeze-drying of the collected fractions provided farnesyl peptide L-**7** as white solid (9 mg).

N-Dodecanoyl-Ile-Leu-Gly-His-Cit-Asp-Tyr-Lys-OH (L-**8**): A dry sample of resin L-**1** (3.04 g, 1 mmol) was swollen in THF (15 mL) in a plastic syringe tube equipped with Teflon™ filter, stopcock and stopper, and treated with lauric acid (613 mg, 3 mmol), DIEA (1.05 mL, 6 mmol) and HBTU (1.14 g, 3mmol), agitated on an orbital shaker for 3 h at room temperature, filtered and washed with DMF (3 × 25 mL), isopropanol (3 × 25 mL), dichloromethane (3 × 25 mL) and THF (1 × 30 mL). The resin was exposed to a mixture of TFA:TES:H_2O (95:2.5:2.5), stirred for 2h, filtered and washed with TFA (1 × 10 mL) and DCM (1 × 10 mL). The filtrate and washing were combined, evaporated to a residue, which was washed with cold ether, and purified by RP-HPLC using 5–50% MeCN (0.1% FA)/H_2O (0.1% FA). Freeze drying of the collected fractions gave L-**8** as a white solid (159 mg).

4.3. Biology

4.3.1. Serum Stability Study

Serum was warmed and kept on ice throughout the procedure. Two blanks were prepared by adding 5 μL of DMSO to 95 μL of serum. These were incubated for 2 h and submitted to the same treatment as the other samples. Two series of vials containing 95 μL of serum were prepared and spiked with either 5 μL of L-**PDC31** [0.4 mM] or L-**4d** [0.4 mM], and incubated for 120, 60, 30, 15, 10 and 5 min, respectively, after which 100 μL of 4% phosphoric acid was added. Two vials were also spiked with 5 μL L-PDC31 and L-**4d**, respectively, and immediately treated with phosphoric acid (time = 0 min). The vials were incubated for 5 min at 95 °C, cooled on ice for 2 min, treated with 600 μL of cold MeCN containing L-**4f** (0.02 mM) as internal standard, and incubated at −20 °C overnight. After the incubation period, the vials were vortexed for 2 min and centrifuged at 4 °C for 15 min. The supernatant was transferred into LC-MS vials and analyzed.

Results were expressed as: $\left(\frac{\frac{AN}{IS}}{\frac{AN_0}{IS_0}}\right) * 100$

AN and IS refer, respectively, to the analyte and internal standard MS signals. Both values are compared with initial injection at which time AN_0 and IS_0 were not incubated.

4.3.2. Ex Vivo Study

Pregnant CD-1 mice (16-17 days gestation, term 19 days) were obtained from Charles River Inc. and used according to a protocol of the Animal Care Committee of Hôpital Sainte-Justine according to the principles of the Guide for the Care and Use of Experimental Animals of the Canadian Council on Animal Care. The animals were maintained on standard laboratory chow under a 12:12 light:dark cycle and allowed free access to chow and water.

The uterus from the CD-1 mouse was obtained from the animal immediately after term delivery under anesthesia (2.5% isoflurane). Briefly, a midline abdominal incision was made and the uterine horns were rapidly excised, cleansed carefully of the surrounding connective tissues, and removed. Longitudinal myometrial strips (2 to 3 mm wide and 1 cm long) were dissected free from the uterus and mounted isometrically in organ tissue baths. The initial tension was set at 2 g. The tissue baths contained 20 mL of Krebs buffer of the following composition (in mM): 118 NaCl, 4.7 KCl, 2.5 $CaCl_2$, 0.9 $MgSO_4$, 1 KH_2PO_4, 11.1 glucose, and 23 $NaHCO_3$ (pH 7.4). The buffer was equilibrated with 95% oxygen/5% carbon dioxide at 37 °C. Isometric tension was measured by a force transducer and recorded by a BIOPAC data acquisition system (BIOPAC MP150, Montreal, PQ, Canada). Experiments were begun after 1 h equilibration. Mean tension of spontaneous contractions was measured using a BIOPAC digital polygraph system (AcqKnowledge); the same parameters were also determined after addition of $PGF_{2\alpha}$ in the presence or the absence of a 20 min-pretreatment with different FP inhibitors. At the start of each experiment, mean tension of spontaneous myometrial contractions was considered as a reference response. Changes in mean tension (g) were expressed as percentages of the initial reference response (% of baseline).

At the start of each experiments, mean tension of spontaneous myometrial contractions was considered as a reference response. Increase in mean tension (%) was expressed as percentages of (X/Y)-100, where X is the change in mean tension (g) induced by $PGF_{2\alpha}$ and Y is the initial reference response (g). Data are representative of 4–6 experiments per treated group. All results are expressed as means ± SEM and were compared by Independent *t*-tests. Statistical tests were performed with GraphPad Prism 4.3 software and $p < 0.05$ was considered statistically significant.

4.3.3. In Vivo Study

Timed-pregnant CD-1 mice at 16 days gestation (normal term is 19.2 days) were anesthetized with isoflurane (2%). Primed osmotic pumps (Alzet pump, Alzet, Cupertino, CA) containing either saline ($n = 4$) or compound L-**4d** (20 mg/day/animal, $n = 5$) were respectively subcutaneously implanted on the backs of the animals; infusion of peptide was immediately preceded by bolus injection of peptide (0.1 mg/animal intraperitoneally). Within 15 min after placement of the pumps, animals were injected with lipopolysaccharide (LPS) *Escherichia coli* endotoxin (10 μg/animal intraperitoneally) to mimic the inflammatory/infectious component of human preterm labor. Animals were inspected every hour for the first 18 h and every 2 h thereafter to document the timing of birth. Results are expressed as percentages of animals delivered following the injection of LPS [57]. All the experiments were approved by the Animal Care Committee of Centre Hospitalier Universitaire Sainte-Justine (Montreal, QC, Canada).

5. Conclusions

Herein, we report effective solid-phase methods for installing alkyl, PEG, farnesyl and alkanoyl *N*-terminal grafts onto small peptides. Evaluation of the peptide derivatives ex vivo has identified that *N*-dodecyl peptide L-**4d** exhibited a significant reduction of PGF2α-induced contractility in post-partum ex vivo assay versus vehicle. Moreover, in mouse plasma, the dodecyl chain prolonged stability of L-**4d** due likely to a protective effect against proteases. Although the strategy proved successful ex vivo and *in vitro*, *N*-dodecyl peptide L-**4d** was inactive in vivo when given by subcutaneous injection to induced mice. Considering the proof that L-PDC31 can exhibit activity when conjugated to a dodecyl chain, further research is merited to study alternative means of administration and conjugation towards the development of a cost-effective tocolytic agent for treating preterm labor.

Author Contributions: Conceptualization, J.P., S.C. and W.D.L.; peptide synthesis, *c*LogP compilation, and stability study, J.P.; ex vivo and in vivo study, X.H.; manuscript writing, J.P.; manuscript revision, W.D.L.; supervision and funding acquisition, S.C. and W.D.L.

Funding: Natural Sciences and Engineering Research Council of Canada (NSERC) Discovery Research Project #04079, and for the Canadian Institutes of Health Research (CIHR) and NSERC Collaborative Health Research Project "Treatment of Preterm Birth with ProstaglandinF2alpha Receptor Modulators" No. 337381, the Fonds de recherche nature et technologie Quebec for the Centre in Green Chemistry and Catalysis (FRQNT-2020-RS4-265155-CCVC).

Acknowledgments: We thank the respective funding agencies, and the Université de Montréal. We thank Alexandra Fürtös, Marie-Christine Tang and Karine Venne of the Université de Montréal Mass Spectrometry Facility for mass spectral analyses. Professor Huy Ong (Université de Montréal) and his group are thanked for help in acquiring the mice serum.

Conflicts of Interest: The authors declare no conflict of interest.

References

1. Slattery, M.M.; Morrison, J.J. Preterm delivery. *Lancet* **2002**, *360*, 1489–1497. [CrossRef]
2. Russell, R.B.; Green, N.S.; Steiner, C.A.; Meikle, S.; Howse, J.L.; Poschman, K.; Dias, T.; Potetz, L.; Davidoff, M.J.; Damus, K.; et al. Cost of hospitalization for preterm and low birth weight infants in the United States. *Pediatrics* **2007**, *120*, e1–e9. [CrossRef] [PubMed]
3. Hack, M.; Flannery, D.J.; Schluchter, M.; Cartar, L.; Borawski, E.; Klein, N. Outcomes in Young Adulthood for Very-Low-Birth-Weight Infants. *N. Engl. J. Med.* **2002**, *346*, 149–157. [CrossRef] [PubMed]
4. O'Connor, A.R.W.; David, C.M.; Fielder, A.R. Ophthalmological problems associated with preterm birth. *Eye* **2007**, *21*, 1254–1260. [CrossRef] [PubMed]
5. Marlow, M.W.; Wolke, D.; Bracelwell, M.A.; Samara, M. Neurologic and developmental disability at six years of age after extremely preterm birth. *New Engl. J. Med. Chem.* **2005**, *352*, 9–19. [CrossRef] [PubMed]
6. Rich-Edwards, J.W.; Stampfer, M.J.; Manson, J.E.; Rosner, B.; Hankinson, S.E.; Colditz, G.A.; Hennekens, C.H.; Willet, W.C. Birth weight and risk of cardiovascular disease in a cohort of women followed up since 1976. *BMJ* **1997**, *315*, 396–400. [CrossRef]
7. Blencowe, H.; Cousens, S.; Oestergaard, M.; Chou, D.; Moller, A.B.; Narwal, R.; Adler, A.; Garcia, C.V.; Rohde, S.; Say, L.; et al. National, regional and worldwide estimates of preterm birth. *Lancet* **2012**, *379*, 2126–2172.
8. Papatsonis, D.; Flenady, V.; Cole, S.; Liley, H. Oxytocin receptor antagonists for inhibiting preterm labour. *Cochrane Database Syst. Rev.* **2005**.
9. King, F.J.; Flenady, V.; Papatosnis, D.; Dekker, G.; Carbonne, B. Calcium channel blockers for inhibiting preterm labour; a systematic review of the evidence and a protocol for administration of nifedipine. *Aust. N. Z. J. Obstet. Gynaecol.* **2003**, *43*, 192–198. [CrossRef]
10. Meidahl Petersen, K.; Jimenez-Solem, E.; Andersen, J.T.; Petersen, M.; Brødbæk, K.; Køber, L.; Torp-Pedersen, C.; Poulsen, H.E. β-Blocker treatment during pregnancy and adverse pregnancy outcomes: A nationwide population-based cohort study. *BMJ Open* **2012**, *2*, e001185. [CrossRef]
11. Crowther, C.A.; Hillier, J.E.; Doyle, L.W. Magnesium sulphate for preventing preterm birth in threatened preterm labour. *Cochrane Database Syst. Rev.* **2002**.
12. Loudon, J.A.Z.; Groom, K.A.; Bennett, R. Prostaglandin inhibitors in preterm labour. *Best Pract. Res. Clin. Obstet. Gynaecol.* **2003**, *17*, 731–744. [CrossRef]
13. Haas, D.M. Tocolytic therapy: A meta-analysis and decision analysis. *Obstet. Gynecol.* **2009**, *113*, 585–594.
14. Simhan, H.N.; Caritis, S.N. Prevention of preterm delivery. *N. Engl. J. Med.* **2007**, *357*, 477–487. [CrossRef]
15. Olson, D.M. The role of prostaglandins in the initiation of parturition. *Best Pr. Res. Clin. Obs. Gynaecol.* **2003**, *17*, 717–730. [CrossRef]
16. Olson, D.M.; Zaragoza, D.B.; Shallow, M.C.; Cook, J.L.; Mitchell, B.F.; Grigsby, P.; Hirst, J. Myometrial activation and preterm labour: Evidence supporting a role for the prostaglandin F receptor—a review. *Placenta* **2003**, *24*, 47–54. [CrossRef]
17. Sugimoto, Y.; Yamasaki, A.; Segi, E.; Tsuboi, K.; Aze, Y.; Nishimura, T.; Oida, H.; Yoshida, N.; Tanaka, T.; Katsuyama, M.; et al. Failure of parturition in mice lacking the prostaglandin F receptor. *Science* **1997**, *277*, 681–683. [CrossRef]
18. Peri, K.G.; Quiniou, C.; Hou, X.; Abran, D.; Varma, D.R.; Lubell, W.D.; Chemtob, S. THG113: A novel selective FP antagonist that delays preterm labor. *Semin. Perinatol.* **2002**, *26*, 389–397. [CrossRef]
19. Peri, K.; Polyak, F.; Lubell, W.D.; Thouin, E.; Chemtob, S. Peptides and peptidomimetics useful for inhibiting the activity of prostaglandin F2a receptor. WO 2003104266A2, 18 December 2002.
20. Böttcher, B.; Laterza, R.M.; Wildt, L.; Seufert, R.J.; Buhling, K.J.; Singer, C.F.; Hill, W.; Griffin, P.; Jilma, B.; Schulz, M.; et al. A first-in-human study of PDC31 (prostaglandin F2α receptor inhibitor) in primary dysmenorrhea. *Hum. Rreprod.* **2014**, *29*, 2465–2473. [CrossRef]
21. Presland, J. Identifying novel modulators of G protein-coupled receptors via interaction at allosteric sites. *Curr. Opin. Drug Discovery Dev.* **2005**, *8*, 567–576.
22. Gokarn, Y.R.; McLean, M.; Laue, T.M. Effect of PEGylation on protein hydrodynamics. *Mol. Pharm.* **2012**, *9*, 762–773. [CrossRef] [PubMed]

23. Moosmann, A.B.; Blath, J.; Lindner, R.; Muller, E.; Bottinger, H. Aldehyde PEGylation kinetics: A standard protein versus a pharmaceutically relevant single chain variable fragment. *Bioconjug. Chem.* **2011**, *22*, 1545–1558. [CrossRef] [PubMed]
24. Roberts, M.J.B.; Harris, J.M. Chemistry for peptide and protein PEGylation. *Adv. Drug Del. Rev.* **2002**, *54*, 459–476. [CrossRef]
25. Ryan, S.M.; Mantovani, G.; Wang, X.; Haddleton, D.M.; Brayden, D.J. Advances in PEGylation of important biotech molecules: Delivery aspects. *Exoert Opin. Drug Deliv.* **2008**, *5*, 371–383. [CrossRef] [PubMed]
26. Bailon, P.; Palleroni, A.; Schaffer, C.A.; Spence, C.L.; Fung, W.J.; Porter, J.E.; Ehrlich, G.K.; Pan, W.; Xu, Z.X.; Modi, M.W.; et al. Rational design of a potent, long lasting form of interferon: A 40kDa branched poly-ethylene glycol-conjugated interferon alpha-2a for the treatment of hepatitis C. *Bioconjug. Chem.* **2001**, *12*, 195–202. [CrossRef]
27. Trainer, J.; Drake, W.M.; Katznelson, L.; Freda, P.U.; Herman-Bonert, V.; van der Lely, A.J.; Dimaraki, E.V.; Stewart, P.M.; Friend, K.E.; Vance, M.L.; et al. Treatment of Acromegaly with the Growth Hormone-Receptor Antagonist Pegvisomant. *N. Engl. J. Med.* **2000**, *342*, 1171–1177. [CrossRef]
28. Knudsen, L.B.; Lau, J. The discovery and development of liraglutide and semaglutide. *Front. Endocrinol.* **2019**, *10*. [CrossRef]
29. Blundell, J.; Finlayson, G.; Axelsen, M.; Flint, A.; Gibbons, C.; Kvist, T.; Hjerpsted, J.B. Effects of once-weekly semaglutide on appetite, energy intake, control of eating, food preference and body weight in subjects with obesity. *Diabetes. Obes. Metab.* **2017**, *19*, 1242–1251. [CrossRef]
30. Wang, J.H.; Hogenkam, D.J.; Tran, M.; Li, W.Y.; Yoshimura, R.F.; Johnstone, T.B.C.; Shen, W.C.; Gee, K.W. Reversible Lipidization for the Oral Delivery of leu-enkephalin. *J. Drug Target.* **2006**, *14*, 127–136. [CrossRef]
31. Al-Obeidi, F.; Hruby, V.; Yaghoubi, N.; Marwan, M.M.; Hadley, M.E. Synthesis and biological activities of fatty acid conjugates of a cyclic lactam alpha-melanotropin. *J. Med. Chem.* **1992**, *35*, 118–123. [CrossRef] [PubMed]
32. Ward, B.P.; Ottaway, N.L.; Perez-Tilve, D.; Ma, D.; Gelfanov, V.M.; Tschöp, M.H.; Dimarchi, R.D. Peptide lipidation stabilizes structure to enhance biological function. *Mol. Metab.* **2013**, *2*, 468–479. [CrossRef] [PubMed]
33. Baltz, R.H.; Miao, V.; Wrigley, S.K. Natural products to drugs, daptomycin and related lipopeptide antibiotics. *Nat. Proc. Re* **2005**, *22*, 717–741. [CrossRef] [PubMed]
34. Fung, S.; Hruby, V.J. Design of cyclic and other templates for potent and selective peptide α-MSH analogues. *Curr. Opini. Chem. Biol.* **2005**, *9*, 352–358. [CrossRef]
35. Hadley, M.E.; al-Obeidi, F.; Hruby, V.J.; Weinrach, J.C.; Freedberg, D.; Jiang, J.W.; Stover, R.S. Biological Activities of Melanotropic Peptide Fatty Acid Conjugates. *Pigment Cell Res.* **1991**, *4*, 180–185. [CrossRef]
36. Wright, T.H.; Brooks, A.E.; Didsbury, A.J.; Williams, G.M.; Harris, W.; Dunbar, R.; Brimble, M.A. Direct peptide lipidation through thiol-ene coupling enables rapid synthesis and evaluation of self-adjuvanting vaccine candidates. *Angew. Chem. Int. Ed. Engl.* **2013**, *52*, 10616–10619. [CrossRef]
37. Rezler, E.M.; Khan, D.R.; Lauer-Fields, J.; Cudic, M.; Baronas-Lowell, D.; Fields, G.B. Targeted Drug Delivery Utilizing Protein-Like Molecular Architecture. *J. Am. Chem. Soc.* **2007**, *129*, 4961–4972. [CrossRef]
38. Versluis, F.; Voskuhl, J.; van Kolck, B.; Zope, H.; Bremmer, M.; Albregtse, T.; Kros, A. In situ modification of plain liposomes with lipidated coiled coil forming peptides induces membrane fusion. *J. Am. Chem. Soc.* **2013**, *135*, 8057–8062. [CrossRef]
39. Johannessen, L.; Remsberg, J.; Gaponenko, V.; Adams, K.M.; Barchi, J.J., Jr.; Tarasov, S.G.; Jiang, S.; Tarasova, N.I. Peptide structure stabilization by membrane anchoring and its general applicability to the development of potent cell-permeable inhibitors. *Chembiochem.* **2011**, *12*, 914–921. [CrossRef]
40. Cox, A.D.; Der, C.D. Protein prenylation, more than just glue? *Curr. Opin. Cell Biol.* **1992**, *4*, 1008–1016. [CrossRef]
41. Lane, K.T.; Beese, L.S. Thematic review series, lipid posttranslational modifications. Structural biology of protein farnesyltransferase and geranylgeranyltransferase type I. *J. Lipid Res.* **2006**, *47*, 681–699. [PubMed]
42. London, N.; Lamphear, C.L.; Hougland, J.L.; Fierke, C.A.; Schueler-Furman, O. Identification of a novel class of farnesylation targets by structure-based modeling of binding specificity. *PLOS Comput. Biol.* **2011**, *7*, e1002170. [CrossRef] [PubMed]

43. Marshell, C.J. Protein prenylation: A mediator of protein-protein interactions. *Science* **1993**, *259*, 1865–1866. [CrossRef] [PubMed]
44. Ochocki, J.D.; Igbavboa, U.; Gibson Wood, W.; Wattenberg, E.V.; Distefano, M.D. Enlarging the scope of cell-penetrating prenylated peptides to include farnesylated 'CAAX' box sequences and diverse cell types. *Chem. Biol. Drug Des.* **2010**, *76*, 107–115. [CrossRef]
45. Shen, G.; Huhman, D.; Lei, Z.; Snyder, J.; Sumner, L.W.; Dixon, R.A. Characterization of an isoflavonoid-specific prenyltransferase from Lupinus albus. *Plant Physiol.* **2012**, *159*, 70–80. [CrossRef]
46. Benfenati, E.; Gini, G.; Piclin, N.; Roncaglioni, A.; Varì, M.R. Predicting logP of pesticides using different software. *Chemosphere* **2003**, *53*, 1155–1164. [CrossRef]
47. Medic-Saric, M.; Ana Mornar, A.; Badovinac-Črnjević, T.; Jasprica, I. Experimental and Calculation Procedures for Molecular Lipophilicity: A Comparative Study for 3,3′-(2-Methoxybenzylidene)bis(4-hydroxycoumarin). *Croatica Chemica Acta.* **2004**, *77*, 367–370.
48. Veronese, F.M. Peptide and protein PEGylation: A review of problems and solutions. *Biomaterials.* **2001**, *22*, 405–417. [CrossRef]
49. Lubell, W.D.; Blankenship, J.W.; Fridkin, G.; Kaul, R. *"Peptides," in Science of Synthesis*; Weinreb, S.M., Ed.; Thieme: Stuttgart, Germany, 2005; pp. 713–809.
50. Arya, W.; Barnes, C.Q.; Daroswska, M.L. A Solid Phase Library Synthesis of Hydroxyindoline-Derived Tricyclic Derivatives by Mitsunobu Approach. *J. Comb. Chem.* **2004**, *6*, 65–72. [CrossRef]
51. Bisegger, P.; Manov, N.; Bienz, S. Solid-phase synthesis of cyclic polyamines. *Tetrahedron* **2008**, *64*, 7531–7536. [CrossRef]
52. Lencina, C.L.; Dassonville-Klimpt, A.; Sonnet, P. New efficient enantioselective synthesis of 2-oxopiperazines: A practical access to chiral 3-substituted 2-oxopiperazines. *Tet. Asymmetry* **2008**, *19*, 1689–1697. [CrossRef]
53. Tumkevicius, S.; Masevicius, V.; Petraityte, G. 4-Amino-5-(arylaminomethyl)-2-(methylthio)furo [2,3-d]pyrimidines via Mitsunobu Reaction of 4-Amino-5-(hydroxymethyl)-2-(methylthio)furo [2,3-d]pyrimidine with *N*-Mesyl- and *N*-Nosylarylamines. *Synthesis* **2012**, *44*, 1329–1338. [CrossRef]
54. Mir, F.M.; Atmuri, N.D.P.; Bourguet, C.B.; Fores, J.R.; Hou, X.; Chemtob, S.; Lubell, W.D. Paired Utility of Aza-Amino Acyl Proline and Indolizidinone Amino Acid Residues for Peptide Mimicry: Conception of Prostaglandin F2α Receptor Allosteric Modulators That Delay Preterm Birth. *J. Med. Chem.* **2019**, *62*, 4500–4525. [CrossRef] [PubMed]
55. Sakai, M.; Tanebe, K.; Sasaki, Y.; Momma, K.; Yoneda, S.; Saito, S. Evaluation of the tocolytic effect of a selective cyclooxygenase-2 inhibitor in a mouse model of lipopolysaccharide-induced preterm delivery. *Mol. Hum. Reprod.* **2001**, *7*, 595–602. [CrossRef]
56. Tahara, M.; Kawagishi, R.; Sawada, K.; Morishige, K.; Sakata, M.; Tasaka, K.; Murata, Y. Tocolytic effect of a Rho-kinase inhibitor in a mouse model of lipopolysaccharide-induced preterm delivery. *Am. J. Obstet. Gynecol.* **2005**, *192*, 903–908. [CrossRef]
57. Goupil, E.; Tassy, D.; Bourguet, C.; Quiniou, C.; Wisehart, V.; Pétrin, D.; Le Gouill, C.; Devost, D.; Zingg, H.H.; Bouvier, M.; et al. A novel biased allosteric compound inhibitor of parturition selectively impedes the prostaglandin F2alpha-mediated Rho/ROCK signaling pathway. *J. Biol. Chem.* **2010**, *285*, 25624–25636. [CrossRef]
58. O'Brien, M.; Morrison, J.J.; Smith, T.J. Expression of prothrombin and protease activated receptors in human myometrium during pregnancy and labor. *Biol. Reprod.* **2008**, *78*, 20–26. [CrossRef]
59. Pham, W.; Kircher, M.F.; Weissleder, R.; Tung, C.H. Enhancing membrane permeability by fatty acylation of oligoarginine peptides. *Chembiochem.* **2004**, *5*, 1148–1151. [CrossRef]
60. Friedrich, H.B.; Singh, N. The very efficient oxidation of alcohols by poly (4-vinylpyridine)-supported sodium ruthenate. *Tet. Lett.* **2000**, *41*, 3971–3974. [CrossRef]
61. Vidal, D.M.; Fávaro, C.F.; Guimarães, M.M.; Zarbin, P.H.G. Identification and synthesis of the male-produced sex pheromone of the soldier beetle Chauliognathus fallax (Coleoptera: Cantharidae). *J. Brazilian Chem. Soc.* **2016**, *27*, 1678–4790.
62. Han, X.; Dong, L.; Geng, C.; Jiao, P. Catalytic Asymmetric Synthesis of Isoxazolines from Silyl Nitronates. *Org. Lett.* **2015**, *17*, 3194–3197. [CrossRef] [PubMed]
63. Matuszewska, I.; Leniewski, A.; Roszkowski, P.; Czarnocki, Z. Synthesis of a novel class of fatty acids-derived isoquinolines. *Chem. Phys. Lipids* **2005**, *135*, 131–145. [CrossRef] [PubMed]

64. Mao, W.; Shi, W.; Li, J.; Su, D.; Wang, X.; Zhang, L.; Pan, L.; Wu, X.; Wu, H. Organocatalytic and Scalable Syntheses of Unsymmetrical 1, 2, 4, 5-Tetrazines by Thiol-Containing Promotors. *Angew. Chem Int. Ed.* **2019**, *58*, 1106–1109. [CrossRef] [PubMed]
65. Eissler, S.; Kley, M.; Bächle, D.; Loidl, G.; Meier, T.; Samson, D. Substitution determination of Fmoc-substituted resins at different wavelengths. *J. Peptide Sci.* **2017**, *23*, 757–762. [CrossRef] [PubMed]

Sample Availability: Samples not available.

molecules

MDPI

Article

Structure–Activity Relationships of 7-Substituted Dimethyltyrosine-Tetrahydroisoquinoline Opioid Peptidomimetics

Deanna Montgomery [1], Jessica P. Anand [2,3], Mason A. Baber [1], Jack J. Twarozynski [2], Joshua G. Hartman [2], Lennon J. Delong [2], John R. Traynor [2,3] and Henry I. Mosberg [1,3,*]

[1] Department of Medicinal Chemistry, College of Pharmacy, University of Michigan, Ann Arbor, MI 48109, USA; dmontg@umich.edu (D.M.); mbaber@rollins.edu (M.A.B.)

[2] Department of Pharmacology, Medical School, University of Michigan, Ann Arbor, MI 48109, USA; janand@umich.edu (J.P.A.); jactwaro@umich.edu (J.J.T.); hartjosh@umich.edu (J.G.H.); delongl@umich.edu (L.J.D.); jtraynor@umich.edu (J.R.T.)

[3] Edward F. Domino Research Center, Medical School, University of Michigan, Ann Arbor, MI 48109, USA

* Correspondence: him@umich.edu; Tel.: +1-734-764-8117

Academic Editor: Derek J. McPhee
Received: 2 November 2019; Accepted: 21 November 2019; Published: 26 November 2019

check for updates

Abstract: The opioid receptors modulate a variety of biological functions, including pain, mood, and reward. As a result, opioid ligands are being explored as potential therapeutics for a variety of indications. Multifunctional opioid ligands, which act simultaneously at more than one type of opioid receptor, show promise for use in the treatment of addiction, pain, and other conditions. Previously, we reported the creation of bifunctional kappa opioid receptor (KOR) agonist/mu opioid receptor (MOR) partial agonist ligands from the classically delta opioid receptor (DOR) antagonist selective dimethyltyrosine-tetrahydroisoquinoline (Dmt-Tiq) scaffold through the addition of a 7-benzyl pendant on the tetrahydroisoquinoline ring. This study further explores the structure–activity relationships surrounding 7-position pendants on the Dmt-Tiq scaffold. Some analogues maintain a KOR agonist/MOR partial agonist profile, which is being explored in the development of a treatment for cocaine addiction. Others display a MOR agonist/DOR antagonist profile, which has potential to be used in the creation of a less addictive pain medication. Ultimately, we report the synthesis and in vitro evaluation of novel opioid ligands with a variety of multifunctional profiles.

Keywords: peptidomimetic; structure-activity; opioids; multifunctional ligands

1. Introduction

Opioids have one of the longest known histories of any drug class. The use of opium for ritual, medicinal, and/or recreational purposes dates back to ancient civilizations [1,2]. In the early 1800s, Friedrich Sertürner isolated the primary active ingredient of opium and named it morphine [1]. This began the chemical exploration of the opiates, and ultimately, led to discovery of the opioid receptors and their endogenous ligands. It is widely accepted that there are three major types of opioid receptors—the kappa opioid receptor (KOR), the mu opioid receptor (MOR), and the delta opioid receptor (DOR). These receptors have high sequence and structural homology, and they are all Class A GPCRs [3,4]. The structure and function of this type of receptor have been thoroughly reviewed [5,6]. Though most well-known for its role in regulating pain, the opioid system is also involved in many other biological processes, including mood [7–9] and reward [8,10]. As such, opioids remain an important and promising class of molecules for the development of therapeutics for a variety of indications.

Functions of the opioid receptors are modulated by both endogenous and exogenous opioid ligands. In the two centuries since the discovery of morphine, many semi-synthetic and synthetic opioids have been developed for this purpose. As the complex pharmacology of the opioid system continues to be revealed, it has been posited that unwanted effects and desired effects may result from the same interaction of an opioid agonist or antagonist with its target. As a result, the development of selective agents has declined, and the development of multifunctional ligands, compounds that act simultaneously at multiple opioid receptor types, has gained popularity as a strategy for the design of therapeutics [11,12]. The current state of multifunctional opioid ligands has recently been reviewed [13].

Our group [14] and others [15–19] have shown that the dimethyltyrosine-tetrahydroisoquinoline (Dmt-Tiq) scaffold can be used in the development of multifunctional opioid ligands (Figure 1). This scaffold, originally developed as a selective DOR antagonist, has been extensively explored through synthesis of many analogues. However, the confines of traditional peptide synthesis have limited substitution on the tetrahydroisoquinoline (Tiq) ring. Nearly two decades ago, minor substitutions were reported at the 6-, 7-, and 8- positions, but all of these compounds displayed a DOR antagonist profile similar to that of the parent peptide [17,20]. Recently, we reported that installation of a 7-benzyl pendant on the Tiq could alter the profile of this series to KOR agonism/MOR partial agonism [14].

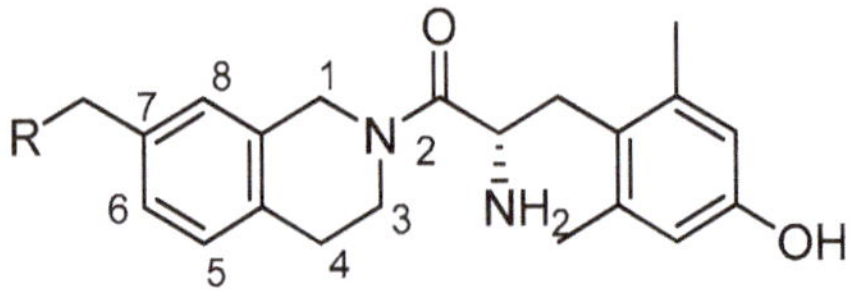

Figure 1. A variety of pendants were introduced at the 7-position of the tetrahydroisoquinoline of the dimethyltyrosine-tetrahydroisoquinoline (Dmt-Tiq) scaffold.

KOR agonists have shown potential for use in the treatment of cocaine addiction because of their reward-modulating properties. Specifically, administration of a KOR agonist can reduce cocaine self-administration in non-human primates [21,22]. However, KOR agonism is also associated with dysphoria, an intense feeling of unease or dissatisfaction [7]. As a result, selective KOR agonists have limited therapeutic potential. It is well known that MOR agonism is associated with euphoria. Therefore, a bifunctional KOR agonist/MOR agonist offers a potential alternative to a selective KOR agonist that may result in a more favorable side effect profile. In fact, there is evidence to suggest that a KOR agonist/MOR agonist may be useful in the treatment of cocaine addiction [23,24].

The aim of this work was to explore structure–activity relationships around the 7-benzyl pendant which introduced KOR agonism to the Dmt-Tiq scaffold. Novel analogues reported here reveal that substitution on the benzyl ring can maintain a KOR agonist/MOR partial agonist profile while analogues with other 7-position pendants show varied results. Overall, this work demonstrates the development of novel Dmt-Tiq peptidomimetics that display a range of multifunctional opioid profiles.

2. Results

A series of novel Dmt-Tiq compounds with substitution at the Tiq 7-position were prepared and evaluated in vitro for opioid activity.

2.1. Synthesis

All compounds were prepared from commercial starting materials according to one of the synthetic routes shown in Scheme 1. In the first route, commercially available carboxylic acid **1** was reduced to the corresponding secondary alcohol **2** using borane dimethylsulfide. An Appel reaction was performed to convert alcohol **2** to benzyl bromide **3**. The pendant was then attached via Suzuki coupling of intermediate **3** with the corresponding boronic acid or S_N2 reaction with the corresponding nucleophile.

In the second route, Boc-protected tetrahydroisoquinoline **5** was prepared from commercially available 7-bromotetrahydroisoquinoline (**4**). This intermediate was converted to boronic ester **6**, and the appropriate pendant was attached by Suzuki coupling with the corresponding benzyl bromide. In each case, after the pendant was attached, the Boc group was removed from intermediate **7a–z** with acid, and the deprotected tetrahydroisoquinoline intermediate was coupled with diBoc-protected dimethyltyrosine. Finally, the Boc groups were removed to yield the final peptidomimetic **8a–z**.

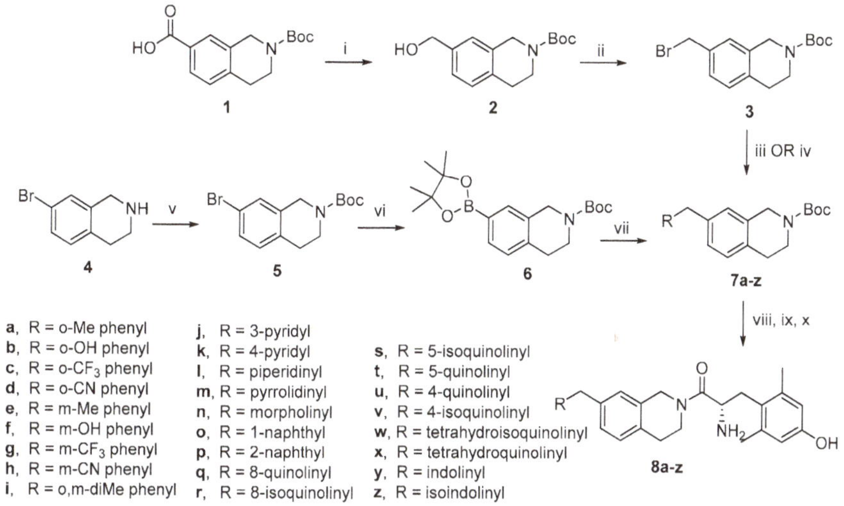

Scheme 1. Preparation of Dmt-Tiq peptidomimetics. *Reagents and conditions*: (i) BH_3 SMe_2, THF; (ii) CBr_4, PPh_3, DCM; (iii) substituted aryl boronic acid, Pd(dppf)Cl_2, K_2CO_3, 3:1 acetone:water; (iv) amine, K_2CO_3, DMF; (v) Boc_2O, microwave; (vi) bis(pinacolato)diboron, Pd(dppf)Cl_2, CH_3CO_2K, DMSO; (vii) substituted benzyl bromide, Pd(dppf)Cl_2, K_2CO_3, 3:1 acetone/water; (viii) HCl, 1,4-dioxane or TFA, DCM; (ix) diBoc-Dmt, PyBOP, 6Cl-HOBt, DIEA, DMF; (x) TFA, DCM.

2.2. Pharmacological Evaluation

Each novel compound was evaluated for binding to and stimulation of KOR, MOR, and DOR. Binding affinity (K_i) was determined by competitive displacement of [^{3}H]-diprenorphine, a non-selective opioid receptor antagonist with similar affinity for each of the three receptors. Potency (EC_{50}) and efficacy, expressed as percent stimulation compared to a standard agonist at each receptor, were determined by a [^{35}S]-GTPγS binding assay.

Building on our previous work [14], several ortho and meta substituents on the benzyl ring were investigated as well as the *o*-,*m*-dimethyl analogue. The results of the pharmacological evaluation of these compounds are shown in Table 1. Data for the previously reported 7-benzyl analogue **4c** is shown for comparison. Previously, this compound was evaluated at human KOR, rat MOR, and rat DOR. The profile shown here differs slightly from that previously reported because all compounds in this study were evaluated only at human receptors. All ortho- and meta-substituted analogues reported here display single digit nanomolar or subnanomolar binding at all three opioid receptors. In general, ortho analogues show the highest affinity for KOR compared to the other receptors, while most meta analogues show the highest affinity for DOR. Compared to standard agonists, each of these analogues retains moderate (54%) to high (89%) efficacy at KOR and low (29%) to high efficacy (81%) at MOR. Most analogues show no DOR agonism, but the ortho trifluoromethyl analogue **8c** shows low DOR efficacy and potency. Potency for these compounds remains primarily in the double or triple digit nanomolar range. The balance of potencies varies for ortho analogues, while meta analogues and the disubstituted analogue are consistently more potent at MOR than KOR.

Table 1. Substituted 7-benzyl pendants on the Dmt-Tiq scaffold. [1]

Compound	R	Ki (nM)			EC$_{50}$ (nM)			% Stimulation		
		KOR	MOR	DOR	KOR	MOR	DOR	KOR	MOR	DOR
4c	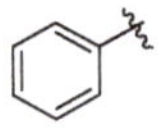	2.3 (0.3)	5.3 (0.5)	2.2 (0.7)	97 (24)	68 (15)	5.7 (2.0)	82 (6)	39 (4)	20 (3)
8a	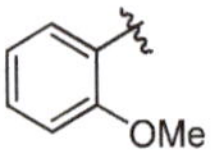	3.1 (0.9)	3.7 (0.6)	2.7 (0.7)	130 (41)	92 (26)	dns *	72 (11)	37 (8)	dns *
8b	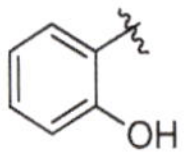	0.32 (0.01)	1.2 (0.1)	2.5 (0.3)	11 (1)	43 (13)	dns *	89 (6)	60 (5)	dns *
8c	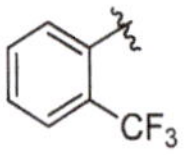	2.6 (0.6)	4.3 (1.3)	4.9 (2)	173 (55)	53 (11)	342 (32)	81 (11)	76 (6)	24 (3)
8d	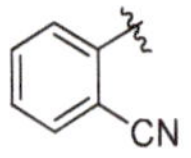	0.5 (0.1)	6.8 (0.2)	3.6 (0.8)	3.7 (0.8)	664 (515)	dns	80 (9)	31 (9)	dns
8e	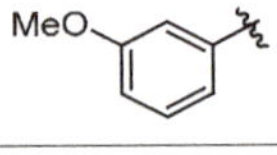	3.0 (0.9)	2.7 (0.6)	1.7 (0.4)	148 (38)	24 (3)	dns	74 (4)	48 (6)	dns
8f	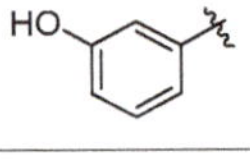	0.8 (0.2)	0.6 (0.2)	1.4 (0.1)	148 (53)	18 (3)	dns *	83 (5)	81 (9)	dns *
8g	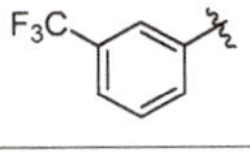	5.4 (1.1)	4.1 (1.1)	1.6 (0.5)	319 (115)	205 (96)	dns	68 (8)	45 (3)	dns
8h	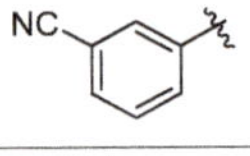	5.9 (0.9)	3.4 (1.3)	1.4 (0.2)	287 (61)	53 (6)	dns	60 (8)	29 (3)	dns
8i	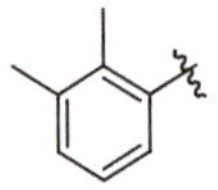	5.8 (1.2)	5.2 (1.4)	3.6 (0.6)	1030 (50)	380 (187)	dns *	54 (9)	34 (3)	dns *

[1] Binding affinity (K_i) values determined by competitive displacement of [^{3}H]-diprenorphine in membrane preparations from CHO cells expressing human KOR, MOR, or DOR. Potency (EC$_{50}$) and efficacy values determined by [^{35}S]-GTPγS binding in the same membrane preparations. Efficacy expressed as percent stimulation versus standard agonists—U69,593 (KOR), DAMGO (MOR), or DPDPE (DOR). All values expressed as mean (SEM) of three or more separate assays run in duplicate unless otherwise noted. * $n = 2$; dns = does not stimulate, average maximal stimulation <10% at concentrations up to 10 μM.

Next, we explored the incorporation of nitrogen into the aromatic ring of the pendant. In place of the benzyl pendant, 3- and 4-pyridyl pendants were added at the 7-position of the tetrahydroisoquinoline ring with a methylene spacer (Table 2). Due to well-known synthetic difficulties [25], the 2-pyridyl analogue was not successfully synthesized. Evaluation of the pyridyl analogues revealed a loss in binding and a drastic loss of potency at KOR with low efficacy at MOR and no agonism at DOR, compared to their carbocyclic counterparts.

Non-aromatic pendants were also explored. Table 3 shows pharmacological data for analogues with saturated, cyclic amine pendants. For this series, all KOR agonism was lost, and only weak potency and low efficacy at MOR were observed.

Table 2. Pyridyl 7-position pendants on the Dmt-Tiq scaffold. [1]

Compound	R	Ki (nM)			EC_{50} (nM)			% Stimulation		
		KOR	MOR	DOR	KOR	MOR	DOR	KOR	MOR	DOR
8j	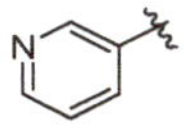	56 (0.9)	5.4 (0.3)	1.5 (0.2)	988 (277)	145 (30)	dns	40 (7)	23 (1)	dns
8k	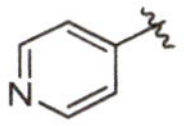	44 (12)	42 (18)	2.6 (1.0)	1180 (287)	179 (17)	dns	44 (9)	28 (1)	dns

[1] Binding affinity (K_i) values determined by competitive displacement of [^{3}H]-diprenorphine in membrane preparations from CHO cells expressing human KOR, MOR, or DOR. Potency (EC_{50}) and efficacy values determined by [^{35}S]-GTPγS binding in the same membrane preparations. Efficacy expressed as percent stimulation versus standard agonists—U69,593 (KOR), DAMGO (MOR), or DPDPE (DOR). All values expressed as mean (SEM) of three or more separate assays run in duplicate unless otherwise noted. dns = does not stimulate, average maximal stimulation <10% at concentrations up to 10 μM.

Table 3. Aliphatic 7-position pendants on the Dmt-Tiq scaffold. [1]

Compound	R	Ki (nM)			EC_{50} (nM)			% Stimulation		
		KOR	MOR	DOR	KOR	MOR	DOR	KOR	MOR	DOR
8l	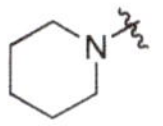	29 (11)	4.7 (0.9)	87 (15)	dns	845 (97)	dns	dns	34 (5)	dns
8m	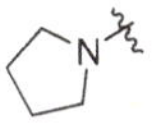	69 (3)	17 (11)	175 (9)	dns	639 * (162)	dns *	dns	40 * (22)	dns *
8n	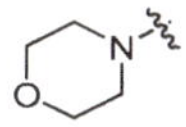	43 (17)	39 (27)	5.6 (1.6)	dns	860 (200)	dns	dns	38 (14)	dns

[1] Binding affinity (K_i) values determined by competitive displacement of [^{3}H]-diprenorphine in membrane preparations from CHO cells expressing human KOR, MOR, or DOR. Potency (EC_{50}) and efficacy values determined by [^{35}S]-GTPγS binding in the same membrane preparations. Efficacy expressed as percent stimulation versus standard agonists—U69,593 (KOR), DAMGO (MOR), or DPDPE (DOR). All values expressed as mean (SEM) of three or more separate assays run in duplicate unless otherwise noted. * $n = 2$; dns = does not stimulate, average maximal stimulation <10% at concentrations up to 10 μM.

To test whether opioid activity could be maintained in the presence of larger pendants, 1- and 2-naphthyl analogues were synthesized. These results are shown in Table 4. The 1-naphthyl pendant displays a KOR agonist/MOR partial agonist profile, while the 2-naphthyl pendant results in a drastic loss in KOR binding and a complete loss of KOR agonism.

Given the MOR/KOR profile of analogue **8o**, a nitrogen scan was conducted to further explore the structure–activity relationships around this pendant (Table 5). Similar to the pyridyl analogues, synthetic difficulties prevented the synthesis and evaluation of the 1-isoquinolinyl analogue. With few exceptions, single digit nanomolar or stronger binding is observed at all three receptors, and these analogues favor binding to DOR over MOR and KOR. All of these compounds show MOR agonism, and all except analogue **8u** display partial to full KOR agonism. However, only compounds **8q** and **8v** shows DOR agonism. Ultimately, the addition of a single nitrogen to this ring results in compounds that show a range of multifunctional opioid profiles.

Finally, bicyclic pendants with one saturated ring and one aromatic ring were explored. This subset of analogues displays two distinct profiles (Table 6). Compounds **8x** and **8y** show balanced affinity and efficacy at KOR and MOR, while compounds **8w** and **8z** display a loss in KOR binding and no KOR agonism. However, the latter two compounds show potent, moderate to high efficacy at MOR and strong binding but no agonism at DOR.

Table 4. Naphthyl 7-position pendants on the Dmt-Tiq scaffold. [1]

Compound	R	Ki (nM)			EC_{50} (nM)			% Stimulation		
		KOR	MOR	DOR	KOR	MOR	DOR	KOR	MOR	DOR
8o	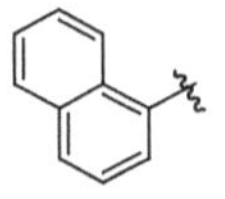	4.7 (0.5)	5.2 (1.0)	3.2 (0.6)	349 (112)	132 (76)	dns	83 (14)	59 (1)	dns
8p	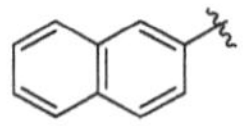	142 (23)	5.8 (1.6)	3.5 (0.7)	dns	176 (59)	dns	dns	51 (9)	dns

[1] Binding affinity (K_i) values determined by competitive displacement of [^{3}H]-diprenorphine in membrane preparations from CHO cells expressing human KOR, MOR, or DOR. Potency (EC_{50}) and efficacy values determined by [^{35}S]-GTPγS binding in the same membrane preparations. Efficacy expressed as percent stimulation versus standard agonists—U69,593 (KOR), DAMGO (MOR), or DPDPE (DOR). All values expressed as mean (SEM) of three or more separate assays run in duplicate unless otherwise noted. dns = does not stimulate, average maximal stimulation <10% at concentrations up to 10 μM.

Table 5. Nitrogen scan of 7-position 1-naphthyl pendant on the Dmt-Tiq scaffold. [1]

Compound	R	Ki (nM)			EC_{50} (nM)			% Stimulation		
		KOR	MOR	DOR	KOR	MOR	DOR	KOR	MOR	DOR
8q	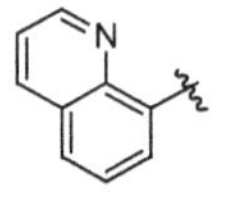	19 (2)	1.4 (0.3)	0.46 (0.08)	258 (16)	24 (4)	1.2 (0.8)	25 (3)	63 (8)	23 (4)
8r	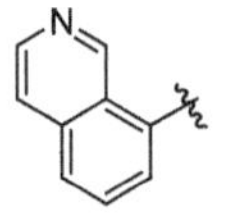	2.7 (0.7)	1.8 (0.3)	0.69 (0.24)	65 (19)	24 (6)	dns *	42 (15)	36 (5)	dns *
8s	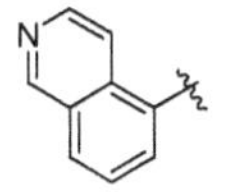	10 (1)	9.7 (1.4)	1.2 (0.2)	609 (226)	43 (21)	dns	24 (2)	28 (8)	dns
8t	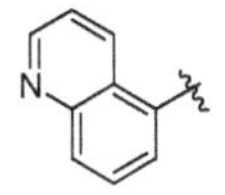	1.5 (0.5)	4.6 (0.5)	1.2 (0.4)	58 (11)	54 (15)	dns *	69 (1)	31 (6)	dns *
8u	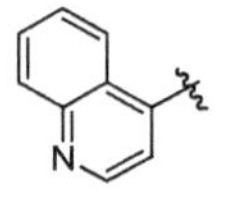	8.6 (0.4)	6.6 (1.0)	0.79 (0.25)	dns	54 (19)	dns *	dns	45 (12)	dns *
8v	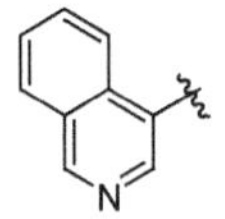	0.73 (0.03)	1.4 (0.2)	0.30 (0.04)	14 (1)	12 (3)	19 (10)	71 (16)	81 (7)	39 (7)

[1] Binding affinity (K_i) values determined by competitive displacement of [^{3}H]-diprenorphine in membrane preparations from CHO cells expressing human KOR, MOR, or DOR. Potency (EC_{50}) and efficacy values determined by [^{35}S]-GTPγS binding in the same membrane preparations. Efficacy expressed as percent stimulation versus standard agonists—U69,593 (KOR), DAMGO (MOR), or DPDPE (DOR). All values expressed as mean (SEM) of three or more separate assays run in duplicate unless otherwise noted. * $n = 2$; dns = does not stimulate, average maximal stimulation <10% at concentrations up to 10 μM.

Table 6. Bicyclic aliphatic 7-position pendants on the Dmt-Tiq scaffold. [1]

Compound	R	Ki (nM)			EC_{50} (nM)			% Stimulation		
		KOR	MOR	DOR	KOR	MOR	DOR	KOR	MOR	DOR
8w	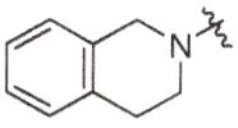	42 (8)	0.6 (0.1)	2.3 (0.6)	dns	8.2 (1.0)	dns *	dns	85 (9)	dns *
8x	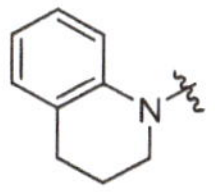	7.1 (1.4)	7.2 (1.6)	6.6 (1.0)	375 (109)	73 (22)	dns *	67 (3)	65 (10)	dns *
8y	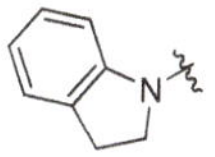	2.6 (0.6)	2.2 (0.6)	1.7 (0.5)	106 (20)	42 (10)	dns *	66 (8)	65 (5)	dns *
8z	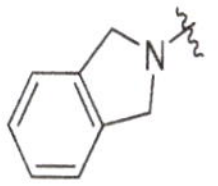	65 (23)	1.5 (0.2)	1.3 (0.4)	dns	27 (0.3)	dns *	dns	63 (10)	dns *

[1] Binding affinity (K_i) values determined by competitive displacement of [^{3}H]-diprenorphine in membrane preparations from CHO cells expressing human KOR, MOR, or DOR. Potency (EC_{50}) and efficacy values determined by [^{35}S]-GTPγS binding in the same membrane preparations. Efficacy expressed as percent stimulation versus standard agonists—U69,593 (KOR), DAMGO (MOR), or DPDPE (DOR). All values expressed as mean (SEM) of three or more separate assays run in duplicate unless otherwise noted. * $n = 2$; dns = does not stimulate, average maximal stimulation <10% at concentrations up to 10 μM.

3. Discussion

Previous work by our group [14] and others [15–19] has indicated that the classically DOR antagonist selective dimethyltyrosine-tetrahydroisoquinoline (Dmt-Tiq) scaffold can be used as a starting point for the development of multifunctional opioid ligands. Building on our previous work, this study further explores installation of a 7-position pendant on the tetrahydroisoquinoline ring as a means of developing ligands with pharmacologically useful, multifunctional profiles. Previously, we reported that introduction of ortho and meta substituents onto a 7-benzyl pendant could produce ligands that demonstrate KOR agonism and MOR partial agonism [14], a bifunctional profile which has shown promise for the treatment of addiction to cocaine and other drugs of abuse. Here, we further explore the structure–activity relationships surrounding this novel series of opioid ligands and report compounds with this and other multifunctional opioid profiles.

Based on previously reported initial results from this series [14], we believed ortho and meta substituents on a 7-benzyl pendant to be promising structural modifications for the development of KOR agonist/MOR partial agonist ligands. A series of additional ortho and meta substitutions were evaluated to confirm whether they would exhibit the anticipated profile (Table 1). As expected, ortho and meta substitutions on the 7-benzyl pendant are favorable for the development of KOR/MOR ligands. Because di-substitution (compound **8i**) results in a notable drop in KOR potency, it shows no advantage over a single ortho or meta substituent. A few of the ligands in this series, including analogue **8c**, show DOR agonism, which represents a problem for the development of a therapeutically useful KOR/MOR ligand because DOR agonism is associated with problematic side effects, including convulsions [9,26,27]. On the other hand, DOR antagonism may be beneficial for the development of a treatment for addiction since it has been shown to lower the addiction potential of MOR agonists in preclinical models [28–30]. The strong MOR agonism of some compounds in this series (compounds **8c** and **8f**) is also a concern for the development of a therapy, as this activity would likely impart greater abuse potential. The most promising compound in this series for the development of a KOR agonist/MOR partial agonist for treatment of cocaine addiction, analogue **8b**, shows high potency and efficacy at KOR, high potency and low efficacy at MOR, and is devoid of DOR agonism. This compound also has higher affinity for KOR and MOR than for DOR (eight-fold and two-fold, respectively), making it a promising candidate for further evaluation.

The introduction of a nitrogen to the 7-benzyl ring was not favorable for the development of a KOR/MOR ligand (Table 2). Rather, these analogues are selective for DOR over KOR and MOR and display low potency and efficacy at KOR and MOR. Replacement of the benzyl pendant with a saturated, cyclic amine pendant likewise decreases MOR potency drastically and eliminates KOR agonism altogether (Table 3). Unlike many of the compounds reported here, these analogues do not show particularly useful opioid profiles.

To explore the potential of installing larger pendants at the Tiq 7-position, we first synthesized analogues with 1- and 2-naphthyl pendants (Table 4). Though the high clogP (5.6) and associated insolubility of these compounds is a problem for the ultimate development of a therapeutic, they were prepared as useful probes to further explore what might be tolerated in this series. Based on our previous observations from ortho, meta, and para substitutions [14], we hypothesized that the 1-naphthyl pendant would be favorable for the development of a KOR agonist while the 2-naphthyl pendant would not. The 1-naphthyl pendant points in the same direction as ortho and meta substituents, where there is room for additional steric bulk to be accommodated in the active configuration of the KOR orthosteric site. The 2-naphthyl pendant, on the other hand, points in the direction of meta and para substituents, where it clashes with the receptor. As expected, the 1-naphthyl analogue **8o** shows the desired KOR/MOR profile, while the 2-naphthyl analogue **8p** shows a drastic decrease in KOR binding and a complete loss of KOR agonism.

Based on these findings, we conducted a nitrogen scan of the 1-naphthyl pendant. The introduction of a single nitrogen drops the clogP by approximately 1.5 units, making these analogues much more promising candidates for use in animal studies and clinical settings. The profile of these analogues differed based on the placement of the nitrogen. Most of these compounds (analogues **8q**–**8v**) show some degree of KOR agonism and MOR agonism, but only analogue **8t** displays the desired KOR agonist/MOR partial agonist profile. Notably, this compound is equipotent at KOR and MOR and is a promising candidate for further study. It is approximately 3-fold selective for KOR and DOR over MOR which may lower the abuse potential of such a compound. Analogue **8u** displays partial agonism only at MOR but high affinity for DOR, a profile most similar to that of previously reported Dmt-Tiq compounds. On the other hand, compound **8v** has a potent KOR agonist/MOR agonist/DOR partial agonist profile and is weakly selective for KOR and DOR over MOR. While interesting, this profile is likely clinically irrelevant.

Finally, we explored bicyclic pendants with a cyclic amine attached to an aromatic ring. The profile differs, likely due to the placement of the second ring within the receptor binding site. As expected, those that would most closely mimic the 1-naphthyl pendant, compounds **8w** and **8z**, exhibit a KOR agonist/MOR agonist profile. The binding and efficacy profile at KOR and MOR for these two compounds is remarkably balanced, though they are more potent at MOR (five-fold and two-fold, respectively). As discussed above, the higher MOR efficacy and potency of these compounds compared to others would likely impart greater addiction potential. On the other hand, those compounds which more closely mimic the 2-naphthyl pendant, analogues **8w** and **8z**, show no KOR agonism, as expected. However, these analogues exhibit MOR agonism and DOR antagonism, a bifunctional profile being explored in the development of a less addictive treatment for pain [13,31,32]. Both compounds display potent MOR agonism and selectivity for MOR and DOR over KOR (18-fold and 43-fold, respectively). In addition, compound **8z** shows balanced affinity at MOR and DOR, a quality previously explored by our group as a way to mitigate addiction potential [33]. These compounds represent a starting point for further study for the development of a MOR agonist/DOR antagonist.

In conclusion, this work reports novel opioid ligands with a variety of multifunctional profiles. We have further elucidated structure–activity relationships surrounding the 7-position pendant on the tetrahydroisoquinoline ring of the classically DOR antagonist selective Dmt-Tiq scaffold. Ortho substituted analogues and select bicyclic pendant analogues show promise for the development of a

KOR agonist/MOR partial agonist, a profile being investigated for the treatment of cocaine addiction. Compounds **8w** and **8z** exhibit a balanced MOR agonist/DOR antagonist profile and have potential to be investigated as a treatment for pain with lowered addiction potential. Future work will examine the pharmacokinetic properties of these compounds and explore the in vivo activity of interesting compounds from this series.

4. Materials and Methods

4.1. Chemistry

The chemical methods used were the same as those previously described [14] with any changes noted below. Unless otherwise noted, all reagents and solvents were purchased from commercial sources and used without additional purification. DiBoc-DMT was prepared from commercially available DMT according to standard procedures as previously reported [14]. Microwave reactions were performed in a Discover SP microwave synthesizer (CEM Corp., Matthews, NC, USA) in a closed vessel with maximum power input of 300 W. Column chromatography was carried out on silica gel cartridges using an Isolera One flash purification system (Biotage AB, Uppsala, Sweden) with a linear gradient of 100% hexanes to 100% ethyl acetate. Before chromatographic purification, crude reaction mixtures were analyzed by thin layer chromatography in hexanes/ethyl acetate. Purification of final compounds was performed using asemipreparative HPLC (Waters Technologies Corp., Milford, MA, USA) with a Vydac protein and peptide C18 reverse phase column using a linear gradient of 100% solvent A (water with 0.1% TFA) to 100% solvent B (acetonitrile with 0.1% TFA) at a rate of 1% per minute with UV absorbance monitored at 230 nm. Purity of final compounds was determined on an Alliance 2690 analytical HPLC (Waters Technologies Corp., Milford, MA, USA) with a Vydac protein and peptide C18 reverse phase column using the same gradient with UV absorbance monitored at 230 nm. Purity of final compounds used for testing was ≥95% as determined by HPLC. ^{1}H-NMR data for intermediates and final compounds in $CDCl_3$ or CD_3OD was obtained on a 400 MHz or 500 MHz Varian spectrometer (Agilent Technologies Inc., Santa Clara, CA, USA). EIMS data was obtained using an Agilent 6130 HPLC-MS (Agilent Technologies Inc., Santa Clara, CA, USA) in positive ion mode. HREIMS data was obtained using an Agilent QTOF HPLC-MS (Agilent Technologies Inc., Santa Clara, CA, USA) in positive ion mode.

4.1.1. General Procedure A for Microwave Suzuki Coupling of Benzyl Bromide 3 and Pendant Boronic Acid

Benzyl bromide **3** (1.0 eq), the appropriate boronic acid (1.5 eq), Pd(dppf)Cl_2 (0.1 eq), and K_2CO_3 (3.0 eq) were combined in a microwave vessel equipped with a teflon stirbar. The system was flushed with argon. A degassed mixture of 3:1 acetone:water (3 mL) was added, and the reaction was heated in a microwave to 100 °C for 30 min. The product was purified via silica gel chromatography in ethyl acetate/hexanes.

4.1.2. General Procedure B for HCl Boc Deprotection, Peptide Coupling, and TFA Boc Deprotection

The appropriate Boc-protected amine intermediate was dissolved in 1,4-dioxane (2–5 mL) and excess concentrated HCl (100–500 μL) was added. The reaction mixture stirred at room temperature for 1–3.5 h. The solvent was removed under vacuum to yield the deprotected amine. The amine intermediate (1.0 eq), diBoc-DMT (1.05 eq), PyBOP (1.0 eq), and 6Cl-HOBt (1.0 eq) were combined, and the reaction flask was flushed with argon. Dry DMF (3–12 mL) and DIEA (10 eq) were added. The reaction mixture stirred at room temperature for 6–24 h. The solvent was removed under vacuum, and the coupled product was purified via silica gel chromatography in ethyl acetate/hexanes. The Boc-protected compound was dissolved in DCM (2–2.5 mL). An equal volume of TFA was added, and the reaction mixture stirred at room temperature for 1–1.5 h. The solvent was removed under vacuum, and the product was purified by semi-preparative HPLC and lyophilized.

4.1.3. General Procedure C for Microwave Suzuki Coupling of Boronic Ester **6** and Pendant Benzyl Bromide

The appropriate benzyl bromide (1.5–2.0 eq), intermediate **6** (1.0 eq), Pd(dppf)Cl_2 (0.1 eq), and K_2CO_3 (3.0 eq) were combined in a microwave vessel equipped with a teflon stirbar. The system was flushed with argon. A degassed mixture of 3:1 acetone:water (2–3 mL) was added, and the reaction was heated in a microwave to 100 °C for 30 min. The product was purified via silica gel chromatography in ethyl acetate/hexanes.

4.1.4. General Procedure D for Microwave Suzuki Coupling of Boronic Ester **6** and Pendant Benzyl Bromide

The appropriate benzyl bromide (1.0 eq), intermediate **6** (1.5 eq), Pd(dppf)Cl_2 (0.1 eq), and K_2CO_3 (3.0 eq) were combined in a microwave vessel equipped with a teflon stirbar. The system was flushed with argon. A degassed mixture of 3:1 acetone:water (2–3 mL) was added, and the reaction was heated in a microwave to 100 °C for 30 min. The product was purified via silica gel chromatography in ethyl acetate/hexanes.

4.1.5. General Procedure E for S_N2 reaction of Benzyl Bromide **3** and Pendant Amine

Benzyl bromide **3** (1.0 eq), the appropriate nucleophile (1.2 eq), and K_2CO_3 (1.2 eq) were dissolved in dry DMF (3 mL) under an inert atmosphere. The reaction stirred at room temperature overnight. The reaction mixture was partitioned between 2 M NaOH and ethyl acetate. The aqueous layer was extracted with additional ethyl acetate. Combined organic layers were dried over $MgSO_4$, filtered, and concentrated under vacuum to obtain the product.

4.1.6. General Procedure F for TFA Boc Deprotection, Peptide Coupling, and TFA Boc Deprotection

The appropriate Boc-protected amine intermediate was dissolved in DCM (1–3 mL). An equal volume of TFA was added, and the reaction mixture stirred at room temperature for 1–1.5 h. The solvent was removed under vacuum to yield the deprotected amine. The amine intermediate (1.0 eq), diBoc-DMT (1.05 eq), and PyBOP (1.0 eq) were combined, and the reaction flask was flushed with argon. Dry DMF (3–12 mL) and DIEA (10 eq) were added. The reaction mixture stirred at room temperature for 6–24 h. The solvent was removed under vacuum, and the coupled product was purified via silica gel chromatography in ethyl acetate/hexanes. The Boc-protected compound was dissolved in DCM (2–2.5 mL). An equal volume of TFA was added, and the reaction mixture stirred at room temperature for 1–1.5 h. The solvent was removed under vacuum, and the product was purified by semi-preparative HPLC and lyophilized.

Tert-butyl 7-(hydroxymethyl)-3,4-dihydroisoquinoline-2(1H)-carboxylate (**2**). To a solution of compound **1** in dry THF (15 mL), a 2.0 M solution of borane dimethyl sulfide in THF (2.7 mL, 5.41 mmol, 3.0 eq) was added dropwise over 15 min under inert atmosphere. The reaction mixture stirred at room temperature overnight. The reaction was quenched by the addition of methanol (20 mL). The solvent was removed under vacuum. The crude product was dissolved in ethyl acetate and washed with saturated aqueous $NaHCO_3$ and brine. The combined aqueous layers were extracted with ethyl acetate. The combined organic layers were dried over $MgSO_4$, filtered, and concentrated under vacuum to yield the product as a colorless oil (475 mg, 100%). ^{1}H-NMR ($CDCl_3$, 500 MHz) δ 7.16 (d, J = 7.9 Hz, 1H), 7.13 (d, J = 5.8 Hz, 1H), 7.12 (s, 1H), 4.65 (s, 2H), 4.57 (s, 2H), 3.63 (t, J = 5.9 Hz, 2H)), 2.82 (t, J = 5.8 Hz, 2H), 1.49 (s, 9H).

Tert-butyl 7-(bromomethyl)-3,4-dihydroisoquinoline-2(1H)-carboxylate (**3**). To a solution of compound **2** (950 mg, 3.61 mmol, 1.0 eq) in DCM (40 mL), CBr_4 (1.32 g, 3.97 mmol, 1.1 eq) and a solution of PPh_3 (1.14 g, 4.33 mmol, 1.2 eq) in DCM (5 mL) were added. The reaction stirred at room temperature for 2 h. The product was purified via silica gel chromatography in ethyl acetate/hexanes to yield a white solid (1.08 g, 92%). ^{1}H-NMR ($CDCl_3$, 500 MHz) δ 7.19 (d, J = 8.3 Hz, 1H), 7.14 (s, 1H), 7.11 (d, J = 7.8 Hz, 1H), 4.56 (s, 2H), 4.47 (s, 2H), 3.64 (t, J = 6.0 Hz, 2H), 2.82 (t, J = 5.9 Hz, 2H), 1.49 (s, 9H).

Tert-butyl 7-bromo-3,4-dihydroisoquinoline-2(1H)-carboxylate (**5**). 7-bromo-1,2,3,4-tetrahydroisoqui noline **4** (75 μL, 0.50 mmol, 1.0 eq) and di-tert-butyl dicarbonate (120 mg, 0.55 mmol, 1.1 eq) were combined in a microwave vessel equipped with a teflon stirbar. The system was flushed with argon, and the reaction was heated in a microwave to 100 °C for 15 min. The reaction mixture was diluted with DCM and washed with saturated aqueous $NaHCO_3$ and brine. The organic layer was dried over $MgSO_4$, filtered, and concentrated under vacuum to obtain the product as a pale orange oil (145 mg, 99%). ^{1}H-NMR ($CDCl_3$, 500 MHz) δ 7.25 (m, 2H), 6.98 (d, *J* = 8.0 Hz, 1H), 4.52 (s, 2H), 3.61 (t, *J* = 5.7 Hz, 2H), 2.75 (t, *J* = 6.0 Hz, 2H), 1.48 (s, 9H).

Tert-butyl 7-(4,4,5,5-tetramethyl-1,3,2-dioxaborolan-2-yl)-3,4-dihydroisoquinoline-2(1H)-carboxylate (**6**). Intermediate **5** (945 mg, 3.03 mmol, 1.0 eq), bis(pinacolato)diboron (1.54 g, 6.06 mmol, 2.0 eq), Pd(dppf)Cl_2 (222 mg, 0.303 mmol, 0.1 eq), and potassium acetate (892 mg, 9.09 mmol, 3.0 eq) were combined in DMSO (20 mL), and the system was flushed with argon. The reaction was heated to 90 °C overnight. The reaction mixture was concentrated under vacuum to remove most DMSO. The remaining mixture was diluted with water and extracted with three portions of DCM. The combined organic layers were washed with water and brine, dried over $MgSO_4$, filtered, and concentrated under vacuum. The product was purified via silica gel chromatography in ethyl acetate/hexanes to yield a pale yellow oil (1.05 g, 96%). ^{1}H-NMR ($CDCl_3$, 500 MHz) δ 7.59 (d, *J* = 5.7 Hz, 1H), 7.14 (d, *J* = 5.5 Hz, 1H), 4.58 (s, 2H), 3.63 (br s, 2H), 2.84 (br s, 2H), 1.48 (s, 9H), 1.34 (s, 12H).

Tert-butyl 7-(2-methoxybenzyl)-3,4-dihydroisoquinoline-2(1H)-carboxylate (**7a**). Compound **7a** was synthesized following General Procedure A from compound **3** (60 mg, 0.18 mmol, 1.0 eq), (2-methoxyphenyl)boronic acid (42 mg, 0.28 mmol, 1.5 eq), Pd(dppf)Cl_2 (13 mg, 0.02 mmol, 0.1 eq), and K_2CO_3 (76 mg, 0.55 mmol, 3.0 eq) to yield the product as a colorless oil (37 mg, 57%). ^{1}H-NMR ($CDCl_3$, 500 MHz) δ 7.21 (t, *J* = 7.6 Hz, 1H), 7.07 (d, *J* = 7.2 Hz, 1H), 7.03 (s, 2H), 6.95 (s, 1H), 6.88 (t, *J* = 8.2 Hz, 2H), 4.52 (s, 2H), 3.93 (s, 2H), 3.83 (s, 3H), 3.63 (s, 2H), 2.79 (t, *J* = 5.8 Hz, 2H), 1.49 (s, 9H).

(S)-2-amino-3-(4-hydroxy-2,6-dimethylphenyl)-1-(7-(2-methoxybenzyl)-3,4-dihydroisoquinolin-2(1H)-yl) propan-1-one (**8a**). Following General Procedure B, intermediate **7a** (37 mg, 0.10 mmol) was deprotected to yield the amine intermediate as a colorless oil. This intermediate was coupled to diBoc-DMT (45 mg, 0.10 mmol, 1.05 eq) in the presence of PyBOP (54 mg, 0.10 mmol, 1.0 eq), and DIEA (142 μL, 1.04 mmol, 10 eq) to yield the product as a brown oil. No 6Cl-HOBt was used. TFA deprotection yielded the product as a white solid. ^{1}H-NMR (CD_3OD, 500 MHz, rotamers) δ 7.17 (t, *J* = 7.9 Hz, 2H), 7.05 (t, *J* = 7.4 Hz, 2H), 6.97 (d, *J* = 7.7 Hz, 1H), 6.94–6.90 (m, 4H), 6.89–6.82 (m, 4H), 6.50 (d, *J* = 3.9 Hz, 1H), 6.39 (s, 2H), 6.33 (s, 2H), 4.59–4.45 (m, 4H), 4.15 (d, *J* = 15.7 Hz, 1H), 3.86 (d, *J* = 3.7 Hz, 2H), 3.85 (d, *J* = 2.8 Hz, 2H), 3.78 (d, *J* = 1.6 Hz, 3H), 3.78 (d, *J* = 1.2 Hz, 3H), 3.71–3.65 (m, 1H), 3.65–3.58 (m, 1H), 3.33 (d, *J* = 15.7 Hz, 1H), 3.25–3.17 (m, 2H), 3.09 (d, *J* = 11.4 Hz, 1H), 2.72–2.65 (m, 1H), 2.65–2.58 (m, 1H), 2.55–2.45 (m, 1H), 2.24 (s, 6H), 2.18 (s, 6H), 1.98–1.87 (m, 1H). HPLC retention time: 39.1 min. HREIMS *m*/*z* 445.2494 (calcd. for C28H32N2O3, 445.2486).

Tert-butyl 7-(2-hydroxybenzyl)-3,4-dihydroisoquinoline-2(1H)-carboxylate (**7b**). Compound **7b** was synthesized following General Procedure A from compound **3** (60 mg, 0.18 mmol, 1.0 eq), (2-hydroxyphenyl)boronic acid (38 mg, 0.28 mmol, 1.5 eq), Pd(dppf)Cl_2 (13 mg, 0.02 mmol, 0.1 eq), and K_2CO_3 (76 mg, 0.55 mmol, 3.0 eq) to yield the product as a yellow oil (33 mg, 53%). ^{1}H-NMR ($CDCl_3$, 500 MHz) δ 7.16–7.10 (m, 2H), 7.08–7.01 (m, 2H), 6.96 (s, 1H), 6.89 (t, *J* = 7.5 Hz, 1H), 6.79 (d, *J* = 7.9 Hz, 1H), 4.51 (s, 2H), 3.95 (s, 2H), 3.62 (s, 2H), 2.78 (t, *J* = 5.9 Hz, 2H), 1.48 (s, 9H).

(S)-2-amino-3-(4-hydroxy-2,6-dimethylphenyl)-1-(7-(2-hydroxybenzyl)-3,4-dihydroisoquinolin-2(1H)-yl) propan-1-one (**8b**). Following General Procedure B, intermediate **7b** (33 mg, 0.10 mmol) was deprotected to yield the amine intermediate as an off-white solid. This intermediate was coupled to diBoc-DMT (42 mg, 0.10 mmol, 1.05 eq) in the presence of PyBOP (50 mg, 0.10 mmol, 1.0 eq), and DIEA (132 μL, 0.97 mmol, 10 eq) to yield the product as a brown oil. No 6Cl-HOBt was used. TFA deprotection yielded the product as a white solid. ^{1}H-NMR (CD_3OD, 500 MHz, rotamers) δ 7.01 (ddt, *J* = 10.9, 5.1, 1.8 Hz, 4H), 6.97 (d, *J* = 7.6 Hz, 3H), 6.92 (d, *J* = 7.9 Hz, 1H), 6.88 (d, *J* = 7.9 Hz, 1H), 6.78–6.70 (m, 4H), 6.55 (s, 1H), 6.40 (s, 2H), 6.33 (s, 2H), 4.61 (d, *J* = 16.9 Hz, 1H), 4.58–4.49 (m, 2H), 4.47 (d, *J* = 16.5 Hz,

1H), 4.16 (d, *J* = 15.6 Hz, 1H), 3.87 (s, 2H), 3.86 (s, 2H), 3.75–3.68 (m, 1H), 3.66–3.59 (m, 1H), 3.34 (d, *J* = 15.8 Hz, 1H), 3.26–3.17 (m, 3H), 3.10–3.05 (m, 2H), 2.72–2.65 (m, 2H), 2.65–2.59 (m, 2H), 2.55–2.45 (m, 1H), 2.24 (s, 6H), 2.19 (s, 6H), 2.03–1.95 (m, 2H). HPLC retention time: 32.8 min. HREIMS *m/z* 431.2337 (calcd. for C27H30N2O3, 431.2329).

tert-Butyl 7-(2-(trifluoromethyl)benzyl)-3,4-dihydroisoquinoline-2(1H)-carboxylate (**7c**). Compound **7c** was synthesized following General Procedure C from intermediate **6** (100 mg, 0.278 mmol, 1.0 eq), 1-(bromomethyl)-2-(trifluoromethyl)benzene (133 mg, 0.556 mmol, 2.0 eq), Pd(dppf)Cl_2 (20 mg, 0.028 mmol, 0.1 eq), and K_2CO_3 (115 mg, 0.834 mmol, 3.0 eq) to yield a colorless oil (27 mg 25%). ^{1}H-NMR ($CDCl_3$, 400 MHz) δ 7.67 (d, *J* = 7.9 Hz, 1H), 7.43 (t, *J* = 7.5 Hz, 1H), 7.31 (t, *J* = 7.7 Hz, 1H), 7.18 (d, *J* = 7.9 Hz, 1H), 7.06 (d, *J* = 7.8 Hz, 1H), 6.95 (d, *J* = 7.0 Hz, 1H), 6.89 (s, 1H), 4.52 (s, 2H), 4.14 (s, 2H), 3.63 (t, *J* = 5.4 Hz, 2H), 2.80 (t, *J* = 5.9 Hz, 2H), 1.48 (s, 9H).

(S)-2-amino-3-(4-hydroxy-2,6-dimethylphenyl)-1-(7-(2-(trifluoromethyl)benzyl)-3,4-dihydroisoquinolin-2(1H)-yl)propan-1-one (**8c**). Following General Procedure B, intermediate **7c** (27 mg, 0.069 mmol, 1.0 eq) was deprotected to yield the amine intermediate as a white solid. This intermediate was coupled to diBoc-DMT (30 mg, 0.074 mmol, 1.05 eq) in the presence of PyBOP (36 mg, 0.070 mmol, 1.0 eq) and DIEA (98 μL, 0.700 mmol, 10 eq) to yield the product as a brown oil. No 6Cl-HOBt was used. TFA deprotection yielded the product as an off-white solid (24 mg, 57%, 3 steps). ^{1}H-NMR (CD_3OD, 500 MHz, rotamers) δ 7.70–7.66 (m, 2H), 7.54–7.48 (m, 2H), 7.40–7.35 (m, 2H), 7.28–7.22 (m, 2H), 6.98 (d, *J* = 7.8 Hz, 1H), 6.95–6.91 (m, 2H), 6.89 (s, 1H), 6.86 (d, 1H), 6.47 (s, 1H), 6.41 (s, 2H), 6.31 (s, 2H), 4.61 (d, *J* = 17.0 Hz, 1H), 4.58–4.51 (m, 2H), 4.49 (d, *J* = 17.0 Hz, 1H), 4.18 (d, *J* = 15.8 Hz, 1H), 4.12 (s, 2H), 4.11 (s, 2H), 3.86–3.80 (m, 1H), 3.59–3.52 (m, 1H), 3.39 (d, *J* = 15.8 Hz, 1H), 3.26–3.18 (m, 3H), 3.11–3.06 (m, 2H), 2.76–2.69 (m, 2H), 2.68–2.63 (m, 1H), 2.56–2.49 (m, 1H), 2.24 (s, 6H), 2.20 (s, 6H), 2.01–1.92 (m, 1H). ^{19}F-NMR (CD_3OD, 470 MHz, rotamers) δ −60.76, −77.10. HPLC retention time: 42.2 min. HREIMS *m/z* 483.2262 (calcd. for C28H29F3N2O2, 483.2254).

tert-Butyl 7-(2-cyanobenzyl)-3,4-dihydroisoquinoline-2(1H)-carboxylate (**7d**). Compound **7d** was synthesized following General Procedure C from intermediate **6** (75 mg, 0.209 mmol, 1.0 eq), 3-(bromomethyl)phenol (78 mg, 0.418 mmol, 2.0 eq), Pd(dppf)Cl_2 (15 mg, 0.021 mmol, 0.1 eq), and K_2CO_3 (87 mg, 0.627 mmol, 3.0 eq) to yield the product as a colorless oil (26 mg, 37%). ^{1}H-NMR ($CDCl_3$, 500 MHz) δ 7.15 (t, *J* = 7.8 Hz, 1H), 7.04 (d, *J* = 7.8 Hz, 1H), 6.99 (d, *J* = 7.3 Hz, 1H), 6.92 (s, 1H), 6.79–6.74 (m, 1H), 6.69 (d, *J* = 8.1 Hz, 1H), 6.65 (s, 1H), 4.52 (s, 2H), 3.87 (s, 2H), 3.62 (t, *J* = 5.9 Hz, 2H), 2.78 (t, *J* = 5.9 Hz, 2H), 1.49 (s, 9H).

(S)-2-((2-(2-amino-3-(4-hydroxy-2,6-dimethylphenyl)propanoyl)-1,2,3,4-tetrahydroisoquinolin-7-yl)methyl)benzonitrile (**8d**). Following General Procedure B, intermediate **7d** (20 mg, 0.057 mmol, 1.0 eq) was deprotected to yield the amine intermediate as a colorless oil. This intermediate was coupled to diBoc-DMT (24 mg, 0.059 mmol, 1.05 eq) in the presence of PyBOP (29 mg, 0.056 mmol, 1.0 eq) and DIEA (80 μL, 0.560 mmol, 10 eq) to yield the product as a brown oil. No 6Cl-HOBt was used. TFA deprotection yielded the product as a white solid (3 mg, 10%, 3 steps). ^{1}H-NMR (CD_3OD, 500 MHz, rotamers) δ 7.70 (s, 1H), 7.68 (s, 1H), 7.62–7.57 (m, 2H), 7.45–7.35 (m, 4H), 7.03 (d, *J* = 8.1 Hz, 1H), 7.00 (s, 1H), 6.99–6.97 (m, 2H), 6.95 (d, *J* = 7.8 Hz, 1H), 6.56 (s, 1H), 6.39 (s, 2H), 6.29 (s, 2H), 4.62 (d, *J* = 16.9 Hz, 1H), 4.57–4.49 (m, 3H), 4.18 (d, *J* = 15.9 Hz, 1H), 4.15 (s, 2H), 4.13 (d, *J* = 3.1 Hz, 2H), 3.58–3.51 (m, 1H), 3.43 (d, *J* = 16.2 Hz, 0H), 3.26–3.18 (m, 4H), 3.06 (dd, *J* = 13.8, 4.2 Hz, 2H), 2.74–2.69 (m, 2H), 2.69–2.62 (m, 1H), 2.56–2.49 (m, 1H), 2.24 (s, 6H), 2.19 (s, 6H), 2.01–1.95 (m, 1H). HPLC retention time: 34.4 min. HREIMS *m/z* 440.2336 (calcd. for C28H29N3O2, 440.2333).

Tert-butyl 7-(3-methoxybenzyl)-3,4-dihydroisoquinoline-2(1H)-carboxylate (**7e**). Compound **7e** was synthesized following General Procedure D from 3-methoxybenzyl bromide (42 μL, 0.30 mmol, 1.0 eq), intermediate **6** (161 mg, 0.45 mmol, 1.5 eq), Pd(dppf)Cl_2 (22 mg, 0.03 mmol, 0.1 eq), and K_2CO_3 (124 mg, 0.90 mmol, 3.0 eq) to yield the product as a colorless oil (42 mg, 40%). ^{1}H-NMR ($CDCl_3$, 500 MHz) δ 7.22 (t, *J* = 7.8 Hz, 1H), 7.06 (d, *J* = 7.8 Hz, 1H), 7.01 (d, *J* = 7.9 Hz, 1H), 6.94 (s, 1H), 6.79 (d, *J* = 7.5 Hz, 1H), 6.77–6.73 (m, 2H), 4.53 (s, 2H), 3.91 (s, 2H), 3.79 (s, 3H), 3.63 (br s, 2H), 2.80 (t, *J* = 5.9 Hz, 2H), 1.50 (s, 9H).

(S)-2-amino-3-(4-hydroxy-2,6-dimethylphenyl)-1-(7-(3-methoxybenzyl)-3,4-dihydroisoquinolin-2(1H)-yl) propan-1-one (**8e**). Following General Procedure B, intermediate **7e** (42 mg, 0.119 mmol, 1.0 eq) was deprotected to yield the amine intermediate as a white solid. This intermediate was coupled to diBoc-DMT (50 mg, 0.123 mmol, 1.05 eq) in the presence of PyBOP (61 mg, 0.117 mmol, 1.0 eq), 6Cl-HOBt (20 mg, 0.117 mmol, 1.0 eq), and DIEA (164 μL, 1.17 mmol, 10 eq). Silica gel chromatography yielded the coupled product as a colorless oil (66 mg, 88%). TFA deprotection yielded the product as a white solid. ^{1}H-NMR (CD_3OD, 500 MHz, rotamers) δ 7.16 (td, *J* = 7.8, 3.5 Hz, 2H), 6.99 (dd, *J* = 7.7, 1.7 Hz, 1H), 6.97–6.93 (m, 3H), 6.91 (d, *J* = 7.8 Hz, 1H), 6.76–6.70 (m, 6H), 6.49 (s, 1H), 6.40 (s, 2H), 6.32 (s, 2H), 4.61 (d, *J* = 16.9 Hz, 1H), 4.58–4.53 (m, 2H), 4.50 (d, *J* = 16.9 Hz, 1H), 4.17 (d, *J* = 15.7 Hz, 1H), 3.87 (s, 2H), 3.86 (s, 2H), 3.78–3.76 (m, 1H), 3.75 (s, 3H), 3.74 (s, 3H), 3.66–3.53 (m, 1H), 3.37 (d, *J* = 15.8 Hz, 1H), 3.26–3.17 (m, 3H), 3.11–3.05 (m, 2H), 2.70 (q, *J* = 7.3, 6.7 Hz, 2H), 2.67–2.62 (m, 1H), 2.52 (dt, *J* = 16.2, 6.2 Hz, 1H), 2.24 (s, 6H), 2.19 (s, 6H), 2.01–1.94 (m, 1H). HPLC retention time: 37.9 min. EIMS *m*/*z* 445.3 (calcd. for C28H32N2O3, 445.24).

tert-Butyl 7-(3-hydroxybenzyl)-3,4-dihydroisoquinoline-2(1H)-carboxylate (**7f**). Compound **7f** was synthesized following General Procedure C from intermediate **6** (75 mg, 0.209 mmol, 1.0 eq), 3-(bromomethyl)phenol (78 mg, 0.418 mmol, 2.0 eq), Pd(dppf)Cl_2 (15 mg, 0.021 mmol, 0.1 eq), and K_2CO_3 (87 mg, 0.627 mmol, 3.0 eq) to yield the product as a colorless oil (26 mg, 37%). ^{1}H-NMR ($CDCl_3$, 500 MHz) δ 7.15 (t, *J* = 7.8 Hz, 1H), 7.04 (d, *J* = 7.8 Hz, 1H), 6.99 (d, *J* = 7.3 Hz, 1H), 6.92 (s, 1H), 6.79–6.74 (m, 1H), 6.69 (d, *J* = 8.1 Hz, 1H), 6.65 (s, 1H), 4.52 (s, 2H), 3.87 (s, 2H), 3.62 (t, *J* = 5.9 Hz, 2H), 2.78 (t, *J* = 5.9 Hz, 2H), 1.49 (s, 9H).

(S)-2-amino-3-(4-hydroxy-2,6-dimethylphenyl)-1-(7-(3-hydroxybenzyl)-3,4-dihydroisoquinolin-2(1H)-yl) propan-1-one (**8f**). Following General Procedure B, intermediate **7f** (26 mg, 0.077 mmol, 1.0 eq) was deprotected to yield the amine intermediate as a colorless oil. This intermediate was coupled to diBoc-DMT (33 mg, 0.080 mmol, 1.05 eq) in the presence of PyBOP (40 mg, 0.076 mmol, 1.0 eq) and DIEA (110 μL, 0.760 mmol, 10 eq) to yield the crude product as a brown oil. No 6Cl-HOBt was used. The crude product was purified via silica gel chromatography in ethyl acetate/hexanes. Subsequent TFA deprotection yielded the product as a white solid (8 mg, 40%, 3 steps). ^{1}H-NMR (CD_3OD, 500 MHz, rotamers) δ 7.09–7.03 (m, 2H), 6.99 (d, *J* = 8.5 Hz, 1H), 6.96–6.93 (m, 3H), 6.91 (d, *J* = 7.8 Hz, 1H), 6.65 (s, 1H), 6.64 (s, 1H), 6.61–6.57 (m, 3H), 6.49 (s, 1H), 6.40 (s, 2H), 6.32 (s, 2H), 4.62 (d, *J* = 16.9 Hz, 1H), 4.58–4.52 (m, 2H), 4.49 (d, *J* = 16.7 Hz, 1H), 4.17 (d, *J* = 15.7 Hz, 1H), 3.82 (s, 2H), 3.81 (s, 2H), 3.79–3.72 (m, 1H), 3.62–3.56 (m, 1H), 3.37 (d, *J* = 15.8 Hz, 1H), 3.26–3.17 (m, 3H), 3.07 (dd, *J* = 13.7, 4.2 Hz, 2H), 2.75–2.67 (m, 2H), 2.67–2.60 (m, 1H), 2.55–2.48 (m, 1H), 2.24 (s, 6H), 2.20 (s, 6H), 2.02–1.95 (m, 1H). HPLC retention time: 30.9 min. HREIMS *m*/*z* 431.2331 (calcd. for C27H30N2O3, 431.2329).

Tert-butyl 7-(3-(trifluoromethyl)benzyl)-3,4-dihydroisoquinoline-2(1H)-carboxylate (**7g**). Compound **7g** was synthesized following General Procedure D from 3-(trifluromethyl)benzyl bromide (33 μL, 0.21 mmol, 1.0 eq), intermediate **6** (114 mg, 0.32 mmol, 1.5 eq), Pd(dppf)Cl_2 (15 mg, 0.02 mmol, 0.1 eq), and K_2CO_3 (88 mg, 0.64 mmol, 3.0 eq) to yield the product as a colorless oil (28 mg, 34%). EIMS *m*/*z* 414.2 (calcd. for C22H24F3NO2 + Na, 414.17).

(S)-2-amino-3-(4-hydroxy-2,6-dimethylphenyl)-1-(7-(3-(trifluoromethyl)benzyl)-3,4-dihydroisoquinolin-2 (1H)-yl)propan-1-one (**8g**). Following General Procedure B, intermediate **7g** (28 mg, 0.072 mmol, 1.0 eq) was deprotected to yield the amine intermediate as a yellow oil. The crude product was rinsed with two 2 mL portions of diethyl ether to yield a white solid. This intermediate was coupled to diBoc-DMT (56 mg, 0.138 mmol, 1.92 eq) in the presence of PyBOP (68 mg, 0.131 mmol, 1.82 eq), 6Cl-HOBt (22 mg, 0.131 mmol, 1.82 eq), and DIEA (184 μL, 1.31 mmol, 18 eq). Silica gel chromatography yielded the coupled product as a colorless oil (64 mg, 72%). TFA deprotection yielded the product as a white solid. ^{1}H-NMR (CD_3OD, 500 MHz, rotamers) δ 7.50–7.43 (m, 8H), 7.02–6.97 (m, 3H), 6.96–6.93 (m, 2H), 6.48 (s, 1H), 6.39 (s, 2H), 6.30 (s, 2H), 4.62 (d, *J* = 16.9 Hz, 1H), 4.59–4.51 (m, 2H), 4.52 (d, *J* = 17.3 Hz, 1H), 4.18 (d, *J* = 15.8 Hz, 1H), 4.00 (s, 2H), 3.99 (s, 2H), 3.81 (dt, *J* = 12.9, 5.7 Hz, 1H), 3.59–3.52 (m, 1H), 3.40 (d, *J* = 15.8 Hz, 1H), 3.26–3.17 (m, 3H), 3.08 (dt, *J* = 13.8, 4.1 Hz, 2H), 2.71 (q, *J* = 5.4 Hz, 2H), 2.68–2.64 (m, 1H), 2.56–2.49 (m, 1H), 2.23 (s, 6H), 2.19 (s, 6H), 2.00–1.93 (m, 1H). ^{19}F NMR (CD_3OD, 470 MHz,

rotamers) δ −64.03 (d, *J* = 28.1 Hz), −77.17. HPLC retention time: 43.3 min. EIMS *m*/*z* 483.3 (calcd. for C28H29F3N2O2, 483.22).

Tert-butyl 7-(3-cyanobenzyl)-3,4-dihydroisoquinoline-2(1H)-carboxylate (**7h**). Compound **7h** was synthesized following General Procedure D from 3-(bromomethyl)benzonitrile (40 mg, 0.20 mmol, 1.0 eq), intermediate **6** (109 mg, 0.30 mmol, 1.5 eq), Pd(dppf)Cl_2 (15 mg, 0.02 mmol, 0.1 eq), and K_2CO_3 (84 mg, 0.61 mmol, 3.0 eq) to yield the product as a colorless oil (30 mg, 43%). ^{1}H-NMR ($CDCl_3$, 500 MHz) δ 7.50 (dt, *J* = 7.4, 1.5 Hz, 1H), 7.45 (s, 1H), 7.43 (t, *J* = 8.0 Hz, 1H), 7.39 (t, *J* = 7.6 Hz, 2H), 7.08 (d, *J* = 7.8 Hz, 1H), 6.96 (d, *J* = 7.7 Hz, 1H), 6.90 (s, 1H), 4.54 (s, 2H), 3.96 (s, 2H), 3.64 (t, *J* = 5.9 Hz, 2H), 2.81 (t, *J* = 5.9 Hz, 2H), 1.49 (s, 9H).

(S)-2-amino-3-(4-hydroxy-2,6-dimethylphenyl)-1-(7-(3-isocyanobenzyl)-3,4-dihydroisoquinolin-2(1H)-yl) propan-1-one (**8h**). Following General Procedure B, intermediate **7h** (30 mg, 0.086 mmol, 1.0 eq) was deprotected to yield the amine intermediate as an off-white solid (21 mg, 84%). The crude product was rinsed with three small portions of diethyl ether. This intermediate was coupled to diBoc-DMT (32 mg, 0.077 mmol, 1.05 eq) in the presence of PyBOP (39 mg, 0.074 mmol, 1.0 eq), 6Cl-HOBt (13 mg, 0.074 mmol, 1.0 eq), and DIEA (104 μL, 0.74 mmol, 10 eq). Silica gel chromatography yielded the coupled product as a white solid (27 mg, 57%). TFA deprotection yielded the product as a white solid. ^{1}H-NMR (CD_3OD, 500 MHz, rotamers) δ 7.57–7.51 (m, 6H), 7.48–7.43 (m, 2H), 7.03–6.99 (m, 3H), 6.97–6.94 (m, 2H), 6.48 (s, 1H), 6.39 (s, 2H), 6.29 (s, 2H), 4.63 (d, *J* = 17.0 Hz, 1H), 4.59–4.49 (m, 2H), 4.53 (d, *J* = 17.6 Hz, 2H), 4.18 (d, *J* = 15.8 Hz, 1H), 3.98 (s, 2H), 3.97 (s, 2H), 3.83 (dt, *J* = 12.3, 5.6 Hz, 1H), 3.59–3.51 (m, 1H), 3.41 (d, *J* = 15.7 Hz, 1H), 3.27–3.18 (m, 3H), 3.07 (dt, *J* = 13.8, 4.0 Hz, 2H), 2.74–2.70 (m, 2H), 2.69–2.63 (m, 1H), 2.53 (dt, *J* = 16.2, 5.9 Hz, 1H), 2.24 (s, 6H), 2.20 (s, 6H), 1.98 (dt, *J* = 16.0, 5.8 Hz, 1H). HPLC retention time: 35.2 min. EIMS *m*/*z* 440.2 (calcd. for C28H29N3O2, 440.23).

Tert-butyl 7-(2,3-dimethylbenzyl)-3,4-dihydroisoquinoline-2(1H)-carboxylate (**7i**). Compound **7i** was synthesized following General Procedure C from intermediate **6** (100 mg, 0.278 mmol, 1.0 eq), 1-(bromomethyl)-2,3-dimethylbenzene (83 mg, 0.417 mmol, 1.5 eq), Pd(dppf)Cl_2 (20 mg, 0.028 mmol, 0.1 eq), and K_2CO_3 (115 mg, 0.834 mmol, 3.0 eq) to yield the product as a colorless oil (51 mg, 52%). ^{1}H-NMR ($CDCl_3$, 500 MHz) δ 7.09–7.06 (m, 2H), 7.04 (d, *J* = 7.6 Hz, 1H), 6.99 (d, *J* = 6.1 Hz, 1H), 6.93 (d, *J* = 7.9 Hz, 1H), 6.86 (s, 1H), 4.51 (s, 2H), 3.98 (s, 2H), 3.63 (t, *J* = 6.8 Hz, 2H), 2.79 (t, *J* = 6.0 Hz, 2H), 2.30 (s, 3H), 2.15 (s, 3H), 1.50 (s, 9H).

(S)-2-amino-1-(7-(2,3-dimethylbenzyl)-3,4-dihydroisoquinolin-2(1H)-yl)-3-(4-hydroxy-2,6-dimethylphenyl) propan-1-one (**8i**). Following General Procedure B, intermediate **7i** (51 mg, 0.145 mmol) was deprotected to yield the amine intermediate. This intermediate was coupled to diBoc-DMT (63 mg, 0.153 mmol, 1.05 eq) in the presence of PyBOP (76 mg, 0.146 mmol, 1.0 eq), and DIEA (199 μL, 1.46 mmol, 10 eq) to yield the product as a brown oil. No 6Cl-HOBt was used. TFA deprotection yielded the product as a white solid. ^{1}H-NMR (CD_3OD, 500 MHz, rotamers) δ 7.04–6.97 (m, 5H), 6.97–6.92 (m, 2H), 6.90–6.88 (m, 2H), 6.86–6.82 (m, 2H), 6.41 (s, 1H), 6.40 (s, 2H), 6.30 (s, 2H), 4.58 (d, *J* = 17.0 Hz, 1H), 4.62–4.48 (m, 2H), 4.46 (d, *J* = 16.9 Hz, 1H), 4.14 (d, *J* = 15.7 Hz, 1H), 3.95 (d, *J* = 2.8 Hz, 2H), 3.93 (s, 2H), 3.83–3.74 (m, 1H), 3.62–3.49 (m, 1H), 3.36 (d, *J* = 14.8 Hz, 1H), 3.26–3.17 (m, 3H), 3.08 (t, *J* = 4.9 Hz, 1H), 3.05 (t, *J* = 4.9 Hz, 1H), 2.72–2.61 (m, 3H), 2.54–2.47 (m, 1H), 2.25 (s, 3H), 2.25 (s, 3H), 2.23 (s, 6H), 2.19 (s, 6H), 2.09 (d, *J* = 2.2 Hz, 3H), 2.07 (d, *J* = 1.6 Hz, 3H), 2.00–1.93 (m, 1H). HPLC retention time: 43.2 min. HREIMS *m*/*z* 443.2699 (calcd. for C29H34N2O2, 443.2693).

Tert-butyl 7-(pyridin-3-ylmethyl)-3,4-dihydroisoquinoline-2(1H)-carboxylate (**7j**). Compound **7j** was synthesized following General Procedure C from intermediate **6** (104 mg, 0.289 mmol, 1.0 eq), 3-(bromomethyl)pyridine hydrobromide (110 mg, 0.433 mmol, 1.5 eq), Pd(dppf)Cl_2 (21 mg, 0.029 mmol, 0.1 eq), and K_2CO_3 (120 mg, 0.867 mmol, 3.0 eq) to yield the product as a colorless oil (20 mg, 21%).^{1}H-NMR ($CDCl_3$, 500 MHz) δ 8.49 (s, 1H), 8.46 (d, *J* = 4.1 Hz, 1H), 7.46 (d, *J* = 7.7 Hz, 1H), 7.20 (dd, *J* = 7.8, 4.8 Hz, 1H), 7.07 (d, *J* = 7.9 Hz, 1H), 6.97 (d, *J* = 7.9 Hz, 1H), 6.91 (s, 1H), 4.52 (s, 2H), 3.93 (s, 2H), 3.62 (br s, 2H), 2.79 (t, *J* = 6.0 Hz, 2H), 1.48 (s, 9H).

(S)-2-amino-3-(4-hydroxy-2,6-dimethylphenyl)-1-(7-(pyridin-3-ylmethyl)-3,4-dihydroisoquinolin-2(1H)-yl)propan-1-one (**8j**). Following General Procedure B, intermediate **7j** (20 mg, 0.062 mmol, 1.0 eq)

was deprotected to yield the amine intermediate as a colorless oil. The crude product was rinsed with several small portions of diethyl ether. This intermediate was coupled to diBoc-DMT (26 mg, 0.064 mmol, 1.05 eq) in the presence of PyBOP (32 mg, 0.061 mmol, 1.0 eq), 6Cl-HOBt (10 mg, 0.061 mmol, 1.0 eq), and DIEA (86 µL, 0.61 mmol, 10 eq). Silica gel chromatography yielded the coupled product (8 mg, 21%, 2 steps). TFA deprotection yielded the product as a white solid. ^{1}H-NMR (CD_3OD, 500 MHz, rotamers) δ 8.67–8.61 (m, 4H), 8.29 (d, *J* = 8.1 Hz, 1H), 8.26 (d, *J* = 8.0 Hz, 1H), 7.87 (dd, *J* = 8.1, 5.5 Hz, 1H), 7.83 (dd, *J* = 8.0, 5.5 Hz, 1H), 7.09–6.98 (m, 5H), 6.56 (s, 1H), 6.39 (s, 2H), 6.23 (s, 2H), 4.64 (d, *J* = 17.1 Hz, 1H), 4.59–4.52 (m, 2H), 4.53 (d, *J* = 16.6 Hz, 1H), 4.21 (d, *J* = 15.8 Hz, 1H), 4.14 (s, 2H), 4.12 (d, *J* = 3.2 Hz, 2H), 3.97 (dt, *J* = 13.2, 5.3 Hz, 1H), 3.48 (d, *J* = 16.1 Hz, 1H), 3.43 (dd, *J* = 13.0, 6.5 Hz, 1H), 3.26–3.19 (m, 3H), 3.08 (ddd, *J* = 13.7, 6.4, 4.1 Hz, 2H), 2.72 (t, *J* = 6.0 Hz, 2H), 2.69–2.62 (m, 1H), 2.57–2.49 (m, 1H), 2.23 (s, 6H), 2.20 (s, 6H), 1.99 (dt, *J* = 16.1, 6.1 Hz, 1H). HPLC retention time: 16.9 min. EIMS *m*/*z* 416.2 (calcd. for C26H29N3O2, 416.23).

Tert-butyl 7-(pyridin-4-ylmethyl)-3,4-dihydroisoquinoline-2(1H)-carboxylate (**7k**). Compound **7k** was synthesized following General Procedure C from intermediate **6** (112 mg, 0.312 mmol, 1.0 eq), 4-(bromomethyl)pyridine hydrobromide (118 mg, 0.468 mmol, 1.5 eq), Pd(dppf)Cl_2 (23 mg, 0.031 mmol, 0.1 eq), and K_2CO_3 (129 mg, 0.936 mmol, 3.0 eq) to yield the product as a colorless oil (20 mg, 20%). ^{1}H-NMR ($CDCl_3$, 500 MHz) δ 8.49 (d, *J* = 5.4 Hz, 2H), 7.13–7.05 (m, 3H), 6.97 (d, *J* = 7.8 Hz, 1H), 6.91 (s, 1H), 4.53 (s, 2H), 3.91 (s, 2H), 3.63 (s, 2H), 2.80 (t, *J* = 5.0 Hz, 2H), 1.48 (s, 9H).

(S)-2-amino-3-(4-hydroxy-2,6-dimethylphenyl)-1-(7-(pyridin-4-ylmethyl)-3,4-dihydroisoquinolin-2(1H)-yl)propan-1-one (**8k**). Following General Procedure B, intermediate **7k** (20 mg, 0.062 mmol, 1.0 eq) was deprotected to yield the amine intermediate as a cloudy, yellow oil. The crude product was rinsed with several small portions of diethyl ether. This intermediate was coupled to diBoc-DMT (26 mg, 0.064 mmol, 1.05 eq) in the presence of PyBOP (32 mg, 0.061 mmol, 1.0 eq), 6Cl-HOBt (10 mg, 0.061 mmol, 1.0 eq), and DIEA (86 µL, 0.61 mmol, 10 eq). Silica gel chromatography yielded the coupled product (24 mg, 63%, 2 steps). TFA deprotection yielded the product as a white solid. ^{1}H-NMR (CD_3OD, 500 MHz, rotamers) δ 8.69–8.65 (m, 4H), 7.81–7.77 (m, 4H), 7.10–7.07 (m, 2H), 7.06 (d, *J* = 7.8 Hz, 1H), 7.01 (d, 2H), 6.58 (s, 1H), 6.40 (s, 2H), 6.25 (s, 2H), 4.65 (d, *J* = 17.1 Hz, 1H), 4.58–4.55 (m, 2H), 4.53 (d, *J* = 16.8 Hz, 1H), 4.25–4.22 (m, 3H), 4.20 (d, *J* = 3.0 Hz, 2H), 3.96 (dt, *J* = 12.9, 5.3 Hz, 1H), 3.48 (d, *J* = 15.0 Hz, 1H), 3.46–3.42 (m, 1H), 3.27–3.19 (m, 3H), 3.08 (ddd, *J* = 13.7, 6.2, 4.2 Hz, 2H), 2.74 (t, *J* = 6.1 Hz, 2H), 2.70–2.62 (m, 1H), 2.58–2.51 (m, 1H), 2.24 (s, 6H), 2.21 (s, 6H), 2.00 (dt, *J* = 16.2, 5.8 Hz, 1H). HPLC retention time: 17.0 min. EIMS *m*/*z* 416.3 (calcd. for C26H29N3O2, 416.23).

Tert-butyl 7-(piperidin-1-ylmethyl)-3,4-dihydroisoquinoline-2(1H)-carboxylate (**7l**). Compound **7l** was synthesized following General Procedure E from compound **3** (35 mg, 0.107 mmol, 1.0 eq), piperidine (13 µL, 0.129 mmol, 1.2 eq), and K_2CO_3 (18 mg, 0.129 mmol, 1.2 eq) to yield the product as an orange oil (27 mg, 77%). ^{1}H-NMR ($CDCl_3$, 500 MHz) δ 7.10 (d, *J* = 8.0 Hz, 1H), 7.09–7.03 (m, 2H), 4.56 (s, 2H), 3.63 (s, 2H), 3.42 (s, 2H), 2.80 (t, *J* = 5.7 Hz, 2H), 2.36 (s, 4H), 1.57 (p, *J* = 5.5 Hz, 4H), 1.48 (s, 9H), 1.47–1.39 (m, 2H).

(S)-2-amino-3-(4-hydroxy-2,6-dimethylphenyl)-1-(7-(piperidin-1-ylmethyl)-3,4-dihydroisoquinolin-2(1H)-yl)propan-1-one (**8l**). Following General Procedure B, intermediate **7l** (27 mg, 0.082 mmol, 1.0 eq) was deprotected to yield the amine intermediate as an orange oil. The crude product was rinsed with several small portions of diethyl ether. This intermediate was coupled to diBoc-DMT (35 mg, 0.087 mmol, 1.05 eq) in the presence of PyBOP (43 mg, 0.082 mmol, 1.0 eq), 6Cl-HOBt (14 mg, 0.082 mmol, 1.0 eq), and DIEA (115 µL, 0.82 mmol, 10 eq). TFA deprotection yielded the product as a white solid. ^{1}H-NMR (CD_3OD, 500 MHz, rotamers) δ 6.48–6.45 (m, 2H), 6.41 (d, *J* = 7.8 Hz, 1H), 6.35 (d, *J* = 7.8 Hz, 1H), 6.32 (d, *J* = 8.3 Hz, 1H), 5.97 (s, 1H), 5.59 (s, 2H), 5.41 (s, 2H), 3.89 (d, *J* = 17.3 Hz, 1H), 3.82–3.76 (m, 3H), 3.46 (d, *J* = 16.0 Hz, 1H), 3.43–3.32 (m, 4H), 3.24 (dt, *J* = 13.0, 5.2 Hz, 1H), 2.73 (d, *J* = 16.1 Hz, 2H), 2.67–2.56 (m, 5H), 2.46–2.37 (m, 3H), 2.32–2.25 (m, 2H), 2.10 (q, *J* = 10.9 Hz, 4H), 1.97 (t, *J* = 5.7 Hz, 2H), 1.93–1.85 (m, 1H), 1.79 (dt, *J* = 16.4, 6.5 Hz, 1H), 1.43 (s, 6H), 1.40 (s, 6H), 1.21 (dt, *J* = 16.4, 5.4 Hz, 1H), 1.13 (s, 2H), 1.10 (s, 3H), 1.01 (d, *J* = 14.4 Hz, 2H), 0.92 (q, *J* = 13.2 Hz, 4H), 0.74–0.66 (m, 2H). HPLC retention time: 16.7 min. EIMS *m*/*z* 422.3 (calcd. for C26H35N3O2, 422.27).

Tert-butyl 7-(pyrrolidin-1-ylmethyl)-3,4-dihydroisoquinoline-2(1H)-carboxylate (**7m**). Compound **7m** was synthesized following General Procedure E from compound **3** (29 mg, 0.089 mmol, 1.0 eq), pyrrolidine (9 μL, 0.107 mmol, 1.2 eq), and K_2CO_3 (15 mg, 0.107 mmol, 1.2 eq) to yield the product as a dark yellow-orange oil (28 mg, 100%). ^{1}H-NMR ($CDCl_3$, 500 MHz) δ 7.13–7.10 (m, 1H), 7.10–7.06 (m, 2H), 4.56 (s, 2H), 3.67–3.61 (m, 2H), 3.58 (s, 2H), 2.80 (d, *J* = 6.1 Hz, 2H), 2.55–2.47 (m, 4H), 1.79 (p, *J* = 3.0 Hz, 4H), 1.49 (s, 9H).

(S)-2-amino-3-(4-hydroxy-2,6-dimethylphenyl)-1-(7-(pyrrolidin-1-ylmethyl)-3,4-dihydroisoquinolin-2(1H)-yl)propan-1-one (**8m**). Following General Procedure B, intermediate **7m** (28 mg, 0.088 mmol, 1.0 eq) was deprotected to yield the amine intermediate. The crude product was rinsed with several small portions of diethyl ether. This intermediate was coupled to diBoc-DMT (37 mg, 0.091 mmol, 1.05 eq) in the presence of PyBOP (45 mg, 0.087 mmol, 1.0 eq), 6Cl-HOBt (15 mg, 0.087 mmol, 1.0 eq), and DIEA (122 μL, 0.87 mmol, 10 eq). TFA deprotection yielded the product as a white solid. ^{1}H-NMR (CD_3OD, 500 MHz, rotamers) δ 7.31–7.26 (m, 2H), 7.24 (d, *J* = 7.6 Hz, 2H), 7.17 (d, *J* = 7.9 Hz, 1H), 7.13 (d, *J* = 7.8 Hz, 1H), 6.79 (s, 1H), 6.41 (s, 2H), 6.23 (s, 2H), 4.70 (d, *J* = 17.2 Hz, 1H), 4.61 (d, *J* = 17.0 Hz, 1H), 4.62–4.51 (m, 2H), 4.31 (s, 2H), 4.31–4.22 (m, 3H), 4.03 (dt, *J* = 11.7, 5.2 Hz, 1H), 3.53 (d, *J* = 16.0 Hz, 1H), 3.51–3.41 (m, 5H), 3.29–3.25 (m, 1H), 3.26–3.21 (m, 2H), 3.20–3.13 (m, 4H), 3.12–3.06 (m, 2H), 2.79 (t, *J* = 6.0 Hz, 2H), 2.76–2.67 (m, 1H), 2.59 (dt, *J* = 16.4, 6.0 Hz, 1H), 2.24 (s, 6H), 2.22 (s, 6H), 2.19–2.16 (m, 4H), 2.05–1.97 (m, 5H). HPLC retention time: 15.3 min. HREIMS *m*/*z* 408.2649 (calcd. for C25H33N3O2, 408.2646).

tert-butyl 7-(morpholinomethyl)-3,4-dihydroisoquinoline-2(1H)-carboxylate (**7n**). Compound **7n** was synthesized following General Procedure E from compound **3** (31 mg, 0.095 mmol, 1.0 eq), morpholine (10 μL, 0.114 mmol, 1.2 eq), and K_2CO_3 (16 mg, 0.114 mmol, 1.2 eq) to yield the product as a pale yellow oil (32 mg, 100%). ^{1}H-NMR ($CDCl_3$, 500 MHz) δ 7.11 (d, *J* = 7.8 Hz, 1H), 7.08 (s, 2H), 4.56 (s, 2H), 3.70 (t, *J* = 4.7 Hz, 4H), 3.64 (t, *J* = 6.5 Hz, 2H), 3.45 (s, 2H), 2.81 (t, *J* = 5.9 Hz, 2H), 2.43 (t, *J* = 4.6 Hz, 4H), 1.49 (s, 9H).

(S)-2-amino-3-(4-hydroxy-2,6-dimethylphenyl)-1-(7-(morpholinomethyl)-3,4-dihydroisoquinolin-2(1H)-yl) propan-1-one (**8n**). Following General Procedure B, intermediate **7n** (28 mg, 0.088 mmol, 1.0 eq) was deprotected to yield the amine intermediate. The crude product was rinsed with several small portions of diethyl ether. This intermediate was coupled to diBoc-DMT (37 mg, 0.091 mmol, 1.05 eq) in the presence of PyBOP (45 mg, 0.087 mmol, 1.0 eq), 6Cl-HOBt (15 mg, 0.087 mmol, 1.0 eq), and DIEA (122 μL, 0.87 mmol, 10 eq). TFA deprotection yielded the product as a white solid. ^{1}H-NMR (CD_3OD, 500 MHz, rotamers) δ 7.30–7.28 (m, 2H), 7.24 (d, *J* = 7.8 Hz, 1H), 7.17 (d, *J* = 7.6 Hz, 1H), 7.14 (d, *J* = 7.8 Hz, 1H), 6.81 (s, 1H), 6.40 (s, 2H), 6.22 (s, 2H), 4.70 (d, *J* = 17.3 Hz, 1H), 4.63–4.55 (m, 3H), 4.31 (s, 2H), 4.29–4.21 (m, 3H), 4.13–4.05 (m, 1H), 4.08–3.99 (m, 4H), 3.74 (q, *J* = 12.7 Hz, 4H), 3.55 (d, *J* = 16.0 Hz, 1H), 3.42–3.32 (m, 5H), 3.28–3.25 (m, 1H), 3.25–3.20 (m, 2H), 3.21–3.12 (m, 4H), 3.13–3.06 (m, 2H), 2.79 (t, *J* = 6.1 Hz, 2H), 2.75–2.66 (m, 1H), 2.60 (dt, *J* = 16.5, 5.9 Hz, 1H), 2.24 (s, 6H), 2.22 (s, 6H), 2.03 (dt, *J* = 11.1, 5.7 Hz, 1H). HPLC retention time: 14.0 min. HREIMS *m*/*z* 424.2597 (calcd. for C25H33N3O3, 424.2595).

Tert-butyl 7-(naphthalen-1-ylmethyl)-3,4-dihydroisoquinoline-2(1H)-carboxylate (**7o**). Compound **7o** was synthesized following General Procedure C from intermediate **6** (100 mg, 0.278 mmol, 1.0 eq), 1-(bromomethyl)naphthalene (123 mg, 0.556 mmol, 2.0 eq), Pd(dppf)Cl_2 (20 mg, 0.028 mmol, 0.1 eq), and K_2CO_3 (115 mg, 0.834 mmol, 3.0 eq) to yield the product as a yellow oil (41 mg, 39%). ^{1}H-NMR ($CDCl_3$, 500 MHz) δ 8.03–7.98 (m, 1H), 7.89–7.86 (m, 1H), 7.78 (d, *J* = 8.2 Hz, 1H), 7.49–7.45 (m, 2H), 7.43 (d, *J* = 7.7 Hz, 1H), 7.31 (d, *J* = 7.1 Hz, 1H), 7.03 (s, 2H), 6.95 (s, 1H), 4.50 (s, 2H), 4.41 (s, 2H), 3.63 (s, 2H), 2.80 (t, *J* = 5.9 Hz, 2H), 1.49 (s, 9H).

(S)-2-amino-3-(4-hydroxy-2,6-dimethylphenyl)-1-(7-(naphthalen-1-ylmethyl)-3,4-dihydroisoquinolin-2 (1H)-yl)propan-1-one (**8o**). Following General Procedure B, intermediate **7o** (41 mg, 0.110 mmol, 1.0 eq) was deprotected to yield the amine intermediate. This intermediate was coupled to diBoc-DMT (47 mg, 0.115 mmol, 1.05 eq) in the presence of PyBOP (57 mg, 0.110 mmol, 1.0 eq), 6Cl-HOBt (57 mg, 0.330 mmol, 3.0 eq), and DIEA (154 μL, 1.1 mmol, 10 eq). Silica gel chromatography yielded the coupled product (57 mg, 78%, 2 steps). TFA deprotection yielded the product as a white solid.

^{1}H-NMR (CD_3OD, 500 MHz, rotamers) δ 7.98–7.94 (m, 2H), 7.86–7.83 (m, 2H), 7.76 (d, *J* = 8.2 Hz, 2H), 7.46–7.39 (m, 6H), 7.35 (d, *J* = 7.0 Hz, 1H), 7.32 (d, *J* = 6.9 Hz, 1H), 7.00 (d, *J* = 7.8 Hz, 1H), 6.97–6.94 (m, 2H), 6.92 (s, 1H), 6.88 (d, *J* = 7.8 Hz, 1H), 6.47 (s, 1H), 6.38 (s, 2H), 6.32 (s, 2H), 4.55 (d, *J* = 17.1 Hz, 1H), 4.52–4.47 (m, 2H), 4.44 (d, *J* = 16.9 Hz, 1H), 4.38 (s, 4H), 4.10 (d, *J* = 15.8 Hz, 1H), 3.79 (dt, *J* = 11.9, 5.6 Hz, 1H), 3.56–3.49 (m, 1H), 3.36 (d, *J* = 15.8 Hz, 1H), 3.24–3.15 (m, 3H), 3.05 (dt, *J* = 13.7, 5.1 Hz, 2H), 2.68 (t, *J* = 6.2 Hz, 2H), 2.66–2.60 (m, 1H), 2.49 (dt, *J* = 16.0, 6.2 Hz, 1H), 2.21 (s, 6H), 2.16 (s, 6H), 1.94 (dt, *J* = 16.1, 6.0 Hz, 1H). HPLC retention time: 43.3 min. EIMS *m*/*z* 465.2 (calcd. for C31H32N2O2, 465.25).

Tert-butyl 7-(naphthalen-2-ylmethyl)-3,4-dihydroisoquinoline-2(1H)-carboxylate (**7p**). Compound **7p** was synthesized following General Procedure C from intermediate **6** (100 mg, 0.278 mmol, 1.0 eq), 2-(bromomethyl)naphthalene (123 mg, 0.556 mmol, 2.0 eq), Pd(dppf)Cl_2 (20 mg, 0.028 mmol, 0.1 eq), and K_2CO_3 (115 mg, 0.834 mmol, 3.0 eq) to yield the product (42 mg, 40%). ^{1}H-NMR ($CDCl_3$, 500 MHz) δ 7.79 (q, *J* = 8.1, 7.7 Hz, 3H), 7.65 (s, 1H), 7.45 (p, *J* = 7.1, 6.5 Hz, 2H), 7.32 (d, *J* = 8.5 Hz, 1H), 7.06 (s, 2H), 6.97 (s, 1H), 4.53 (s, 2H), 4.11 (s, 2H), 3.64 (s, 2H), 2.81 (t, *J* = 6.0 Hz, 2H), 1.49 (s, 9H).

(S)-2-amino-3-(4-hydroxy-2,6-dimethylphenyl)-1-(7-(naphthalen-2-ylmethyl)-3,4-dihydroisoquinolin-2 (1H)-yl)propan-1-one (**8p**). Following General Procedure B, intermediate **7p** (42 mg, 0.112 mmol, 1.0 eq) was deprotected to yield the amine intermediate. Half of this intermediate (18 mg, 0.058 mmol, 1.0 eq) was coupled to diBoc-DMT (25 mg, 0.061 mmol, 1.05 eq) in the presence of PyBOP (30 mg, 0.058 mmol, 1.0 eq), 6Cl-HOBt (10 mg, 0.058 mmol, 1.0 eq), and DIEA (81 μL, 0.58 mmol, 10 eq). TFA deprotection yielded the product as a brown solid. ^{1}H-NMR (CD_3OD, 500 MHz, rotamers) δ 7.81–7.72 (m, 6H), 7.63 (d, *J* = 6.7 Hz, 2H), 7.46–7.38 (m, 4H), 7.29 (d, *J* = 8.3 Hz, 2H), 7.05 (d, *J* = 8.5 Hz, 1H), 7.02–6.96 (m, 3H), 6.93 (d, *J* = 7.8 Hz, 1H), 6.53 (s, 1H), 6.40 (s, 2H), 6.32 (s, 2H), 4.61 (d, *J* = 16.9 Hz, 1H), 4.57–4.48 (m, 2H), 4.50 (d, *J* = 16.8 Hz, 1H), 4.16 (d, *J* = 15.8 Hz, 1H), 4.07 (s, 2H), 4.06 (s, 2H), 3.77 (dt, *J* = 12.1, 5.7 Hz, 1H), 3.61–3.53 (m, 1H), 3.38 (d, *J* = 15.8 Hz, 1H), 3.24–3.17 (m, 3H), 3.06 (dt, *J* = 13.8, 5.2 Hz, 2H), 2.71 (q, *J* = 5.8 Hz, 2H), 2.67–2.61 (m, 1H), 2.52 (dt, *J* = 15.7, 6.3 Hz, 1H), 2.22 (s, 6H), 2.18 (s, 6H), 1.98 (dt, *J* = 16.2, 5.9 Hz, 1H). HPLC retention time: 43.5 min. EIMS *m*/*z* 465.3 (calcd. for C31H32N2O2, 465.25).

Tert-butyl 7-(quinolin-8-ylmethyl)-3,4-dihydroisoquinoline-2(1H)-carboxylate (**7q**). Compound **7q** was synthesized following General Procedure A from compound **3** (75 mg, 0.23 mmol, 1.0 eq), quinolin-8-ylboronic acid (60 mg, 0.345 mmol, 1.5 eq), Pd(dppf)Cl_2 (17 mg, 0.023 mmol, 0.1 eq), and K_2CO_3 (95 mg, 0.69 mmol, 3.0 eq) to yield the product as a colorless oil (18 mg, 21%). ^{1}H-NMR ($CDCl_3$, 500 MHz) δ 8.97 (dd, *J* = 4.2, 1.8 Hz, 1H), 8.15 (dd, *J* = 8.3, 1.8 Hz, 1H), 7.74–7.65 (m, 1H), 7.46 (s, 1H), 7.44 (s, 1H), 7.41 (dd, *J* = 8.3, 4.2 Hz, 1H), 7.13 (dd, *J* = 7.6, 1.8 Hz, 1H), 7.07 (s, 1H), 7.04 (d, *J* = 7.9 Hz, 1H), 4.64 (s, 2H), 4.52 (s, 2H), 3.62 (s, 2H), 2.79 (t, *J* = 5.3 Hz, 2H), 1.48 (s, 9H).

(S)-2-amino-3-(4-hydroxy-2,6-dimethylphenyl)-1-(7-(quinolin-8-ylmethyl)-3,4-dihydroisoquinolin-2(1H)-yl)propan-1-one (**8q**). Following General Procedure F, intermediate **7q** (18 mg, 0.048 mmol) was deprotected to yield the amine intermediate. This intermediate was coupled to diBoc-DMT (21 mg, 0.05 mmol, 1.05 eq) in the presence of PyBOP (25 mg, 0.048 mmol, 1.0 eq), and DIEA (84 μL, 0.48 mmol, 10 eq) to yield the product. No 6Cl-HOBt was used. TFA deprotection yielded the product as a white solid. ^{1}H-NMR (CD_3OD, 500 MHz, rotamers) δ 9.03 (td, *J* = 4.9, 1.7 Hz, 2H), 8.79 (dd, *J* = 8.3, 1.7 Hz, 1H), 8.75 (dd, *J* = 8.3, 1.7 Hz, 1H), 8.04 (dd, *J* = 8.1, 1.6 Hz, 1H), 8.00 (dd, *J* = 8.1, 1.4 Hz, 1H), 7.81 (ddd, *J* = 13.0, 8.3, 4.9 Hz, 2H), 7.75–7.66 (m, 3H), 7.63 (dd, *J* = 7.3, 1.4 Hz, 1H), 7.04 (dd, *J* = 7.8, 1.8 Hz, 1H), 7.01 (d, *J* = 1.7 Hz, 1H), 6.96 (s, 2H), 6.94 (d, *J* = 7.9 Hz, 1H), 6.58 (s, 1H), 6.38 (s, 2H), 6.24 (s, 2H), 4.61 (d, *J* = 15.8 Hz, 1H), 4.58 (s, 2H), 4.56 (s, 2H), 4.56–4.52 (m, 2H), 4.47 (d, *J* = 17.0 Hz, 1H), 4.17 (d, *J* = 15.9 Hz, 1H), 3.84 (dt, *J* = 12.9, 5.5 Hz, 1H), 3.54–3.47 (m, 1H), 3.38 (d, *J* = 15.9 Hz, 1H), 3.25–3.16 (m, 3H), 3.11–3.05 (m, 2H), 2.69 (q, *J* = 5.5 Hz, 2H), 2.66–2.59 (m, 1H), 2.52 (dt, *J* = 16.2, 7.4, 4.8 Hz, 1H), 2.21 (s, 6H), 2.18 (s, 6H), 1.98 (ddd, *J* = 16.2, 6.4, 4.4 Hz, 1H). HPLC retention time: 25.0 min. EIMS *m*/*z* 466.3 (calcd. for C30H31N3O2, 466.24).

Tert-butyl 7-(isoquinolin-8-ylmethyl)-3,4-dihydroisoquinoline-2(1H)-carboxylate (**7r**). Compound **7r** was synthesized following General Procedure A from compound **3** (77 mg, 0.24 mmol, 1.0 eq), isoquinolin-8-ylboronic acid (49 mg, 0.283 mmol, 1.2 eq), Pd(dppf)Cl_2 (18 mg, 0.024 mmol, 0.1 eq), and K_2CO_3 (98 mg, 0.71 mmol, 3.0 eq) to yield the product as a pale pink oil (55 mg, 62%). ^{1}H-NMR

($CDCl_3$, 500 MHz) δ 9.47 (s, 1H), 8.52 (d, *J* = 5.6 Hz, 1H), 7.73 (d, *J* = 8.3 Hz, 1H), 7.68–7.60 (m, 2H), 7.40 (d, *J* = 7.0 Hz, 1H), 7.02 (q, *J* = 8.0 Hz, 2H), 6.94 (s, 1H), 4.48 (s, 4H), 3.61 (s, 2H), 2.77 (t, *J* = 6.1 Hz, 2H), 1.47 (s, 9H).

(S)-2-amino-3-(4-hydroxy-2,6-dimethylphenyl)-1-(7-(isoquinolin-8-ylmethyl)-3,4-dihydroisoquinolin-2 (1H)-yl)propan-1-one (**8r**). Following General Procedure F, intermediate **7r** (27 mg, 0.072 mmol) was deprotected to yield the amine intermediate. This intermediate was coupled to diBoc-DMT (31 mg, 0.076 mmol, 1.05 eq) in the presence of PyBOP (37 mg, 0.072 mmol, 1.0 eq), and DIEA (125 µL, 0.72 mmol, 10 eq) to yield the product. No 6Cl-HOBt was used. TFA deprotection yielded the product as a white solid. ^{1}H-NMR (CD_3OD, 500 MHz, rotamers) δ 9.73 (s, 1H), 9.72 (s, 1H), 8.54 (t, *J* = 5.0 Hz, 2H), 8.38 (d, *J* = 6.3 Hz, 1H), 8.35 (d, *J* = 6.2 Hz, 1H), 8.17–8.10 (m, 3H), 8.08 (q, *J* = 7.6 Hz, 1H), 7.82 (d, *J* = 6.6 Hz, 1H), 7.76 (d, *J* = 6.9 Hz, 1H), 7.07–7.02 (m, 2H), 7.00–6.94 (m, 3H), 6.53 (s, 1H), 6.36 (s, 2H), 6.17 (s, 2H), 4.61 (s, 2H), 4.60 (s, 2H), 4.57 (d, *J* = 14.3 Hz, 1H), 4.54 (dd, *J* = 11.9, 4.1 Hz, 2H), 4.48 (d, *J* = 17.0 Hz, 1H), 4.16 (d, *J* = 15.8 Hz, 1H), 3.97 (dt, *J* = 12.9, 5.3 Hz, 1H), 3.45 (d, *J* = 15.8 Hz, 1H), 3.38 (dt, *J* = 13.2, 6.7 Hz, 1H), 3.24–3.15 (m, 3H), 3.07 (ddd, *J* = 13.6, 11.5, 4.1 Hz, 2H), 2.69 (t, *J* = 6.0 Hz, 2H), 2.62 (ddd, *J* = 12.5, 7.5, 4.7 Hz, 1H), 2.52 (ddd, *J* = 16.2, 7.5, 4.8 Hz, 1H), 2.19 (s, 6H), 2.17 (s, 6H), 1.96 (ddd, *J* = 16.3, 6.9, 4.7 Hz, 1H). HPLC retention time: 21.4 min. EIMS *m/z* 466.3 (calcd. for C30H31N3O2, 466.24).

Tert-butyl 7-(isoquinolin-5-ylmethyl)-3,4-dihydroisoquinoline-2(1H)-carboxylate (**7s**). Compound **7s** was synthesized following General Procedure A from compound **3** (73 mg, 0.224 mmol, 1.0 eq), isoquinolin-5-ylboronic acid (46 mg, 0.269 mmol, 1.2 eq), Pd(dppf)Cl_2 (16 mg, 0.022 mmol, 0.1 eq), and K_2CO_3 (93 mg, 0.672 mmol, 3.0 eq) to yield the product as a yellow oil (48 mg, 57%). ^{1}H-NMR ($CDCl_3$, 500 MHz) δ 9.26 (s, 1H), 8.50 (d, *J* = 6.0 Hz, 1H), 7.88 (d, *J* = 8.1 Hz, 1H), 7.76 (d, *J* = 6.0 Hz, 1H), 7.55 (t, *J* = 7.6 Hz, 1H), 7.50 (d, *J* = 7.1 Hz, 1H), 7.04 (d, *J* = 7.8 Hz, 1H), 6.97 (s, 1H), 6.91 (s, 1H), 4.49 (s, 2H), 4.36 (s, 2H), 3.62 (t, *J* = 5.9 Hz, 2H), 2.78 (t, *J* = 5.9 Hz, 2H), 1.47 (s, 9H).

(S)-2-amino-3-(4-hydroxy-2,6-dimethylphenyl)-1-(7-(isoquinolin-5-ylmethyl)-3,4-dihydroisoquinolin-2 (1H)-yl)propan-1-one (**8s**). Following General Procedure F, intermediate **7s** (24 mg, 0.064 mmol) was deprotected to yield the amine intermediate. This intermediate was coupled to diBoc-DMT (28 mg, 0.067 mmol, 1.05 eq) in the presence of PyBOP (33 mg, 0.064 mmol, 1.0 eq), and DIEA (111 µL, 0.64 mmol, 10 eq) to yield the product. No 6Cl-HOBt was used. TFA deprotection yielded the product as a white solid. ^{1}H-NMR (CD_3OD, 500 MHz, rotamers) δ 9.67 (d, *J* = 7.1 Hz, 2H), 8.52 (d, *J* = 7.0 Hz, 2H), 8.44 (t, *J* = 7.6 Hz, 2H), 8.35 (t, *J* = 8.9 Hz, 2H), 8.04–7.91 (m, 4H), 7.04–6.92 (m, 5H), 6.51 (s, 1H), 6.37 (s, 2H), 6.23 (s, 2H), 4.58 (d, *J* = 17.4 Hz, 2H), 4.56–4.50 (m, 2H), 4.53 (s, 2H), 4.52 (s, 2H), 4.47 (d, *J* = 17.1 Hz, 1H), 4.15 (d, *J* = 15.8 Hz, 1H), 3.90 (dt, *J* = 12.9, 5.4 Hz, 1H), 3.48–3.39 (m, 1H), 3.41 (d, *J* = 15.8 Hz, 1H), 3.24–3.16 (m, 3H), 3.07 (ddd, *J* = 13.3, 8.5, 4.1 Hz, 2H), 2.69 (t, 2H), 2.62 (ddd, *J* = 12.6, 7.5, 4.7 Hz, 1H), 2.51 (ddd, *J* = 16.2, 7.3, 4.8 Hz, 1H), 2.21 (s, 6H), 2.17 (s, 6H), 1.96 (ddd, *J* = 16.2, 6.9, 4.9 Hz, 1H). HPLC retention time: 21.5 min. EIMS *m/z* 466.3 (calcd. for C30H31N3O2, 466.24).

Tert-butyl 7-(quinolin-5-ylmethyl)-3,4-dihydroisoquinoline-2(1H)-carboxylate (**7t**). Compound **7t** was synthesized following General Procedure A from compound **3** (50 mg, 0.153 mmol, 1.0 eq), quinolin-5-ylboronic acid (32 mg, 0.184 mmol, 1.2 eq), Pd(dppf)Cl_2 (11 mg, 0.015 mmol, 0.1 eq), and K_2CO_3 (63 mg, 0.459 mmol, 3.0 eq) to yield the product as a yellow oil (36 mg, 63%). ^{1}H-NMR ($CDCl_3$, 500 MHz) δ 8.90 (dd, *J* = 4.2, 1.7 Hz, 1H), 8.30 (ddd, *J* = 8.6, 1.7, 0.9 Hz, 1H), 8.04 (d, *J* = 8.5 Hz, 1H), 7.66 (t, *J* = 7.8 Hz, 1H), 7.39–7.33 (m, 2H), 7.03 (d, *J* = 7.6 Hz, 1H), 6.99–6.85 (m, 2H), 4.48 (s, 2H), 4.39 (s, 2H), 3.60 (t, *J* = 6.1 Hz, 2H), 2.77 (t, *J* = 6.0 Hz, 2H), 1.47 (s, 9H).

(S)-2-amino-3-(4-hydroxy-2,6-dimethylphenyl)-1-(7-(quinolin-5-ylmethyl)-3,4-dihydroisoquinolin-2(1H)-yl)propan-1-one (**8t**). Following General Procedure F, intermediate **7t** (36 mg, 0.096 mmol) was deprotected to yield the amine intermediate. This intermediate was coupled to diBoc-DMT (41 mg, 0.100 mmol, 1.05 eq) in the presence of PyBOP (49 mg, 0.095 mmol, 1.0 eq), and DIEA (123 µL, 0.95 mmol, 10 eq) to yield the product. No 6Cl-HOBt was used. TFA deprotection yielded the product as a white solid. ^{1}H-NMR (CD_3OD, 500 MHz, rotamers) δ 9.15 (dd, *J* = 8.5, 5.5 Hz, 2H), 9.10 (td, *J* = 5.1, 1.5 Hz, 2H), 8.13 (t, *J* = 9.1 Hz, 2H), 8.05 (ddd, *J* = 18.3, 8.7, 7.1 Hz, 2H), 7.93 (ddd, *J* = 8.7, 7.4, 5.2 Hz, 2H), 7.78 (d, *J* = 7.1 Hz, 1H), 7.74 (d, *J* = 7.1 Hz, 1H), 7.04–6.92 (m, 5H), 6.50 (s, 1H), 6.36 (s, 2H), 6.23 (s,

2H), 4.59 (d, *J* = 16.4 Hz, 1H), 4.55 (s, 2H), 4.54 (s, 2H), 4.54–4.52 (m, 2H), 4.47 (d, *J* = 17.1 Hz, 1H), 4.15 (d, *J* = 15.8 Hz, 1H), 3.90 (dt, *J* = 12.9, 5.4 Hz, 1H), 3.43 (dt, *J* = 13.1, 6.6 Hz, 1H), 3.41 (d, *J* = 15.9 Hz, 1H), 3.24–3.16 (m, 3H), 3.07 (ddd, *J* = 13.3, 8.5, 4.1 Hz, 2H), 2.69 (t, *J* = 6.0 Hz, 2H), 2.63 (ddd, *J* = 12.5, 7.4, 4.7 Hz, 1H), 2.50 (ddd, *J* = 16.2, 7.4, 4.8 Hz, 1H), 2.20 (s, 6H), 2.17 (s, 6H), 1.94 (ddd, *J* = 16.1, 6.8, 4.6 Hz, 1H). HPLC retention time: 21.6 min. EIMS *m*/*z* 466.3 (calcd. for C30H31N3O2, 466.24).

Tert-butyl 7-(quinolin-4-ylmethyl)-3,4-dihydroisoquinoline-2(1H)-carboxylate (**7u**). Compound **7u** was synthesized following General Procedure A from compound **3** (50 mg, 0.153 mmol, 1.0 eq), quinolin-4-ylboronic acid (32 mg, 0.184 mmol, 1.2 eq), Pd(dppf)Cl_2 (11 mg, 0.015 mmol, 0.1 eq), and K_2CO_3 (63 mg, 0.459 mmol, 3.0 eq) to yield the product as a colorless oil (32 mg, 56%). ^{1}H-NMR ($CDCl_3$, 500 MHz) δ 8.83 (d, *J* = 4.4 Hz, 1H), 8.13 (d, *J* = 8.4 Hz, 1H), 8.03 (dd, *J* = 8.5, 1.3 Hz, 1H), 7.70 (t, *J* = 7.7 Hz, 1H), 7.54 (t, *J* = 7.7 Hz, 1H), 7.15 (d, *J* = 4.2 Hz, 1H), 7.07 (d, *J* = 7.6 Hz, 1H), 7.03–6.88 (m, 2H), 4.50 (s, 2H), 4.40 (s, 2H), 3.63 (t, *J* = 5.4 Hz, 2H), 2.80 (t, *J* = 5.8 Hz, 2H), 1.47 (s, 9H).

(S)-2-amino-3-(4-hydroxy-2,6-dimethylphenyl)-1-(7-(quinolin-4-ylmethyl)-3,4-dihydroisoquinolin-2(1H)-yl)propan-1-one (**8u**). Following General Procedure F, intermediate **7u** (32 mg, 0.085 mmol) was deprotected to yield the amine intermediate. This intermediate was coupled to diBoc-DMT (37 mg, 0.089 mmol, 1.05 eq) in the presence of PyBOP (44 mg, 0.085 mmol, 1.0 eq), and DIEA (148 µL, 0.85 mmol, 10 eq) to yield the product. No 6Cl-HOBt was used. TFA deprotection yielded the product as a white solid. ^{1}H-NMR (CD_3OD, 500 MHz, rotamers) δ 9.07 (dd, *J* = 9.2, 5.6 Hz, 2H), 8.55 (t, *J* = 9.6 Hz, 2H), 8.26 (t, *J* = 8.8 Hz, 2H), 8.18–8.11 (m, 2H), 8.00–7.93 (m, 2H), 7.78 (d, *J* = 5.6 Hz, 2H), 7.12 (dd, *J* = 7.7, 1.8 Hz, 1H), 7.10 (s, 1H), 7.05 (s, 2H), 7.01 (d, *J* = 7.8 Hz, 1H), 6.60 (s, 1H), 6.37 (s, 2H), 6.20 (s, 2H), 4.74 (s, 2H), 4.71 (s, 2H), 4.61 (d, *J* = 17.2 Hz, 1H), 4.55 (dd, *J* = 12.0, 4.1 Hz, 2H), 4.51 (d, *J* = 17.1 Hz, 1H), 4.20 (d, *J* = 15.8 Hz, 1H), 3.99 (dt, *J* = 12.9, 5.3 Hz, 1H), 3.48 (d, *J* = 15.8 Hz, 1H), 3.40 (dt, *J* = 13.2, 6.7 Hz, 1H), 3.25–3.17 (m, 3H), 3.08 (ddd, *J* = 13.9, 9.9, 4.1 Hz, 2H), 2.73 (t, *J* = 6.1 Hz, 2H), 2.65 (ddd, *J* = 12.5, 7.4, 4.8 Hz, 1H), 2.54 (ddd, *J* = 16.4, 7.4, 4.9 Hz, 1H), 2.21 (s, 6H), 2.18 (s, 6H), 1.98 (ddd, *J* = 16.3, 7.0, 4.7 Hz, 1H). HPLC retention time: 21.2 min. EIMS *m*/*z* 466.3 (calcd. for C30H31N3O2, 466.24).

Tert-butyl 7-(isoquinolin-4-ylmethyl)-3,4-dihydroisoquinoline-2(1H)-carboxylate (**7v**). Compound **7v** was synthesized following General Procedure A from compound **3** (50 mg, 0.153 mmol, 1.0 eq), isoquinolin-4-ylboronic acid (32 mg, 0.184 mmol, 1.2 eq), Pd(dppf)Cl_2 (11 mg, 0.015 mmol, 0.1 eq), and K_2CO_3 (63 mg, 0.459 mmol, 3.0 eq) to yield the crude product. Silica gel chromatography yielded a mixture of products. This mixture was used directly in the next step.

(S)-2-amino-3-(4-hydroxy-2,6-dimethylphenyl)-1-(7-(isoquinolin-4-ylmethyl)-3,4-dihydroisoquinolin-2 (1H)-yl)propan-1-one (**8v**). Following General Procedure F, intermediate **7v** (19 mg, 0.051 mmol) was deprotected. The crude product was purified by semi-preparative HPLC to yield the product as a white solid (21 mg, 100%). EIMS calcd. for [C19H18N2 + H]$^+$: 275.15, found: 275.2. The amine was coupled to diBoc-DMT (23 mg, 0.057 mmol, 1.05 eq) in the presence of PyBOP (28 mg, 0.054 mmol, 1.0 eq), and DIEA (94 µL, 0.54 mmol, 10 eq) to yield the product. No 6Cl-HOBt was used. TFA deprotection yielded the product as a white solid. ^{1}H-NMR (CD_3OD, 500 MHz, rotamers) δ 9.65 (d, *J* = 6.0 Hz, 2H), 8.50 (t, *J* = 8.3 Hz, 2H), 8.42–8.35 (m, 4H), 8.22–8.14 (m, 2H), 8.04–7.97 (m, 2H), 7.10 (dd, *J* = 7.8, 1.8 Hz, 1H), 7.07 (s, 1H), 7.02 (s, 2H), 6.97 (d, *J* = 7.9 Hz, 1H), 6.56 (s, 1H), 6.37 (s, 2H), 6.21 (s, 2H), 4.61 (d, *J* = 16.1 Hz, 1H), 4.57 (s, 2H), 4.56 (s, 2H), 4.55–4.52 (m, 2H), 4.49 (d, *J* = 17.2 Hz, 1H), 4.17 (d, *J* = 15.8 Hz, 1H), 3.95 (dt, *J* = 12.9, 5.3 Hz, 1H), 3.45 (d, *J* = 15.5 Hz, 1H), 3.43–3.38 (m, 1H), 3.25–3.17 (m, 3H), 3.07 (ddd, *J* = 13.7, 8.1, 4.1 Hz, 2H), 2.72 (t, *J* = 6.0 Hz, 2H), 2.65 (ddd, *J* = 12.7, 7.3, 4.8 Hz, 1H), 2.52 (ddd, *J* = 16.4, 7.1, 4.8 Hz, 1H), 2.21 (s, 6H), 2.17 (s, 6H), 1.95 (dt, *J* = 16.4, 6.2 Hz, 1H). HPLC retention time: 21.5 min. EIMS *m*/*z* 466.3 (calcd. for C30H31N3O2, 466.24).

Tert-butyl 7-((3,4-dihydroisoquinolin-2(1H)-yl)methyl)-3,4-dihydroisoquinoline-2(1H)-carboxylate (**7w**). Compound **7w** was synthesized following General Procedure E from compound **3** (50 mg, 0.153 mmol, 1.0 eq), 1,2,3,4-tetrahydroisoquinoline (23 µL, 0.184 mmol, 1.2 eq), and K_2CO_3 (25 mg, 0.184 mmol, 1.2 eq) to yield the product as a colorless oil (24 mg, 41%). ^{1}H-NMR ($CDCl_3$, 500 MHz) δ 7.19 (d, *J* = 7.5 Hz, 1H), 7.15 (s, 1H), 7.12–7.08 (m, 4H), 6.99 (d, *J* = 7.0 Hz, 1H), 4.57 (s, 2H), 3.66 (br s, 2H), 3.64 (s, 2H), 3.63 (s, 2H), 2.90 (t, *J* = 6.0 Hz, 2H), 2.83 (t, *J* = 5.9 Hz, 2H), 2.75 (t, *J* = 5.9 Hz, 2H), 1.49 (s, 9H).

(S)-2-amino-1-(7-((3,4-dihydroisoquinolin-2(1H)-yl)methyl)-3,4-dihydroisoquinolin-2(1H)-yl)-3-(4-hydroxy-2,6-dimethylphenyl)propan-1-one (**8w**). Following General Procedure F, intermediate **7w** (24 mg, 0.063 mmol, 1.0 eq) was deprotected to yield the amine intermediate. This intermediate was coupled to diBoc-DMT (27 mg, 0.067 mmol, 1.05 eq) in the presence of PyBOP (33 mg, 0.064 mmol, 1.0 eq), and DIEA (111 μL, 0.64 mmol, 10 eq) to yield the product. No 6Cl-HOBt was used. TFA deprotection yielded the product as a white solid. ^{1}H-NMR (CD_3OD, 500 MHz, rotamers) δ 7.36–7.33 (m, 2H), 7.32–7.23 (m, 7H), 7.21–7.13 (m, 4H), 6.85 (s, 1H), 6.41 (s, 2H), 6.21 (s, 2H), 4.72 (d, *J* = 17.3 Hz, 1H), 4.62 (d, *J* = 17.3 Hz, 1H), 4.64–4.57 (m, 2H), 4.44 (s, 2H), 4.42–4.35 (m, 5H), 4.29 (d, *J* = 16.0 Hz, 1H), 4.10 (dt, *J* = 13.0, 5.0 Hz, 1H), 3.73 (br s, 1H), 3.57 (d, *J* = 16.1 Hz, 1H), 3.46–3.35 (m, 2H), 3.28–3.26 (m, 1H), 3.26–3.15 (m, 6H), 3.15–3.07 (m, 2H), 2.80 (t, *J* = 6.0 Hz, 2H), 2.76–2.67 (m, 1H), 2.62 (dt, *J* = 16.5, 6.0 Hz, 1H), 2.24 (s, 6H), 2.22 (s, 6H), 2.04 (dt, *J* = 6.9, 5.0 Hz, 1H). HPLC retention time: 21.3 min. HREIMS *m/z* 470.2799 (calcd. for C30H35N3O2, 470.2802).

Tert-butyl 7-((3,4-dihydroquinolin-1(2H)-yl)methyl)-3,4-dihydroisoquinoline-2(1H)-carboxylate (**7x**). Compound **7x** was synthesized following General Procedure E from compound **3** (50 mg, 0.153 mmol, 1.0 eq), 1,2,3,4-tetrahydroquinoline (23 μL, 0.184 mmol, 1.2 eq), and K_2CO_3 (25 mg, 0.184 mmol, 1.2 eq). The reaction mixture was diluted with water. The aqueous layer was extracted with several portions of ethyl acetate. Combined organic layers were dried over $MgSO_4$, filtered, and concentrated under vacuum. Silica gel chromatography yielded a mixture of the desired product and 1,2,3,4-tetrahydroquinoline. The product was partitioned between ethyl acetate and 2 M NaOH. The aqueous layer was extracted with ethyl acetate. Some 1,2,3,4-tetrahydroquinoline remained. The mixture was resubmitted to reaction conditions with additional **3** (25 mg, 0.076, 0.5 eq) and K_2CO_3 (25 mg, 0.184 mmol, 1.2 eq). Silica gel chromatography yielded the desired product as a colorless oil (24 mg, 28%).^{1}H-NMR ($CDCl_3$, 500 MHz) δ 7.08 (s, 1H), 7.02 (s, 1H), 6.99 (t, *J* = 6.5 Hz, 2H), 6.59 (t, *J* = 7.3 Hz, 1H), 6.51 (d, *J* = 8.5 Hz, 1H), 4.55 (s, 2H), 4.44 (s, 2H), 3.65 (s, 2H), 3.36 (t, *J* = 5.7 Hz, 2H), 2.92–2.75 (m, 4H), 2.03 (p, *J* = 6.1 Hz, 2H), 1.50 (s, 9H).

(S)-2-amino-1-(7-((3,4-dihydroquinolin-1(2H)-yl)methyl)-3,4-dihydroisoquinolin-2(1H)-yl)-3-(4-hydroxy-2,6-dimethylphenyl)propan-1-one (**8x**). Following General Procedure F, intermediate **7x** (24 mg, 0.063 mmol, 1.0 eq) was deprotected to yield the amine intermediate. This intermediate was coupled to diBoc-DMT (27 mg, 0.067 mmol, 1.05 eq) in the presence of PyBOP (33 mg, 0.064 mmol, 1.0 eq), and DIEA (111 μL, 0.64 mmol, 10 eq) to yield the product. No 6Cl-HOBt was used. TFA deprotection yielded the product as a white solid. ^{1}H-NMR (CD_3OD, 500 MHz, rotamers) δ 7.09 (d, *J* = 7.9 Hz, 1H), 7.04 (d, *J* = 8.1 Hz, 2H), 7.01 (d, *J* = 7.9 Hz, 1H), 6.99–6.89 (m, 5H), 6.64–6.51 (m, 5H), 6.40 (s, 2H), 6.27 (s, 2H), 4.62 (d, *J* = 17.1 Hz, 1H), 4.58–4.53 (m, 2H), 4.51 (d, *J* = 17.0 Hz, 2H), 4.45 (s, 2H), 4.44 (s, 2H), 4.19 (d, *J* = 15.8 Hz, 1H), 3.93 (dt, *J* = 12.9, 5.4 Hz, 1H), 3.51–3.43 (m, 1H), 3.46 (d, *J* = 15.7 Hz, 1H), 3.40–3.34 (m, 4H), 3.26–3.19 (m, 3H), 3.11–3.05 (m, 2H), 2.81 (q, *J* = 5.9 Hz, 4H), 2.73 (t, *J* = 6.2 Hz, 2H), 2.69–2.62 (m, 1H), 2.54 (dt, *J* = 16.3, 6.1 Hz, 1H), 2.23 (s, 6H), 2.20 (s, 6H), 2.06–1.95 (m, 5H). HPLC retention time: 35.9 min. HREIMS *m/z* 470.2800 (calcd. for C30H35N3O2, 470.2802).

Tert-butyl 7-(indolin-1-ylmethyl)-3,4-dihydroisoquinoline-2(1H)-carboxylate (**7y**). Compound **7y** was synthesized following General Procedure E from compound **3** (50 mg, 0.153 mmol, 1.0 eq), indoline (21 μL, 0.184 mmol, 1.2 eq), and K_2CO_3 (25 mg, 0.184 mmol, 1.2 eq) to yield the product as a brown oil (37 mg, 66%). ^{1}H-NMR ($CDCl_3$, 500 MHz) δ 7.18 (d, *J* = 7.9 Hz, 1H), 7.15–7.08 (m, 3H), 7.07 (t, *J* = 7.6 Hz, 1H), 6.69 (t, *J* = 7.3 Hz, 1H), 6.52 (d, *J* = 7.8 Hz, 1H), 4.58 (s, 2H), 4.21 (s, 2H), 3.66 (s, 2H), 3.32 (t, *J* = 8.2 Hz, 2H), 2.99 (t, *J* = 8.3 Hz, 2H), 2.84 (t, *J* = 6.0 Hz, 2H), 1.51 (s, 9H).

(S)-2-amino-3-(4-hydroxy-2,6-dimethylphenyl)-1-(7-(indolin-1-ylmethyl)-3,4-dihydroisoquinolin-2(1H)-yl)propan-1-one (**8y**). Following General Procedure F, intermediate **7y** (37 mg, 0.102 mmol, 1.0 eq) was deprotected to yield the amine intermediate. This intermediate was coupled to diBoc-DMT (43 mg, 0.105 mmol, 1.05 eq) in the presence of PyBOP (52 mg, 0.100 mmol, 1.0 eq), and DIEA (174 μL, 1.0 mmol, 10 eq) to yield the product. No 6Cl-HOBt was used. TFA deprotection yielded the product as a white solid. ^{1}H-NMR (CD_3OD, 500 MHz, rotamers) δ 7.24–7.18 (m, 3H), 7.18–7.11 (m, 4H), 7.06 (d, *J* = 7.9 Hz, 1H), 7.03–6.94 (m, 4H), 6.89 (d, *J* = 8.5 Hz, 1H), 6.67 (s, 1H), 6.41 (s, 2H), 6.27 (s, 2H), 4.63 (d,

J = 16.9 Hz, 1H), 4.60–4.56 (m, 2H), 4.53 (d, J = 17.2 Hz, 1H), 4.40–4.32 (m, 4H), 4.21 (d, J = 15.8 Hz, 1H), 3.89 (dt, J = 12.7, 5.5 Hz, 1H), 3.55–3.50 (m, 1H), 3.50–3.46 (m, 4H), 3.44 (d, J = 15.9 Hz, 1H), 3.28–3.17 (m, 3H), 3.13–3.06 (m, 2H), 2.99 (t, J = 7.6 Hz, 4H), 2.74 (t, J = 4.7 Hz, 2H), 2.72–2.65 (m, 1H), 2.56 (dt, J = 16.3, 6.0 Hz, 1H), 2.23 (s, 6H), 2.20 (s, 6H), 1.98 (dt, J = 16.2, 5.9 Hz, 1H). HPLC retention time: 30.1 min. HREIMS *m/z* 456.2644 (calcd. for C29H33N3O2, 456.2646).

Tert-butyl 7-(isoindolin-2-ylmethyl)-3,4-dihydroisoquinoline-2(1H)-carboxylate (**7z**). Compound **7z** was synthesized following General Procedure E from compound **3** (50 mg, 0.153 mmol, 1.0 eq), isoindoline HCl (29 mg, 0.184 mmol, 1.2 eq), and K_2CO_3 (25 mg, 0.184 mmol, 1.2 eq) to yield the product as an orange oil (22 mg, 39%). ^{1}H-NMR ($CDCl_3$, 500 MHz) δ 7.29 (s, 1H), 7.21 (d, J = 7.8 Hz, 1H), 7.18 (s, 4H), 7.12 (d, J = 7.6 Hz, 1H), 4.58 (s, 2H), 3.93 (s, 4H), 3.88 (s, 2H), 3.65 (t, J = 8.2 Hz, 2H), 2.84 (t, J = 6.2 Hz, 2H), 1.49 (s, 9H).

(S)-2-amino-3-(4-hydroxy-2,6-dimethylphenyl)-1-(7-(isoindolin-2-ylmethyl)-3,4-dihydroisoquinolin-2(1H)-yl)propan-1-one (**8z**). Following General Procedure F, intermediate **7z** (22 mg, 0.060 mmol, 1.0 eq) was deprotected to yield the amine intermediate. This intermediate was coupled to diBoc-DMT (26 mg, 0.063 mmol, 1.05 eq) in the presence of PyBOP (31 mg, 0.060 mmol, 1.0 eq), and DIEA (105 μL, 0.600 mmol, 10 eq) to yield the product. No 6Cl-HOBt was used. TFA deprotection yielded the product as a white solid. ^{1}H-NMR (CD_3OD, 500 MHz, rotamers) δ 7.41–7.38 (m, 8H), 7.37–7.34 (m, 2H), 7.30 (dd, J = 7.9, 1.8 Hz, 1H), 7.19 (dd, J = 7.9, 3.5 Hz, 1H), 7.16 (dd, J = 8.0, 3.7 Hz, 1H), 6.86 (s, 1H), 6.42 (s, 2H), 6.24 (s, 2H), 4.72 (d, J = 17.2 Hz, 1H), 4.70–4.64 (m, 8H), 4.61 (d, J = 15.3 Hz, 1H), 4.65–4.57 (m, 2H), 4.56 (s, 2H), 4.53 (d, J = 10.7 Hz, 2H), 4.29 (d, J = 16.0 Hz, 1H), 4.09 (dt, J = 13.2, 4.9 Hz, 1H), 3.57 (d, J = 15.9 Hz, 1H), 3.44–3.37 (m, 1H), 3.29–3.25 (m, 1H), 3.24 (q, J = 13.0 Hz, 2H), 3.15–3.07 (m, 2H), 2.80 (t, J = 4.3 Hz, 2H), 2.75–2.67 (m, 1H), 2.61 (dt, J = 16.2, 5.6 Hz, 1H), 2.25 (s, 6H), 2.23 (s, 6H), 2.07–2.00 (m, 1H). HPLC retention time: 20.1 min. HREIMS *m/z* 456.2645 (calcd. for C29H33N3O2, 456.2646).

4.2. Pharmacology

The pharmacological methods used were the same as those previously described [14], with any changes noted below. Unless otherwise noted, all tissue culture reagents and radiolabeled ligands were purchased from commercial sources. Cell lines were provided by Professor Lawrence Toll [34].

4.2.1. Cell Lines and Membrane Preparations

Membranes prepared from transfected Chinese Hamster Ovary cells stably expressing human KOR, human MOR, or human DOR were used for all assays. Cells were grown to confluence at 37 °C in 5% CO_2 in 1:1 DMEM:F12 media with 10% *v/v* fetal bovine serum and 5% *v/v* penicillin/streptomycin. Membranes were prepared by washing confluent cells three times with ice cold phosphate-buffered saline (0.9% NaCl, 0.61 mM Na_2HPO_4, 0.38 mM KH_2PO_4, pH 7.4). Cells were detached from the plates by incubation in warm harvesting buffer (20 mM HEPES, 150 mM NaCl, 0.68 mM EDTA, pH 7.4) and pelleted by centrifugation at 200× *g* for 3 min. The cell pellet was suspended in ice-cold 50 mM Tris-HCl buffer, pH 7.4 and homogenized with a Tissue Tearor (Biospec Products, Inc, distributed by Cole-Parmer, Vernon Hills, IL, USA) for 20 s at setting 4. The homogenate was centrifuged at 20,000× *g* for 20 min at 4 °C, and the pellet was rehomogenized in 50 mM Tris-HCl pH 7.4 with a Tissue Tearor for 10 s at setting 2, followed by recentrifugation. The final pellet was resuspended in 50 mM Tris-HCl pH 7.4 and frozen in aliquots at −80 °C. Protein concentration was determined via Pierce BCA protein assay kit using bovine serum albumin as the standard.

4.2.2. Binding Affinity

Binding affinities for all test compounds at KOR, MOR, and DOR were determined by competitive displacement of [^{3}H]-diprenorphine as previously reported [35–38]. In a 96-well plate format, cell membranes (5–10 μg of protein) and [^{3}H]-diprenorphine (0.2 nM) were incubated in Tris-HCl buffer (50 mM, pH 7.4) with various concentrations of test compound at 25 °C for 1 h, allowing the mixture to reach equilibrium. Nonspecific binding was determined using the opioid antagonist naloxone (10 μM), and total binding was determined using vehicle in the absence of competitive ligand. After incubation, membranes were filtered through Whatman GF/C 1.2 micron glass fiber filters and washed with 50 mM Tris-HCl buffer. The radioactivity remaining on the filters was then quantified by liquid scintillation counting after saturation with EcoLume liquid scintillation cocktail in a Microbeta 2450 (Perkin-Elmer, Waltham, MA, USA). Binding affinity (K_i) values were calculated using the Cheng–Prusoff equation via nonlinear regression analysis using GraphPad Prism software from at least three separate binding assays performed in duplicate.

4.2.3. Stimulation of [^{35}S]-GTPγS Binding

Agonist stimulation of KOR, MOR, and DOR by all test compounds was determined by [^{35}S]-guanosine 5′-*O*-[γ-thio]triphosphate ([^{35}S]-GTPγS) binding assays as previously reported [35–38]. In a 96-well plate format, membranes from cells expressing opioid receptors as described above (10 µg of protein), [^{35}S]-GTPγS (0.1 nM), and guanosine diphosphate (30 µM) were incubated in GTPγS buffer (50 mM Tris-HCl, 100 mM NaCl, 5 mM $MgCl_2$, 1 mM EDTA, pH 7.4) with various concentrations of test compound at 25 °C for 1 h. Basal stimulation was determined by incubation in the absence of any ligand. After incubation, membranes were filtered through Whatman GF/C 1.2 micron glass fiber filters and washed with GTPγS buffer with no EDTA. The radioactivity remaining on the filters was then quantified by liquid scintillation counting after saturation with EcoLume liquid scintillation cocktail in a Perkin-Elmer Microbeta 2450. Data are reported as percent stimulation compared to the effects of 10 µM standard agonists—U69,593 (KOR), DAMGO (MOR), or DPDPE (DOR). Percent stimulation and EC_{50} values were determined via nonlinear regression analysis using GraphPad Prism software from at least three separate assays performed in duplicate. Efficacy is expressed as percent stimulation relative to standard agonists.

Author Contributions: Conceptualization, D.M. and H.I.M.; methodology, D.M.; validation, D.M. and J.P.A.; formal analysis, D.M., J.P.A., M.A.B., J.J.T., J.G.H., L.J.D.; investigation, D.M., J.P.A., M.A.B., J.J.T., J.G.H., L.J.D.; resources, J.R.T., H.I.M.; data curation, J.P.A.; writing—original draft preparation, D.M.; writing—review and editing, D.M., H.I.M.; visualization, D.M.; supervision, J.R.T., H.I.M.; project administration, D.M., J.P.A.; funding acquisition, J.R.T., H.I.M.

Funding: This research was funded by NIH, grant number DA003910. Resources were provided by the Edward F. Domino Research Center. D.M. was supported by an ACS MEDI Pre-doctoral Fellowship and an AFPE Pre-doctoral Fellowship. J.P.A. was supported by NIH, grant number DA 048129. M.A.B. was supported by the University of Michigan Interdisciplinary REU grant (NSF DBI #1560096).

Acknowledgments: The authors would like to thank Ashley C. Brinkel for additional in vitro studies.

Conflicts of Interest: The authors declare no conflict of interest. The funders had no role in the design of the study; in the collection, analyses, or interpretation of data; in the writing of the manuscript, or in the decision to publish the results.

References

1. Brownstein, M.J. A brief history of opiates, opioid peptides, and opioid receptors. *Proc. Natl. Acad. Sci. USA* **1993**, *90*, 5391–5393. [CrossRef] [PubMed]
2. Levinthal, C.F. Milk of Paradise/Milk of Hell—The History of Ideas about Opium. *Perspect. Biol. Med.* **1985**, *28*, 561–577. [CrossRef] [PubMed]
3. Dreborg, S.; Sundstrom, G.; Larsson, T.A.; Larhammar, D. Evolution of vertebrate opioid receptors. *Proc. Natl. Acad. Sci. USA* **2008**, *105*, 15487–15492. [CrossRef] [PubMed]
4. Kieffer, B.L.; Evans, C.J. Opioid receptors: From binding sites to visible molecules in vivo. *Neuropharmacology* **2009**, *56*, 205–212. [CrossRef]
5. Erlandson, S.C.; McMahon, C.; Kruse, A.C. Structural Basis for G Protein–Coupled Receptor Signaling. *Annu. Rev. Biophys.* **2018**, *47*, 1–18. [CrossRef]
6. Weis, W.I.; Kobilka, B.K. The Molecular Basis of G Protein–Coupled Receptor Activation. *Annu. Rev. Biochem.* **2018**, *87*, 897–919. [CrossRef]

7. Chavkin, C.; Koob, G.F. Dynorphin, Dysphoria, and Dependence: The Stress of Addiction. *Neuropsychopharmacol. Rev.* **2016**, *41*, 373–374. [CrossRef]
8. Lalanne, L.; Ayranci, G.; Kieffer, B.L.; Lutz, P.-E. The kappa opioid receptor: From addiction to depression, and back. *Front. Psychiatry* **2014**, *5*, 170. [CrossRef]
9. Lutz, P.E.; Kieffer, B.L. Opioid receptors: Distinct roles in mood disorders. *Trends Neurosci.* **2013**, *36*, 195–206. [CrossRef]
10. Le Merrer, J.; Becker, J.A.J.; Befort, K.; Kieffer, B.L. Reward Processing by the Opioid System in the Brain. *Physiol. Rev.* **2009**, *89*, 1379–1412. [CrossRef]
11. Dietis, N.; Guerrini, R.; Calo, G.; Salvadori, S.; Rowbotham, D.J.; Lambert, D.G. Simultaneous Targeting of Multiple Opioid Receptors: A Strategy to Improve Side-effect Profile. *Br. J. Anaesth.* **2009**, *103*, 38–49. [CrossRef]
12. Turnaturi, R.; Arico, G.; Ronsisvalle, G.; Parenti, C.; Pasquinucci, L. Multitarget opioid ligands in pain relief: New players in an old game. *Eur. J. Med. Chem.* **2016**, *108*, 211–228. [CrossRef]
13. Anand, J.P.; Montgomery, D. Multifunctional opioid ligands. *Handb. Exp. Pharmacol.* **2018**, *247*, 21–51.
14. Montgomery, D.; Anand, J.P.; Griggs, N.W.; Fernandez, T.J.; Hartman, J.G.; Sánchez-Santiago, A.A.; Pogozheva, I.D.; Traynor, J.R.; Mosberg, H.I. Novel Dimethyltyrosine–Tetrahydroisoquinoline Peptidomimetics with Aromatic Tetrahydroisoquinoline Substitutions Show in Vitro Kappa and Mu Opioid Receptor Agonism. *ACS Chem. Neurosci.* **2019**. [CrossRef]
15. Balboni, G.; Guerrini, R.; Salvadori, S.; Bianchi, C.; Rizzi, D.; Bryant, S.D.; Lazarus, L.H. Evaluation of the Dmt-Tic pharmacophore: Conversion of a potent delta-opioid receptor antagonist into a potent delta agonist and ligands with mixed properties. *J. Med. Chem.* **2002**, *45*, 713–720. [CrossRef]
16. Balboni, G.; Salvadori, S.; Trapella, C.; Knapp, B.I.; Bidlack, J.M.; Lazarus, L.H.; Peng, X.; Neumeyer, J.L. Evolution of the bifunctional lead mu agonist/delta Antagonist containing the 2′,6′-dimethyl-L-tyrosine-1,2,3,4-tetrahydroisoquinoline-3-carboxylic acid (Dmt-Tic) opioid pharmacophore. *ACS Chem. Neurosci.* **2010**, *1*, 155–164. [CrossRef]
17. Santagada, V.; Balboni, G.; Caliendo, G.; Guerrini, R.; Salvadori, S.; Bianchi, C.; Bryant, S.D.; Lazarus, L.H. Assessment of substitution in the second pharmacophore of Dmt-Tic analogues. *Bioorg. Med. Chem. Lett.* **2000**, *10*, 2745–2748. [CrossRef]
18. Balboni, G.; Salvadori, S.; Guerrini, R.; Negri, L.; Giannini, E.; Bryant, S.D.; Jinsmaa, Y.; Lazarus, L.H. Direct influence of C-terminally substituted amino acids in the Dmt-Tic pharmacophore on delta-opioid receptor selectivity and antagonism. *J. Med. Chem.* **2004**, *47*, 4066–4071. [CrossRef]
19. Pagé, D.; Naismith, A.; Schmidt, R.; Coupal, M.; Labarre, M.; Gosselin, M.; Bellemare, D.; Payza, K.; Brown, W. Novel C-terminus modifications of the Dmt-Tic motif: A new class of dipeptide analogues showing altered pharmacological profiles toward the opioid receptors. *J. Med. Chem.* **2001**, *44*, 2387–2390. [CrossRef]
20. Pagé, D.; McClory, A.; Mischki, T.; Schmidt, R.; Butterworth, J.; St-Onge, S.; Labarre, M.; Payza, K.; Brown, W. Novel Dmt-Tic dipeptide analogues as selective delta-opioid receptor antagonists. *Bioorg. Med. Chem. Lett.* **2000**, *10*, 167–170. [CrossRef]
21. Mello, N.K.; Negus, S.S. Effects of kappa opioid agonists on cocaine- and food-maintained responding by rhesus monkeys. *J. Pharmacol. Exp. Ther.* **1998**, *286*, 812–824. [PubMed]
22. Negus, S.S.; Mello, N.K.; Portoghese, P.S.; Lin, C. Effects of Kappa Opioids on Cocaine Self-Administration by Rhesus Monkeys. *J. Pharmacol. Exp. Ther.* **1997**, *282*, 44–55. [PubMed]
23. Neumeyer, J.L.; Bidlack, J.M.; Zong, R.; Bakthavachalam, V.; Gao, P.; Cohen, D.J.; Negus, S.S.; Mello, N.K. Synthesis and opioid receptor affinity of morphinan and benzomorphan derivatives: Mixed kappa agonists and mu agonists/antagonists as potential pharmacotherapeutics for cocaine dependence. *J. Med. Chem.* **2000**, *43*, 114–122. [CrossRef] [PubMed]
24. Bowen, C.A.; Stevens Negus, S.; Zong, R.; Neumeyer, J.L.; Bidlack, J.M.; Mello, N.K. Effects of Mixed-Action kappa/mu Opioids on Cocaine Self-Administration and Cocaine Discrimination by Rhesus Monkeys. *Neuropsychopharmacology* **2003**, *28*, 1125–1139. [CrossRef]
25. Dick, G.R.; Woerly, E.M.; Burke, M.D. A general solution for the 2-pyridyl problem. *Angew. Chemie Int. Ed.* **2012**, *51*, 2667–2672. [CrossRef]
26. Mabrouk, O.S.; Viaro, R.; Volta, M.; Ledonne, A.; Mercuri, N.; Morari, M. Stimulation of delta Opioid Receptor and Blockade of Nociceptin/Orphanin FQ Receptor Synergistically Attenuate Parkinsonism. *J. Neurosci.* **2014**, *34*, 12953–12962. [CrossRef]

27. Dripps, I.J.; Jutkiewicz, E.M. Delta Opioid Receptors and Modulation of Mood and Emotion. *Handb. Exp. Pharmacol.* **2017**, *247*, 179–197.
28. Abdelhamid, E.E.; Sultana, M.; Portoghese, P.S.; Takemori, A.E. Selective Blockage of the Delta Opioid Receptors Prevents the Development of Morphine Tolerance and Dependence in Mice. *J. Pharmacol. Exp. Ther.* **1991**, *258*, 299–301.
29. Rozenfeld, R.; Abul-Husn, N.S.; Gomes, I.; Devi, L.A. An Emerging Role for the Delta Opioid Receptor in the Regulation of Mu Opioid Receptor Function. *Sci. World J.* **2007**, *7*, 64–73. [CrossRef]
30. Martin, T.J.; Kim, S.A.; Cannon, D.G.; Sizemore, G.M.; Bian, D.; Porreca, F.; Smith, J.E. Antagonism of Delta(2) Opioid Receptors by Naltrindole-5′-isothiocyanate Attenuates Heroin Self-Administration but not Antinociception in Rats. *J. Pharmacol. Exp. Ther.* **2000**, *294*, 975–982.
31. Mosberg, H.I.; Yeomans, L.; Harland, A.A.; Bender, A.M.; Sobczyk-Kojiro, K.; Anand, J.P.; Clark, M.J.; Jutkiewicz, E.M.; Traynor, J.R. Opioid Peptidomimetics: Leads for the Design of Bioavailable Mixed Efficacy mu Opioid Receptor (MOR) Agonist/delta Opioid Receptor (DOR) Antagonist Ligands. *J. Med. Chem.* **2013**, *56*, 2139–2149. [CrossRef] [PubMed]
32. Henry, S.P.; Fernandez, T.J.; Anand, J.P.; Griggs, N.W.; Traynor, J.R.; Mosberg, H.I. Structural Simplification of a Tetrahydroquinoline-Core Peptidomimetic μ-Opioid Receptor (MOR) Agonist/δ-Opioid Receptor (DOR) Antagonist Produces Improved Metabolic Stability. *J. Med. Chem.* **2019**, *62*, 4142–4157. [CrossRef] [PubMed]
33. Nastase, A.F.; Griggs, N.W.; Anand, J.P.; Fernandez, T.J.; Harland, A.A.; Trask, T.J.; Jutkiewicz, E.M.; Traynor, J.R.; Mosberg, H.I. Synthesis and Pharmacological Evaluation of Novel C-8 Substituted Tetrahydroquinolines as Balanced-Affinity Mu/Delta Opioid Ligands for the Treatment of Pain. *ACS Chem. Neurosci.* **2018**, *9*, 1840–1848. [CrossRef] [PubMed]
34. Toll, L.; Berzetei-Gurske, I.P.; Polgar, W.E.; Brandt, S.R.; Adapa, I.D.; Rodriguez, L.; Schwartz, R.W.; Haggart, D.; O'Brien, A.; White, A.; et al. Standard binding and functional assays related to medications development division testing for potential cocaine and opiate narcotic treatment medications. *NIDA Res. Monogr.* **1998**, *178*, 440–466. [PubMed]
35. Traynor, J.R.; Nahorski, S.R. Modulation by mu-opioid agonists of guanosine-5′-O-(3-[^{35}S]thio)triphosphate binding to membranes from human neuroblastoma SH-SY5Y cells. *Mol. Pharmacol.* **1995**, *47*, 848–854. [PubMed]
36. Lee, K.O.; Akil, H.; Woods, J.H.; Traynor, J.R. Differential binding properties of oripavines at cloned mu- and delta-opioid receptors. *Eur. J. Pharmacol.* **1999**, *378*, 323–330. [CrossRef]
37. Harrison, C.; Traynor, J.R. The [^{35}S]GTPgammaS binding assay: Approaches and applications in pharmacology. *Life Sci.* **2003**, *74*, 489–508. [CrossRef]
38. Harland, A.A.; Bender, A.M.; Griggs, N.W.; Gao, C.; Anand, J.P.; Pogozheva, I.D.; Traynor, J.R.; Jutkiewicz, E.M.; Mosberg, H.I. Effects of N-Substitutions on the Tetrahydroquinoline (THQ) Core of Mixed-Efficacy μ-Opioid Receptor (MOR)/δ-Opioid Receptor (DOR) Ligands. *J. Med. Chem.* **2016**, *59*, 4985–4998. [CrossRef]

Sample Availability: Limited samples of most final compounds are available from the authors. Detailed synthetic procedures for all novel compounds are included in the manuscript.

molecules

MDPI

Article

Rigorous Computational and Experimental Investigations on MDM2/MDMX-Targeted Linear and Macrocyclic Peptides

David J. Diller [1,2], Jon Swanson [1,3], Alexander S. Bayden [1,4], Chris J. Brown [5], Dawn Thean [5], David P. Lane [5], Anthony W. Partridge [6,7], Tomi K. Sawyer [7,*] and Joseph Audie [1,8,*]

1. CMDBioscience, 5 Park Avenue, New Haven, CT 06511, USA; djrdiller@gmail.com (D.J.D.); jon@chemmodeling.com (J.S.); alexander@bayden.net (A.S.B.)
2. Venenum BioDesign, LLC, 8 Black Forest Road, Hamilton, NJ 08691, USA
3. ChemModeling, LLC, Suite 101, 500 Huber Park Ct, Weldon Spring, MO 63304, USA
4. Kleo Pharmaceuticals, 25 Science Park, Ste 235, New Haven, CT 06511, USA
5. A*STAR, p53 Laboratory, Singapore 138648, Singapore; cjbrown@p53lab.a-star.edu.sg (C.J.B.); dawn.thean@gmail.com (D.T.); dplane@p53Lab.a-star.edu.sg (D.P.L.)
6. MSD International GmbH, Singapore 138665, Singapore; anthony_partridge@merck.com
7. Merck Research Laboratories, 33 Avenue Louis Pasteur, Boston, MA 02115, USA
8. College of Arts and Sciences, Department of Chemistry, Sacred Heart University, 5151 Park Avenue, Fairfield, CT 06825, USA

* Correspondence: sawyerkrt@aol.com (T.K.S.); audiej@sacredheart.edu (J.A.)

Received: 24 November 2019; Accepted: 12 December 2019; Published: 14 December 2019

Abstract: There is interest in peptide drug design, especially for targeting intracellular protein–protein interactions. Therefore, the experimental validation of a computational platform for enabling peptide drug design is of interest. Here, we describe our peptide drug design platform (CMDInventus) and demonstrate its use in modeling and predicting the structural and binding aspects of diverse peptides that interact with oncology targets MDM2/MDMX in comparison to both retrospective (pre-prediction) and prospective (post-prediction) data. In the retrospective study, CMDInventus modules (CMDpeptide, CMDboltzmann, CMDescore and CMDyscore) were used to accurately reproduce structural and binding data across multiple MDM2/MDMX data sets. In the prospective study, CMDescore, CMDyscore and CMDboltzmann were used to accurately predict binding affinities for an Ala-scan of the stapled α-helical peptide ATSP-7041. Remarkably, CMDboltzmann was used to accurately predict the results of a novel D-amino acid scan of ATSP-7041. Our investigations rigorously validate CMDInventus and support its utility for enabling peptide drug design.

Keywords: peptide design; free energy calculation; d-amino acid scan; alanine scan

1. Introduction

A renaissance in peptide drug discovery is underway, especially as it pertains to selectively targeting disease associated intracellular protein–protein interactions. Not surprisingly, many new chemical and biological technologies have been developed and are being used to enable the design and discovery of peptide research tools and drug candidates. Recent work points to an emerging role for information-based and physics-based computational methods to advance novel linear and macrocyclic peptide drug discovery. Here, we take an important step in that direction and describe the rigorous experimental validation of multiple computational methods and predictions in retrospective and prospective peptide conformational modeling and binding affinity studies on the well-known and clinically important p53-MDM2/MDMX systems. Our study is instructive in that it includes a broad range of MDM2/MDMX associated data—including data from linear peptides, D-peptides, stapled peptides, bicyclic peptides, and N–C cyclized peptides—and includes a prospective binding affinity study with computational predictions made using a range of methods prior to experimental testing. Importantly, the prospective binding affinity study strongly validates the use of our computational methods in guiding the design of α-helical peptides and shows how such computational methods, especially when combined with scientific ingenuity, can be used to model and propose novel peptide synthetic modifications.

For nearly three decades, MDM2 and MDMX have been aggressively pursued as oncology drug targets [1]. Briefly, p53 acts as a tumor suppressor by causing cell-cycle arrest and apoptosis in response to DNA damage. For this reason, it is often referred to as the guardian of the genome [2]. In many forms of cancer, p53 is inactivated either through mutation or through the over-expression of negative regulators, including MDM2 and MDMX. MDM2 and MDMX act to regulate p53 via interaction with its N-terminal transactivation domain, which corresponds approximately to residues 17–29. Thus, blocking the MDMX/MDM2/p53 interactions has been and remains a focal point in cancer drug discovery. Indeed, both biotech and pharma have serious interest in developing stapled α-helical peptide drugs to target the p53 binding sites of MDMX and MDM2. Specifically, Aileron Therapeutics is currently testing ALRN-6924, a dual MDM2/MDMX inhibitor in Phase I/II clinical trials [3].

Due to the intense interest over such a long period of time, a rich and complex data set has emerged around inhibitors of the MDM2/p53 and MDMX/p53 interactions. Collectively, this may represent the most extensive target data set available for novel peptide-based drug discovery. For example, there are at least 19 MDM2 and 9 MDMX crystal structures with co-crystallized peptides available in the Protein Data Bank (PDB). Further, many of the co-crystal structures have corresponding structure activity relationship (SAR) data available in the literature (see Table 1), with many having both MDM2 and MDMX SAR data.

Table 1. Datasets used as starting points for binding affinity scoring calculations.

Article	Peptide Ligand	MDM2	MDMX
Li	PMI	3eqs	3eqy
Li	p53	4hfz	3dab
Liu	D-α-helix	3lnj	3lnj/3eqy *
Sawyer	Stapled α-helix	3v3b	4n5t
Fasan	N–C cyclic peptide	2axi	

* 3lnj peptide docked in 3eqy.

The first major MDM2/MDMX-targeted SAR study used linear α-helical peptides comprised of all L-amino acids. Li and co-workers [4] published an extensive mutational analysis of MDM2 and MDMX binding to both p53 (residues 17–28 ETFSDLWKLLPE) and the more potent linear peptide PMI (TSFAEYWNLLSP). This dataset consists largely of an alanine scan of each peptide along with a handful of truncated peptides. Both peptides have been crystallized with MDM2 (p53 in 1ycr [5] and 4hfz [6], and PMI in 3eqs [7]). PMI has additionally been co-crystallized with MDMX (3eqy [7]).

A noteworthy MDM2/MDMX-targeted SAR dataset with peptide ligands comprised of all D-α-helices is provided by Liu and coworkers [8]. In this work, mirror image phage display was used to find an all D-peptide, referred to as PMI-α, that binds potently to MDM2. Importantly, there are three MDM2 crystal structures with all D-amino acid α-helical peptides (3iwy [8], 3lnj [8] and 3tpx [9]). Interestingly, the SAR for the all D-amino acid α-helices differs markedly from that of the L-amino acid α-helices. For example, while the same three MDM2/MDMX pockets are filled by three critical residues of each peptide, the specific nature of the residues is quite different: F-W-L for the L-α-helices and W-L-L for the D-α-helices (Figure 1). Further, the L-α-helices described in the previous paragraph lose 2–5 fold in binding affinity for MDMX relative to MDM2 whereas the D-α-helical peptides lose nearly 100–1000 fold in binding affinity [9].

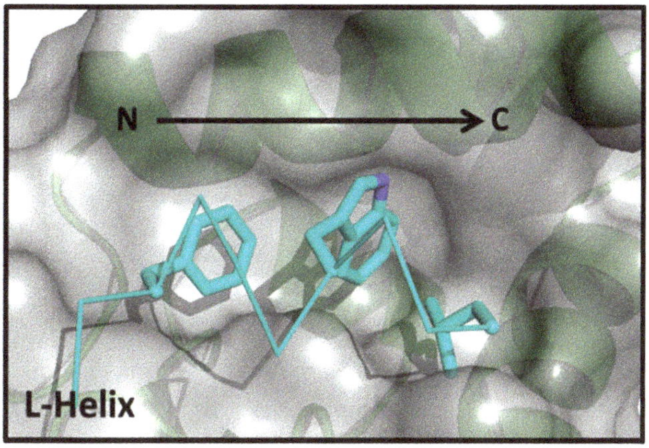

(**A**)

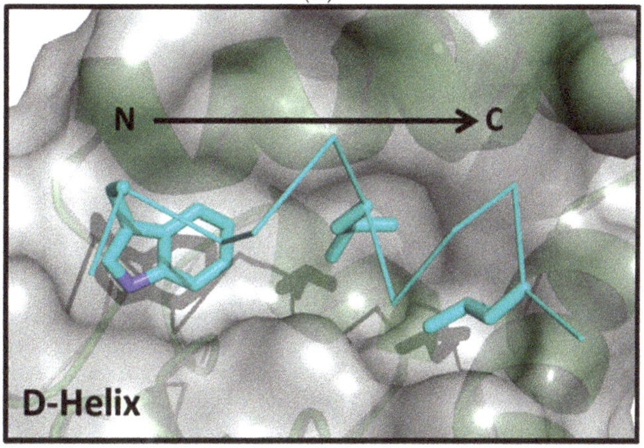

(**B**)

Figure 1. A comparison of the critical binding element of an L-α-helical peptide compare to those of a D-α-helical peptide. (**A**) The L-helical peptide (3jzs [4]). (**B**) The D-helical peptide (3lnj [8]). The preferred residues of the L-α-helix for the three critical pockets are Phe, Trp and Leu whereas the three corresponding interactions of the D-α-helix are Trp, Leu and Leu. In both cases MDM2 is shown in the same orientation.

A significant MDM2/MDMX-targeted α-helical peptide SAR dataset was developed using stapled α-helical peptides. Stapled α-helical peptides are engineered by chemically connecting two side-chains (*i* and *j*) in a helix, typically using an alkyl chain, which can result in stabilization of the α-helical conformation. There are five MDM2/MDMX structures with bound stapled α-helical peptides: (1) 3v3b [10] (1–7 stapled α-helix bound to MDM2), (2) 4ud7/4ue1 [11] (1–4 stapled α-helix bound to MDM2), (3) 4umn [12] (1–7 stapled α-helix bound to the M62A MDM2 mutant), (4) 4n5t [13] (the 1–7 stapled α-helix ATSP-7041 bound to MDMX), and (5) 5afg [14] (a more complicated 1–7 stapled α-helix bound to MDM2). These structures come with excellent SAR, including investigations into the effects of different staples on p53 [15], the impacts of a number of single residue changes, and a full alanine scan around the stapled L-α-helix ATSP3900 [13,16].

In addition to the structures with stapled α-helices, there is a single structure, 3iux [17], with MDM2 bound to a bicyclic peptide with two disulfide bonds, referred to as stingin. Also, there is a single structure of a non-α-helical peptide bound to MDM2, 2axi [18]. This peptide is a 10 residue N–C cyclic peptide adopting a β-hairpin conformation which is capped by a Pro-D-Pro motif. This data set is remarkable in that it includes MDM2 binding data for >70 analogue peptides, many of which contain non-natural amino acids in addition to the invariant D-Pro.

In what follows, we describe the use of several of the computational tools that comprise our integrated computational peptide design platform (CMDInventus) to investigate the extent to which they can reproduce the aforementioned p53/MDM2/MDMX SAR data and prospectively predict the binding effects of conservative and non-conservative peptide ligand modifications. Toward this end, we first describe the use of our physics-based conformational sampling algorithm to successfully model and reproduce the observed bound conformations of several peptide ligands. Second, we describe the utility of our binding free energy estimation methods to reproduce the measured binding and activity trends present in the various data sets. Importantly, all retrospective or post-data collection calculations were performed without explicit fitting or re-parameterization of any kind. Of course, the most demanding test of any method is its accuracy at predicting future observations. Hence, we describe the use of the various computational methods to model and prospectively calculate or blindly predict prior to data collection binding affinities for two series of peptides, one corresponding to an alanine scan and the second to a D-amino acid scan of a stapled α-helical peptide. The prospective all-D scan study is of special importance, as it is experimentally novel and resulted in some nonintuitive computational predictions being confirmed by experiment.

2. Results and Discussion

Because a typical CMDInventus peptide modeling and design work-flow integrates the use of CMDpeptide, CMDescore, CMDyscore and CMDboltzmann, we deemed it important to test all approaches wherever possible in retrospective and prospective analyses. The strength of the retrospective analysis is that it allows the methods to be tested against a large and diverse amount of data. The problem with retrospective testing, however, is that it may suffer from various biases. It is hoped that prospective testing will help mitigate these biases. By testing methods retrospectively and prospectively, it is hoped that information will be gained about the role each method can play in a CMDInventus design work-flow.

2.1. Retrospective Study

Conformational sampling calculations with CMDpeptide. CMDpeptide calculations start from peptide sequences and, when appropriate, inter-residue bonding information such as disulfide bonds. In particular, they do not employ any structural information. The results of the peptide conformational analysis are shown in Table 2 and Figure 2. All RMSDs reported are calculated over the backbone atoms and C_β atoms. This provides a more demanding measure of structural similarity than does the more typical RMSDs over just C_α atoms because including the C_β atom captures side-chain orientation. An assumption behind CMDpeptide is that calculated ensembles will include a broad range of biologically relevant peptide conformations, including protein binding conformations. As will be shown below, this assumption is validated by our results.

In all cases studied, there is at least one peptide conformation among the low-energy conformations (within 15 kcal/mol of the lowest energy conformation) within an RMSD < 1.6 Å of the co-crystallized peptide ligand conformation with an overall average RMSD of 1.12 Å. In fact, for seven of the sixteen cases conformations with RMSDs < 1.0 Å were identified. Hence, CMDpeptide can be used to consistently sample conformations close to the bound conformation observed in MDM2/MDMX cocrystal structures. This is an encouraging result, especially given that a range of peptide lengths (8–18 resides) and chemical types (L-linear, N–C cyclized, bicyclic, D-linear, and L-stapled) were studied and that much of the calculated RMSD values result from conformational deviations at N and C termini. Similarly, it is worth pointing out that there is a relatively weak but non-trivial correlation between peptide length and best low-energy RMSD ($R \approx 0.46$). In fact, a simple two term regression model that includes peptide length and the presence or absence of a staple as independent descriptors can be used to account for ≈ 68% of the measured variation in lowest RMSD.

Table 2. CMDpeptide results: Here, we summarize the full results of the CMDpeptide conformational analysis calculations. Each of these calculations begins with only sequence and inter-residue bonding information, i.e., only topological information. The "Number of AA" column lists the number of amino acids (not including the capping groups) and in parentheses lists the number of non-standard amino acids. The "Min RMSD" column gives the minimum RMSD conformation (Å) relative to the corresponding X-ray conformation of all conformations within 15 kcal/mol of the lowest energy conformation. Finally, the results from clustering with a radius of 1.0 Å are shown, including the total number of clusters (Size) and the lowest RMSD conformations within the top 25, 100 and 500 ranked clusters. All RMSDs are calculated over backbone atoms plus the C_β atoms. Average values are provided (the average value for cluster size has been rounded up to a whole number).

PDB	Description	Number of AA	Min RMSD (Å)	Cluster 1.0 Å			
				Size	25 (RMSD)	100 (RMSD)	500 (RMSD)
1ycr	L-α-helix (p53 17-29)	13 (0)	1.29	9547	2.9	2.2	2.1
2axi	N–C cyclic β-hairpin	10 (1)	0.77	744	1.4	1.3	1.3
2gv2	L-α-helix	8 (4)	1.17	3595	1.9	1.4	1.4
3eqs	L-α-helix	11 (0)	0.75	11,112	1.7	1.7	1.4
3g03	L-α-helix	11 (0)	0.94	9175	2.5	2.1	1.4
3iux	Stingin–2 disulfide bonds	18 (0)	1.34	4721	2.3	2.2	1.7
3iwy	D-α-helix	12 (12)	0.95	8074	2.1	1.8	1.5
3jzo	L-α-helix	12 (0)	1.02	7743	2.6	2.2	1.3
3jzs	L-α-helix	12 (0)	0.92	5368	2.6	2.6	1.5
3lnj	D-α-helix	11 (11)	0.88	3091	2.8	1.5	1.0
3tpx	D-α-helix	11 (11)	0.88	4784	2.4	1.7	1.1
3v3b.	Stapled α-helix	13 (2)	1.40	3674	2.5	2.3	1.8
4n5t	Stapled α-helix	14 (3)	1.44	4310	2.6	2.0	1.5
4ud7	Stapled α-helix	14 (2)	1.32	6484	3.2	2.5	1.5
4umn	Stapled α-helix	11 (2)	1.54	3201	2.2	1.9	1.7
5afg	Stapled α-helix	12 (2)	1.36	4354	2.4	1.5	1.5
		Average	1.12	5624	2.38	2.16	1.48

Not surprisingly, the average best peptide conformation RMSD trends down from 2.38 Å, to 2.16 Å, to 1.48 Å as the number of as the number of conformations allows increases from 25, to 100, to 500. Importantly, even at 500 clusters the best low-energy RMSD peptide identified is never present. So, while the results are encouraging, they suggest that the improvements in the scoring strategy are still needed for identifying and ranking best RMSD peptide binding conformations. This conclusion is reinforced by the fact that our current force field scoring and clustering protocols failed to pick out best RMSD conformations where sampling does not appear to be an issue (sampled conformations within ≈ 0.8 Å of X-ray). It remains a possibility, however, that incomplete sidechain sampling failed to identify a sidechain interaction that would have led to the ranking of those conformation close to the X-ray conformation near to the top of the ensemble. Indeed, the combination of the large sampling space with the scoring problem makes the peptide conformational analysis a difficult challenge.

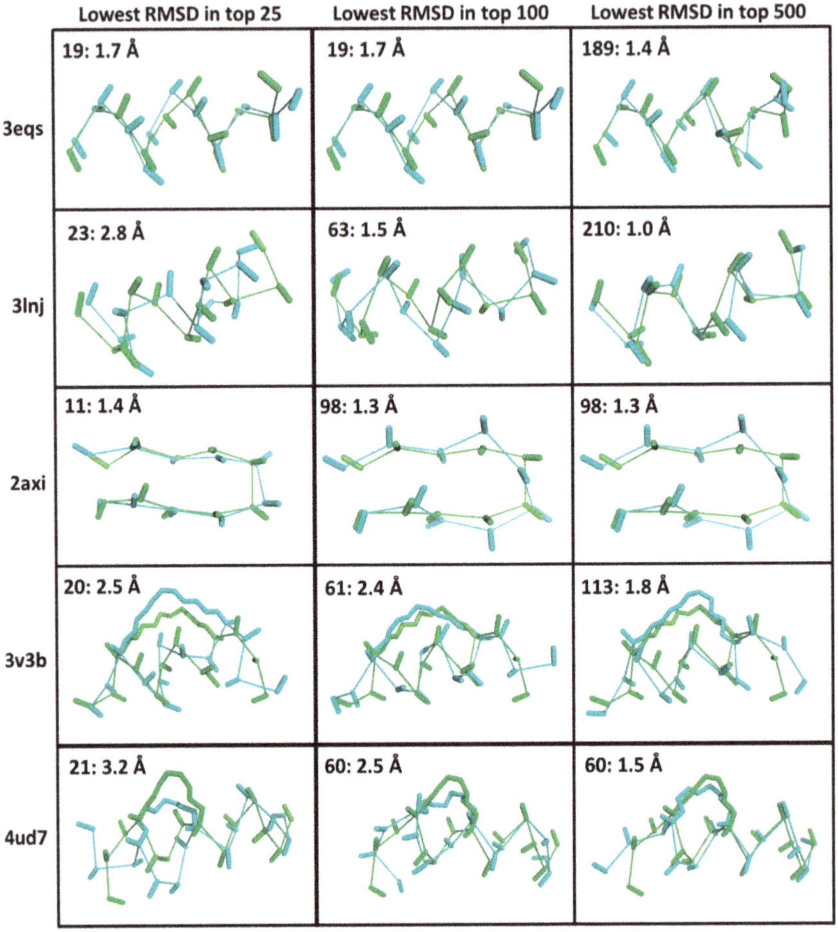

Figure 2. Selected conformations from CMDpeptide calculations. Here, we show select results from Table 2. For this figure, we took the peptides from the PDB structures below. The first column of images shows the conformations in the top 25 ranked conformations with the lowest RMSDs to the bound conformations. The second column of images shows the conformations in the top 100 ranked conformations with the lowest RMSDs. The third column of images shows the conformations in the top 500 ranked conformations with the lowest RMSDs. In each case a conformational ensemble was generated starting from a sequence using the default parameters of CMDpeptide. In each case, the bound conformation is shown in green and the CMDpeptide conformation in cyan. Each peptide is shown as a ribbon with the C_α-C_β bond. Additionally, for the stapled helices the staple is shown.

MDM2-peptide binding affinity calculations with CMDboltzmann. As described in detail in the Materials and Methods section, CMDboltzmann is a tool for estimating the binding affinity of a peptide given knowledge of the binding mode of a portion of its backbone. It particular, it locally samples a peptide conformation in the binding site of a protein producing a calculated binding affinity that is based on numerous similar binding modes of the peptide. As a result, it tends to be less sensitive to the exact details of the starting binding mode. The results of the CMDboltzmann calculations on the various data sets are shown in Figure 3. In all, six MDM2/MDMX SAR datasets were analyzed: (1) p53 L-helix variants, (2) PMI L-α-helix variants, (3) PMI-α D-α-helix variants, (4) ATSP-3900 stapled L-α-helix ala scan variants, (5) p53 L-α-helix staple variants, and (6) N–C cyclized variants. Hence, the

CMDboltzmann binding affinity calculations cover diverse peptide chemistries and topologies. The CMBboltzmann calculations were all performed using the 3eqs structure of MDM2 using the binding mode extracted from the corresponding co-crystal structures with the respective peptide.

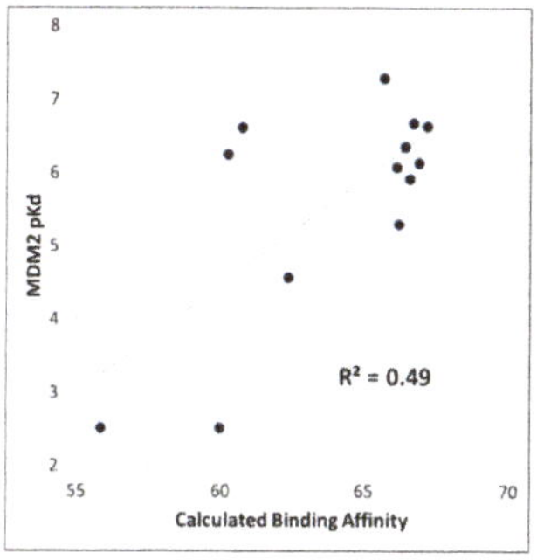

(**A**) Boltzmann calculations on p53 L-α-helix variants

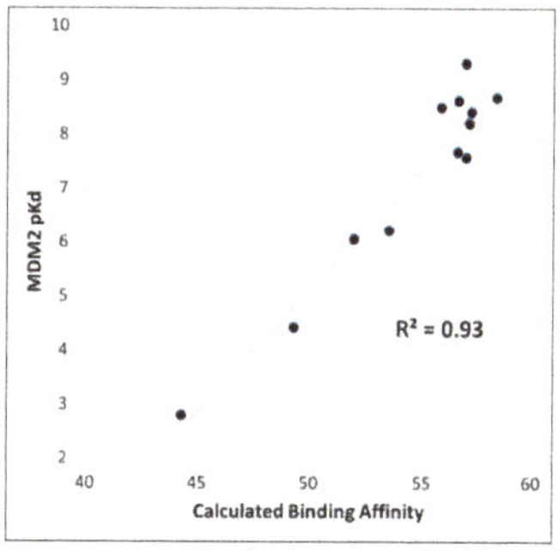

(**B**) Boltzmann calculations on PMI L-α-helix variants

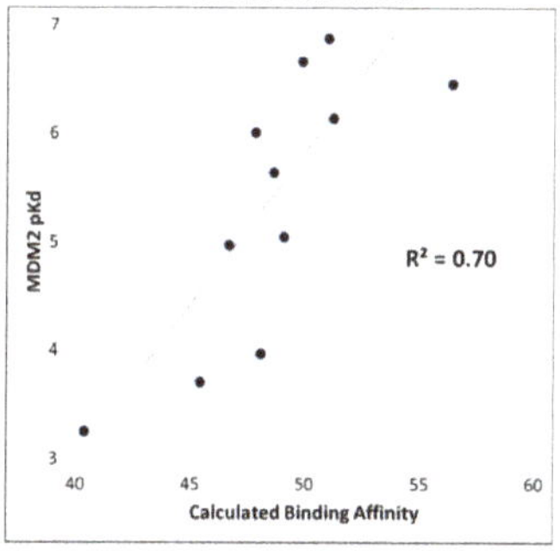

(**C**) Boltzmann calculations on PMI D-α-helix variants

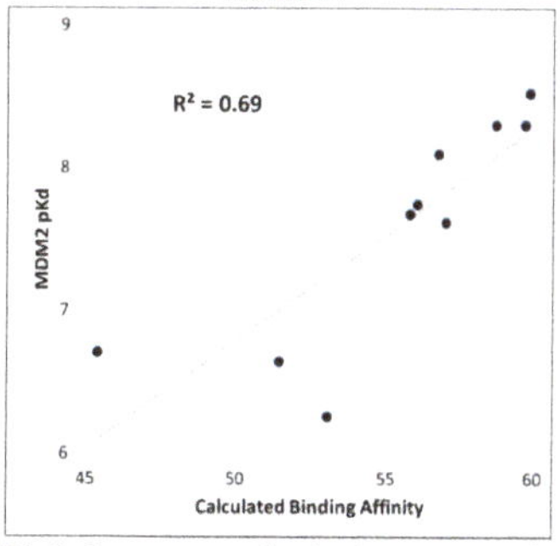

(**D**) Boltzmann calculations on ATSP-3900 stapled L-α-helix variants

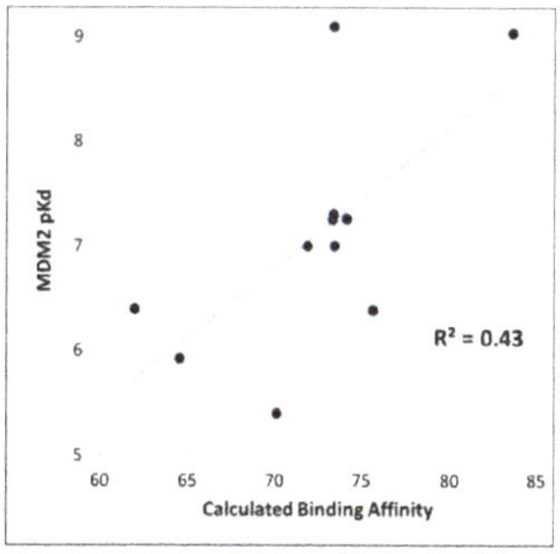

(**E**) Boltzmann calculations on p53 L-α-helix staple variants

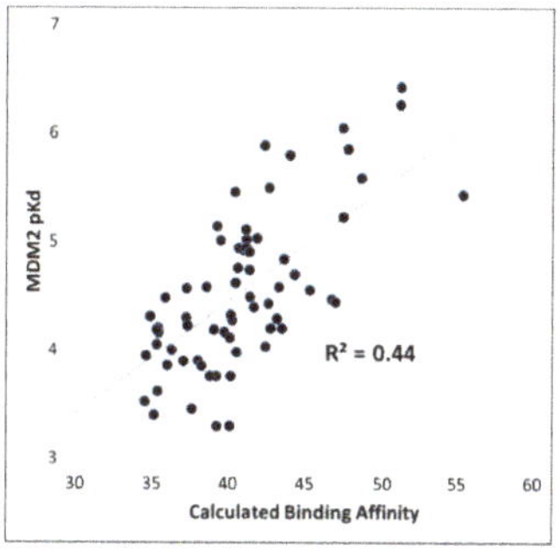

(**F**) N–C cyclic peptides

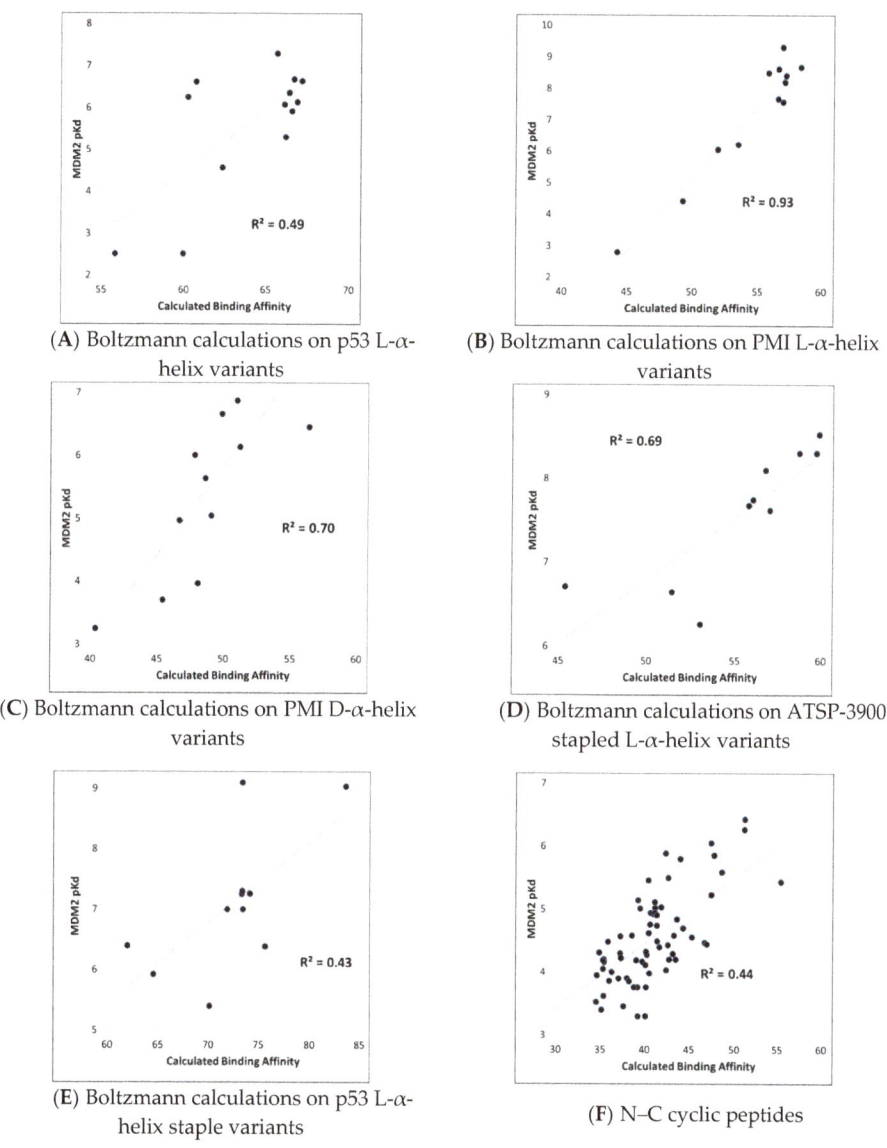

Figure 3. The CMDboltzmann calculations on the individual data sets—All figures show CMDboltzmann calculated binding affinities recorded on the X-axis and experimental binding affinities (typically pKd) recorded on the Y-axis. (**A**) Structure activity relationship (SAR) around the L-α-helix p53 [4]. (**B**) SAR around the L-α-helix PMI [4]. (**C**) SAR around the D-helix PMI-α [8]. (**D**) SAR around the stapled L-α-helix ATSP-3900 [16]. (**E**) SAR around L-α-helix p53 stapled variants SAR [15]. (**F**) SAR around the N–C cyclic peptide from the 2axi structure [18].

As can be seen from Figure 3, the R^2s between calculated and experimental binding affinities vary from 0.43 to 0.93. Hence, the CMDboltzmann calculations can account for some 43%–93% of the measured binding affinity variation. This is an encouraging result, especially given the diverse sizes and topologies of the peptides studied and the large changes in amino acids found in the data sets particularly the N–C cyclized variants.

Further, Figure 4 shows calculated binding affinities versus measured pK_d values for all peptides studied, color coded by data set. Once again, the results are encouraging, as a fairly straight line can be drawn through the calculated and measured binding affinities for all of the PMI L-α-helix, PMI-α D-α-helix, ATSP-3900 stapled L-α-helix, and N–C cyclized peptides. With just these four data sets, i.e., omitting the p53 peptide analogs, the overall R^2 is 0.75. By including the p53 peptide analogs, the R^2 falls to 0.48. The p53 peptide analogs show higher calculated binding affinities than expected, suggesting that a penalty contribution of some kind is missing from the CMDboltzmann model. The missing penalty contribution likely derives from two missing factors. The first factor is the inability of the solvation model to adequately counter balance the electrostatic binding interactions. P53 is a highly negatively charged peptide, as it contains four charged residues and both termini are free and ionized, and the high charge may pose a serious challenge to the EEF1 solvation model. In essence, CMDboltzmann overestimates the electrostatic contributions from charged amino acids. The second missing factor has to do with the conformational penalty associated with the p53 peptide "climbing" into its binding conformation. Indeed, p53 and direct analogs are known to be disordered in water and only adopt an α-helical conformation in the context of MDM2/MDMX binding sites. In fact, p53 has been shown to be approximately 11% α-helical in solution [15]. By comparison, PMI has been shown to readily adopt an α-helical conformation in water as well. Hence, it is reasonable to assume that p53 will suffer a greater free energy cost upon binding when compared to the other peptide ligands. Thus, future work might focus on improving the CMDboltzmann electrostatic solvation model and extending CMDboltzmann to include sampling of unbound conformations to better estimate the free energy penalties associated with burying charged groups and flexible ligand binding.

Calculating MDM2/MDMX binding selectivity with CMDboltzmann. As a final test of the CMDboltzmann procedure for estimating binding affinities, we examined the differences in MDM2 and MDMX binding affinities. The MDMX calculations were all performed using the MDMX structure from 3jzo [19]. For the PMI analogs [4] and L-α-helices the differences in binding affinities are modest. In particular, on average the PMI analogs show two-fold more affinity for MDM2 over MDMX (see Figure 5). Encouragingly, with the exception of a single peptide, our calculations qualitatively agree with experiment as they show very small differences between calculated binding affinities between PMI and MDM2 and MDMX. In contrast, the two most potent of the D-α-helical peptides have been shown to be essentially inactive versus MDM2 [9]. As can be seen in Figure 5, we find substantial differences between the calculated MDM2 and MDMX binding affinities for the D-α-helical peptides. Thus, the MDM2/MDMX affinity selectivity calculations are in encouraging qualitative agreement with the available experimental data for the D-α-helical peptides as well.

Calculating binding affinities from single structures using CMDescore and CMDyscore. CMDescore and CMDyscore, as described in the Materials and Methods section, score peptide binding modes based on a single fixed complex structure. All CMDescore and CMDyscore scoring methods were used to calculate MDM2/MDMX-peptide binding affinities for the datasets summarized in Table 3. For comparative purposes, the Vina and X-score scoring functions and simple surface area and packing empirical functions were also used on the same datasets. Binding affinity and binding energy calculations are shown either ignoring inactive peptides or accounting for them by giving them a very low binding affinity with results summarized in Table 3A,B, respectively. The latter only affects the Li p53 data, but adds information on the ability of the methods to distinguish good from very poor binders. Hence, our focus will be more focused on analyzing the results from Table 3B.

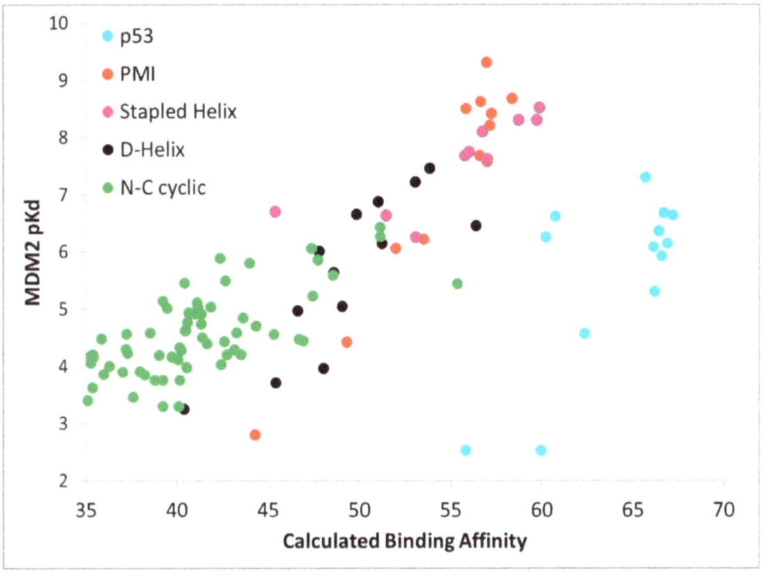

Figure 4. Boltzmann calculations on the entire MDM2 data set. Each of the four data sets shown in Figure 3 above is plotted as a separate color. As is apparent the Li-p53 data set stands out as having higher than expected calculated binding affinities in comparison to the other data sets. There are two reasonable explanations for why the affinity of the p53 analogs is generally overestimated relative to the rest of the peptides. First, these peptides are highly negatively charged while MDM2 has a net positive charge and the empirical solvation model used may not be adequate to address the difference in charge. Second, p53 is known to be highly disordered in solution thereby encurring a large free energy penalty upon binding in the α-helical conformation whereas the other peptide families are known to be more stable and structured in solution.

As indicated in Table 3B, CMDescore generated useful binding affinity estimates for all seven datasets, resulting in an average R^2 of ≈ 0.69. This is an encouraging result, especially given its simplicity, physical intuitiveness, and rapid speed of calculation. Comparing the various CMDyscore results (Table 3B), one can see the clear benefit of adding a solvation term to the force field. Indeed, CMDyscore, when combined with solvation, posted some good correlations and, with two exceptions, consistently outperformed all other scoring procedures resulting in an impressive average R^2 of 0.81. Using uncharged amino acids with CMDyscore resulted in an average R^2 of ≈ 0.73. The simple implementation of CMDyscore produced an R^2 of ≈ 0.62. This pattern suggests the hypothesis that mitigating the impact of charged residues on binding is of considerable importance and that, in the present study, this is best achieved with an implicit solvation model. Our attempt to consider strain in the bound conformation with CMDyscore calculations resulted in the poorest average CMDyscore result (R^2 ≈ 0.60).

It is interesting to note how well the simple packing scoring function performed, yielding an average R^2 of ≈ 0.75 (Table 3B). The packing score is a quality metric available in YASARA [5]. It is a weighted average of three individual metrics: normality of dihedral angles (0.145), normality of 1D distance-dependent packing interactions (0.390), and normality of 3D direction-dependent packing interactions (0.465). The metrics are knowledge-based potentials. The dihedral potential is based on the probability of finding the observed dihedral in a reference PDB database. The 1D potential is based on probabilities of finding specific atom–atom distances. The 3D potential is based on probabilities of finding atoms in a specific direction where the coordinate system is based on a central heavy atom and two of its bonded neighbors. All probabilities are converted to energies which are then converted to

Z-scores. Perhaps this is not too surprising for the MDMX and MDM2 systems, as binding to both targets is dominated by the three hydrophobic hot spot residues. Moreover, success for a simple packing scoring function reproducing affinity trends for known binders to known interfaces does not entail success at predicting hypothesized binders to hypothesized interfaces—a key aspect of computational peptide drug design—where tight packing can be offset or reinforced by electrostatic and desolvation effects, etc. Considerations like these caution against generalization and justify the continued development and use of more complicated multi-term scoring functions, even when correlations prove to be similar on specific datasets.

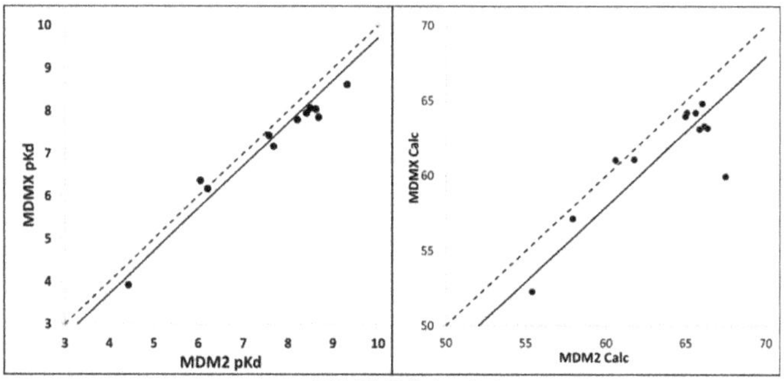

(**A**) PMI Selectivity

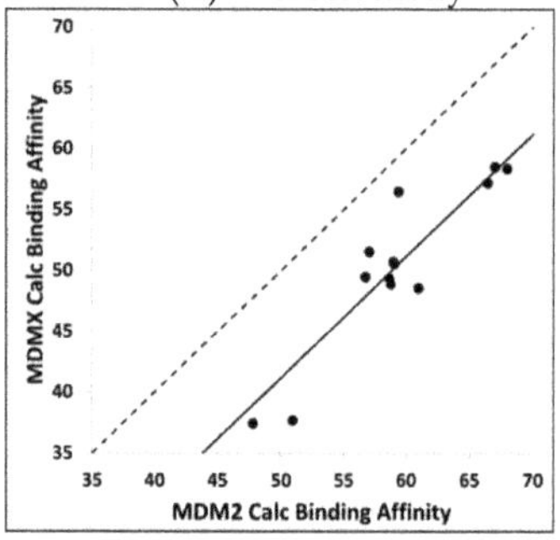

(**B**) D-α-helix selectivity

Figure 5. Selectivity Calculations with CMDboltzmann—Here, we compare measured MDM2/MDMX selectivity to calculated selectivity. (**A**) The left panel shows the experimental pKd of MDM2 versus the experimental MDMX pKd for PMI analogs [4]. The dashed line shows the line where the MDM2 and MDMX are identical. The solid line shows the best fit line to the MDM2/MDMX data. Clearly, the MDM2 and MDMX binding affinities are very close to one another. The right panel shows the comparison of the MDM2 and MDMX calculated binding affinities for the same peptides. Again, the dash line shows where the MDM2 and MDMX calculated binding affinities are identical and the solid line is the best fit between the two. In the calculated case, we see a slight preference for MDM2 over MDMX. (**B**) This panel shows a comparison of the MDM2 and MDMX calculated binding affinities for the D-α-helical analogs [8]. Here, we see a large preference for MDM2 over MDMX. In this case, the experimental binding affinities are not known for all of the peptides. It is known, however, that the two that are most potent for MDM2 are much weaker for MDMX [9]. Thus, the selectivity calculations are in encouraging qualitative agreement with the available experimental data for the D-α-helical peptides as well.

Table 3. Retrospective single pose scoring results.

A. Mutation + scoring (exluding inactives).

	R^2 MDM2					R^2 MDMX			Statistics	
Method	**Li PMI**	**Li p53**	**Liu D-α**	**Guerlavais Stpl-α**	**Fasan Stpl-α**	**Li PMI**	**Li p53**	**Guerlavais Stpl-α**	**Avg**	**Stdev**
CMDescore	0.831	0.031	**0.933**	0.556	0.420 [1]	0.799	0.245	0.829	0.581	0.325
CMDyscore (minimize)	0.775	0.033	0.445	0.475	0.683	0.906	*0.013*	0.823	0.519	0.345
CMDyscore	0.837	0.027	0.463	0.507	**0.705**	0.908	*0.007*	0.837	0.536	0.357
CMDyscore (uncharged)	0.920	0.374	0.574	0.484	0.624	0.884	0.005	0.831	0.587	0.306
CMDyscore (solvation)	**0.930**	**0.485**	0.775	**0.609**	0.518	**0.958**	**0.575**	0.884	**0.717**	**0.193**
Xscore	0.890	0.290	0.726	0.540	0.442	0.850	0.434	0.816	0.624	0.226
VINA	0.912	0.300	0.682	0.493	0.534	0.893	0.233	0.833	0.610	0.263
Packing	0.870	0.330	0.677	0.551	0.418 [1]	0.804	0.566	**0.921**	0.642	0.213
Buried SA	0.795	0.001	0.537	0.289	0.338	0.747	0.022	0.548	0.410	0.301

Bold means the largest in each column; Italics mean an inverse correlation; best prediction in bold; [1] CMDescore and packing interface score are not parameterized for non-canonical amino acids and so these were not included in the correlation; "Stpl-α" stands for stapled alpha helical peptide and "D-α" stands for D alpha helical peptide.

B. Mutation + scoring (including inactives).

	R^2 MDM2					R^2 MDMX			Statistics	
Method	**Li PMI**	**Li p53**	**Liu D-α**	**Guerlavais Stpl-α**	**Fasan Stpl-α**	**Li PMI**	**Li p53**	**Guerlavais Stpl-α**	**Avg**	**Stdev**
CMDescore	0.831	0.466	**0.933**	0.556	0.420 [1]	0.799	0.692	0.829	0.690	0.189
CMDyscore (minimize)	0.775	0.334	0.445	0.475	0.683	0.906	0.317	0.823	0.595	0.230
CMDyscore	0.837	0.332	0.463	0.507	**0.705**	0.908	0.328	0.837	0.615	0.236
CMDyscore (uncharged)	0.920	0.815	0.574	0.484	0.624	0.884	0.717	0.831	0.731	**0.157**
CMDyscore (solvation)	**0.930**	**0.891**	0.775	**0.609**	0.518	**0.958**	**0.909**	0.884	**0.809**	0.163
Xscore	0.890	0.835	0.726	0.540	0.442	0.850	0.863	0.816	0.745	0.166
VINA	0.912	0.835	0.682	0.493	0.534	0.893	0.801	0.833	0.748	0.161
Packing	0.870	0.859	0.677	0.551	0.418 [1]	0.804	0.883	**0.921**	0.748	0.182
Buried SA	0.795	0.523	0.537	0.289	0.338	0.747	0.545	0.548	0.540	0.174

Bold means the largest in each column; Italics mean an inverse correlation; best prediction in bold; [1] CMDescore and packing interface score are not parameterized for non-canonical amino acids and so these were not included in the correlation; "Stpl-α" stands for stapled alpha helical peptide and "D-α" stands for D alpha helical peptide.

Also, worth commenting on is that the scoring functions provide quantitative binding affinity values for all peptides, whereas in the Li dataset some peptides are only listed as qualitatively 'inactive'. In order to include information from inactive peptides, the K_d for these peptides was set to −2.0 kcal/mol. A comparison of the results summarized in Table 3A,B shows that this addition significantly affects the calculated R^2 values for the p53 dataset, illustrating that it is much easier for a scoring function to determine active from inactive compounds than it is to quantitatively discriminate among a set of active compounds.

A plot of the PMI, p53, D-α-helix, and stapled α-helix predictions for the best single scoring function (CMDyscore with solvation) and a consensus scoring function are shown in Figure 6. The consensus score was created by combining the predictions of CMDescore, CMDyscore, VINA, and Xscore. For each score, the values were normalized between zero (worst score) and one (best score). The consensus score then was taken as the mean of these four normalized scores. This consensus score was then plotted against the normalized binding energies. In the case of MDM2, the best single function outperformed the consensus. For MDMX, however, the consensus score proved to be superior. Note also that the overall correlation across the data sets is not as strong as with any individual dataset. This is not surprising, given the data was collected by different groups.

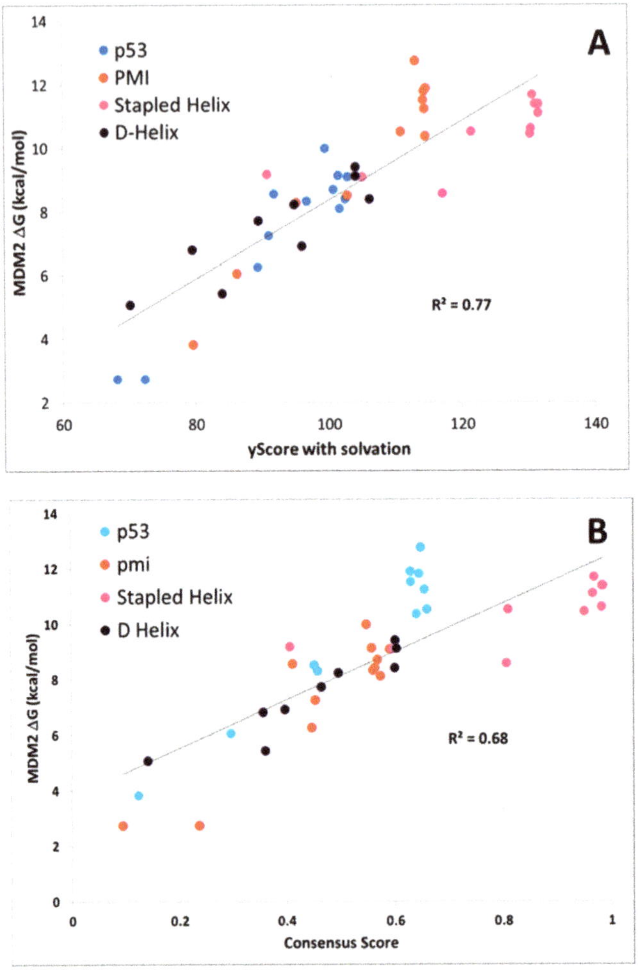

Figure 6. Single pose scoring results with CMDyscore with solvation (**A**) and the consensus score (**B**).

Unlike CMDescore, CMDyscore is parameterized for non-standard amino acids. Hence, a plot of the CMDyscore results with N–C cyclized mutants included was also prepared and is provided in Figure 7. Including the cyclic peptides, with the primarily alanine, scanning results of the other datasets (PMI, p53, D-α-helix, and stapled α-helix), adds a number of complications for making realistic comparisons using single point calculations. One complication is that for the earlier calculations, only a single residue was mutated and, in general, the mutation was to a residue smaller in size than the original. All the cyclic peptides were built from a single starting template and multiple mutations involving both larger and smaller residues were required. As a result, more extensive minimization of the starting structure was carried out. The cyclic peptides also involved more variation in the number and type of charged residues.

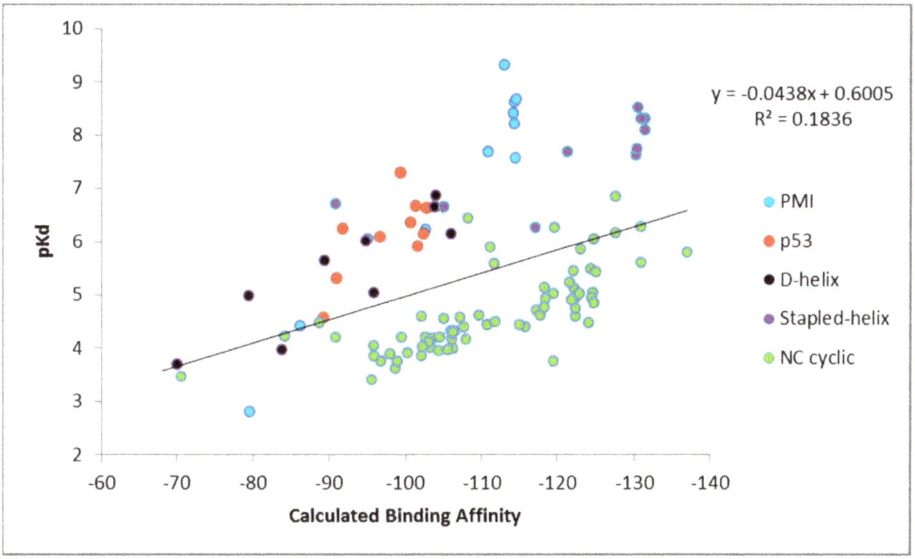

(**A**)

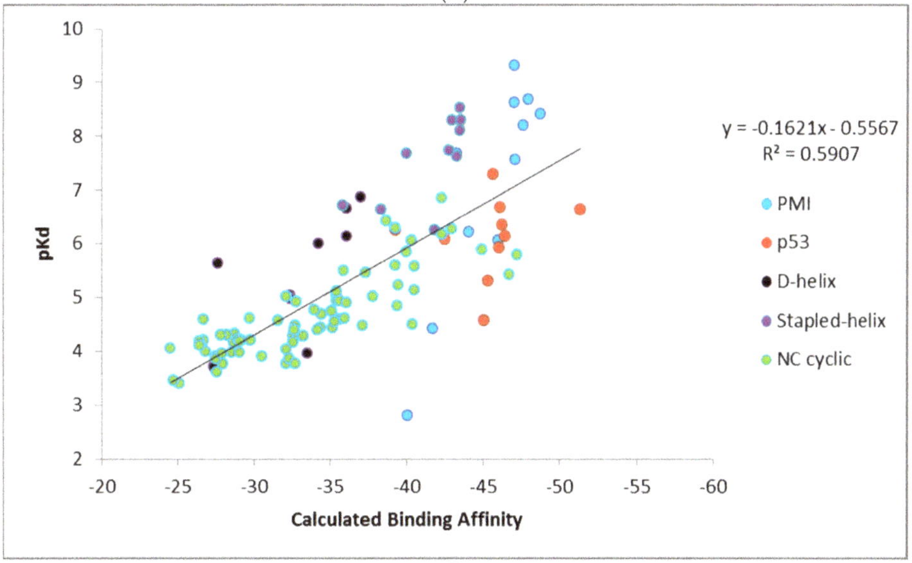

(**B**)

Figure 7. *Cont.*

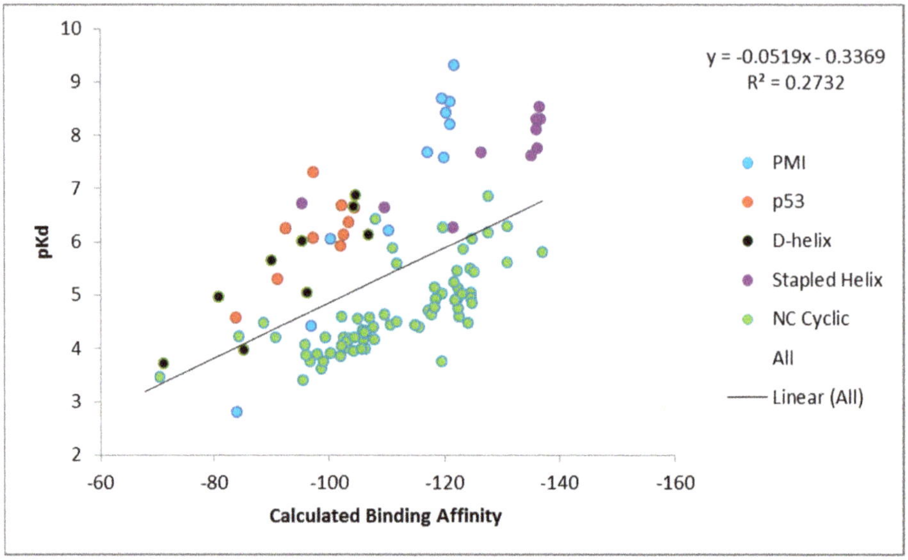

(**C**)

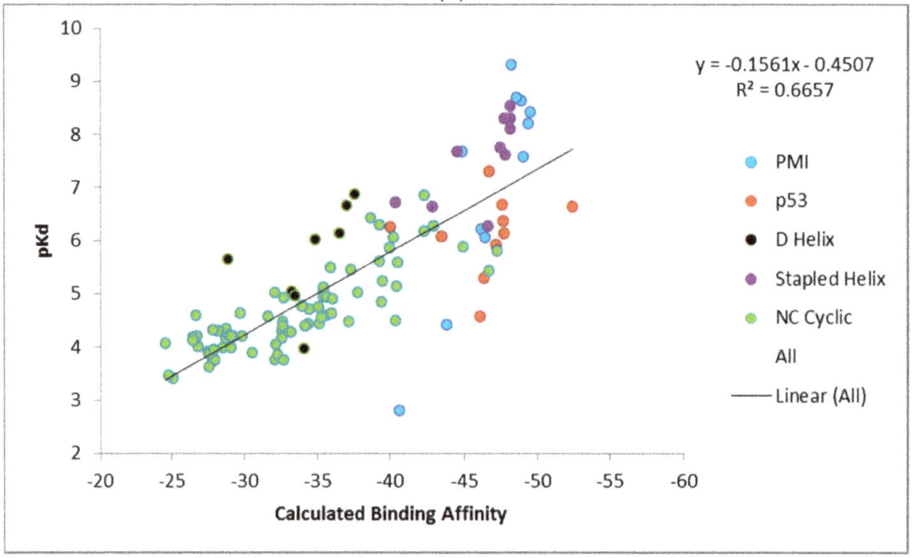

(**D**)

Figure 7. CMDyscore with solvation on the full data set. (**A**) CMDyscore with solvation with default CMDyscore settings. (**B**) CMDyscore after more extensive minimization of all datasets using solvation (**C**) or default settings (**D**).

Figure 7 summarizes the CMDyscore results with the combined datasets. It is apparent in Figure 7A that despite reasonable correlations in the individual datasets, cyclic peptides are shifted to the right with respect to the other datasets, i.e., their calculated affinities are over estimated relative to the helical peptides. In the combined dataset, the default CMDyscore parameters show good correlation with the combined data set. It was thought that part of the problem was that different protocols were used to minimize the complexes. All complexes were therefore run through another series of minimizations and rescored. First all but the peptide side chains were fixed and the complex minimized. A second minimization step was done allowing all side chains to relax. Finally, a third minimization was done with the protein fixed and the peptide completely free. The correlations did improve. The R^2 for CMDyscore with solvation improved from 0.18 to 0.27. More impressive was the performance of the default CMDyscore, which improved from an already respectable R^2 of 0.59 to 0.67. To a large extent, this is because the default method better predicts the large cyclic peptide data set, but one can also see from the graph for the default method, that the cyclic peptides are no longer shifted to the right.

The most likely reason for the observed results is that the PBSA in YASARA uses a somewhat ad hoc value for scaling the surface area. When used on data sets of similar size and composition, it improves the correlation. For a more diverse data set it is not helpful. The results may improve by better parameterization of the SA term. However, the focus of the article is on a rigorous examination of the existing methods and exploring methods to improve the results after the fact is outside the scope. Nevertheless, mutation and single point energy calculations following a mild minimization protocol do provide reasonably good correlation with experiment.

2.2. Prospective Study

In addition to the retrospective calculations, the same methods were used to prospectively estimate or to blindly predict the binding affinities of a series of analogs of ATSP-7041 (A8Q, Q9L) to MDM2. In particular, the calculations were performed on an Ala scan and novel D-amino acid scan of an ATSP-7041 analog (having A8Q and Q9L modifications) prior to synthesis and experimental binding affinity measurements. Undoubtedly, putting blind predictions in jeopardy of observational falsification provides a more rigorous test of a computational method.

The predictions made using the sampling-based CMDboltzmann method and the single pose scoring functions CMDyscore and CMDescore are shown in Table 4 and Figure 8. Importantly, all three computational binding affinity prediction methods produced generally good agreement with the experimentally measured Ala scan data of the ATSP-7041 analog binding to MDM2, with the R^2s for CMDescore, CMDyscore and CMDboltzmann being 0.67, 0.84 and 0.82, respectively.

Surprisingly, all three methods predicted that the mutation of Trp7 to dTrp7 would lead to only a modest drop in potency. This prediction was eventually confirmed by experimental measurements. Interestingly, CMDescore and CMDyscore were used to predict that the Phe3 to dPhe3 mutation would have a small effect, while the application of CMDboltzmann predicted a strongly destabilizing effect. The CMDboltzmann prediction was later confirmed by experimental measurement. Subsequently, a crystal structure, 6aaw [20], was solved further validating the fit of the dTrp sidechain. The differential prediction successes of CMDescore, CMDyscore and CMDboltzmann on the Phe3 and Trp7 mutants helps to account for the R^2 values and trend obtained for the full MDM2-ATSP7041 D-amino acid scan results (0.30, 0.09 and 0.38 for CMDescore, CMDyscore and CMDboltzmann, respectively).

When Phe3 is mutated to dPhe3, the aromatic rings of the two cases overlap almost completely. It is thus not surprising that the empirical CMDescore scoring function displays problems here, as the number of carbon–carbon contacts is identical. The dPhe3 mutation does result in short van der Waals contacts with two residues in the protein, which ideally a physics-based force-field would identify as unfavorable. As part of the CMDyscore binding energy calculation, however, the peptide was fully minimized in the binding site which may have removed the bad contacts, resulting in a failed prediction. Interestingly, the correlation obtained with CMDyscore without the minimization step is significantly better (0.74) and still predicts that a mutation to dTrp will have little effect. The differences between the minimized and un-minimized predictions might be because the strain in dPhe3 is propagated to the backbone upon minimization, where it will not have an effect on a single point binding energy calculation. It must be admitted, however, that all of this may be coincidence, as the un-minimized correlation result is not the result of a blind study. It does, however, suggest that generating affinity predictions from a conformational ensemble, as is done with CMDboltzmann, captures more subtle structural effects and can be worth the extra computational expenditure. The sub-optimal R^2 obtained with CMDboltzmann on the D-scan data stems from the Thr2 to dThr mutation, where the measured drop in potency is just over a log unit whereas the CMDboltzmann prediction is of a slight increase in binding affinity. Recall that the CMDboltzmann procedure allows the two residues at the N- and C-termini to be fully flexible (they are not constrained whatsoever). Indeed, this might have allowed too much flexibility to be incorporate into the simulation, resulting in the poor Thr2 to dThr2 prediction results.

Table 4. Prospective Testing Data.

Residue	Experimental MDM2		Experimental MDMX		Calculated MDM2 Calculated Binding *		
	Kd (nM)	ΔΔG (kcal)	Kd (nM)	ΔΔG (kcal)	CMDescore ΔΔG (kcal)	CMDyscore ΔΔG (kcal)	CMDboltzmann ΔΔG
WT	18.6		12.5				
L1A	19.3	0.03	9.6	−0.16	0.2	−0.30	1.2
T2A	155.3	1.73			−0.2	−0.91	1.3
F3A	9585.9	5.09	4873	3.53	1.8	27.28	7.8
E5A	29.8	0.38	45.6	0.75	0.0	1.81	−1.4
Y6A	51.5	0.83	130.3	1.37	0.7	9.42	0.4
W7A	5145.9	4.58	11161	4.02	3.8	36.41	11.6
Q8A	32.6	0.46	57.1	0.88	0.3	1.71	−1.0
L9A	15.8	−0.13	13.4	0.00	0.2	0.42	−0.7
Cba10A	413.7	2.53	94.7	1.18	0.8	10.74	7.1
S12A	20.4	0.08	43.9	0.73	0.2	−2.29	1.3
L1dL	27.5	0.23	21.8	0.31	0.0	−1.90	−1.3
T2dT	217.8	1.46			0.3	−2.24	−2.6
F3dF [b]	6385.1	3.47	7397	3.77	−0.2	−4.04	5.7
E5dE	36.8	0.41			−0.5	−2.44	1.5
Y6dY	365.1	1.77	921.2	2.53	0.7	5.91	0.7
W7dW [b]	32.9	0.34	63.4	0.94	0.2	−1.73	2.2
Q8dQ	26.5	0.20	36.6	0.62	0.2	−0.93	2.3
L9dL	32.2	0.32	38.8	0.65	0.0	−1.08	−2.5
Cba10dCba	3809.5	3.17	805.1	2.45	1.3	8.21	3.5
S12dS	10.7	−0.31	36.9	0.62	−0.5	−2.45	0.1
A13dA	17.2	−0.05	34.9	0.59	0.3	−0.69	0.0
A14dA	18.4	−0.02	4.9	−0.57	−0.3	4.31	−1.9

* The MDM2 and MDMX data are very similar; MDMX data is excluded to avoid redundancy and minimize clutter. [b] All three methods were used to make the successful but surprising prediction that the chiral amino acid substitution W7 → dW7 would be weakly destabilizing; only CMDboltzmann was used to successfully predict the strongly destabilizing effect of F3 → dF7. This nicely illustrates the important role a more computationally expensive algorithm like CMDboltzmann can play in prospective peptide ligand candidate design and optimization.

In summary, the Ala scan data of the ATSP-7041 analog (see Table 4) closely mirrored that of ATSP-3900 [16], with large losses in potency for any of the F3A, W7A or Cba10A mutations and modest to no loss in potency when other residues are mutated to Ala. Importantly, CMDescore, CMDyscore and CMDboltzmann were used to generate Ala scan predictions that were ultimately shown to agree nicely with experimental measurements.

The corresponding D-amino acid scan of the ATSP-7041 analog, however, produced an experimental surprise, namely that the change of Trp7 to dTrp7 led to a small drop in binding affinity. Based on Figure 8C it is apparent that the drop in calculated affinity with CMDBoltzmann for W7dW is within the range of the majority of other changes that led to relatively small experimental affinity changes. On the other hand, the changes F3dF, F3dA, W7A and Cba10A all showed large drops in calculated and experimental affinity. Finally, CMDboltzmann showed a modest drop in calculated affinity for the Cba10dCba change whereas the experimental drop in affinity was comparable to that of the F3dF, F3dA, W7A, and Cba10A changes. While the change in CMDescore and CMDyscore, Figure 8A,B respectively, is indeed small for W7dW, these scoring functions also do not change with the F3dF and Cba10dCba changes. This highlights the value of including the computationally more demanding sampling when making more complex changes. Indeed, the poorer agreement with the d-Amino Acid scan when compared to the Ala-scan may in part be to a larger difference in the solution behavior when the amino acids are change to their D counterpart.

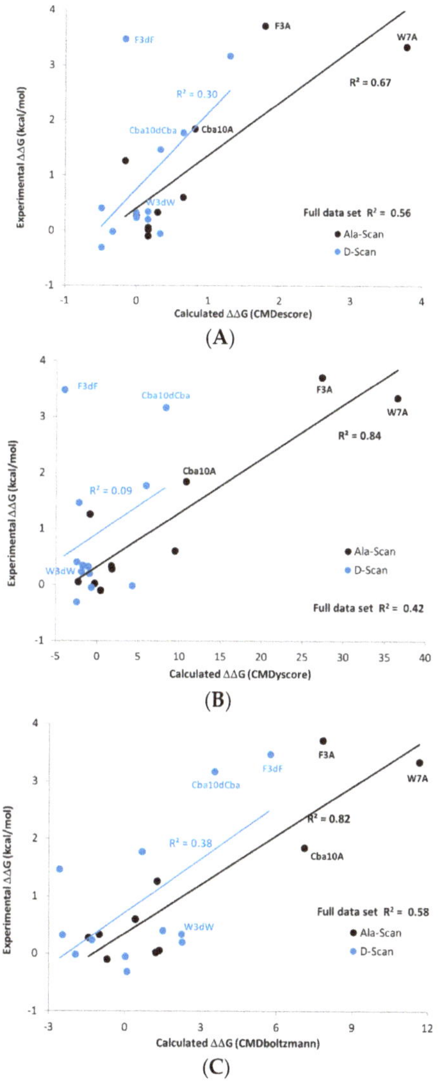

Figure 8. Scoring results on the prospective data. (**A**) CMDescore. (**B**) CMDyscore (**C**) CMDboltzmann.

Comparison of Single Point Results with CMDBoltzmann Results. In general, calculation of relative binding affinities using either a single point low-energy conformation or an ensemble of low-energy conformations and an appropriate scoring function has proven fairly effective for the MDM2/MDMX target. The single point calculations have the advantage of being fast, allowing screening of large numbers of peptides. The ensemble-based approach has the advantage of more fully defining the conformational space of the peptides and appears more robust. The single point method, if not given an appropriate starting conformation, can fail completely. No one conformation is likely to dominate in the Boltzmann ensemble.

Importance of solvation model to adequately complement electrostatics. A good solvation model should account for two situations which are not adequately represented using a simple 'gas-phase' implementation of a force field. The first is the affinity gain from associating hydrophobic surfaces in the complex and the affinity loss from desolvating polar groups involved in binding. The second is a better treatment of attenuation of charge–charge interactions in a polar medium. When molecular dynamics is used to calculate an ensemble of low-energy conformations, the overall charge of the system can be neutralized by the addition of counter ions and explicit solvent can be used to attenuate the Coulombic interactions. One challenge of accurately scoring protein–peptide interactions is that it is not feasible to include counter ions or explicit solvent when comparing the energy of two protein–peptide complexes. One thus needs to handle the problems of charge neutralization and attenuation using more ad hoc methods.

In this study, several techniques were used. Neutralizing the charged groups was tried as a method of both obtaining charge balance and attenuating Coulombic interactions. The problem with this approach is that ionic interactions become hydrogen bond interactions. An alternate approach was used in CMDyscore. In that case, charges were adjusted so as to provide an overall neutral complex and the PBSA method was used to account for polar and nonpolar solvation terms.

To handle attenuation of the Coulombic interactions several methods were used: scaling the charges, using a distant-dependent dielectric constant and using a PBSA implicit solvent model. Comparing CMDyscore variations, the simplest approach (scaled charges) shows poorer correlation with experiment than either using neutral groups or the PBSA solvation model. The best average correlation on the linear helical data was achieved when using the PBSA implicit solvent model. The reason may be the more accurate treatment of the hydrophobic effect. The MDM2/MDMX system is perhaps not the best test for methods for implicitly handling charges. The binding is entirely due to hydrophobic interactions with the charged residues largely being solvent exposed. We have found that in general that implicit solvation models have problems when there are multiple charged groups not involved in binding. These charged groups should be balanced by a nearby counter ion, but in an implicit model, they are not. The summation of these unbalanced long-range interactions can significantly affect the calculated energy, distorting the results. Thus, correlation of binding affinity with calculated binding energy in our experience is much better with peptides that primarily consist of polar and nonpolar amino acids, as is the case with MDM2/MDMX.

dTrp7 results. The comparison of the predictions for dPhe3 and dTrp7 are particularly interesting. At first glance, the D and L conformations are quite similar. In both cases, the aromatic rings overlap almost completely. In essence, the β-carbon is either above or below the plane of the backbone, with the aromatic rings angled into the same region of space.

In the case of Trp7, there are two features which distinguish it from Phe3: the tryptophan makes a hydrogen bond to Met50 in the protein (the Trp N are almost exactly superimposed) and the pocket containing the Trp7 is not quite as tight as for Phe-3. In the single point (minimized) mutations the larger dTrp has six contacts closer than 3 angstroms, the closest being 2.1 angstroms, while dPhe has seven contacts, the closest being 1.6 angstroms. In addition, when the complexes are aligned on the protein, the C alpha carbons in Trp7 and dTrp7 are 0.57 angstroms apart, whereas the C_α carbons in Phe3 and 0.94 angstroms apart. These are subtle differences and it is remarkable and highly encouraging that CMDBoltzmann was able to detect the difference and correctly predict that only Trp7 mutating to dTrp would not show a significant loss in affinity.

Implications for CMDInventus work-flow approach to peptide modeling and design. Our approach to computational peptide drug design employs multiple methods in a hierarchical and integrated fashion. In a typical work-flow, CMDpeptide can be used to model the solution and binding conformations of a peptide scaffold which can then be systematically mutated and evaluated for its binding affinity to a protein target using methods that range from computationally fast and un-rigorous (CMDescore) to slower and more rigorous (CMDyscore) to very slow and highly rigorous (CMDboltzmann). Hence, all three binding affinity prediction methods (and by implication CMDpeptide, as it is used in CMDboltzmann calculations) were tested retrospectively (using previously published data) and prospectively (using novel data collected after computational predictions had been made).

The results presented here validate the use of CMDpeptide to model biologically relevant conformations for diverse MDM2/MDMX peptides, as it yielded X-ray like conformations for all cases tested. Future work will focus on developing an improved scoring strategy for identifying relevant conformations from calculated conformational ensembles. Also, while CMDpeptide was indirectly tested in the prospective CMDboltzmann study, a direct test of CMDpeptide in a prospective study would also be desirable.

Our results also validate the integrated use of CMDescore and CMDboltzmann without the need for re-calibration, as both produced consistently encouraging results across multiple data sets in both the retrospective and prospective studies and with CMDboltzmann producing overall better results than CMDescore. Having said that, additional research is needed to parameterize and test CMDescore on the 2axi cyclized multiple mutation data asset and for use with non-standard amino acids more generally. Similarly, more research is needed to develop an optimized force field and solvation model for use with constrained CMDboltzmann (and CMDpeptide) dihedral space Monte Carlo and minimization calculations. CMDyscore with solvation produced the best overall results in the retrospective analysis of the linear peptide/helical datasets. To obtain good results on the multi-mutation cyclized 2axi data, however, required the use of a more extensive minimization protocol or the substitution of the default CMDyscore for CMDyscore with solvation. Similarly, CMDyscore with solvation produced nice results in the alanine scanning prospective study but poor results in the prospective D-scanning study that were improved ad hoc by eliminating any minimization prior to scoring. This suggests that the best CMDyscore flavor and minimization procedure should, whenever possible, be calibrated, selected and applied on a case-by-case basis. In the absence of training data, it seems the best choice would be CMDyscore with solvation using the standard minimization protocol. Future work will focus on developing a more generally useful flavor of CMDyscore or on developing a general and systematic procedure for selecting the best flavor of CMDyscore to apply to a particular protein–peptide system.

The results presented here suggest a robust role for CMDinventus in a structure-based drug design project. Given the vast sequence space accessible around a binding mode for even a modestly sized peptide, fast simple scoring functions such as CMDescore and CMDyscore are necessary. Particularly, by considering side-chain changes one at a time, these scoring functions can be used to rapidly search 1000s of possible side chains per position ultimately narrowing the list to a handful that are the most promising. Depending on computing resources, CMDboltzmann can be used to further and more accurately prioritize 100s to 1000s of the sequences of greatest interest. Indeed, the results of these calculations could be used to prioritize further synthesis or could be used for more computationally expensive methods such as molecular dynamics [21,22], free energy perturbation [23,24] or thermodynamic integration [25,26].

3. Materials and Methods

CMDInventus is a proprietary platform for computer-aided peptide drug design. CMDInventus consists of self-contained computational tools or modules for solving specific biophysical problems. The various modules can be strung together and integrated to form project-specific peptide drug design work-flows. The present study focused on the use of several CMDInventus modules to run retrospective and prospective calculations for various MDM2/MDMX datasets.

All retrospective and prospective calculations either involved explicit sampling of peptide conformational space and/or configurational (conformational + translational + rotational) space or were derived from single crystal structures. In the present study, we employed two modules that use the same code base for peptide conformational and configurational sampling. The first application, called CMDpeptide, is for physics-based peptide conformational sampling from sequence information alone. Here the goal is to start with a peptide sequence, and where applicable inter-residue bonding information, and generate an ensemble of three-dimensional peptide structures that contains all biologically relevant conformations. The ensemble of conformations should include those relevant for binding target proteins, those that are cleaved by proteases, those that traverse cell membranes, etc. For most peptides of interest (5–20 amino acids), the ensembles contain thousands of low-energy conformations that can be further reduced through RMSD-based clustering. The second application, which we refer to as CMDboltzmann, is for estimating the binding affinity of a peptide sequence around a given backbone binding mode. It involves local peptide configurational sampling, subject to user provided constraints, to optimize a peptide binding mode with its protein target and the calculation of a predicted binding affinity from the resulting configurational ensemble. The chief difference between CMDpeptide and CMDboltzmann is that the latter involves placement of a peptide in a binding site, which requires inclusion of protein–peptide energetic interactions in any scoring function and explicit sampling of conformational and rigid-body coordinates. Additionally, while CMDpeptide assumes nothing about the structure of the peptide, CMDboltzmann uses different constraints to direct the peptide into the protein binding site. Fundamentally, both algorithms can be broken down into two loosely independent parts: sampling and scoring. Each of these is briefly described below, with particular emphasis on the differences between them.

In addition to the sampling-based methods, we describe several empirical and force field-based scoring functions for estimating protein–peptide binding affinities from single protein–peptide poses. These include our in-house empirical scoring function (CMDescore) and force field-based scoring function (CMDyscore). For comparative purposes, we also provide results obtained using the widely employed Xscore and Vina scoring functions along with protein–peptide surface area (SA) burial and interface packing (IP) calculations. The chief difference between these approaches and CMDboltzmann is that they are used to estimate the binding affinity from a single protein–peptide pose, whereas binding affinity estimates obtained using CMDboltzmann involve sampling thousands of softly constrained peptide backbone structures in the protein binding site. Because they only require a single pose the scoring functions are computationally much more efficient, making it possible to rapidly estimate binding affinities for thousands or even millions of peptide ligand sequences or binding poses in relatively short order.

The main goal of a typical peptide drug design project is to narrow the vast theoretical peptide sequence space down to a manageable number of viable candidate sequences that are predicted to bind a protein target of interest. A standard CMDInventus work-flow for accomplishing this would begin with combinatorial sequence scanning with a fixed peptide backbone, and rapid free energy scoring and ranking with CMDescore. Promising sequences would then be scored and prioritized using CMDyscore. The most promising peptide ligand sequences would then be scored for their protein binding affinities using the computationally expensive CMDboltzmann module. In addition, CMDboltzmann is useful for examining larger discrete changes to a peptide structure when the assumption of a fixed binding mode for the peptide ligand may no longer be valid and is somewhat relaxed (cyclization, large changes in side chains, changes in stereochemistry, etc.).

Full peptide conformational sampling with CMDpeptide. The purpose of CMDpeptide is the calculation of biologically relevant peptide conformational ensembles. All CMDpeptide conformational sampling is done in dihedral space, with fixed bond lengths and angles, using a multiple copy simulated annealing with minimization (MCSAM) algorithm [27–29]. Each run begins by initializing a stack of conformations by generating 100 conformations at random followed by energy minimization. During the run, the stack is allowed to grow to 200 conformations according to previously describe rules for maintaining the conformational stack [27]. For conformational sampling with CMDpeptide, only topological information, that is sequence information and any inter-residue bonds such as disulfide bonds, is used. Each run consists of 10,000 Monte Carlo w/Minimization (MCM) steps performed as described previously [27]. To ensure complete coverage, 500 independent runs are typically performed per peptide. In addition, Phi/Psi biasing is performed using pre-calculated Ramachandran plots. The plot for residue n within a given sequence (A_1-A_2- … -A_n- … -A_{N-1}-A_N) is calculated by thoroughly sampling the tri-peptide Ac-A_{n-1}-A_n-A_{n+1}-NH2. The reason for creating the plots in this fashion, rather than using plots derived from PDB structures, is the need for chemical and conformational generality. In particular, relying solely on PDB derived Ramachandran plots would effectively limit one to using the standard 20 amino acids. This would seriously limit the development and use of CMDInventus as a general computational framework for enabling peptide-based drug design using such things as non-natural side chains, D-amino acids, β-amino acids, α-di-substituted amino acids, and so forth.

Estimating binding affinities from conformational ensembles with CMDboltzmann. The primary goal of a CMDboltzmann calculation is to estimate the binding affinity of a protein–peptide binding mode where the peptide ligand is treated as semi-flexible. The binding mode for the peptide backbone would ideally derive from a co-crystal structure but can be derived from a docked or theoretically calculated binding mode. Importantly, CMDboltzmann can be used to calculate binding affinities as peptide sequences are mutated around a given binding mode. Thus, for CMDboltzmann calculations the simulation begins with a peptide backbone positioned in a binding site. While it is desirable for the peptide backbone to qualitatively maintain its binding configuration, significant changes in a side chain might require some movement of the peptide backbone. Hence, the backbone is permitted a limited range of softly constrained motions. To accomplish this, the same MCSAM algorithm described above is used with the following differences. The first and largest difference is the presence of the protein which greatly affects the scoring and subsequent ranking of each peptide configuration; the scoring of the protein–peptide interactions is described below in the sampling energy function section. For the calculations described here, the protein is held rigid, though in many cases we allow side-chain flexibility for residues of the protein in the binding site. The second difference is the presence of a constraint, described below in the sampling energy function section, that is applied to prevent the peptide backbone from deviating too greatly from its starting position. Typically, the backbone is constrained so that its atoms can move 1.0 Å without penalty. If a backbone atom moves more than 1.0 Å a harmonic penalty is applied. The third and final differences are details in the runs, including the number of steps per run (2000) and the total number of runs (100). Fewer steps and runs are needed because the conformational space being searched is far smaller due to the backbone constraints and the presence of the protein.

Force field used in calculations involving sampling. The Amber99sb force field provides all bonded interactions; because the sampling is done in dihedral space, this entails the use of only the Amber99sb dihedral energy terms. All nonbonded interactions within a peptide and between a protein and peptide are calculated as the sum of the Van der Waals interactions, the electrostatic interactions, and an empirical solvation term. The Van der Waals parameters are taken from Amber99sb [30]. For solvation, the EEF1 continuum model [31] is used, as it provides a reasonable balance between accuracy and speed. The electrostatic contribution to the system energy is calculated using a distance dependent dielectric function consistent with the recommendations of the EEF1 solvation model, i.e., the effective dielectric constant between two atoms is 4d where d is the distance between the two atoms. The atomic charges used for the electrostatic calculation are generated for each amino acid via the RESP [32,33] procedure applied to individual amidated and acylated amino acid building blocks using the quantum chemistry package GAMESS [34,35] at the B3LYP/6-31 G** level of theory. The final score calculated for a configuration of the peptide is simply the sum of these terms without any reweighting.

For the CMDboltzmann calculations, a constraint is applied to each heavy atom of the peptide ligand backbone (excluding the 2 terminal residues). The constraint is implemented as a harmonic well with a distance tolerance of 1.0 Å inside of which no penalty is applied. This allows the backbone to sample locally around the starting binding mode without deviating too much from the desired binding mode. Thus, for a CMDboltzmann calculation the MCSAM algorithm works to optimize the combination of backbone constraints + peptide internal energy + protein–peptide interaction energy. The final score for a given peptide sequence is the Boltzmann weighted, using the total energy, average of the protein–peptide interaction energy over the minimum energy pose from each of the 100 runs. In the present study, no attempt was made to estimate relative strain energies for different sequences, the assumption being that this is a minor contributor. In some cases, particularly with the linear α-helices, this may be poor assumption. In fact, recent work suggests that optimizing a sequence to stabilize a conformation is a viable option to improving potency [36–43].

Estimating binding affinities with CMDescore and CMDyscore from single pose structures. CMDescore [44–47] is a simple empirical scoring function for predicting binding affinities. It comes in a variety of flavors depending on the number of terms in the function. All flavors are premised on rigid-body binding and are parameterized for use on protein–protein and protein–peptide complexes composed of standard amino acids. For the present study, the flavor used has been described previously and is a linear combination of four regression weighted terms that quantify hydrophobic and charged group burial at a given protein–ligand interface and hydrogen bonding and salt bridge interactions across a given interface and is given by the following equation for binding affinity (BA) [47].

$$BA = -1.94 + 0.16 \cdot \Delta X_H - 0.68 \cdot \Delta X_C - 0.52 \cdot X_{HB} - 0.41 \cdot \Delta X_{SB} \quad (1)$$

The first term, X_H, refers to the free energy change associated with hydrophobic group burial (carbon and sulfur atoms). The second term, X_C, refers to the free energy change associated with charge group burial (nitrogen and oxygen atoms of charged D, E, K and R side chains). The third, X_{HB}, and fourth terms, X_{SB}, refer to the total number of conventional hydrogen bonds and net number of salt bridges calculated across a given protein–peptide interface.

CMDyscore [6,48,49] is a force-field-based scoring function based on the YASARA modeling and simulation package. As part of the scoring process, the mutated complexes were subjected to two rounds of minimization. During the first round all backbone atoms in the protein and peptide were fixed, and side chains in the protein that were less than four angstroms from the peptide and all side chains in the peptide were permitted to move. During the second round the entire protein is fixed and the entire peptide to allowed to move.

Four flavors of CMDyscore were used to calculate binding affinities: (1) simple, (2) unbound ligand minimized to apply a pseudo 'strain' penalty, (3) charged residues neutralized, and (4) implicit solvation model. The CMDyscore methods are implemented using YASARA [50]. Before calculating the scores, the complex was minimized using the NOVA force field [51]. The first method calculates the binding energy according to the formula:

$$Energy(complex) - Energy(protein) - Energy(peptide) \quad (2)$$

The NOVA force field was used for the calculation of the energies of the individual protein, peptide and the protein–peptide complex. The complex was first minimized using the NOVA force field [51]. The NOVA force field was chosen because it is optimized for in vacuo minimizations, as necessitated for a fast scoring function. The energies for protein and peptide were calculated according to the rigid-body binding assumption, i.e., by extracting each in turn from the complex in the exact conformation that they assume in the complex.

The pseudo 'strain' penalty was originally implemented to handle the scoring of docking poses. One concern with docking is that in an attempt to maximize the docking protein interaction energy terms, the peptide ligand will be placed in an unrealistically high energy or strained conformation. This method introduces moderate peptide ligand flexibility into the binding energy calculation by minimizing the peptide after it is extracted from the complex:

$$Energy(complex) - Energy(protein) - Energy(peptide,\ minimized) \quad (3)$$

If the binding conformation is not a low-energy conformation, the binding energy will be reduced, possibly significantly. This approach has been used in small molecule docking studies; Greenidge and coworkers, for example, included a similar term in when docking the PDBbind data set [52]. They did MM/GBSA calculations and found the best correlation ($R^2 = 0.63$) with the strain energy term included and explicit waters excluded.

The latter two flavors represent alternate methods of damping the charge effects in the absence of explicit solvent. We have observed that peptides with charged residues are particularly hard to score. Even with the NOVA force field, peptides with charged side chains can appear as outliers. One way this problem was addressed was by neutralizing all the charged groups in the protein and peptide. The other way that this problem was addressed was to use a PBSA implicit solvent model. The PBSA model adds two terms to the energy: the polar and non-polar contributions to the solvation free energies. The former is determined by solving the Poisson-Boltzmann equation [53]. The latter is estimated from the solvent accessible surface area (SASA). A scaling factor of 0.65 was used for converting the surface area to free energy. The scaling factor comes from the YASARA manual. It was decided not to optimize the parameter based on the current data set, as it was felt that the initial results were reasonable and optimizing the value with a small data set would introduce undue bias.

In addition to CMDescore and CMDyscore, the docking score used by VINA [54], the Xscore [55] scoring function, and very simple scoring functions based solely on packing interface (PI) potential and buried surface area (SA) were also used. All were used according to their default settings and parameters.

Structure preparation for CMDescore and CMDyscore: In general, MDM2 and MDMX X-ray structures bound to reference peptides were prepared for subsequent calculations using standard cleaning and optimization procedures. This was followed by mutation or mutation and minimization of a reference peptide according to the relevant SAR data set. This, in turn, was followed by free energy scoring of all reference and mutated MDM2/MDMX targeting peptides.

Both the Li-p53 and Li-PMI datasets are alanine scanning datasets. Crystal structures for the Li-PMI data set are available for MDM2 and MDMX (3eqs and 3eqy). There are also crystal structures for the Li-p53 data set (4hfz and 1ycr for MDM2 and 3dab for MDMX). These crystal structures were used after applying a standard clean up routine (remove waters and counter ions, remove all but one of each chain, and add hydrogens).

For the Liu D-α-helical PMI-α alanine scanning peptide data set there are two relevant MDM2 crystal structures (3iwy and 3lnj). 3lnj was selected as the starting point. Because Asn2 has a seriously distorted geometry, it was removed and rebuilt. Because it was absent from the structure, Thr1 was built with standard α-helical Phi/Psi angles and an optimized side chain. There is no MDMX structural data for the Liu D-α-helical peptides.

There are crystal structures of stapled peptides bound to MDM2 and MDMX (3v3b and 4n5t). These were used as the starting points for mutation of the bound reference peptides to the sequence used in the Guerlavais ATSP-3900 stapled L-α-helix data set.

The cyclic peptides were all built from a single reference structure (2axi). A similar procedure to that used for the single residue mutations for the preceding data sets was used with the modification that mutations were done sequentially, the result of the previous single residue mutation serving as the input for the next mutation. The process was continued until the desired sequence was produced. As a result, the binding site was more fully minimized for the cyclic peptides than for the other data sets.

Several scoring functions were used to calculate binding affinities from the X-ray poses produced using the above-described procedures. In particular, two in house scoring functions were used:

To apply these scoring functions to the various MDM2 and MDMX data sets, co-crystal structures of reference peptides bound to MDM2 or MDMX binding sites were used as starting points. Peptide ligand residues were then either (1) mutated or (2) mutated and refined through a constrained minimization procedure according to the above-described data sets. Finally, all mutated structures were scored using all available single-point affinity estimation methods. More theoretical and computational details are provided below in the Results and discussion section.

Mdm2 Competitive Fluorescence Anisotropy Assay and K_d Determination Purified MDM2 (1-125) protein was titrated against 50 nM carboxyfluorescein (FAM)-labeled 12/1 peptide [56] (FAM-RFMDYWEGL-NH_2). Dissociation constants for titration of MDM2 against FAM-labeled 12/1 peptide were determined by fitting the experimental data to a 1:1 binding model equation shown below: [57,58].

$$r = r_0 + (r_b - r_0)\left(\frac{(K_d + [L]_t + [P]_t) - \sqrt{(K_d + [L]_t + [P]_t)^2 - 4[L]_t[P]_t}}{2[L]_t}\right) \tag{4}$$

$[P]$ is the protein concentration (MDM2), $[L]$ is the labeled peptide concentration, r is the anisotropy measured, r_o is the anisotropy of the free peptide, r_b is the anisotropy of the MDM2–FAM-labeled peptide complex, K_d is the dissociation constant, $[L]_t$ is the total FAM-labeled peptide concentration, and $[P]_t$ is the total MDM2 concentration. The determined apparent K_d value of FAM-labeled 12/1 peptide (13.0 nM) was used to determine the apparent K_d values of the respective competing ligands in subsequent competition assays.

Apparent K_d values were determined for a variety of molecules via competitive fluorescence anisotropy experiments. Titrations were carried out with the concentration of MDM2 held constant at 250 nM and the labeled peptide at 50 nM. The competing molecules were then titrated against the complex of the FAM-labeled peptide and protein. Apparent K_d values were determined by fitting the experimental data to the equations shown below: [58,59].

$$\begin{aligned}
r &= r_0 + (r_b - r_0)\left(\frac{2\sqrt{(d^2-3e)}\cos\left(\frac{\theta}{3}\right)-9}{3K_{d1}+2\sqrt{(d^2-3e)}\cos\left(\frac{\theta}{3}\right)-d}\right)\\
d &= K_{d1} + K_{d2} + [L]_{st} + [L]_t - [P]_t\\
e &= ([L]_t - [P]_t)K_{d1} + ([L]_{st} - [P]_t)K_{d2} + K_{d1}K_{d2}\\
f &= -K_{d1}K_{d2}[P]_t\\
\theta &= \cos^{-1}\left(\frac{-2d^3+9de-27f}{2\sqrt{(d^2-3e)^3}}\right)
\end{aligned} \tag{5}$$

$[L]_{st}$ and $[L]_t$ denote labeled ligand and total unlabeled ligand input concentrations, respectively. K_{d2} is the dissociation constant of the interaction between the unlabeled ligand and the protein. In all competitive types of experiments, it is assumed that $[P]_t > [L]_{st}$, otherwise considerable amounts of free labeled ligand would always be present and would interfere with measurements. K_{d1} is the apparent K_d for the labeled peptide used in the respective experiment, which has been experimentally determined as described in the previous paragraph. The FAM-labeled peptide was dissolved in dimethyl sulfoxide (DMSO) at 1 mM and diluted into experimental buffer. Readings were carried out with an Envision Multilabel Reader (PerkinElmer). Experiments were carried out in PBS (2.7 mM KCl, 137 mM NaCl, 10 mM Na_2HPO_4 and 2 mM KH_2PO_4 (pH 7.4)) and 0.1% Tween 20 buffer. All titrations were carried out in triplicate. Curve-fitting was carried out using Prism 4.0 (GraphPad, San Diego, CA, USA).

To validate the fitting of a 1:1 binding model we carefully determined that the anisotropy value at the beginning of the direct titrations between MDM2 and the FAM-labeled peptide did not differ significantly from the anisotropy value observed for the free fluorescently labeled peptide. Negative control titrations of the ligands under investigation were also carried out with the fluorescently labeled peptide (in the absence of MDM2) to ensure no interactions were occurring between the ligands and FAM-labeled peptide. In addition, we ensured that the final baseline in the competitive titrations did not fall below the anisotropy value for the free FAM-labeled peptide, which would otherwise indicate an unintended interaction between the ligand and the FAM-labeled peptide to be displaced from the MDM2 binding site.

4. Conclusions

CMDInventus is a modular computational package for performing peptide drug modeling calculations. The modules CMDpeptide and CMDboltzmann involve the explicit sampling of peptide conformational or configurational space and can be used to model and predict peptide conformations and protein–peptide binding affinities, respectively. CMDescore and CMDyscore are empirical and force field-based scoring functions, respectively, that can be used to rapidly predict protein–peptide binding affinities from single complex structures. All six methods were used to retrospectively reproduce diverse MDM2/MDMX-peptide data sets with an encouraging degree of success. CMDescore, CMDyscore and CMDboltzmann were used to prospectively and accurately predict the experimentally measured binding affinity results for an Ala-scan of the pharmaceutically relevant stapled peptide ATSP-7041. Remarkably, CMDboltzmann was used to successfully and accurately predict the results of a novel D-scan of ATSP-7041. All results were obtained without any re-fitting or re-parameterization. Collectively, our results suggest that CMDInventus is useful for retrospectively modeling and prospectively predicting the conformational and binding behavior for diverse and pharmaceutically relevant linear and macrocyclic α-helical peptides and that CMDInventus can serve as computational platform for enabling novel peptide drug design and discovery.

Author Contributions: J.A., J.S., D.J.D. and T.K.S. conceived and designed the study. Under J.A.'s guidance, D.J.D., A.S.B. and J.S. performed all computational calculations; all four authors participated in data analysis and interpretation. T.K.S., A.W.P., D.P.L., C.J.B. and D.T. coordinated and performed experimental work (i.e., chemistry, biology and data analysis) of the stapled peptides shown in Table 4. J.A., D.J.D. and J.S. took the lead on writing the manuscript; T.K.S. provided invaluable feedback and helped to edit the manuscript.

Funding: This research received no external funding.

Conflicts of Interest: At the time of the study and some of the writing, Joseph Audie and David Diller were employed by CMDBioscience and Jon Swanson worked as a consultant for CMDBioscience. CMDBioscience has since gone out of business, but at the time hoped to get a peptide drug design deal with Merck.

References

1. Wade, M.; Li, Y.C.; Wahl, G.M. MDM2, MDMX and p53 in oncogenesis and cancer therapy. *Nat. Rev. Cancer* **2013**, *13*, 83–96. [CrossRef]
2. Zhang, Q.; Zeng, S.X.; Lu, H. Targeting p53-MDM2-MDMX loop for cancer therapy. *Sub-Cell. Biochem.* **2014**, *85*, 281–319. [CrossRef]
3. Carvajal, L.A.; Neriah, D.B.; Senecal, A.; Benard, L.; Thiruthuvanathan, V.; Yatsenko, T.; Narayanagari, S.R.; Wheat, J.C.; Todorova, T.I.; Mitchell, K.; et al. Dual inhibition of MDMX and MDM2 as a therapeutic strategy in leukemia. *Sci. Transl. Med.* **2018**, *10*, eaao3003. [CrossRef]
4. Li, C.; Pazgier, M.; Yuan, W.; Liu, M.; Wei, G.; Lu, W.Y.; Lu, W. Systematic mutational analysis of peptide inhibition of the p53-MDM2/MDMX interactions. *J. Mol. Biol.* **2010**, *398*, 200–213. [CrossRef]
5. Kussie, P.H.; Gorina, S.; Marechal, V.; Elenbaas, B.; Moreau, J.; Levine, A.J.; Pavletich, N.P. Structure of the MDM2 oncoprotein bound to the p53 tumor suppressor transactivation domain. *Science* **1996**, *274*, 948–953. [CrossRef]
6. Anil, B.; Riedinger, C.; Endicott, J.A.; Noble, M.E. The structure of an MDM2-Nutlin-3a complex solved by the use of a validated MDM2 surface-entropy reduction mutant. *Acta Crystallogr. Sect. DBiol. Crystallogr.* **2013**, *69*, 1358–1366. [CrossRef]
7. Pazgier, M.; Liu, M.; Zou, G.; Yuan, W.; Li, C.; Li, J.; Monbo, J.; Zella, D.; Tarasov, S.G.; Lu, W. Structural basis for high-affinity peptide inhibition of p53 interactions with MDM2 and MDMX. *Proc. Natl. Acad. Sci. USA* **2009**, *106*, 4665–4670. [CrossRef]
8. Liu, M.; Pazgier, M.; Li, C.; Yuan, W.; Lu, W. A left-handed solution to peptide inhibition of the p53-MDM2 interaction. *Angew. Chem. Int. Ed. Engl.* **2010**, *49*, 3649–3652. [CrossRef]
9. Zhan, C.; Zhao, L.; Wei, X.; Wu, X.; Chen, X.; Yuan, W.; Lu, W.Y.; Pazgier, M.; Lu, W. An ultrahigh affinity d-peptide antagonist Of MDM2. *J. Med. Chem.* **2012**, *55*, 6237–6241. [CrossRef]
10. Baek, S.; Kutchukian, P.S.; Verdine, G.L.; Huber, R.; Holak, T.A.; Lee, K.W.; Popowicz, G.M. Structure of the stapled p53 peptide bound to Mdm2. *J. Am. Chem. Soc.* **2012**, *134*, 103–106. [CrossRef]

11. Tan, Y.S.; Reeks, J.; Brown, C.J.; Thean, D.; Ferrer Gago, F.J.; Yuen, T.Y.; Goh, E.T.; Lee, X.E.; Jennings, C.E.; Joseph, T.L.; et al. Benzene Probes in Molecular Dynamics Simulations Reveal Novel Binding Sites for Ligand Design. *J. Phys. Chem. Lett.* **2016**, *7*, 3452–3457. [CrossRef]
12. Chee, S.M.; Wongsantichon, J.; Soo Tng, Q.; Robinson, R.; Joseph, T.L.; Verma, C.; Lane, D.P.; Brown, C.J.; Ghadessy, F.J. Structure of a stapled peptide antagonist bound to nutlin-resistant Mdm2. *PLoS ONE* **2014**, *9*, e104914. [CrossRef]
13. Chang, Y.S.; Graves, B.; Guerlavais, V.; Tovar, C.; Packman, K.; To, K.H.; Olson, K.A.; Kesavan, K.; Gangurde, P.; Mukherjee, A.; et al. Stapled alpha-helical peptide drug development: A potent dual inhibitor of MDM2 and MDMX for p53-dependent cancer therapy. *Proc. Natl. Acad. Sci. USA* **2013**, *110*, E3445–E3454. [CrossRef]
14. Lau, Y.H.; Wu, Y.; Rossmann, M.; Tan, B.X.; de Andrade, P.; Tan, Y.S.; Verma, C.; McKenzie, G.J.; Venkitaraman, A.R.; Hyvonen, M.; et al. Double Strain-Promoted Macrocyclization for the Rapid Selection of Cell-Active Stapled Peptides. *Angew. Chem. Int. Ed. Engl.* **2015**, *54*, 15410–15413. [CrossRef]
15. Bernal, F.; Tyler, A.F.; Korsmeyer, S.J.; Walensky, L.D.; Verdine, G.L. Reactivation of the p53 tumor suppressor pathway by a stapled p53 peptide. *J. Am. Chem. Soc.* **2007**, *129*, 2456–2457. [CrossRef]
16. Guerlavais, V.; Darlak, K.; Graves, B.; Tovar, C.; Packman, K.; Olson, K.; Kesavan, K.; Gangurde, P.; Horstick, J.; Mukherjee, A.; et al. (Eds.) *Design, Synthesis, Biophysical and Structure-Activity Properties of a Novel Dual MDM2 and MDMX Targeting Stapled α-Helical Peptide, ATSP-7041 that Exhibits Potent In Vitro and In Vivo Efficacy in Xenograft Models of Human Cancer*; American Peptide Society: San Diego, CA, USA, 2013.
17. Li, C.; Pazgier, M.; Liu, M.; Lu, W.Y.; Lu, W. Apamin as a template for structure-based rational design of potent peptide activators of p53. *Angew. Chem. Int. Ed. Engl.* **2009**, *48*, 8712–8715. [CrossRef]
18. Fasan, R.; Dias, R.L.; Moehle, K.; Zerbe, O.; Obrecht, D.; Mittl, P.R.; Grutter, M.G.; Robinson, J.A. Structure-activity studies in a family of beta-hairpin protein epitope mimetic inhibitors of the p53-HDM2 protein-protein interaction. *ChemBioChem* **2006**, *7*, 515–526. [CrossRef]
19. Phan, J.; Li, Z.; Kasprzak, A.; Li, B.; Sebti, S.; Guida, W.; Schonbrunn, E.; Chen, J. Structure-based design of high affinity peptides inhibiting the interaction of p53 with MDM2 and MDMX. *J. Biol. Chem.* **2010**, *285*, 2174–2183. [CrossRef]
20. Partridge, A.W.; Kaan, H.Y.K.; Juang, Y.C.; Sadruddin, A.; Lim, S.; Brown, C.J.; Ng, S.; Thean, D.; Ferrer, F.; Johannes, C.; et al. Incorporation of Putative Helix-Breaking Amino Acids in the Design of Novel Stapled Peptides: Exploring Biophysical and Cellular Permeability Properties. *Molecules* **2019**, *24*, 2292. [CrossRef]
21. Colizzi, F.; Perozzo, R.; Scapozza, L.; Recanatini, M.; Cavalli, A. Single-molecule pulling simulations can discern active from inactive enzyme inhibitors. *J. Am. Chem. Soc.* **2010**, *132*, 7361–7371. [CrossRef]
22. De Vivo, M.; Masetti, M.; Bottegoni, G.; Cavalli, A. Role of Molecular Dynamics and Related Methods in Drug Discovery. *J. Med. Chem.* **2016**, *59*, 4035–4061. [CrossRef]
23. Jiang, W.; Chipot, C.; Roux, B. Computing Relative Binding Affinity of Ligands to Receptor: An Effective Hybrid Single-Dual-Topology Free-Energy Perturbation Approach in NAMD. *J. Chem. Inf. Model.* **2019**, *59*, 3794–3802. [CrossRef]
24. Steinbrecher, T.B.; Dahlgren, M.; Cappel, D.; Lin, T.; Wang, L.; Krilov, G.; Abel, R.; Friesner, R.; Sherman, W. Accurate Binding Free Energy Predictions in Fragment Optimization. *J. Chem. Inf. Model.* **2015**, *55*, 2411–2420. [CrossRef]
25. Zou, J.; Tian, C.; Simmerling, C. Blinded prediction of protein-ligand binding affinity using Amber thermodynamic integration for the 2018 D3R grand challenge 4. *J. Comput. Aided Mol. Des.* **2019**, *33*, 1021–1029. [CrossRef]
26. Garton, M.; Corbi-Verge, C.; Hu, Y.; Nim, S.; Tarasova, N.; Sherborne, B.; Kim, P.M. Rapid and accurate structure-based therapeutic peptide design using GPU accelerated thermodynamic integration. *Proteins* **2019**, *87*, 236–244. [CrossRef]
27. Abagyan, R.; Totrov, M. Biased probability Monte Carlo conformational searches and electrostatic calculations for peptides and proteins. *J. Mol. Biol.* **1994**, *235*, 983–1002. [CrossRef]
28. Liu, Y.; Beveridge, D.L. Exploratory studies of ab initio protein structure prediction: Multiple copy simulated annealing, AMBER energy functions, and a generalized born/solvent accessibility solvation model. *Proteins* **2002**, *46*, 128–146. [CrossRef]
29. Abagyan, R.A.; Totrov, M. Ab InitioFolding of Peptides by the Optimal-Bias Monte Carlo Minimization Procedure. *J. Comput. Phys.* **1999**, *151*, 402–421. [CrossRef]

30. Hornak, V.; Abel, R.; Okur, A.; Strockbine, B.; Roitberg, A.; Simmerling, C. Comparison of multiple Amber force fields and development of improved protein backbone parameters. *Proteins* **2006**, *65*, 712–725. [CrossRef]
31. Lazaridis, T.; Karplus, M. Effective energy function for proteins in solution. *Proteins* **1999**, *35*, 133–152. [CrossRef]
32. Singh, U.C.; Kollman, P.A. An approach to computing electrostatic charges for molecules. *J. Comput. Chem.* **1984**, *5*, 129–145. [CrossRef]
33. Besler, B.H.; Merz, K.M.; Kollman, P.A. Atomic charges derived from semiempirical methods. *J. Comput. Chem.* **1990**, *11*, 431–439. [CrossRef]
34. Schmidt, M.W.; Baldridge, K.K.; Boatz, J.A.; Elbert, S.T.; Gordon, M.S.; Jensen, J.H.; Koseki, S.; Matsunaga, N.; Nguyen, K.A.; Su, S.; et al. General atomic and molecular electronic structure system. *J. Comput. Chem.* **1993**, *14*, 1347–1363. [CrossRef]
35. Gordon, M.S.; Schmidt, M.W. Advances in electronic structure theory: GAMESS a decade later A2—Dykstra, Clifford E. In *Theory and Applications of Computational Chemistry*; Frenking, G., Kim, K.S., Scuseria, G.E., Eds.; Elsevier: Amsterdam, The Netherlands, 2005; pp. 1167–1189. [CrossRef]
36. Bellows, M.L.; Floudas, C.A. Computational methods for de novo protein design and its applications to the human immunodeficiency virus 1, purine nucleoside phosphorylase, ubiquitin specific protease 7, and histone demethylases. *Curr. Drug Targets* **2010**, *11*, 264–278. [CrossRef]
37. Bellows, M.L.; Fung, H.K.; Taylor, M.S.; Floudas, C.A.; Lopez de Victoria, A.; Morikis, D. New compstatin variants through two de novo protein design frameworks. *Biophys. J.* **2010**, *98*, 2337–2346. [CrossRef]
38. Bellows, M.L.; Taylor, M.S.; Cole, P.A.; Shen, L.; Siliciano, R.F.; Fung, H.K.; Floudas, C.A. Discovery of entry inhibitors for HIV-1 via a new de novo protein design framework. *Biophys. J.* **2010**, *99*, 3445–3453. [CrossRef]
39. Bellows-Peterson, M.L.; Fung, H.K.; Floudas, C.A.; Kieslich, C.A.; Zhang, L.; Morikis, D.; Wareham, K.J.; Monk, P.N.; Hawksworth, O.A.; Woodruff, T.M. De novo peptide design with C3a receptor agonist and antagonist activities: Theoretical predictions and experimental validation. *J. Med. Chem.* **2012**, *55*, 4159–4168. [CrossRef]
40. Fung, H.K.; Floudas, C.A.; Taylor, M.S.; Zhang, L.; Morikis, D. Toward full-sequence de novo protein design with flexible templates for human beta-defensin-2. *Biophys. J.* **2008**, *94*, 584–599. [CrossRef]
41. Gorham, R.D., Jr.; Forest, D.L.; Khoury, G.A.; Smadbeck, J.; Beecher, C.N.; Healy, E.D.; Tamamis, P.; Archontis, G.; Larive, C.K.; Floudas, C.A.; et al. New compstatin peptides containing N-terminal extensions and non-natural amino acids exhibit potent complement inhibition and improved solubility characteristics. *J. Med. Chem.* **2015**, *58*, 814–826. [CrossRef]
42. Halai, R.; Bellows-Peterson, M.L.; Branchett, W.; Smadbeck, J.; Kieslich, C.A.; Croker, D.E.; Cooper, M.A.; Morikis, D.; Woodruff, T.M.; Floudas, C.A.; et al. Derivation of ligands for the complement C3a receptor from the C-terminus of C5a. *Eur. J. Pharmacol.* **2014**, *745*, 176–181. [CrossRef]
43. Smadbeck, J.; Peterson, M.B.; Zee, B.M.; Garapaty, S.; Mago, A.; Lee, C.; Giannis, A.; Trojer, P.; Garcia, B.A.; Floudas, C.A. De novo peptide design and experimental validation of histone methyltransferase inhibitors. *PLoS ONE* **2014**, *9*, e95535. [CrossRef] [PubMed]
44. Audie, J. Development and validation of an empirical free energy function for calculating protein-protein binding free energy surfaces. *Biophys. Chem.* **2009**, *139*, 84–91. [CrossRef] [PubMed]
45. Audie, J. Continued development of an empirical function for predicting and rationalizing protein-protein binding affinities. *Biophys. Chem.* **2009**, *143*, 139–144. [CrossRef] [PubMed]
46. Audie, J.; Scarlata, S. A novel empirical free energy function that explains and predicts protein-protein binding affinities. *Biophys. Chem.* **2007**, *129*, 198–211. [CrossRef] [PubMed]
47. Swanson, J.; Audie, J. An unexpected way forward: Towards a more accurate and rigorous protein-protein binding affinity scoring function by eliminating terms from an already simple scoring function. *J. Biomol. Struct. Dyn.* **2018**, *36*, 83–97. [CrossRef] [PubMed]
48. Krieger, E.; Darden, T.; Nabuurs, S.B.; Finkelstein, A.; Vriend, G. Making optimal use of empirical energy functions: Force-field parameterization in crystal space. *Proteins* **2004**, *57*, 678–683. [CrossRef] [PubMed]
49. Krieger, E.; Joo, K.; Lee, J.; Raman, S.; Thompson, J.; Tyka, M.; Baker, D.; Karplus, K. Improving physical realism, stereochemistry, and side-chain accuracy in homology modeling: Four approaches that performed well in CASP8. *Proteins* **2009**, *77* (Suppl. 9), 114–122. [CrossRef]
50. Krieger, E.; Vriend, G. YASARA View—molecular graphics for all devices—from smartphones to workstations. *Bioinformatics* **2014**, *30*, 2981–2982. [CrossRef]

51. Krieger, E.; Koraimann, G.; Vriend, G. Increasing the precision of comparative models with YASARA NOVA–a self-parameterizing force field. *Proteins* **2002**, *47*, 393–402. [CrossRef]
52. Greenidge, P.A.; Kramer, C.; Mozziconacci, J.C.; Wolf, R.M. MM/GBSA binding energy prediction on the PDBbind data set: Successes, failures, and directions for further improvement. *J. Chem. Inf. Model.* **2013**, *53*, 201–209. [CrossRef]
53. Baker, N.A.; Sept, D.; Joseph, S.; Holst, M.J.; McCammon, J.A. Electrostatics of nanosystems: Application to microtubules and the ribosome. *Proc. Natl. Acad. Sci. USA* **2001**, *98*, 10037–10041. [CrossRef] [PubMed]
54. Trott, O.; Olson, A.J. AutoDock Vina: Improving the speed and accuracy of docking with a new scoring function, efficient optimization, and multithreading. *J. Comput. Chem.* **2010**, *31*, 455–461. [CrossRef] [PubMed]
55. Wang, R.; Lai, L.; Wang, S. Further development and validation of empirical scoring functions for structure-based binding affinity prediction. *J. Comput. Aided Mol. Des.* **2002**, *16*, 11–26. [CrossRef] [PubMed]
56. Bottger, V.; Bottger, A.; Howard, S.F.; Picksley, S.M.; Chene, P.; GarciaEcheverria, C.; Hochkeppel, H.K.; Lane, D.P. Identification of novel mdm2 binding peptides by phage display. *Oncogene* **1996**, *13*, 2141–2147.
57. Lai, Z.; Auger, K.R.; Manubay, C.M.; Copeland, R.A. Thermodynamics of p53 Binding to hdm2(1–126): Effects of Phosphorylation and p53 Peptide Length. *Arch. Biochem. Biophys.* **2000**, *381*, 278–284. [CrossRef] [PubMed]
58. Roehrl, M.H.A.; Wang, J.Y.; Wagner, G. A general framework for development and data analysis of competitive high-throughput screens for small-molecule inhibitors of protein-protein interactions by fluorescence polarization. *Biochemistry* **2004**, *43*, 16056–16066. [CrossRef] [PubMed]
59. Wang, Z.-X. An exact mathematical expression for describing competitive binding of two different ligands to a protein molecule. *FEBS Lett.* **1995**, *360*, 111–114. [CrossRef]

Sample Availability: All data used in the preparation of this manuscript will be made available upon request.

molecules

MDPI

Review

Current Mechanistic and Pharmacodynamic Understanding of Melanocortin-4 Receptor Activation

Shubh Sharma, Alastair S. Garfield, Bhavik Shah, Patrick Kleyn, Ilia Ichetovkin, Ida Hatoum Moeller, William R. Mowrey and Lex H.T. Van der Ploeg *

Rhythm Pharmaceuticals, Boston, MA 02116, USA; ssharma@rhythmtx.com (S.S.); agarfield@rhythmtx.com (A.S.G.); bshah@rhythmtx.com (B.S.); pkleyn@rhythmtx.com (P.K.); ichetov@rhythmtx.com (I.I.); imoeller@rhythmtx.com (I.H.M.); bmowrey@rhythmtx.com (W.R.M.)

* Correspondence: lvanderploeg@rhythmtx.com; Tel.: +1-857-264-4287

Academic Editors: Henry Mosberg, Tomi Sawyer and Carrie Haskell-Luevano
Received: 21 April 2019; Accepted: 15 May 2019; Published: 16 May 2019

check for updates

Abstract: In this work we summarize our understanding of melanocortin 4 receptor (MC4R) pathway activation, aiming to define a safe and effective therapeutic targeting strategy for the MC4R. Delineation of cellular MC4R pathways has provided evidence for distinct MC4R signaling events characterized by unique receptor activation kinetics. While these studies remain narrow in scope, and have largely been explored with peptidic agonists, the results provide a possible correlation between distinct ligand groups and differential MC4R activation kinetics. In addition, when a set of small-molecule and peptide MC4R agonists are compared, evidence of biased signaling has been reported. The results of such mechanistic studies are discussed.

Keywords: melanocortin-4 receptor; obesity; peptide agonist; cardiovascular profile; GαS signaling; receptor desensitization; receptor internalization

1. Introduction

It is with great pleasure we dedicate this review article to Prof. Victor J. Hruby, in honor of his 80th birthday. Prof. Hruby has been a seminal leader in several areas of peptide research. His research has blazed the trail for melanocortin research efforts, including building understanding of chemistry, biology and pharmacology of melanocortins. Prof. Hruby has made many pivotal contributions to the scientific community, by creating widely used melanocortin receptor agonists, MT-I (NDP-α-MSH), MT-II, and the melanocortin receptor-3 and -4 antagonist SHU9119. These reagents have been instrumental in unraveling the function of melanocortin receptors including their roles in pigmentation, energy homeostasis, body weight regulation and sexual arousal. Prof. Hruby continues to make powerful contributions to the melanocortin research field, through the development of potent and selective agonists and antagonists for various melanocortin receptor subtypes.

The central hypothalamic melanocortin-4 receptor (MC4R) is a uniquely validated therapeutic target for the treatment of obesity based on both pharmacologic and human genetic evidence [1–4]. Acting in concert with leptin (a satiety hormone), ghrelin (a hunger hormone) and their receptors, the MC4R holds a key position in the regulation of energy homeostasis and body weight. The MC4R and leptin receptor are key components of the MC4R pathway, which, when disrupted by genetic defects in any of these contributing receptor/ligand systems, causes impaired energy balance [1,5–7]. A variety of peptide and small molecule MC4R agonists have been developed over the past nearly three decades and have been shown in rodent models to elicit decreases in food intake and body weight. However, the diverse nature of MC4R-driven pharmacological efficacy has posed challenges in developing an MC4R agonist for the treatment of obesity. These hurdles include MC4R-related sympathetic activation leading to elevation of blood pressure (BP) and heart rate (HR), as well as activation of sexual arousal [8–12]. As a result, the feasibility of targeting the MC4R for treating obesity by peptides and small molecules ligands has been called into question, despite intense drug discovery and development activity which started in the 1990s. There have been some notable successes in creating MC4R agonist compositions, including orally bioavailable leads (for example, Merck compounds MK-0493 and MB243; Pfizer compound-13; and several Neurocrine NBI compounds described in MacNeil et al. [13]; Palucki et al. [14]; Ujjainwalla and Sebhat [15]; Chen et al. [16]; Krishna et al. [17]; He et al. [18]; and Lansdell et al. [19] and reviewed in Todorovic and Haskell-Luevano [20] and Ericson et al. [21]. MK-0493 evaluated in a phase-1 human study was shown to be ineffective in controlling food intake or body weight meaningfully [17]. A few peptide MCR agonist compositions, including LY2112688, MC4R-NN2-0453, and AZD2820, were also explored in early clinical studies for the treatment of obesity (Table 1). However, their development was stopped due to several adverse effects, including increased HR and BP, hyperpigmentation (melanocortin receptor-1 (MC1R)-driven), and sexual arousal, which were seen in early clinical trials. Similarly, development of bremelanotide, an MC4R peptide agonist for the treatment of male erectile dysfunction, was halted following adverse effects, including BP and HR elevation, as well as nausea and vomiting [22]. However, bremelanotide is currently being investigated for the treatment of hypoactive sexual dysfunction in pre-menopausal women [23].

Table 1. Structures of various melanocortin-4 receptor (MC4R) agonists evaluated in human clinical studies.

Setmelanotide:	Ac-Arg-cyclo(Cys-D-Ala-His-D-Phe-Arg-Trp-Cys)-amide
LY2112688:	Ac-D-Arg-cyclo(Cys-Glu-His-D-Phe-Arg-Trp-Cys)-amide
MC4-NN-0453:	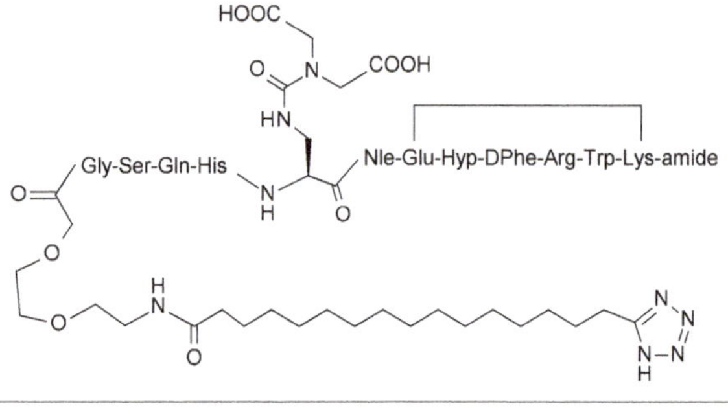
MK-0493:	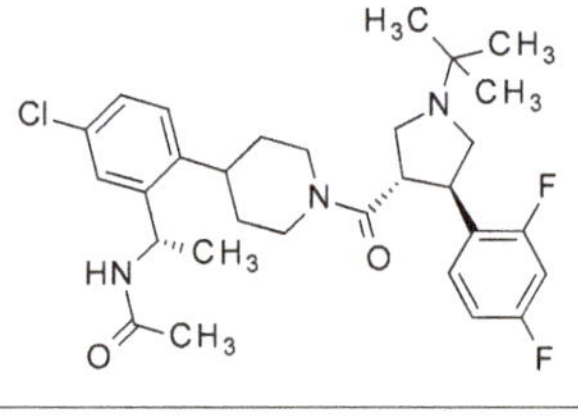
AZD2820:	Structure undisclosed

Setmelanotide, an eight amino acid cyclic MC4R agonist peptide (Table 1), is being investigated in several clinical studies for the treatment of obesity, including rare genetic disorders of obesity. These genetic deficiencies include subjects with pro-opiomelanocortin (*POMC*) deficiency, proprotein-convertase (*PCSK1*) deficiency, leptin receptor (*LEPR*) deficiency, Prader-Willi syndrome (*PWS*), Bardet-Biedl syndrome (*BBS*), Alström syndrome (*AS*), and selected other genetic forms of early-onset severe obesity arising from defects that impair the MC4R pathway. Earlier results indicate that setmelanotide is generally well tolerated in humans and holds promise for treating obesity and hyperphagia in subjects with these rare genetic disorders of obesity.

This review compares the unique pharmacological and mechanistic profiles of several MC4R agonists based on a series of in vivo and in vitro studies. Special emphasis is placed on comparative pharmacological data obtained for the MC4R agonist peptides setmelanotide and LY2112688 [11]. While both setmelanotide and LY2112688 are potent MC4R agonists which can elicit decreases in food intake and body weight in animal models, only setmelanotide lacks adverse increases in cardiovascular activity (HR and BP) in non-human primates and humans [3,24,25]. Studies highlighting key differentiating features among these two agonists are discussed.

2. Agonist Induced Signaling, Desensitization, and Internalization of MC4R

Recent investigations which may help differentiate various in vivo pharmacological profiles of certain MC4R agonists have revealed an agonist-based bias for the activation of distinct MC4R intracellular signaling pathways. Studies probing differential MC4R signaling have included assays performed under equilibrium ligand binding conditions or temporally dynamic activation of the MC4R followed by the measurement of their impact on internalization and desensitization of the MC4R. Various intracellular pathways that could be invoked in neural MCR signaling, along with biased signaling ligands, have recently been reviewed by Yang and Tao [26]. Various signaling pathways explored with MC4R include the use of different G-proteins, including Gαs, Gαi/Gαo, Gαq, and G-protein dependent mitogen-activated protein kinases/extracellular signal-regulated kinases (MAPK/ERK) activation, as well as G-protein independent effects on the potassium channel Kir7.1 on MC4R neurons. These are discussed in more detail in the following sections.

The most ubiquitous MC4R signaling events described are mediated through Gαs activation, leading to the production of intracellular cyclic adenosine monophosphate (cAMP). However, recent studies using surrogate reporter systems in MC4R-expressing cells have produced indirect evidence for the involvement of a Gαq signaling pathway leading to the activation of phospholipase-C (PLC) and calcium mobilization [4]. Some investigators have explored the involvement of the Gi/o-mediated pathway, without, however, clear evidence of its involvement [27]. This initial evidence of possible divergence in signaling pathways downstream of MC4R is of interest and requires in depth follow-up to understand its impact in physiologically relevant signaling events. The results of these studies are summarized here and include evaluations of setmelanotide, a related compound RM-511 [28], and the LY2112688 MC4R agonist peptide.

2.1. Equilibrium Binding and Activation

It is well established that MC4R signals through Gαs under equilibrium ligand binding conditions using human embryonic kidney (HEK), Chinese hamster ovary (CHO), or monkey kidney tissue derived fibroblast-like cell (COS) cell-based systems stably transfected with MC4R [3,4,14,19,24,28–31]. Under these equilibrium conditions, receptor activation by both peptide and small molecule agonists can be antagonized by MC4R antagonists like SHU9119 or Agouti gene-related peptide (AgRP). While AgRP is an endogenous antagonist of MC4R mediated GαS signaling, it has also been shown in in vitro systems to function as an inverse agonist by decreasing basal levels of cAMP [32,33]. Table 2 summarizes the effective concentration for 50% stimulation (EC_{50}) values for cAMP stimulation and Ki (binding constant) values for receptor binding for setmelanotide, LY2112688, Melanotan-II (MT-II) and alpha-melanocyte stimulating hormone (α-MSH, an endogenous agonist) in CHO cells stably transfected with human (h)MC1R, hMC3R, hMC4R, or hMC5R (these agonists do not interact with the MC2R). In these experiments, setmelanotide, MT-II, and LY2112688 displayed approximately similar binding affinities for the MC4R. In cAMP functional assays performed under equilibrium conditions, the potencies for each of these three agonists were also equivalent when compared between setmelanotide and LY2112688 or MT-II, with setmelanotide being about three times less active.

Table 2. Inhibitory constants and 50% effective concentrations of peptide agonists in CHO-K1 cells expressing human melanocortin receptors (data from Kievit et al. [24]).

Compound	Binding Assay Ki [nM]				cAMP Assay EC_{50} [nM]			
	hMC1R	hMC3R	hMC4R	hMC5R	hMC1R	hMC3R	hMC4R	hMC5R
α-MSH	0.32	15.5	41.4	332	1.01	1.04	4.7	10.5
MT-II	0.27	24	2.66	23.1	0.2	0.51	0.05	5.33
Setmelanotide	3.9	10	2.1	430	5.8	5.3	0.27	1600
LY2112688	4	35.1	1.84	5160	8.12	10.3	0.09	5760

2.2. *Dynamic Signaling upon Exposure to MC4R Agonists*

In prior studies using time-resolved signaling conditions, LY-2112688, MT-II, THIQ, and a setmelanotide analog, RM-511, were shown to differentiate in their dynamic effects during MC4R signaling or antagonism by AgRP [34].

These studies by Molden et al. [34] employed acute exposure to the MC4R agonist and applied cell-based reporter moiety and receptor tags for tracking receptor activation kinetics. Using a temporally-resolved Förster resonance energy transfer (FRET) based cAMP assay with $Neuro2A_{HA\text{-}MC4R\text{-}GFP}$ cells (stably expressing epitope-tagged hemagglutinin-MC4R-green fluorescent protein along with endogenous MC4R), Molden et al. [34] revealed evidence of biased signaling dynamics with this set of MC4R agonists, as measured by Gαs mediated cAMP induction. These studies were performed at ≥10 fold the respective EC_{50} concentrations of the agonists and investigated agonist stimulated receptor internalization and desensitization. In these assays, cAMP induction by either α-MSH (200 nM) or LY2112688 (100 nM) could be quickly reversed upon withdrawal of the ligand from the incubation medium and washing the cells free of ligand. These observations contrasted with the remarkable robust stimulation of signaling by MT-II (2 nM), THIQ (1 μM), or RM-511 (100 nM), which persisted for the 1 hr observation period following withdrawal of the respective agonists from the medium and washing of the cells. Furthermore, continued MT-II-induced stimulation could not be reversed by treatment with AgRP. The prolonged non-antagonizable cAMP stimulation may have been due to the presence of internalized constitutively active MC4R. Agonist-induced internalization of MC4R was further studied with an α-MSH (500 nM) re-challenge following initial ligand exposure and wash off (Table 3). In this experiment the cells were treated with the MC4R agonist for 10 min, followed by its withdrawal (washing off) and immediate re-challenge with α-MSH (500 nM) to observe the kinetics of re-accumulation of cAMP. After the wash off, the cAMP stimulation initiated by both α-MSH and LY2112688 was fully reversed, while THIQ stimulation was only partially reversed. The stimulation initiated by MT-II and RM-511 could not be reversed upon washing. Therefore, both MT-II and RM-511 were argued to induce receptor internalization and continued signaling, while α-MSH and LY2112688 were ineffective, and THIQ was able to induce this only partially. Interestingly, Garnell et al. [35] have previously shown that intracellularly targeted α-MSH to intracellular MC4R at the endoplasmic reticulum (by co-transfecting both in neuroblastoma N2A cells) can lead to cAMP stimulation. These activated MC4Rs do not desensitize and can cycle to the cell surface. The level of this intracellular MC4R stimulation is comparable to cAMP activation achieved by acute exposure of the MC4R transfected N2A cells to α-MSH.

Table 3. Dynamic cAMP stimulation upon ligand incubation, washout, and α-MSH re-challenge, showing persistent signaling by certain MC4R ligands (adapted from Molden et al. [34]).

MC4R Ligands and Incubation Concentration	Dynamic cAMP Response				Comment
	Time = 0 min	Time = 10–20 min	Time = 20–50 min	Time = 55–60 min	
	Initial (time 0–10 min)	Ligand challenge at 10 min	Ligand washed out after 10 min incubation and measured cAMP 20–30 min post washing	cAMP following 500 nM α-MSH re-challenge at 55 min	
α-MSH, 200 nM	–	++++	–	++++	Full reversal of signal upon washing out
LY2112688, 100 nM	–	++++	–	++++	Full reversal of signal upon washing out
THIQ, 1 μM	–	++++	++	++++	Partial reversal upon washout
MT-II, 200 nM	–	++++	++++	++++	No reversal upon washout
RM-511, 100 nM	–	++++	++++	++++	No reversal upon washout

– represents a zero or basal level response, or response without any ligand exposure; ++ represents about half the maximal cAMP stimulation response; ++++ represents a 100% cAMP stimulation response.

Earlier investigations of agonist-induced time-dependent internalization of MC4R expressed in HEK cells and COS cells have also been reported by Shinyama et al. [29]. However, unlike the acute exposure studies of Molden et al. [34], the studies of Shinyama et al. [29] reported that chronic exposure to α-MSH (0.1–1000 μM) in GT1-7 mouse hypothalamic cells caused loss of MC4R activity. This desensitization was interpreted to be due to MC4R internalization in the absence of constitutive signaling. This conclusion was based on the observation that impaired cAMP stimulation resulted after the washing off of the agonist, followed by a re-challenge with 100 μM α-MSH. Useful mechanistic insights on receptor internalization have also been developed. Shinyama et al. [29] found that internalization of the MC4R was dependent on β-arrestin and dynamin, as well as partly dependent on protein kinase-A (PKA) activation. Using a specific phosphorylation inhibitor, H89, the authors showed that Thr312 and Ser329/330 residues in the c-terminal tail of the MC4R are potential phosphorylation sites upon activation of the receptor by α-MSH. These phosphorylation sites were observed to be critical for the recruitment of β-arrestin and subsequent internalization of the receptor. Based on these studies, Shinyama et al. [29] concluded that agonist-induced phosphorylation at the c-terminus of the MC4R is manifested by an agonist-induced conformational change in the receptor needed for its internalization. For example, forskolin increased cAMP but did not induce receptor internalization [29]. Interestingly, low concentrations of α-MSH causing only a small increase in cAMP were enough to cause acute receptor internalization and desensitization [29]. Based on these results, as well as the observation that haploinsufficiency of MC4R can cause obesity, Shinyama et al. [29] have suggested that the MC4R can be activated following low receptor occupancy, where subtle changes in activation or MC4R numbers may be sufficient to exert control over energy homeostasis. Furthermore, in their studies, AgRP (1–10 nM), an endogenous antagonist of MC4R, caused a concentration-dependent increase in cell surface expression of the MC4R. Synthetic small molecule antagonists are also known to facilitate trafficking and rescue intracellularly held mutated MC4R [36]. Based on these results it was proposed that AgRP may be involved in the cell surface trafficking of the MC4R, whereas the endogenous agonist α-MSH brings about the agonist-induced conformational transition needed for phosphorylation and subsequent internalization and desensitization. Studies by Gao et al. [37] and Cai et al. [38] using MC4R transfected HEK293 cells have provided similar evidence for peptide agonist induced internalization of MC4R with no evidence of associated involvement of PKA, probably due to a different host cell system. Further, peptide antagonists used in these studies failed to induce internalization.

Similar findings have also been reported by Nickolls et al. [31], who studied a set of peptide and non-peptide agonists for cAMP accumulation, calcium mobilization (using a fluorescence imaging plate reader (FLIPR) system), and MC4R internalization (FLAG-tagged MC4R by fluorescence-activated cell sorting) assays. While all the agonists were able to stimulate cAMP accumulation, only the peptidic agonists caused strong responses in the calcium mobilization and internalization assays. In these studies, small molecule agonists were observed to be impaired in both the calcium mobilization and internalization assays (Table 4). This study therefore suggested that the subset of peptide agonists capable of causing internalization were distinct in their signaling mechanism over the non-peptides, which were not able to similarly effect receptor internalization. The peptide agonists included in this study were α-MSH, β-MSH, γ-MSH, des-acetyl-α-MSH, and NDP-α-MSH. The small molecule agonists were THIQ and similarly related analogs, as shown in Table 4.

Table 4. Data from Nickolls et al. [31] showing impaired internalization of MC4R by small molecule agonists as compared with the peptide agonists. The general structure of these small molecules is given directly below.

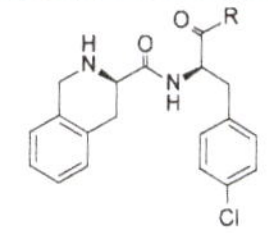

Ligand	R	MC4R Binding Ki (nM)	MC4R EC_{50} (nM) *(Intrinsic Activity)*		
			cAMP Accumulation	Calcium Mobilization	Internalization
α-MSH *	Acetyl-SYSMEHFRWGKPV-amide	50.1	21.4 *(100)*	129 *(100)*	28.8 *(100)*
β-MSH *	DEGPYRMEHFRWGSPPKD	18.6	11.2 *(83)*	174 *(94)*	43.7 *(118)*
γ-MSH *	YVMGHFRWDRFG	589	631 *(80)*	>1000 *(62)*	>1000 *(75)*
des-acetyl-α-MSH	SYSMEHFRWGKPV-amide	30.2	17.4 *(84)*	110 *(96)*	30.2 *(107)*
NDP-α-MSH	Acetyl-SYS(Nle)H(D-Phe)-RWGKPV-amide	3.98	1.38 *(112)*	120 *(80)*	7.24 *(89)*
THIQ	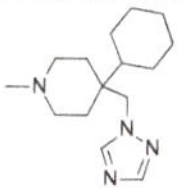	10.7	1.32 *(98)*	692 *(7)*	0.81 *(29)* **
NBI-55886	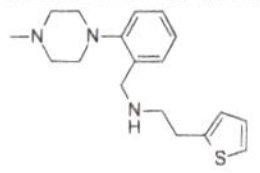	9.55	331 *(73)*	>1000 *(40)*	3.47 *(16)* **
NBI-56297	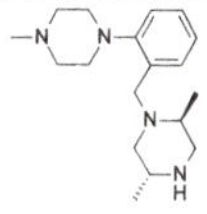	20	129 *(81)*	>1000 *(23)*	7.94 *(−5)* **
NBI-56453	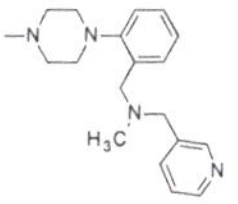	74.1	513 *(103)*	45.7 *(7)*	5.25 *(27)* **
NBI-58702	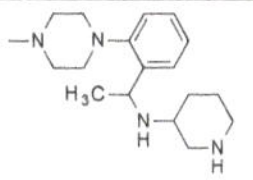	6.31	43 *(110)*	2.4 *(20)*	7.59 *(38)* **
NBI-58704	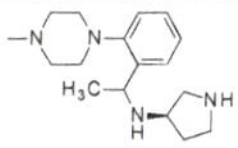	13.5	204 *(149)*	17.8 *(23)*	145 *(34)* **

* Endogenous melanocortin receptor-4 agonist. ** For all the small molecules, the intrinsic activity for internalization was significantly different and lower than that in the cAMP accumulation assay.

2.3. *Evidence for Gαq Signaling*

With the widely used cell systems employed for measuring MC4R activation, it has been challenging to show the engagement of other G-protein signaling pathways, including Gαq and Gαi/o. Clément et al. [4] have recently provided evidence using HEK293 cell-based systems that incorporated reporter gene systems, such as cAMP binding response element (CREB) and nuclear factor of activated T-cells (NFAT) reporters, that MC4R agonists can exhibit a differential preference for MC4R signaling through one or the other G-protein coupled pathways. For example, when comparing EC_{50} values of three peptide agonists, α-MSH, setmelanotide, and LY2112688, in the reporter gene-based cAMP (Gαs) and phospholipase C-β(PLC) measured through NFAT reporter assay (a possible surrogate of Gαq and/or Gβγ of Gi/o signaling), interesting observations were made. All the EC_{50} data in this study were obtained under equilibrium stimulation conditions and for the Gαs signaling the EC_{50} values were: α-MSH 23 ± 7 nM; setmelanotide 3.9 ± 1.7 nM, and LY2112688 14 ± 4 nM. In the NFAT signaling assay the EC_{50} values were: α-MSH 480 ± 260 nM; setmelanotide 5.9 ± 1.8 nM; and LY2112688 330 ± 190 nM. While the Gαs signaling (cAMP measurement) among these three ligands was found to be comparable to that observed in the CHO cell-based system with endogenous Gαs-coupled signaling protein, the NFAT reporter system (PLC activity measurement) revealed differences in the ability of these ligands to activate the MC4R measured through NFAT signaling. In this assay, setmelanotide was about 80 times more potent than α-MSH and about 55 times more potent than LY2112688. Clément et al. [4] further provided evidence that the potent setmelanotide induced PLC-β activation through MC4R could be due to Gαq activation, as this effect could not be blocked by pertussis toxin (PTX), which inhibits Gi/o signaling. Li et al. [39] have also shown the presence of MC4R-coupled Gαq/11 signaling in the paraventricular nucleus (PVN) of mice, which upon PLC activation leads to MT-II-induced decrease in feeding without impacting cardiovascular response. It remains to be seen, however, if similar results can be confirmed with a more diverse set of MC4R agonists in similar cell-based assay systems.

Antagonism of setmelanotide-induced cAMP and PLC by AgRP, as seen in a study by Clément et al. [4], provides further evidence for potential differences in the MC4R signaling ability when compared between α-MSH, setmelanotide, and LY2112688. In the cAMP antagonism assay, AgRP was about three times less efficient in inhibiting setmelanotide-related stimulation (AgRP IC_{50} 9.24 nM) than LY2112688 (AgRP IC_{50} 3.56 nM). However, in the PLC assay (through the NFAT reporter gene), 100 nM AgRP could not antagonize setmelanotide-stimulated activation while the stimulation by either α-MSH or LY2112688 was completely antagonized. Therefore, when compared to α-MSH and LY2112688, it was shown that not only can setmelanotide activate the PLC-related signaling pathway more robustly but also that this effect cannot be efficiently antagonized by AgRP.

In summary, the complexity of MC4R intracellular signaling is profound and while the physiological relevance of in vitro identified systems remains to be determined, it seems plausible that agonist-induced MC4R internalization could be critical for MC4R-mediated physiological control in energy homeostasis. It is important to note that the MC4R is proposed to be a constitutively active receptor and its activation at low receptor occupancy with α-MSH is proposed to cause its acute internalization. By contrast, AgRP binds the MC4R and causes its upregulation and translocation to, or retention at, the cell surface. Based on our comparator data, it is possible that the peptidic MC4R agonists capable of inducing MC4R internalization may be considered suitable drug candidates for therapeutic intervention for the treatment of obesity. This finding is of interest as all the small molecules studied were ineffective in causing MC4R internalization. Similarly, selected other drug candidates, including the peptidic lead LY2112688 in comparison to RM-511 and MT-II, activate and desensitize the MC4R differently. While there is no published report on its ability to induce MC4R internalization, one small molecule drug candidate lead, MK0493, was found to be ineffective in inducing weight loss in human clinical evaluation [17].

In addition to the above described G-protein related intracellular signaling of MC4R, there have been reports of additional direct mechanisms for the regulation of MC4R neurons in the PVN of the hypothalamus by G-protein independent mechanisms. For example, Ghamari-Langroudi et al. [40] have indicated the involvement of an inwardly rectifying potassium channel (Kir7.1) that closes upon binding of α-MSH to MC4R to depolarize the MC4R neurons, while the binding of the antagonist AgRP causes hyperpolarization by opening the channel. This α-MSH-induced Kir7.1 signaling was proposed as being central to melanocortin-mediated regulation of energy homeostasis within the PVN, with AgRP acting as an agonist in opening this channel [40]. Additionally, Vongs et al. [41] have shown that NDP-α-MSH can intracellularly activate MAPK/ERK1/2 in MC4R-transfected CHO-K1 cells, an effect that is likely dependent on inositol triphosphate IP3. However, as discussed by Yang and Tao [26], the activation of the MAPK/ERK pathway appears to be much more diverse as, in addition to IP3, it can also be shown to involve PKA and protein kinase-C (PKC)/calcium and to be dependent on the cell systems and the MC4R activation ligand used. Rather than functioning as an antagonist in the GαS-mediated cAMP stimulation, AgRP induced phosphorylation in the ERK pathway. Further studies are needed to sort through the signaling diversity associated with the MAPK/ERK activation pathway.

3. Feeding and Weight Loss Studies in Rodents

The efficacy of setmelanotide and other MC4R agonists has been studied in diverse preclinical models, including mouse models of diet-induced obesity (DIO) and Sprague-Dawley rats [28]. In an acute study in DIO mice, 6.4 μmole of setmelanotide (identified in this study as BIM-22493) administered as a single intraperitoneal injection 30 min prior to food presentation strongly and significantly inhibited food intake during refeeding following an overnight fast. These effects appear MC4R-mediated, as in the Kumar et al. study [28] there was no impact on food intake observed in the MC4R-knockout mice, while the MC3R knockout mice responded like wild-type mice, thereby establishing that the setmelanotide effect is dependent on a functional MC4R and does not require MC3R in this model system. Similarly, setmelanotide also reduced food intake during refeeding after an overnight fast in male Sprague–Dawley rats at 100 or 500 nmol/kg administered subcutaneously [28]. Furthermore, in chronic studies performed in DIO mice, setmelanotide (300 nmol/kg/day for 14 days, administered by subcutaneous (SC) osmotic pump) was also shown to reduce body weight and improve glucose homeostasis and dyslipidemia. The suppression of food intake and weight loss was most pronounced during days 1–4 of treatment, and by day 12 the effect on food intake was no longer significant, although food intake still appeared lower compared to controls [28].

In a comparative study with MC4R-homozyogus knockout ($MC4R^{-/-}$), MC4R-heterozygous ($MC4R^{+/-}$), and wild-type mice maintained on a high fat diet (45% kcal fat) and implanted with subcutaneous osmotic pumps containing either 1.34 mg/kg/day setmelanotide or the vehicle, Collet et al. [3] reported that wild-type mice were most sensitive to the treatment emergent weight loss. The $MC4R^{-/-}$ null mice did not respond in this study and the heterozygous $MC4R^{+/-}$ mice exhibited an intermediate response to setmelanotide. This study therefore reinforced the finding that the weight loss effects induced by setmelanotide are fully dependent on the presence of a functional MC4R.

LY2112688 was also shown to be efficacious in a diet-induced obese rat model of food intake and weight loss [30]. In this study, a dose-dependent decrease in cumulative food intake and cumulative body weight loss was observed at doses of 0.075 μmol/kg/day and 0.299 μmol/kg/day administered subcutaneously for 14 days. The impact of the top dose on daily food intake, however, lasted only for the first five days of dosing, as food intake was not different from the vehicle-treated group thereafter. There was also a significant lowering of fat mass seen at the higher dosages, with no impact on lean body mass during this 14-day testing period. Therefore, these MC4R agonists reduce food intake and body weight in rodent models by activating the MC4R, in keeping with the physiological function of the MC4R pathway.

4. Body Weight Effects in Obese Non-Human Primates

The effects of SC infusion of setmelanotide (0.50 mg/kg/day for eight weeks) on body weight have been reported for a group of twelve male Rhesus monkeys maintained on high-fat diet (HFD) for approximately 1.5 years before initiation of these setmelanotide dosing studies [24]. The LY2112688 peptide was used in this study as a comparator. Nine of the 12 animals were obese, insulin-resistant, and hypertensive at baseline, and the remaining three animals, classified as diet- resistant, had normal body weight, adiposity, and blood pressure.

After treatment with setmelanotide for one week, there was a significant decrease in food intake (~35%). Similar to the findings in rodents as discussed above, this effect was reported as transient, with food intake normalizing by weeks 4 through 7 of treatment, with a moderate increase in food intake during week 8 of drug treatment. Upon cessation of setmelanotide treatment, a significant increase in food intake was reported over the pretreatment baseline level, followed by normalization of food intake by 12 weeks post-treatment, when the animals had returned to their pretreatment body weight.

Interestingly, following cessation of the setmelanotide treatment, body weight remained suppressed for about 2–4 weeks in all study animals before rebounding, as if a post-treatment therapeutic benefit was retained. A significant decrease in food intake was also reported with LY2112688 at the same dose of 0.5 mg/kg/day; however, the decrease was significantly smaller than that seen with a comparable dose of setmelanotide.

Consistent with the significant decrease in food intake, the obese animals were reported to have lost ~0.75 kg (~5% of their body weight) after treatment with setmelanotide for two weeks and ~1 kg after treatment for four weeks. It is interesting to note that even after food intake increased, the animals were reported to continue to lose weight during setmelanotide treatment, leading to a mean peak weight loss of ~13.5%. After cessation of setmelanotide treatment, the animals began to regain body weight (0.5 kg by four weeks post-treatment) and a return to baseline weight by 10–12 weeks post-treatment, by which time food intake had also returned to baseline.

Activation of MC4R pathway has also been associated with several non-feeding related activities, including increased yawning, muscular stiffness, stretching, and penile erections [9]; however, none of these effects were observed in these experiments with setmelanotide.

5. Effect of Setmelanotide and LY2112688 on Cardiovascular Function

Comparative cardiovascular effects of setmelanotide and LY2112688 have been reported [24]. Briefly, in this study the groups of obese and lean Rhesus monkeys maintained on an HFD were the same as those used in the weight loss studies described above [24]. The animals received setmelanotide 0.50 mg/kg/day via SC bolus injection for four days, with telemetric measurements of the BP and HR. Following a washout period, the same group of animals received setmelanotide (0.50 mg/kg/day) or LY2112688 (0.17 or 0.50 mg/kg/day) via SC infusion for seven days. Setmelanotide (0.50 mg/kg) administered via an acute SC injection resulted in a mild increase in HR, though the obese Rhesus, in contrast to the rat, exhibited a compensatory drop in BP that persisted for 6–7 h post-dose. Upon subsequent daily bolus SC injections in the Rhesus, the heart rate response was reported to decline on days 2 and 3, and was nearly absent by day 4, while associated reduction in food intake persisted for four days of setmelanotide administrations.

In contrast to the findings reported with setmelanotide administered via SC injection, no acute increase in HR was reported after continuous SC infusion of setmelanotide at 0.50 mg/kg/day for seven days. In fact, a significant decrease in mean HR was reported, primarily in obese animals. HR remained significantly lower in the obese animals four weeks post-dose. Paralleling the decrease in HR, a significant decrease in diastolic BP was also reported in both obese and lean animals. In a follow-up study in the cynomolgus monkey, setmelanotide continuously infused at a 50-fold higher dose of 25 mg/kg/day for three days did not cause any biologically significant changes in systolic pressures, HR, or electrocardiogram (ECG) interval duration or waveforms [25]. By contrast, after SC infusion of LY2112688, increases in BP and HR were observed in the obese Rhesus. Significant mean increases of 15.5 and 16.5 beats per minute (bpm) at 0.17 mg/kg/day of LY2112688 for day 1 and 2, respectively, and 14.4 bpm at 0.5 mg/kg/day on day 2, were observed [24].

In the Sprague-Dawley rat model the HR and mean blood pressure effects of setmelanotide and LY2112688 and diverse other MC4R agonists were studied after single and multiple dose subcutaneous administration, which was were found to induce sustained increases in HR and mean blood pressure [25]. It is therefore interesting to note that while both setmelanotide and LY2112688 induced increased HR and BP in the rat model of cardiovascular (CV) activity, only setmelanotide was devoid of these same effects in the monkey cardiovascular model. The observed effects in the rat model for these MC4R agonists do not differ from previously reported cardiovascular effects revealing increases in blood pressure and heart rate in rodents with the MC4R pan-agonist MT-II [42–44]. Interestingly, α-MSH administered intravenously (IV) has been shown to fail to increase HR and BP in mice and rabbits but has been observed to elicit CV effects when administered directly into the circumventricular system, suggesting that limiting central nervous system (CNS) exposure may overcome adverse sympathetic CV sequela in preclinical models [45,46].

6. Perspective

MC4R agonists are linked to an increase in sympathetic tone, which is anticipated to directly impact heart rate and mean blood pressure. These effects can be blunted by a co-administration of α and β blockers, outlining the classical activation of sympathetically mediated CV control [10]. Most of these MC4R agonists have been shown to induce increases in mean arterial blood pressure and heart rate, even at anorexigenic doses [47], indicating that MC4R is involved in regulating CV function [9]. The CV activity data obtained to date with setmelanotide and other MC4R agonists suggest a species specific response when compared between rodents and non-human primates. Thus, although an effect on heart rate and blood pressure has been seen in rats, results of studies of non-human primates and CV data obtained for humans [3,24,25] has shown that subcutaneously infused setmelanotide or subcutaneously injected setmelanotide [3] has no effect on heart rate and blood pressure. Furthermore, LY2112688 studied in the same group of Rhesus induced both robust heart rate and blood pressure responses at similar infused dosage levels. These results point to the unique cardiovascular safety of setmelanotide when compared to the LY2112688 peptide. Furthermore, at the same dosage levels, setmelanotide has been associated with a more robust response in weight loss when compared to LY2112688, which is indicative of a favorable therapeutic index for setmelanotide in the treatment of obesity. While the mechanistic reasons for these differences are being studied, earlier studies in rodents have shown that some degree of brain penetration may be needed for the CV response, as shown in studies reporting increased CV effects upon intracerebroventricular (ICV) administration as compared to the IV administration of α-MSH in rodents and rabbits, which has been shown to fail to elicit CV responses [44–46]. It is interesting to note that brain penetration of MT-II and other ligands may not be required to elicit beneficial effects in the control of food intake and obesity in rodents [48]. However, exposure below analytically detectable levels of CNS exposure cannot be excluded [48]. Combining these data suggests that apparently poorly brain penetrant MC4R agonists (below analytical detection levels) with a unique receptor activation pharmacology profile may show promise for the treatment of obesity without the CV side effects.

The in vitro MC4R signaling studies discussed show that setmelanotide and LY2112688 diverge in their receptor activation kinetics in transfected MC4R cell reporter systems. In accordance with cell-based observations, we speculate that setmelanotide binding to MC4R is conducive to causing conformational change in the MC4R, which Shinyama et al. [29] have shown to be critical for agonist-induced receptor internalization. Based on the studies summarized above, we speculate that LY2112688, like α-MSH, is not able to trigger this same conformational change and consequently fails to elicit MC4R internalization and constitutive signaling. While the significance of the agonist-induced internalization of the MC4R to its pharmacological profile is yet to be established, additional receptor dynamics, such as homo- or hetero-receptor dimerization states, could be considered as playing a role. In addition, differences in brain penetration or distribution within the brain of each agonist may contribute to the diverse physiological effects observed. For example, it has been reported that the disruption of Gαs signaling, while maintaining Gαq/11 signaling in the PVN of mice, can abolish the cardiovascular effects of pan-agonist MT-II [39]. Furthermore, in humans with gain-of-function MC4R mutations, Lotta et al. [49] have shown that such mutations can present biased MC4R-signaling through MAPK activation and recruitment of β-arrestin, which correlates with their lower body mass index and protection against obesity, type-2 diabetes, and coronary artery disease. Further studies on biased signaling and unique receptor desensitization kinetics of the MCRs are anticipated to provide further insights into the diverse pharmacology of the melanocortin agonists currently in development.

Author Contributions: Conceptualization, S.S. and L.V.d.P.; writing—original and draft preparation, S.S. and L.V.d.P.; writing—review and editing, all authors.

Funding: The writing of this review received no external funding.

Acknowledgments: We thank all our Rhythm colleagues and numerous collaborators for their helpful discussion.

Conflicts of Interest: All authors are employees of Rhythm Pharmaceuticals.

References

1. Marks, D.L.; Cone, R.D. Central melanocortins and the regulation of weight during acute and chronic disease. *Recent Prog. Horm. Res.* **2001**, *56*, 359–375. [CrossRef]
2. Cone, R.D. The central melanocortin system and its role in energy homeostasis. *Ann. Endocrinol.* **1999**, *60*, 3–9.
3. Collet, T.H.; Dubern, B.; Mokrosinski, J.; Connors, H.; Keogh, J.M.; Mendes de Oliveira, E.; Henning, E.; Poitou-Bernert, C.; Oppert, J.M.; Tounian, P.; et al. Evaluation of a melanocortin-4 receptor (MC4R) agonist (Setmelanotide) in MC4R deficiency. *Mol. Metab.* **2017**, *6*, 1321–1329. [CrossRef] [PubMed]
4. Clément, K.; Biebermann, H.; Farooqi, I.S.; Van der Ploeg, L.; Wolters, B.; Poitou, C.; Puder, L.; Fiedorek, F.; Gottesdiener, K.; Kleinau, G.; et al. MC4R agonism promotes durable weight loss in patients with leptin receptor deficiency. *Nat. Med.* **2018**, *24*, 551–555. [CrossRef]
5. Balthasar, N.; Coppari, R.; McMinn, J.; Shun, M.; Liu, S.M.; Charlotte, E.; Lee, C.E.; Tang, V.; Kenny, C.D.; McGovern, R.A.; et al. Leptin receptor signaling in POMC neurons is required for normal body weight homeostasis. *Neuron* **2004**, *42*, 983–991. [CrossRef] [PubMed]
6. Lee, Y.S. The Role of Leptin-Melanocortin System and Human Weight Regulation: Lessons from Experiments of Nature. *Ann. Acad. Med. Singapore* **2009**, *38*, 34–44.
7. Van der Klaauw, A.A.; Farooqi, I.S. The hunger genes: Pathways to obesity. *Cell* **2015**, *161*, 119–132. [CrossRef]
8. Van der Ploeg, L.H.T.; Martin, W.J.; Martin, A.D.; Nargund, R.P.; Austin, C.P.; Guan, X.-M.; Drisko, J.; Cashen, D.; Sebhat, I.; Patchett, A.A.; et al. A role for the melanocortin 4 receptor in sexual function. *Proc. Natl. Acad. Sci. USA* **2002**, *99*, 11381–11386. [CrossRef]
9. Martin, W.J.; MacIntyre, D.E. Melanocortin receptors and erectile function. *Eur. Urol.* **2004**, *45*, 706–713. [CrossRef]
10. Kuo, J.J.; da Silva, A.A.; Tallam, L.S.; Hall, J.E. Role of adrenergic activity in pressor responses to chronic melanocortin receptor activation. *Hypertension* **2006**, *43*, 370–375. [CrossRef]
11. Greenfield, J.R.; Miller, J.W.; Keogh, J.M.; Henning, E.; Satterwhite, J.H.; Cameron, G.S.; Astruc, B.; Mayer, J.P.; Brage, S.; See, T.C.; et al. Modulation of blood pressure by central melanocortinergic pathways. *N. Engl. J. Med.* **2009**, *360*, 44–52. [CrossRef]
12. Tao, Y.-X. The melanocortin-4 receptor: Physiology, pharmacology, and pathophysiology. *Endocr. Rev.* **2010**, *31*, 506–543. [CrossRef]
13. MacNeil, D.J.; Howard, A.D.; Guan, X.-M.; Fong, T.M.; Nargund, R.P.; Bednarek, M.A.; Goulet, M.T.; Weinberg, D.H.; Strack, A.M.; Marsh, D.J.; et al. The role of melanocortins in body weight regulation: Opportunities for the treatment of obesity. *Eur. J. Pharmacol.* **2002**, *450*, 93–109. [CrossRef]
14. Palucki, B.L.; Park, M.K.; Nargund, R.P.; Ye, Z.X.; Sebhat, I.K.; Pollard, P.G.; Kalyani, R.N.; Tang, R.; MacNeil, T.; Weinberg, D.H.; et al. Discovery of (2S)-N-[(1R)-2-[4-cyclohexyl-4-[[(1,1-dimethylethyl)amino] carbonyl]-1-piperidinyl]-1-[(4-fluorophenyl)methyl]-2-oxoethyl]-4-methyl-2-piperazinecarboxamide (MB243), a potent and selective melanocortin subtype-4 receptor agonist. *Bioorg. Med. Chem. Lett.* **2005**, *15*, 171–175. [CrossRef]
15. Ujjainwalla, F.; Sebhat, I.K. Small molecule ligands of the human melanocortin-4 receptor. *Curr. Top. Med. Chem.* **2007**, *7*, 1068–1084. [CrossRef]
16. Chen, C.; Jiang, W.; Tran, J.A.; Tucci, F.C.; Fleck, B.A.; Markison, S.; Wen, J.; Madan, A.; Hoare, S.R.; Foster, A.C.; et al. Identification and characterization of pyrrolidine diastereoisomers as potent functional agonists and antagonists of the human melanocortin-4 receptor. *Bioorg. Med. Chem. Lett.* **2008**, *18*, 129–136. [CrossRef]
17. Krishna, R.; Gumbiner, B.; Stevens, C.; Musser, B.; Mallick, M.; Suryawanshi, S.; Maganti, L.; Zhu, H.; Han, T.H.; Scherer, L.; et al. Potent and selective agonism of the melanocortin receptor 4 with MK-0493 does not induce weight loss in obese human subjects: Energy intake predicts lack of weight loss efficacy. *Clin. Pharmacol. Ther.* **2009**, *86*, 659–666. [CrossRef]

18. He, S.W.; Ye, Z.X.; Dobbelaar, P.H.; Sebhat, I.K.; Guo, L.Q.; Liu, J.; Jian, T.Y.; Lai, Y.J.; Franklin, C.L.; Bakshi, R.K.; et al. Discovery of a spiroindane based compound as a potent, selective, orally bioavailable melanocortin subtype-4 receptor agonist. *Bioorg. Med. Chem. Lett.* **2010**, *20*, 2106–2110. [CrossRef]
19. Lansdell, M.I.; Hepworth, D.; Calabrese, A.; Brown, A.D.; Blagg, J.; Burring, D.J.; Wilson, P.; Fradet, D.; Brown, T.B.; Quinton, F.; et al. Discovery of a selective small-molecule melanocortin-4 receptor agonist with efficacy in a pilot study of sexual dysfunction in humans. *J. Med. Chem.* **2010**, *53*, 3183–3197. [CrossRef]
20. Todorovic, A.; Haskell-Luevano, C. A review of melanocortin receptor small molecule ligands. *Peptides* **2005**, *26*, 2026–2036. [CrossRef]
21. Ericson, M.D.; Lensing, C.J.; Fleming, K.A.; Schlasner, K.N.; Doering, S.R.; Haskell-Luevano, C. Bench-top to clinical therapies: A review of melanocortin ligands from 1954 to 2016. *Biochim. Biophys. Acta Mol. Basis Dis.* **2017**, *1863*, 2414–2435. [CrossRef] [PubMed]
22. White, W.B.; Myers, M.G.; Jordan, R.; Lucas, J. Usefulness of ambulatory blood pressure monitoring to assess the melanocortin receptor agonist bremelanotide. *J. Hypertens.* **2017**, *35*, 761–768. [CrossRef] [PubMed]
23. Clayton, A.H.; Althof, S.E.; Kingsberg, S.; DeRogatis, L.R.; Kroll, R.; Goldstein, I.; Kaminetsky, J.; Spana, C.; Lucas, J.; Jordan, R.; et al. Bremelanotide for female sexual dysfunctions in premenopausal women: A randomized, placebo-controlled dose-finding trial. *Womens Health (Lond)* **2016**, *12*, 325–337. [CrossRef] [PubMed]
24. Kievit, P.; Halem, H.; Marks, D.L.; Dong, J.Z.; Glavas, M.M.; Sinnayah, P.; Pranger, L.; Cowley, M.A.; Grove, K.L.; Culler, M.D. Chronic treatment with a melanocortin-4 receptor agonist causes weight loss, reduces insulin resistance, and improves cardiovascular function in diet-induced obese rhesus macaques. *Diabetes* **2013**, *62*, 490–497. [CrossRef] [PubMed]
25. Van der Ploeg, L.H.T. Rhythm Pharmaceuticals, Boston, MA, USA. Unpublished work. 2012.
26. Yang, L.K.; Tao, Y.X. Biased signaling at neural melanocortin receptors in regulation of energy homeostasis. *Biochim. Biophys. Acta Mol. Basis Dis.* **2017**, *1863*, 2486–2495. [CrossRef] [PubMed]
27. Büch, T.R.; Heling, D.; Damm, E.; Gudermann, T.; Breit, A. Pertussis toxin-sensitive signaling of melanocortin-4 receptors in hypothalamic GT1-7 cells defines agouti-related protein as a biased agonist. *J. Biol. Chem.* **2009**, *284*, 26411–26420. [CrossRef]
28. Kumar, K.G.; Sutton, G.M.; Dong, J.Z.; Roubert, P.; Plas, P.; Halem, H.A.; Culler, M.D.; Yang, H.; Dixit, V.D.; Butler, A.A. Analysis of the therapeutic functions of novel melanocortin receptor agonists in MC3R- and MC4R-deficient C57BL/6J mice. *Peptides* **2009**, *30*, 1892–1900. [CrossRef] [PubMed]
29. Shinyama, H.; Masuzaki, H.; Fang, H.; Flier, J.S. Regulation of melanocortin-4 receptor signaling: Agonist-mediated desensitization and internalization. *Endocrinology* **2003**, *144*, 1301–1314. [CrossRef]
30. Mayer, J.P.; Hsiung, H.M.; Flora, D.B.; Edwards, P.; Smith, D.P.; Zhang, X.Y.; Gadski, R.A.; Heiman, M.L.; Hertel, J.L.; Emmerson, P.J.; et al. Discovery of a beta-MSH-derived MC-4R selective agonist. *J. Med. Chem.* **2005**, *48*, 3095–3098. [CrossRef] [PubMed]
31. Nickolls, S.A.; Fleck, B.; Hoare, S.R.; Maki, R.A. Functional selectivity of melanocortin 4 receptor peptide and nonpeptide agonists: Evidence for ligand-specific conformational states. *J. Pharmacol. Exp. Ther.* **2005**, *313*, 1281–1288. [CrossRef]
32. Haskell-Luevano, C.; Monck, E.K. Agouti-related protein functions as an inverse agonist at a constitutively active brain melanocortin-4 receptor. *Regul. Pept.* **2001**, *99*, 1–7. [CrossRef]
33. Nijenhuis, W.A.; Oosterom, J.; Adan, R.A. AgRP(83-132) acts as an inverse agonist on the human melanocortin-4 receptor. *Mol. Endocrinol.* **2001**, *15*, 164–171. [CrossRef]
34. Molden, B.M.; Cooney, K.A.; Wes, T.K.; Van Der Ploeg, L.H.; Baldini, G. Temporal cAMP Signaling Selectivity by Natural and Synthetic MC4R Agonists. *Mol. Endocrinol.* **2015**, *29*, 1619–1633. [CrossRef]
35. Granell, S.; Molden, B.M.; Baldini, G. Exposure of MC4R to agonist in the endoplasmic reticulum stabilizes an active conformation of the receptor that does not desensitize. *Proc. Natl. Acad. Sci. USA* **2013**, *110*, E4733–E4742. [CrossRef]
36. Huang, H.; Wang, W.; Tao, Y.X. Pharmacological chaperones for the misfolded melanocortin-4 receptor associated with human obesity. *Biochim. Biophys. Acta Mol. Basis Dis.* **2017**, *1863*, 2496–2507. [CrossRef]
37. Gao, Z.; Lei, D.; Welch, J.; Le, K.; Lin, J.; Feng, S.; Duhl, D. Agonist-dependent internalization of the human melanocortin-4 receptors in human embryonic kidney 293 cells. *J. Pharm. Exp. Ther.* **2003**, *307*, 870–877. [CrossRef]

38. Cai, M.; Varga, E.V.; Stankova, M.; Mayorov, A.; Perry, J.W.; Yamamura, H.I.; Trivedi, D.; Hruby, V.J. Cell signaling and trafficking of human melanocortin receptors in real time using two-photon fluorescence and confocal laser microscopy: Differentiation of agonists and antagonists. *Chem. Biol. Drug Des.* **2006**, *68*, 183–193. [CrossRef]
39. Li, Y.Q.; Shrestha, Y.; Pandey, M.; Chen, M.; Kablan, A.; Gavrilova, O.; Offermanns, S.; Weinstein, L.S. G(q/11)α and G(s)α mediate distinct physiological responses to central melanocortins. *J. Clin. Investig.* **2016**, *126*, 40–49. [CrossRef]
40. Ghamari-Langroudi, M.; Digby, G.J.; Sebag, J.A.; Millhauser, G.L.; Palomino, R.; Matthews, R.; Gillyard, T.; Panaro, B.L.; Tough, I.R.; Cox, H.M.; Denton, J.S.; et al. G-protein-independent coupling of MC4R to Kir7.1 in hypothalamic neurons. *Nature* **2015**, *520*, 94–98. [CrossRef]
41. Vongs, A.; Lynn, N.M.; Rosenblum, C.I. Activation of MAP kinase by MC4-R through PI3 kinase. *Regul. Pept.* **2004**, *120*, 113–118. [CrossRef]
42. Kuo, J.J.; da Silva, A.A.; Hall, J.E. Hypothalamic melanocortin receptors and chronic regulation of arterial pressure and renal function. *Hypertension* **2003**, *41*, 768–774. [CrossRef]
43. Ni, X.-P.; Butler, A.A.; Cone, R.D.; Humphreys, M.H. Central receptors mediating the cardiovascular actions of melanocyte stimulating hormones. *J. Hypertension* **2006**, *24*, 2239–2246. [CrossRef]
44. Humphreys, M.H.; Ni, X.-P.; Pearce, D. Cardiovascular effects of melanocortins. *Eur. J. Pharmacol.* **2011**, *600*, 43–52. [CrossRef]
45. Hill, C.; Dunbar, J.C. The effects of acute and chronic alpha melanocyte stimulating hormone (alphaMSH) on cardiovascular dynamics in conscious rats. *Peptides* **2002**, *23*, 1625–1630. [CrossRef]
46. Matsumura, K.; Tsuchihashi, T.; Abe, I.; Iida, M. Central alpha-melanocyte-stimulating hormone acts at melanocortin-4 receptor to activate sympathetic nervous system in conscious rabbits. *Brain Res.* **2002**, *948*, 145–148. [CrossRef]
47. Nordheim, U.; Nicholson, J.R.; Dokladny, K.; Dunant, P.; Hofbauer, K.G. Cardiovascular responses to melanocortin 4-receptor stimulation in conscious unrestrained normotensive rats. *Peptides* **2006**, *27*, 438–443. [CrossRef]
48. Trivedi, P.; Jiang, M.; Tamvakopoulos, C.C.; Shen, X.; Yu, H.; Mock, S.; Fenyk-Melody, J.; Van der Ploeg, L.H.T.; Guan, X.M. Exploring the site of anorectic action of peripherally administered synthetic melanocortin peptide MT-II in rats. *Brain Res.* **2003**, *977*, 221–230. [CrossRef]
49. Lotta, L.A.; Mokrosin'ski, J.; de Oliveira, E.M.; Li, C.; Sharp, S.J.; Luan, J.; Brouwers, B.; Ayinampudi, V.; Bowker, N.; Kerrison, N.; et al. Human Gain-of-Function *MC4R* Variants. *Cell* **2019**, *177*, 597–607. [CrossRef] [PubMed]

molecules

MDPI

Review

Peptide Conjugates with Small Molecules Designed to Enhance Efficacy and Safety

Rongjun He [1,*], Brian Finan [1], John P. Mayer [2] and Richard D. DiMarchi [1,3,*]

1 Novo Nordisk Research Center, Indianapolis, IN 46241, USA; bfin@novonordisk.com
2 Department of Molecular, Developmental & Cell Biology, University of Colorado, Boulder, CO 80309, USA; John.Mayer@Colorado.edu
3 Department of Chemistry, Indiana University, Bloomington, IN 47405, USA
* Correspondence: rjhe@novonordisk.com (R.H.); rdimarch@indiana.edu (R.D.D.)

Academic Editors: Henry Mosberg, Tomi Sawyer and Carrie Haskell-Luevano
Received: 27 April 2019; Accepted: 12 May 2019; Published: 14 May 2019

check for updates

Abstract: Peptides constitute molecular diversity with unique molecular mechanisms of action that are proven indispensable in the management of many human diseases, but of only a mere fraction relative to more traditional small molecule-based medicines. The integration of these two therapeutic modalities offers the potential to enhance and broaden pharmacology while minimizing dose-dependent toxicology. This review summarizes numerous advances in drug design, synthesis and development that provide direction for next-generation research endeavors in this field. Medicinal studies in this area have largely focused upon the application of peptides to selectively enhance small molecule cytotoxicity to more effectively treat multiple oncologic diseases. To a lesser and steadily emerging extent peptides are being therapeutically employed to complement and diversify the pharmacology of small molecule drugs in diseases other than just cancer. No matter the disease, the purpose of the molecular integration remains constant and it is to achieve superior therapeutic outcomes with diminished adverse effects. We review linker technology and conjugation chemistries that have enabled integrated and targeted pharmacology with controlled release. Finally, we offer our perspective on opportunities and obstacles in the field.

Keywords: peptide; peptide-drug conjugate; mixed-mode pharmacology; GLP-1; GnRH; LHRH; chemical linker; cancer; diabetes; obesity; drug discovery

1. Introduction

Peptides represent a powerful class of medicine that currently serves multiple diseases and often constitutes indispensable, life-preserving pharmacology [1–4]. They often display exquisite affinity and specificity for a unique molecular target. This coupled with straightforward endogenous metabolism to constituent amino acids typically translates to high potency medicines, with minimal off-target adverse effects. Being of modest molecular size and certainly much smaller than most proteins enables the relationship of peptide structure to function to be rapidly interrogated by synthetic methods that have matured over the last fifty years [5–10]. These synthetic methods have also evolved to achieve success at a commercial scale which is a significant advantage as it enables molecular diversity that is not readily achieved in larger molecules, facilitates translation to clinical studies and yet often nicely integrates with biosynthetic approaches for larger production and reduced cost. Prominent examples include insulin and related analogs, glucagon-like peptide 1 agonists (GLP-1), somatostatins and many others [1–4,11–14]. Accordingly, peptide-based drug candidates much like proteins have recorded a higher success rate in commercial development relative to classical small molecules. Novo-Nordisk and Amgen, which have heavily focused on peptide and protein drugs, reported the highest clinical success rates relative to similarly-sized peer companies in 2016 [15]. Multiple factors, however, influence these results, such as disease selection, portfolio decision making and executive appetite for risk [16,17].

More than sixty peptide-based drugs are commercially marketed globally, with more than a hundred in various stages of commercial development and many, many more in preclinical research. Virtually all disease areas are touched at some level with endocrinology, cancer, infectious and cardiovascular diseases being most prevalent [1–4]. The global sales for peptide-based medicines in 2015 were in excess of fifty billion U.S. dollars and forecasted to reach seventy in 2019 [1]. Among these, insulin-related medicines are by far the largest given the global epidemic of maturity-onset diabetes [18]. There are many billion-dollar drugs and notably, the use of multiple GLP-1 agonists is accelerating rapidly [19]. It is clear that peptides fulfill a unique therapeutic need where traditional small molecules have not.

Similar to drug discovery directed at small molecules, peptide research has evolved in the direction of multimode pharmacology, [20–22] where single molecules activate multiple receptors in an additive and occasionally in a synergistic manner to achieve superior efficacy often at reduced dose [1–4,23–25]. This type of pharmacology is exemplified in purposefully integrated, dual agonism at amylin and calcitonin, GLP-1 and glucagon, or with gastric inhibitory peptide (GIP), and triple agonism at GLP-1, glucagon and GIP in treatment of the metabolic syndrome [26–35]. The sequence of these multi-action peptides largely derives from intermixing resides from each native hormone to achieve balanced, full agonism at the respective cognate receptors. It is the inherent structural similarity within these related receptors and their natural ligands that enables the discovery of chimeric peptides that can promiscuously bind more than once receptor with similar affinity. Consequently, there are limits to where this approach can be successfully applied as hormones of a more distant sequence will prove increasingly difficult, if not impossible to successfully integrate to a single common binding face. In those instances where the respective receptors are too distant to assemble a single ligand that can fulfill high-affinity binding more traditional approaches to functionate through chemical conjugation to heterodimeric and higher polymeric forms have been applied. This approach is commonly employed in antibody-based drug candidates where more than one receptor is blocked [36–38]. Although less elegant in their molecular design and resulting in appreciably increased molecular size, such polypeptide conjugates can similarly bestow the pharmacological benefits of peptides with a single hybridized binding site.

Conjugates of peptides and small molecules empower the virtues of peptide-based pharmacology with traditional medicinal chemistry [1–3,39–46]. The result is a macromolecule, and as such the biophysical character of the drug candidate and the resultant properties for patient use have paralleled what has been advanced in peptide and protein therapeutics. Consequently, the progression of this form of medicinal chemistry has evolved more from the large molecule side to embrace small molecules, than vice versa. In this review, we focus on peptide-drug conjugates that promote the integrated benefits of peptides and smaller, non-peptide pharmacophores. The presentation is intended to supplement reviews focusing exclusively on peptide-based therapeutics [1–3] and complement those that specifically emphasize applications in cancer [40,41]. The reader is also directed to other reviews with an emphasis on physiochemical properties of peptide-drug conjugates [42] and those predominantly employed for optimizing pharmacokinetic performance [43]. Finally, protein-based drug conjugates other than antibodies are not reviewed but can be found elsewhere [44], and similarly so conjugates for diagnostic purposes with imagining agents or organometallic entities [45,46]. We have selectively cited prominent examples of peptide-drug conjugates as representatives of the class to offer our perspective in molecular design, selection of covalent linkers, and other aspects that influence performance.

2. Why Peptide-Drug Conjugates?

Peptide-based therapeutics historically represented a small fraction of conventional pharmaceutical discovery research where the emphasis has been on small molecules that prioritized the convenience in oral administration nearly as much as the efficacy of the drug. This has resulted in an excessive investment on a finite number of high-profile drug targets that have constrained the broader exploration of human pathology [47,48]. Peptides as a molecular class are well recognized to often provide unprecedented efficacy and the attempts to reduce them to structural mimetics that could be orally administered have largely failed, despite sizable investment to do so. The advent of rDNA-based protein drugs, and in particular antibodies have demonstrated the importance of drug efficacy, especially when applied to life-altering diseases to dominate the convenience of oral administration. Tangential to the popularity of protein-based therapeutics has been increased attention for peptide therapeutics. As a result, notable successes such as parathyroid hormone (PTH), GLP-1, GLP-2 agonists complement the historical importance of such peptides as insulin, gonadotropin-releasing hormone, somatostatin, calcitonin and numerous other less prominent entities such as glucagon, vasopressin and oxytocin. Nonetheless, there is a general sense within the peptide community of there being too few validated drug targets. The integration of peptides with traditional small molecules provides a venue to advance novel macromolecular therapeutics that provide supplemental efficacy but also addresses intracellular drug targets as it has constituted a central limitation in peptide and protein-based pharmacology.

Small molecule drug candidates have historically recorded a higher attrition rate in clinical development, which partially results from suboptimal physicochemical properties [16,17,49]. Conjugation to peptides is an approach to address poor aqueous solubility, untimely metabolism and potentially facilitate cell permeability. It has provided targeted delivery of small molecules to diseased tissue to enhance local drug concentration, and mitigate toxic effects arising from systemic exposure and accumulation in non-diseased tissues [1–4,50,51]. Drug-Drug Interactions (DDI) constitute a common cause of adverse drug reactions that undermines efficacy and with the increased use of multiple drugs in the treatment of complex diseases has emerged as something of elevated importance in drug development [52]. Peptide-drug conjugates by design can minimize DDI by lessening accumulation in tissues where inappropriate biological action is adversely increasing pharmacology arising from other drugs. In this regard, peptide-drug conjugates are largely confined to the extracellular space and as such have been reported to minimize inappropriate hepatic metabolism [2,51].

The origin in the design of molecular conjugates can be traced as far back as a century ago when the German physician-scientist Paul Ehrlich coined the term 'magic bullet' in characterizing a cytotoxic drug to be selectively delivered to a tumor via a targeting agent [53,54]. It was in the second half of the last century when several examples were reported [55–58], with the first instance employing methotrexate (MTX) conjugation to an antibody directed against leukemia cells [55]. The first clinical trial of such an antibody-directed cytotoxic agent (ADC) was reported in 1983 [59], in which an anti-carcinoembryonic antigen (CEA) antibody directed a vinca-alkaloid in treatment of advanced stage cancer. Nearly two decades later as we entered this century the first ADC was FDA-approved and named gemtuzumab ozogamicin [60]. With a commercial trade name of Mylotarg, this chemical conjugate consists of an anti-CD33 antibody linked with calicheamicin, a drug of high systemic toxicity for the treatment of acute myeloid leukemia (AML). The extended period from Paul Ehrlich's time to first drug registration of an ADC was to an appreciable degree due to the relative immaturity of antibody-based therapeutics, until the advent of the last decade of the twentieth century [61]. The first ADC employed polyclonal antibodies with cytotoxic agents non-covalently associated, with human sequence antibodies emerging, with maturation of rDNA-based expression [61]. Subsequent to Mylotarg, brentuximab vedotin (Adcetris) received regulatory approval in 2011 for treatment of Hodgkin lymphoma and systemic anaplastic large cell lymphoma [62,63], and trastuzumab emtansine (Kadcyla) was similarly approved in 2013 for the treatment of HER2-positive metastatic breast cancer [61,64]. Mylotarg was subsequently withdrawn from distribution in 2010 for safety concerns and the absence of proven clinical benefit in a follow-up clinical trial [65]. It was successfully reintroduced as Besponsa in 2017 for treatment of AML and in addition treatment of relapsed or refractory acute lymphoblastic leukemia (ALL) [66]. Currently, there are more than one hundred registered clinical studies that employ some form of ADC [67].

Despite the initial clinical successes, multiple challenges exist in the development of next-generation ADCs. Issues pertaining to the continued identification and validation of disease-specific target antigens remain a central biological challenge to the approach. Advances in site-specific chemical conjugation, often employing novel orthogonal conjugation chemistries with linkers designed for improved therapeutic index continue to provide more homogenous drug candidates. The large molecular size of antibodies has raised questions pertaining to efficient distribution and delivery to disease tissues with subsequent cellular transport. In these last domains, peptide conjugates given their inherently smaller size possess an inherent advantage in comparison to antibodies. The increased molecular diversity and accuracy in chemical synthesis of peptides provide structural precision and optimization that exceeds what is possible with antibodies [60–63,68,69]. As such medicinal chemistry has been employed to enhance potency, drug distribution, pharmacokinetics and metabolism. This approach also simplifies commercial synthesis and compliance with regulatory demands for registration and subsequent requirements in drug manufacture [70]. Peptide-based drug conjugates bind to cell surface targets with high-affinity that parallels that of antibodies and recognize a broad spectrum of biological targets, most notably G protein-coupled receptors (GPCRs), receptor tyrosine kinases (RTKs), and integrins. Being of significantly reduced molecular size relative to ADCs, there is potential for more efficient delivery to sequestered-targets leading to enhanced efficacy, and reduced immunogenicity [1,2]. It should be noted that peptide-drug conjugates are pharmacokinetically distinct from antibodies with a much-reduced circulation time. This can be of particular advantage in the delivery of highly toxic reagents where extended exposure is unwarranted. However, it initially proved a disadvantage as treatment of solid tumors more often required sustained pharmacokinetics, of the type inherent to antibodies. The maturation in chemical approaches to alter and even tailor time-action of peptides with chemical lipidation, pegylation and a host of other technologies has largely eliminated this difference relative to antibodies. While the comparisons will continue, it is less a question of which molecular platform is superior than celebrating diversity as a tool to be employed in achieving superior disease outcomes, conveniently administered at a suitable financial cost.

3. Approved Peptide-Drug Conjugates

Somatostatin (growth hormone-inhibiting hormone, GHIH) is a peptide produced by paracrine cells in the gastrointestinal tract, pancreatic delta cells, and hypothalamic neurons to control multiple endocrine functions [71,72]. It inhibits secretion of growth hormone, thyroid stimulating hormone, and other pituitary-derived hormones, as well as hormone secretion from pancreatic and gastrointestinal cells. Somatostatin exhibits many direct and indirect effects to suppress growth and differentiation in several different cancer cells. Somatostatin analogs such as Octreotide, Lanreotide, and Pasireotide are clinically used in the treatment of acromegaly, as well as hormone-dependent tumors such as pancreatic, and vasoactive intestinal peptide-secreting tumors [72,73]. Somatostatin analogs have also been clinically studied in breast, lung, prostate and gastrointestinal cancers [73].

Somatostatin biologically functions through a family of related receptors in the GPCR superfamily [71]. There are five somatostatin receptors subtypes (SSTR1-5) that are differentially expressed in brain cortex, pituitary, adrenals, pancreas, heart, and gastrointestinal tract [72,74]. The SSTR2 is reported to be overexpressed in many tumors and undergoes ligand-induced internalization. This latter property renders SSTR2 a potential target for intracellularly delivering cytotoxic and other growth suppressive agents to tumor cells [71]. Various somatostatin analogs have been conjugated to radioactive chemotherapeutic agents to induce tumor death by a process termed peptide receptor radionuclide therapy (PRRT) [75,76]. Targeted radioisotope therapy complements the inherent anticancer pharmacology of somatostatin, while simultaneously reducing the systemic radioactive toxicity. Radioactive isotopes conjugated to somatostatin include beta-emitter nuclide 90Y, gamma-emitter 111In, beta and gamma emitter 177Lu, and other more commonly employed nuclear medicines [75,76]. PRRT inhibits tumor progression [77–79], and recently a 177Lu Dotatate conjugate was approved as for treatment of gastroenteropancreatic neuroendocrine tumors [80,81]. 177Lu as a beta-emitter exhibits maximal tissue penetration less than 2 mm, which renders it a good irradiation choice for small tumors. The Lutetium isotope has a reasonable physical half-life of 6.7 days, which makes it favorable from a therapeutic and safety perspective as 99% of the drug is eliminated within two weeks [82–84]. The 177Lu is chelated to octreotide, a somatostatin analog through a DOTA high-affinity binder that is covalently linked to the hormone (Figure 1) [76,85]. The peptide exhibits high potency (IC_{50}: 1.5 nM) at SSTR2 with greater than a hundredfold selectivity over SSTR5 (IC_{50}: 547 nM) and SSTR3 (IC_{50}: >1000 nM) [86]. In a single-arm clinical trial in 310 patients with gastroenteropancreatic cancer, 177Lu-Dotatate treatment provided partial tumor remissions in 28% of patients and complete remissions in 2%. The median progression-free survival was 33 months [87]. In a recent phase 3 trial in progressing, advanced midgut neuroendocrine tumors 177Lu-Dotatate treatment resulted in a progression-free survival rate of 65.2% versus 10.8% at twenty months relative to continuing somatostatin treatment alone [88]. The 177Lu-Dotatate exhibited limited hemato-toxicity, but without renal toxicity. These results in advanced refractory cancer demonstrate the much-improved therapeutic efficacy and safety of the peptide-drug conjugate in comparison to somatostatin or radioisotope therapy alone.

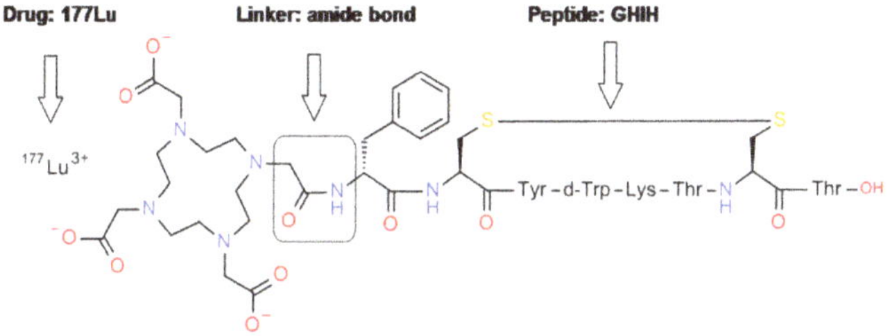

Figure 1. Chemical structure of growth hormone-inhibiting hormone (GHIH)-177Lu conjugate (177Lu-Dotatate).

4. Representative Peptide-Drug Conjugates in Clinical Development

4.1. GnRH-Doxorubicin Conjugate

Gonadotropin-releasing hormone (GnRH or LHRH) is a hypothalamic peptide hormone that binds to receptors in the anterior pituitary to stimulate the release of the follicle-stimulation hormone and luteinizing hormone, two hormones seminal to reproduction [89,90]. GnRH also stimulates gonadotropin release and subsequent steroid hormone release, which are purported stimulants to many forms of cancer [91,92]. Continuous GnRH receptor activation causes down-regulation and desensitization to reduce endogenous steroid hormone biosynthesis and release [93]. Consequently, GnRH super-agonists have been successfully employed in hormone-dependent cancers in what is termed androgen deprivation therapy (ADT) [92,94].

The GnRH receptor is expressed in many endocrine cancers, including breast, ovarian, endometrial, and prostate tumors. Its presence provides the means to target oncolytic drugs to these cancer cells to supplement the clinical benefits currently achieved with ADT alone [90,95]. Zoptarelin Doxorubicin (AN-152, AEZS-108, Zoptrex^{TM}) is a peptide-drug conjugate composed of a GnRH analog and doxorubicin through an ester bond with a glutaric acid spacer (Figure 2) [96]. The conjugate proved more effective than doxorubicin in inhibiting cell proliferation in GnRH receptor positive cancer cell lines [96]. It also was more potent than either agent alone in several xenograft mouse tumor models [97]. These results validate the virtue of targeted, complementary GnRH and doxorubicin pharmacology. Phase 1 studies in endometrial, ovarian and prostate cancer established Zoptarelin Doxorubicin's safety, pharmacokinetics, and maximum tolerated dose [98–100]. In several phase 2 studies the drug-conjugate exhibited promising clinical activity with low systemic toxicity in castration and taxane-resistant prostate cancer [101], advanced or recurrent endometrial cancer [102], and platinum refractory ovarian cancer [103]. In a recent large phase 3 registration trial in advanced endometrial cancer Zoptarelin

Doxorubicin disappointedly failed to improve median overall survival, or progression-free survival when compared to standard doxorubicin therapy [104]. The basis of the failure is unknown but given that doxorubicin at highest dose did not significantly improve patient survival there is a suspicion that deficiencies specific to doxorubicin might be the primary cause, as opposed to something inherent to the drug-conjugate.

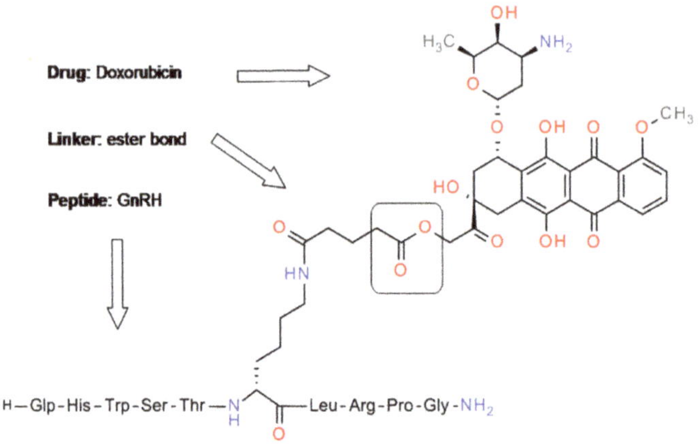

Figure 2. Chemical structure of gonadotropin-releasing hormone (GnRH) or luteinizing hormone-releasing hormone (LHRH)-doxorubicin conjugate (Zoptarelin Doxorubicin, AN-152, AEZS-108).

4.2. *Angiopep-2-Paxlitaxel Conjugate*

Paclitaxel is a potent oncolytic drug that has been widely used in several different cancers [105,106]. However, its low blood–brain barrier (BBB) permeability coupled with multidrug resistance efflux by P-glycoprotein pump (P-gp) has resulted in limited activity in primary and metastatic brain tumors. Angiopep-2 is a peptide that binds the low-density lipoprotein receptor-related protein 1 (LPR1) and it is upregulated in many tumors, including glioma [107,108]. ANG1005 (also named GRN1005) (Figure 3) is a drug conjugate composed of angiopep-2 and paclitaxel designed to increase brain transport through LPR1 mediated transcytosis [109]. The ANG1005 conjugate includes as many as three molar equivalents of paclitaxel relative to a peptide with intent to maximally increase cytotoxic drug concentration [110,111]. ANG1005 demonstrated excellent cytotoxicity against glioblastoma, lung and ovarian cancer cells. Furthermore, ANG1005 was effectively transported to the brain in an LPR1-dependent manner [112] and appeared unaffected by P-gp efflux that would otherwise impair therapeutic efficacy. The efficacy was established through in vivo studies where ANG1005 significantly prolonged survival in mice bearing xenografted glioblastoma or lung carcinoma cells [109]. In phase 1 clinical trials in recurrent malignant glioma tumors [110,111], ANG1005 exhibited plasma half-life of 3.6 h and was well tolerated with a toxicity similar to paclitaxel. Importantly, ANG1005 is designed to cross the BBB to deliver therapeutic concentrations of paclitaxel to the tumor site. A phase 2 study in breast cancer patients with brain metastases demonstrated in a subpopulation of patients a favorable median survival time of eight months as compared to four with standard treatment achieved with other forms of therapy, or two months without treatment [113]. Several additional phase 2 studies with ANG1005 have completed, and include recurrent high-grade glioma, non-small cell lung and brain metastases [114]. Currently, ANG1005 has been successfully registered as an orphan drug for the treatment of multiform glioblastoma [115], and a phase 3 clinical trial with ANG1005 against leptomeningeal disease from breast cancer is reported to be in recruitment phase [116].

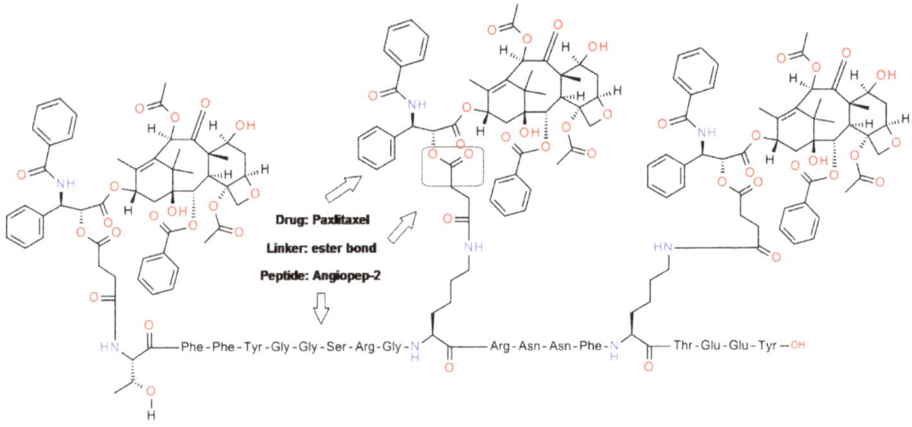

Figure 3. Chemical structure of angiopep-2-paxlitaxel conjugate (ANG1005, GRN1005).

4.3. Tetrapeptide-Thapsigargin Conjugate

Thapsigargin is a highly potent cytotoxic natural product that induces apoptosis in mammalian cells by binding the sarco/endoplasmic reticulum calcium ATPase (SERCA) to disrupt the Ca^{2+} gradient across cytosolic and reticulum compartments [117]. Unlike other cytotoxic agents which inhibit rapidly proliferating cells, thapsigargin kills in a less specific manner given its mechanism, and this has undermined its potential as a chemotherapeutic agent. Chemical conjugation of thapsigargin to a tetrapeptide yields a charged conjugate termed G202 (Mipsagargin) (Figure 4) that is unable to cross the cell membrane to reach SERCA [118–120]. The tetrapeptide is a substrate of the membrane-bound proteolytic enzyme prostate-specific membrane antigen (PSMA), which is overexpressed in prostate cancer and other tumors, but much less so in normal tissues [121,122]. The tetrapeptide is processed by PSMA to provide an analog that is now cell permeable, cytotoxic, and extracellularly concentrated adjacent to cancerous prostate cells [118–120]. By in vitro assessment, G202 was reported to be 57-fold more potent in cell proliferation assays in human prostate cancer cells expressing PMSA, implying PSMA-mediated cytotoxicity [118,119]. Subsequent in vivo studies demonstrated potent anti-tumor activity in mouse xenograft models with human prostate and breast cancer cells, and importantly with much reduced systemic toxicity [118,119]. A Phase 1 clinical trial was completed in patients with refractory, advanced or metastatic solid tumors. G202 was found to be well tolerated in patients at doses up to 88 mg/m^2 (or 2.4 mg/kg) and determined to have a favorable pharmacokinetic profile with a terminal half-life of 21 h, and distribution equivalent to plasma volume [123]. Several Phase 2 clinical trials have completed in prostate cancer, renal cell carcinoma, hepatocellular carcinoma, and glioblastoma but clinical results have not yet been reported [124].

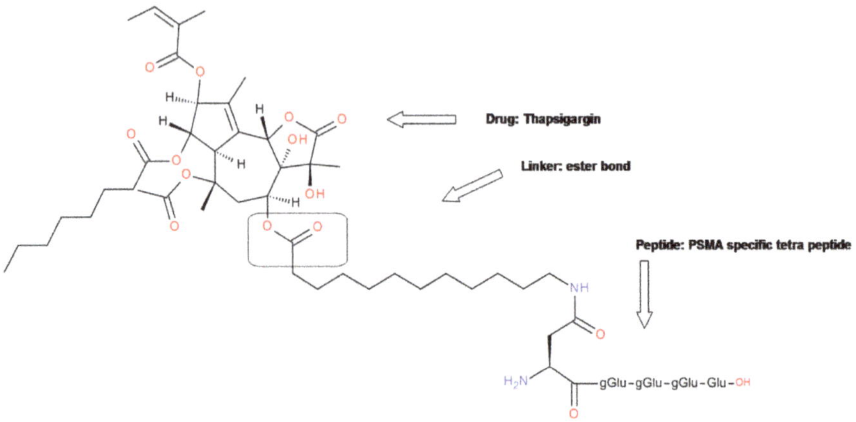

Figure 4. Chemical structure of tetrapeptide-thapsigargin conjugate G202 (Mipsagargin).

4.4. Miscellaneous Peptide-Drug Conjugates

Doxorubicin has been chemically conjugated to a number of other peptides, including cell penetrating peptides (CPP) [125,126], tumor homing peptide Lyp-1 [127], RGD peptides [40], somatostatin [128–130], and bombesin/gastrin-releasing peptide (BN/GRP) [128,131,132], and broadly studied. BIM-23A760, a conjugate of somatostatin and dopamine is in clinical stage development for the treatment of pituitary adenomas [133–135]. A list of peptide-drug conjugates that have progressed into clinical development is summarized in Table 1. Given the sizable unmet medical need in many cancers, it has been the dominant disease for exploring the potential for selectively delivering toxic substances. Nonetheless, the potential for targeted therapy and synergistic efficacy between peptides and small molecules is clear and extends to forms of pharmacology beyond cytotoxicity. Recent applications of peptide-drug conjugates are emerging in other diseases areas, specifically cardiometabolic diseases where multi-mode pharmacology has been a traditional hallmark for successful disease management.

Table 1. Peptide-drug conjugates in various clinical development stages.

Generic Name	Indication	Peptide	Drug	Linker	Mechanism	Status	Reference
Lu177-dotatate	Dastroenteropancreatic neuroendocrine tumors	Somatostatin analogue Octreotide	Radio therapeutic agent Lu177	Amide (Lu177 chelating to metalchelating molecule DOTA)	Somatostatin receptor 2 SSTR2 mediated delivery of nucleotide 177Lu	Approved by FDA and EMA	[76,85–99]
[111In-DTPA-D-Phe1]-octreotide	Imaging/diagnostic	Somatostatin analogue Octreotide	Radio therapeutic agent 111In	Amide (111In chelating to metalchelating molecule DOTA)	Somatostatin receptor 2 SSTR2 mediated tumor scintigraphic imaging	Phase 1 completed	[136,137]
Zoptarelin Doxorubicin, AN-152, AEZS-108	Endometrial cancer Ovarian cancer	GnRH/LHRH	Doxorubicin	Ester	GnRH mediated delivery of doxorubicin to cancer cells	Phase 3 completed	[96,98–103]
ANG1005 GRN1005	Metastases brain cancer	Angiopep-2	Paclitaxel	Ester	Low-density lipoprotein receptor-related protein 1 (LPR1) mediated brain uptake	Orphan drug for glioblastoma multiform, Several phase 2 ongoing	[109–116]
Mipsagargin G202	Various Cancer	Tetrapeptide	Thapsigargin	Ester	Extracellularly tumor-activated prodrug of Thapsigargin	Phase 2 completed	[118–120,123]
Paclitaxel poliglumex CT2103	Various cancer	Poliglumex	Paclitaxel	Ester	Enhanced permeability of tumor vasculature and lack of lymphatic drainage prolonged tumor exposure to the active drug while minimizing systemic exposure	Phase 3 completed	[138–142]
EP-100	Cancer	GnRH/LHRH	CLIP71	Amide	GnRH receptor-mediated cancer cell membrane lysis	Phase 2 completed	[143–145]
BIM-23A760	Pituitary adenomas	Somatostatin	Dopamine	Amide/Thioether	Somatostatin/dopaminethe dual action inhibit the expression/secretion of several pituitary hormones (especially GH/PRL)	Phase 2 terminated	[133–135]
CGC 1072	Psoriasis	Heptaarginine	Cyclosporin A	Ester	CPP mediated topical delivery and inhibition of inflammation	Phase 2, discontinued	[146,147]

Table 1. *Cont.*

Generic Name	Indication	Peptide	Drug	Linker	Mechanism	Status	Reference
KAI-1455	Ischemic organ injury	TAT47-57	εPKC activator	Disulfide	CPP mediated εPKC activator delivery	Phase 1	[148]
KAI-1678	Neuropathic and inflammatory pain	TAT47-57	δ-Protein kinase C inhibitor peptide	Disulfide	CPP mediated εPKC inhibitor delivery	Phase 2 completed	[149–151]
KAI-9803	Myocardial infarction & Cardiovascular disease	TAT47-57	δ-Protein kinase C inhibitor peptide	Disulfide	CPP mediated εPKC inhibitor delivery to reduce the injury to myocardial and endothelial cells during a heart attack	Phase 2 completed	[152–154]
XG-102	Post-cataract surgery, intraocular inflammation and Pain	Tat48-57	31-mer peptide JNK inhibitor	Disulfide	CPP mediated JNK inhibitor delivery to reduce pain and inflammation upon cataract surgery	Phase 3 completed	[155–158]
DTS-108	Cancer	DPV1047 Vectocell peptide	SN38	Ester	CPP DPV1047 mediated delivery of chemotherapeutic drug SN38	Phase 1 completed	[159,160]
DTS-201	Cancer	Tetra peptide	Doxorubicin	Amide	Extracellularly tumor-activated prodrug of doxorubicin	Phase 2 completed	[161–163]
BT-1718	Cancer	Bicyclic peptide	Maytansinoid	Disulfide	Membrane type 1-matrixmetalloprotease mediated toxin delivery	Phase 1	[164]
177Lu- PSMA-617	Cancer	Glutamate-urea-lysine	Radio therapeutic agent Lu177	Amide (Lu177 chelating to metalchelating molecule DOTA)	Prostate-specific membrane antigen (PSMA) mediated delivery of nucleotide 177Lu	Phase 3	[165]

5. Representative Peptide-Drug Conjugates in Preclinical Space

5.1. GLP-1-Estrogen Conjugate

Estrogens are a group of steroid hormones which are commonly used in contraception and hormone replacement therapy. Estrogens also have notable beneficial effects on insulin signaling, glucose production, appetite, and energy expenditure to promote their potential use in the treatment of diabetes, obesity, and associated metabolic diseases [166–169]. However, the chronic use of estrogens has been complicated by oncogenic propensity in gynecological tissues and the increased risk for cardiovascular diseases (CVD) [170]. It has been suggested that tissue-targeted estrogens that selectively function in liver, adipose, pancreas, hypothalamus, but not in ovaries, uterus, and breast could prove efficacious and safe [171,172]. This has long been a priority in the search for small molecule selective estrogen receptor modulators [173,174].

The prospect of using a peptide hormone to target and supplement estrogen pharmacology was advanced by Finan et al. [175]. GLP-1 agonists have emerged as powerful therapy in the treatment of type 2 diabetes, obesity with proven CV benefits. It exerts its effects at specific receptors enriched in the endocrine pancreas and hypothalamic control centers of metabolism [176,177]. A GLP-1 estrogen conjugate formed by an ether link between 17β-estradiol and a lysine side chain amine at position 40 of GLP-1 was synthesized and evaluated in vitro and in vivo (Figure 5) [175]. This conjugate was fully active at the GLP-1 receptor in cell-based assays, and proteolytically stable in human plasma under physiological conditions for at least 120 h, reducing the prospect for premature plasma release. The conjugate demonstrated additive metabolic benefits of GLP-1 and estrogen to reverse obesity, hyperglycemia, and dyslipidemia in diet-induced obese (DIO) mice. Importantly there was no sign of estrogen associated gynecological toxicity or oncogenicity in the conjugate relative to what was observed in unstable conjugates that released systemically acting estrogen [175]. The anorexigenic effects of GLP-1 results from central action and the conjugate delivered estrogenic action to neurons in the dorsal raphe nuclei in female mice and suppressed binge-like eating behavior [178]. Further, it can activate both GLP-1 and estrogen receptors in the supra-mammillary nucleus in rats, resulting in superior effects on food intake and reward, to reduce body weight [179]. Moreover, the conjugate improves insulin sensitivity and glucose homeostasis in non-diabetic mice [180], attenuates hyperphagia and protects beta cell health in New Zealand Obese mice [181]. All these benefits were observed to be much superior to what GLP-1 alone or an untargeted combination provided. These studies demonstrate the enhanced therapeutic efficacy and safety of a GLP-1-estrogen conjugate, which justifies translational study in clinical diabetes and obesity. Similarly, a GLP-1-dexamethasone conjugate was also recently synthesized [182], and its combined therapeutic benefits characterized in metabolically compromised mice. Such a conjugate delivered potent effects in obese mice to lower body weight, improve glucose tolerance, and enhance insulin sensitivity with a reduction in hypothalamic and systemic inflammation. This conjugate was devoid of the adverse effects on glucose handling, bone and body weight typified by chronic systemic action of dexamethasone.

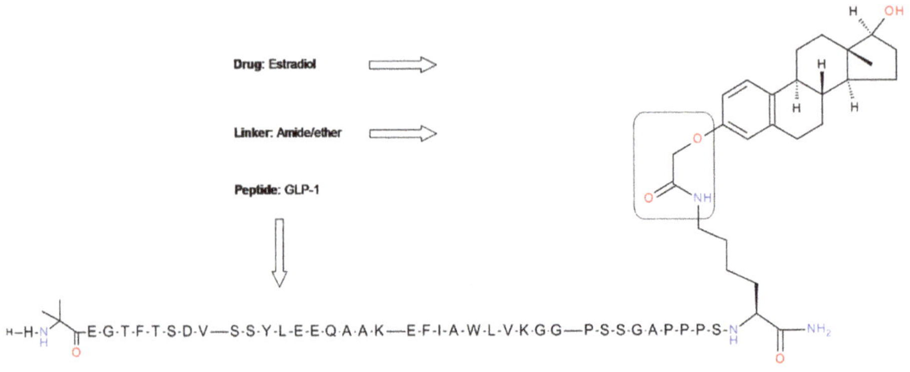

Figure 5. Chemical structure of GLP-1-estradiol conjugate.

5.2. Glucagon-T3 Conjugate

Thyroid hormones are iodinated tyrosine-based amino acids produced by the thyroid gland and are widely prescribed for the treatment of thyroid hormone deficiency [183]. Thyroid hormones have profound effects on metabolism, increasing energy expenditure, fat oxidation, and cholesterol metabolism via multiple pathways to promote therapeutic potential in metabolic diseases [184,185]. However, like estrogens, thyroid hormones are associated with many adverse effects including increased heart rate, muscle wasting, and reduced bone density [186]. Liver-targeted thyromimetics have revealed that it is possible to impact hepatic lipids and atherogenic lipoproteins without the associated adverse effects [187]. Therefore, targeting thyroid hormone action to the liver and adipose tissues and away from the cardiovascular system might also constitute a viable approach to safely harness the metabolic benefits. Glucagon is a hormone well recognized as a counter-regulatory hormone to insulin in its hepatic action to stimulate glucose production. Less well appreciated are the other attributes of glucagon pharmacology which includes body weight lowering, lipid-lowering and cardiovascular protection [188]. These effects derive from the direct and indirect hepatic action of glucagon to promote lipolysis and thermogenesis. It was envisioned that conjugation of thyroid hormone and glucagon could complement one another in improving body weight while mitigating the ability of thyroid hormone to elevate plasma cholesterol [189].

A chemical conjugate of glucagon and the most bioactive form of thyroid hormone, 3,3,5-triiodothyronine (T3), was synthesized and biologically characterized (Figure 6) [189]. The conjugate has a DPP4 resistant d-serine at the second amino acid residue, a solubility enhancing eleven amino acid extension sequence at the C-terminus, and a gamma glutamic acid (gGlu) spacer linking the C-terminal lysine side chain amine and the carboxylate of T3. The conjugate preserved full glucagon in vitro potency at its receptor (EC_{50}: 50 pM). The conjugate demonstrated dramatic metabolic benefits such as body weight lowering via increased energy expenditure, improved plasma cholesterol and triglyceride management, and much reduced hepatic liver stores in a mouse model of NASH [189]. The T3 was documented to be enriched in the liver, but not in pancreas or heart where glucagon receptor expression is less prominent. Analogous experiments in glucagon receptor knockout mice, as well as employment of peptide-conjugates devoid of one or the other hormonal activity, demonstrated that the metabolic benefits were the result of glucagon pharmacology and its targeting of thyroid hormone activity predominantly to the liver. Importantly, concurrent T3 activity counteracted the adverse diabetogenic effects of glucagon while glucagon lessened T3 elevation of cholesterol and its hepatic-targeting eliminated any apparent adverse cardiovascular or bone effects. Hence, pairing glucagon and thyroid hormones as a peptide-drug conjugate provides efficacious management of multiple elements in the metabolic syndrome, including hyperglycemia, obesity, fatty liver disease, and atherosclerosis.

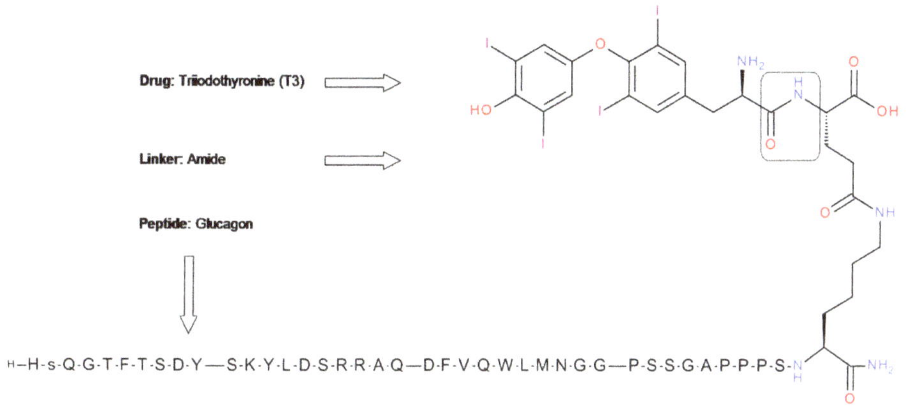

Figure 6. Chemical structure of glucagon-T3 conjugate.

5.3. Knotting Peptide Gemcitabine Conjugate

Integrins are a class of cell adhesion transmembrane receptors that regulate cell growth and function and are associated with several diseases including cancer, infection, and autoimmune diseases [190]. Integrin overexpression is linked to tumor proliferation and migration, which promotes disease progression and reduced patient survival [191,192]. Therefore, integrin antagonists are being clinically developed as therapeutics against cancer [193]. Integrins also provide opportunities for targeted peptide-drug conjugates. Several integrin targeting peptides were conjugated to cytotoxic agents for targeted tumor delivery. These include an RGD-doxorubicin conjugate, an RGD-Pt(iv) complex conjugate, and recently an integrin targeting knottin peptide gemcitabine conjugate [39,40,50,194]. Gemcitabine is a nucleoside based chemotherapeutic agent that blocks DNA replication and is used in the treatment of multiple cancers [195,196]. Like many other cancer drugs, gemcitabine is unrestricted in its action and can kill normal cells. To selectively target tumor cells, gemcitabine was conjugated to an integrin binding knottin peptide named ecballium elaterium trypsin inhibitor (EETI)-2.5Z. It has three intramolecular disulfide bonds to confer high thermal and proteolytic stability (Figure 7) [194]. EETI-2.5Z has low nanomolar binding affinity at integrins expressed on tumor cells, and conjugation with gemcitabine did not measurably affect its activity. Among various chemical conjugates that included an ester, carbamate, amide, and cathepsin B cleavable Val-Ala-PABC linkers, the EETI-2.5Z-Val-Ala-PABC-gemcitabine was observed to be highly stable in cell culture, with minimal premature drug release. More importantly, this conjugate exhibited very potent growth inhibition (ED_{50} of 1–10 nM) against a variety of cancer cells, including glioblastoma, breast, ovarian, and pancreatic cancer cells. The growth inhibition was abolished by the addition of excess unconjugated EETI-2.5Z, suggesting integrin-mediated internalization of gemcitabine pharmacology. PANC-1 pancreatic cancer cells have very high resistance to gemcitabine because of the diminished nucleoside transporter activity in these cells. Nonetheless, EETI-2.5Z-Val-Ala-PABC- gemcitabine was able to overcome the resistance and exhibited a 25-fold enhanced inhibitory activity relative to that of gemcitabine. Hence this peptide-drug conjugate further validated integrin as a therapeutic target for cancer and confirmed that peptides can successfully serve as an alternative to antibody targeted drug delivery. Of course, further preclinical animal studies and eventually human studies must be completed to prove its therapeutic efficacy and safety. It is noteworthy that gemcitabine has also been conjugated to a GnRH agonist [197], similar to the conjugate of GnRH with doxorubicin as discussed previously.

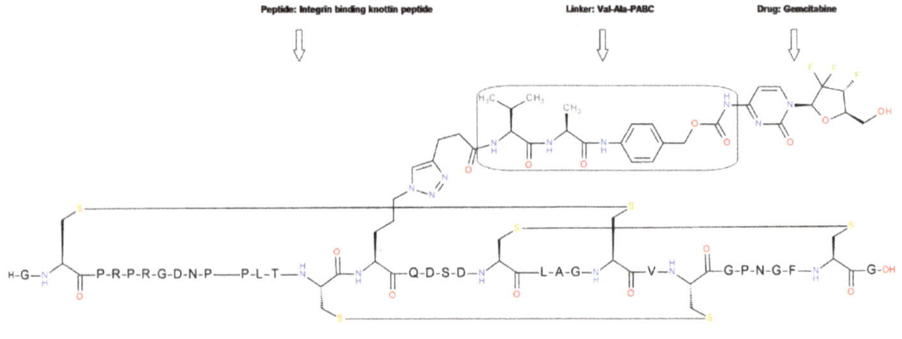

Figure 7. Chemical structure of knotting peptide ecballium elaterium trypsin inhibitor (EETI)-2.5Z-gemcitabine conjugate.

6. Linker and Conjugation Chemistry

The linker is a critical part of a peptide-drug conjugate that integrates the peptide and small molecule medicinal agents. The linker in concert with the peptide and the drug acts to maintain structural integrity during plasma circulation for a sufficient time and preventing premature release of the drug that might result in off-target adverse effects. Nonetheless, the linker should efficiently and specifically release the drug once tissue-targeted to enable a pharmacological effect. Linker technology has largely matured in the neighboring field of ADCs [198–200], where esters, amides, hydrazones, disulfides, and cathepsin B cleavable dipeptides have emerged as the preferred choices (Figure 8). This work has resulted in the development of three marketed drugs (Mylotarg, Adcetris, and Kadcyla), and a score of ADCs currently in clinical assessment [61,68,69,201–204]. These linkers and others have been extensively reviewed elsewhere as referenced. Briefly, hydrazones are relatively stable in plasma, but readily cleaved under acidic conditions, including endosomes and lysosomes where pH resides between 4.5–6.0. Ester bonds are widely used for conjugating drugs to peptides given their relatively straightforward synthesis and well-characterized cleavage by esterases, or under acidic conditions [198–200]. Carbamates perform similar to esters with comparable cleavage mechanisms, but typically with somewhat enhanced chemical and plasma stability. Although esters do not provide high plasma stability, it is still possible to successfully target oncolytic agents. If the goal is to develop a drug candidate of extended duration where the therapeutic index is appreciably increased, an amide bond may be preferable given the much-enhanced chemical and enzymatic plasma stability. Amide bonds are typically processed in lysosomes by multiple proteases to release the conjugated small molecules in a biologically active form [26,120,175]. If cleavage is not observed, dipeptide linkers such as Val-Cit and related dipeptides should be considered, as these can be cleaved by intracellular cathepsin B and other proteases [205]. A recent advance in peptide-based linkers combines Val-Cit with tertiary and heteroaryl amines to achieve traceless release [206]. This overcomes the challenges to employ tertiary amine bioactive molecules as payloads. The tripeptide linker Glu-Val-Cit was reported to further enhance stability and efficacy in mice when compared to the dipeptide linker Val-Cit [207]. It is known that Val-Cit linker, although stable in human plasma, is unstable in mouse plasma due to the cleavage by extracellular carboxylesterases, which causes translational inconsistency when comparing clinical and preclinical data. Thus, the amide bond seems to confer suitable chemical and plasma stability. Another enzyme cleavable linker is the β-glucuronide-based linker such as glucuronide-MABC, this linker offers benefits of high aqueous solubility, serum stability, and facile drug release. The cleavage is promoted by β-glucuronidase which is abundantly present in lysosomes and overexpressed in certain tumors [208,209]. Finally, disulfide bonds are extensively employed in peptide-drug conjugates, owing to what can be high plasma stability, and yet well-known intracellular cleavage by disulfide reduction. Their stability can be further enhanced through the addition of one or two methyl groups adjacent to the disulfide bond. Hence, hydrazone, ester, amide, disulfide, dipeptide, tripeptide, and glucuronide-based linkers provide a diverse set of linkers that can meet most needs in the assembly of peptide-drug conjugates for targeted delivery (Figure 8).

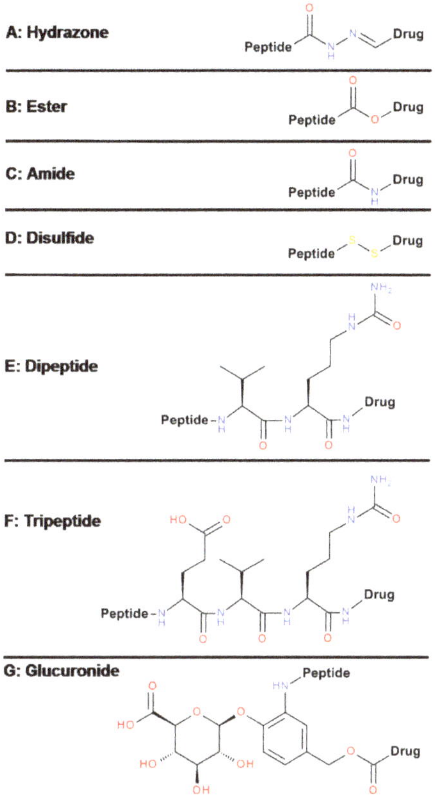

Figure 8. Linker technologies in peptide-drug conjugates.

In ADCs, the linker is installed by conjugation of the linker-drug moiety to the antibody which most often occurs on the reactive surface residues of antibodies such as cysteine and lysine residues [68,200,210–213]. The conjugation is a very critical step in ADC synthesis since typically there are multiple cysteine and lysine residues and without optimization results in a heterogeneous distribution in site and number of drugs that are loaded to the antibody. Molecular engineering and enzymatic modification have provided non-native amino acids to facilitate site-specific conjugation, but there remain technical challenges in commercial-scale production of homogenous ADCs [60,214–216]. Peptide-drug conjugates benefit in employing total chemical synthesis that involves orthogonal side chain protection to control product integrity. Appropriately functionalized amino acids (natural and non-natural) can be utilized for conjugation and examples include alkylation [217–219], Suzuki coupling [220,221], Glaser reaction [222], Diels-Alder reaction [223], CH activation [224], and oxime ligation [225,226]. The single requirement is that the peptide, the small molecule and the conjugated products are chemically stable under the conditions for synthesis and purification. In practice, most of the conjugation reactions still employ a cysteine and lysine residue, but with methods that govern selective modification. Additionally, click-based conjugation has been widely used given its orthogonal and relatively mild reaction conditions [227,228].

6.1. Amide Bond Formation

Amide bond formation is the most straightforward way to attach drug molecules to peptides [1–4,50,51]. In an Fmoc-based peptide assembly on a solid support, a lysine is typically orthogonally protected with Mtt. This protecting group once selectively removed can be coupled to a carboxylic acid of amino acid or small molecule under standard peptide coupling protocols [229,230]. This approach is demonstrated in the synthesis of glucagon-T3, where selectively de-protected lysine side chain amino at position 40 on glucagon backbone first reacted with amino acid Fmoc-gGlu-OH, and then with Boc protected T3 (Scheme 1) [189]. The carboxylic acids of protected T3 could also be pre-activated to something such as a succinate ester to allow direct reaction with the amine without coupling reagents [213,231–233]. Obviously, the linker and drug molecules must tolerate the conditions employed in peptide-resin cleavage (95% TFA with 2.5% TIS, and 2.5% water). Alternatively, selective conjugation can occur with unprotected peptides, employing the enhanced nucleophilic nature of the ε-amino group, as shown in the synthesis of GnRH-doxorubicin conjugate in Scheme 2 [234]. A dipeptide Val-Cit/Ala linker can be inserted using a similar synthetic approach, and an acidic acid such as Asp with orthogonal protection can also be used to conjugate with amine-containing drugs [7,235,236]. In summary, an amide bond is the most conventional and versatile approach to peptide-drug conjugates of suitable chemical and biological stability.

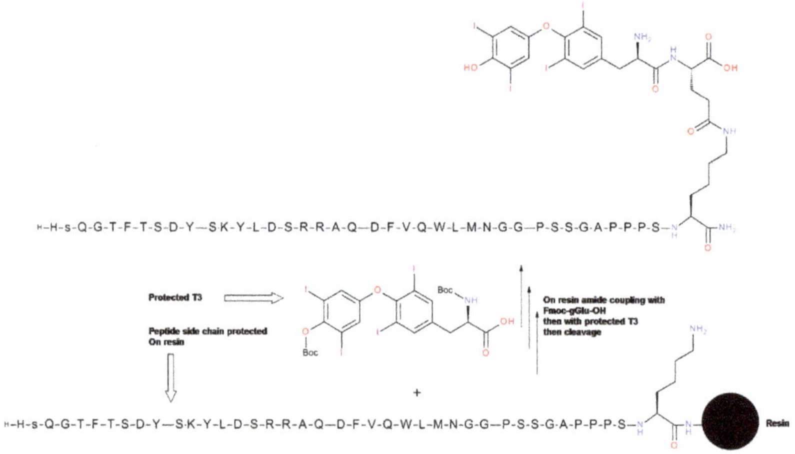

Scheme 1. Conjugation of glucagon and T3 via an amide bond. Amide bond was formed between T3 and protected peptide glucagon with a spacer gGlu on resin [189].

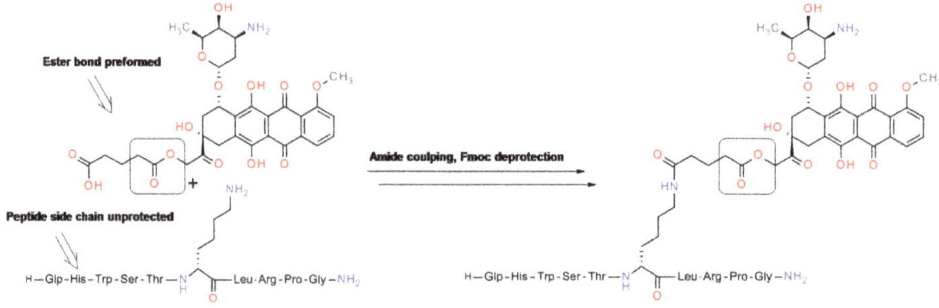

Scheme 2. Conjugation of GnRH peptide and doxorubicin (Zoptarelin Doxorubicin, AN-152, AEZS-108). Amide bond was formed between doxorubicin and unprotected peptide GnRH [234].

6.2. Disulfide Bond Formation

Disulfide bonds have been extensively used in the conjugation of peptides to drugs given the selective nature in formation and the intracellular reduction-mediated release of the drug [210,211,213,237]. Typically, a cysteine residue or a similar thiol is introduced to a noncritical region of the peptide, which is subsequently coupled through a sulfhydryl pre-activated drug (via 2-thiopyridine or DTNP). This reaction often proceeds very quickly and selectively to yield conjugated drug-products (Scheme 3) [238]. The inverse approach is also commonly employed where a peptide cysteine once activated is coupled to a thiol-containing drug to form a conjugated drug-product. There are also several other ways to form a disulfide bond if the more common methods fail, which collectively constitute a diverse set of reactions to construct disulfide bonds [239,240]. Relative to amide bond formation the increased orthogonality of cysteine lessens the need to introduce the drug to a protected peptide, which constitutes a sizable advantage when there are lysines and when the small molecule drug is not suitable for use in standard peptide synthetic protocols. It is worth noting that synthesis of disulfide bonds with adjacent gem-dimethyl groups are better achieved by pre-activating the gem-dimethyl containing sulfhydryl group to react with the less hindered sulfhydryl group. This is a consequence of steric hinderance that serves to reduce the reactivity of sulfhydryl groups surrounded by a gem-dimethyl group.

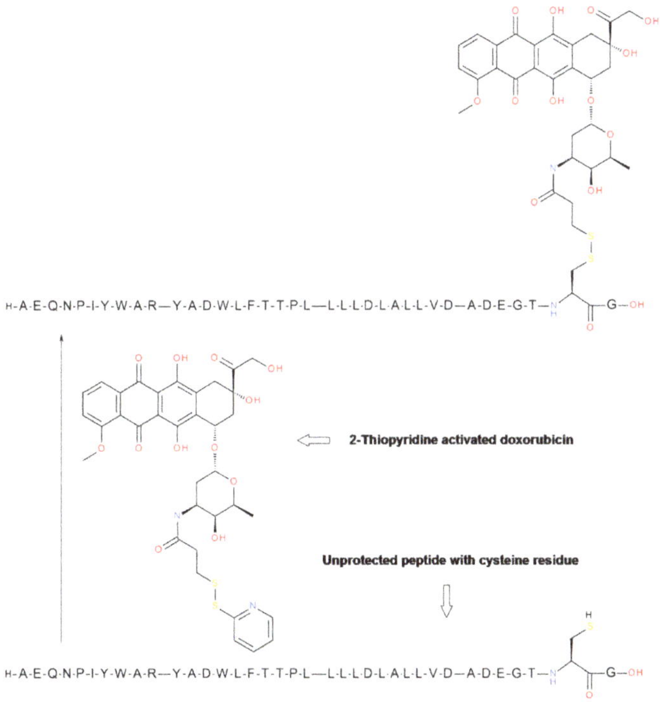

Scheme 3. Conjugation of pH low insertion peptide (pHLIP) and doxorubicin via a disulfide bond. Disulfide bond was formed between 2-thiopyridine activated doxorubicin and unprotected peptide pHLIP via a cysteine residue [238].

6.3. Thioether Formation

The thiol-maleimide reaction is a widely used method to conjugate peptides and drugs, where a peptide sulfhydryl group reacts with a pre-installed maleimide group on the drug (Scheme 4) [201,203,204,241–243]. The reaction is selective and efficient across a variety of solvents across a wide pH range, and the thioether bond offers reasonable chemical stability. Given the Michael reaction mechanism, the product is reversed under alkaline conditions and thiol exchange is reported in storage or in the presence of serum [60,216,244]. This serves to shorten the drug product shelf-life and often the circulating half-life in plasma. Recently, a ring opening stabilization strategy [245–247] or next-generation maleimide (NGM) strategy [248–250] was reported to convert the thiol-maleimide bond to a more stable thioether. In addition to the thiol-maleimide reaction, thiol alkylation is also commonly utilized to form thioether conjugated peptides and drugs. Peptide cysteine residues are typically alkylated through a bromo or iodo acetamide group in the drug, or vice versa [210,211,217–219]. Given the higher reactivity of cysteine towards these alkylating groups under slightly basic conditions, there is no competing amine alkylation, which makes it highly useful in the assembly of chemically and biologically stable peptide-drug conjugates.

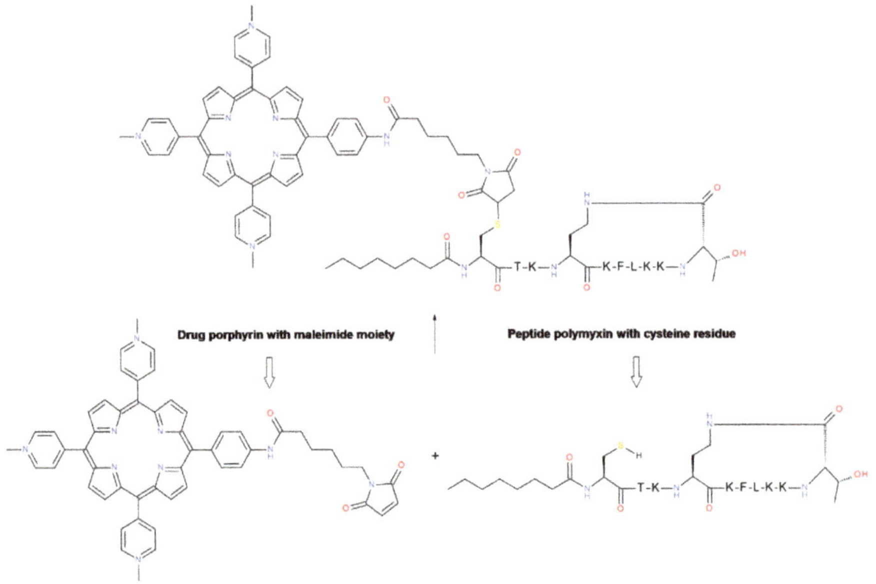

Scheme 4. Conjugation of Polymyxin B and antimicrobial porphyrin via a thiol-maleimide bond. Thiol-maleimide bond was formed between maleimide containing porphyrin and unprotected peptide polymyxin B with a cysteine residue [241].

6.4. Click Reaction

The so-called click reaction between an alkyne and azide (1,3 dipolar cycloaddition) is a widely used method for bioconjugation that is independent of cysteine and lysine residues [214,227,228]. This is a very attractive approach for connecting peptides and drugs when there are multiple lysine or cysteine residues in the peptide. The reaction occurs under mild conditions. It is efficient and devoid of any cross-reaction with natural amino acids, making it an excellent method to make homogenous peptide-drug conjugates. An example is shown in Scheme 5, where the azide group is stable in conventional methods of peptide synthesis, cleavage, and purification. The alkyne group is incorporated into the drug with an additional linker, and the peptide and drug fragments are joined together under a classical Cu-catalyzed reaction. Recent applications of click reaction in peptide-drug conjugate synthesis include EphA2-paclitaxel, GLP-1-vitamin B12, and peptide-glycolipid [251–255].

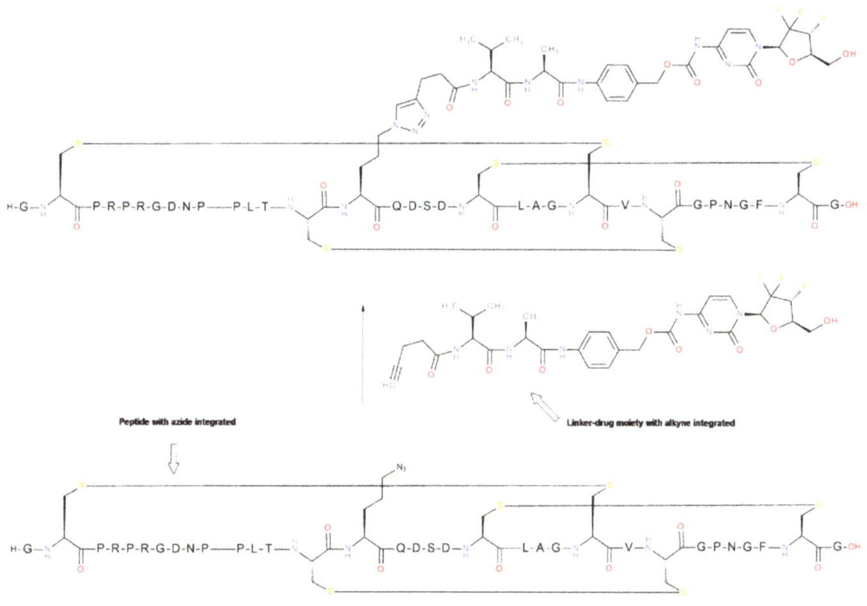

Scheme 5. Conjugation of knotting peptide and gemcitabine via click chemistry. The triazole was formed between the alkyne-containing gemcitabine and an unprotected azide-containing knotting peptide [194].

7. Peptide-Drug Conjugate Design Considerations

It is relatively straightforward to make peptide-drug conjugates, given the established synthetic conjugation strategies but there are a few central considerations that must be addressed to enhance the chance for pharmacological success. First and foremost, there must be a strong biological basis for the specific combination of the two molecular entities that compose the conjugate. Ideally, the drug and peptide operate biologically on different pathways that complement and better yet synergistically provide superior therapeutic outcomes than either operating alone. This is observed in a conjugate such as Zoptarelin Doxorubicin where GnRH functions in androgen deprivation therapy (ADT) for prostate cancer and doxorubicin is a proven oncolytic for multiple cancers. A second consideration pertains to drug targeting, where small molecule-based agents are inherently efficacious but with liabilities usually pertaining to toxicity resulting from systemic exposure. Conjugation to a suitable peptide can provide tissue-specific delivery to concentrate the pharmacology at a preferred site and lessen off-target adverse effects. This is exemplified by the somatostatin conjugate with 177Lu (177Lu-Dotatate). A third consideration is the efficiency in drug transport as peptides typically exhibit therapeutic effects at an extracellular target receptor, and a small molecule drug via an intracellular target. The conjugation targets the small molecule but places a restriction in its performance that is dependent upon the peptide-mediated internalization and subsequent intracellular release. The extracellular peptide receptor must be of sufficient capacity to internalize enough small molecule in a ligand-dependent manner for the drug to render a pharmacological effect. Peptide receptor agonists are more likely to fulfill this requirement as they are proficiently internalized and return to the plasma membrane for reuse in a manner that is more certain than peptide-based antagonists. A fourth consideration pertains to potency and the need to align them across the delivery peptide and small molecule drug. Peptide agonists are often very potent molecules operating at nanomolar or lower concentrations at their target receptors and small molecule drugs are often challenged to match this inherent potency. Increasing the drug payload by a stoichiometric ratio relative to the peptide is one way to achieve potency alignment, but this requires a minimal potency difference in the constituents since there is a practical limit to the molar equivalents of a small molecule that can be attached to a peptide before it loses its biological and physical properties. Increasing the dose to levels beyond that which is necessary for full peptide agonism may be possible if the peptide is devoid of adverse effects when used at super-pharmacological levels. This is a property that is specific to each peptide, as some such as insulin have a narrow therapeutic index with life-threatening consequences for overdosing, while others are more forgiving. Lastly, many small molecules have an appreciable affinity towards plasma proteins such as albumin and conjugation to a peptide can significantly alter the pharmacokinetic profile. This effect can alter the biology of the peptide or incorrectly suggest that an altered activity is a function of the combined biology of the drug candidate. PTH is a hormone where it is well appreciated that pulsatile administration can potently build bone mass and strength, while sustained delivery is known to be bone catabolic. Consequently, it would be a dangerous targeting peptide for any small molecule that alters its pharmacokinetics, independent of any direct change in its interaction with a target receptor. Similarly, nuclear hormones constitute excellent small molecules for tissue targeting but often possess high-affinity plasma protein binding and as such, any peptide conjugate needs to be shown unaltered time-action to attribute additive biology from two supplemental pharmacological mechanisms. In summary, the synthetic chemistry is relatively straightforward, but the design considerations are of utmost importance in selecting matching pairs that are capable of providing supplemental efficacy and selectivity.

8. Outlook and Perspective

Peptide-drug conjugates are a unique class of molecules that integrate peptides and small molecule drugs to achieve increased therapeutic outcomes. They represent an important field in drug discovery that is related in principle to antibody-directed drug targeting. These molecular conjugates leverage the inherent and unique pharmacological abilities of the peptide and the small molecule. A variety of conjugates have been discovered and developed in several therapeutic areas including numerous diseases of endocrine, infectious, and autoimmune origins. Several drug candidates have demonstrated promising preclinical results, and a few have progressed to registered medicines, most notably in the treatment of various cancers. The most powerful examples are those where the macromolecular native of the peptide is used to target small molecule effects to those tissues where the peptide is biologically active. In such instances where the peptide provides supplemental pharmacology to the small molecule the biological outcomes are enhanced, and often with far less off-target toxicity. In addition, conjugation to peptides can diminish common physical challenges in the development of small molecule drugs, and in particular, those pertaining to high lipophilicity, poor solubility and cell impermeability. The recent regulatory approval for GHIH-177Lu conjugate (177Lu-Dotatate) is a notable example of success and provides strong momentum for further applications. The research pertaining to tissue-specific delivery of nuclear hormones in the treatment of the metabolic syndrome broadens the conceptual approach beyond the delivery of cytotoxic agents to achieve mixed-mode agonism of small and large pharmacophores with different mechanisms of action.

Nevertheless, sizable challenges remain and there have been more failures than successes. The obstacles are numerous, and they pertain to both biological and chemical aspects of the strategy. The latter seems more manageable and to a finite degree are related to the biological uncertainties. Specificity remains an elusive goal as it is a rare occurrence when an extracellular target is found at only a single tissue rendering the approach more suitable for improving therapeutic index than engendering absolute specificity. This is a great obstacle when the objective is the elimination of metastatic disease as the destruction of the last percent or less of diseased cells requires dose intensity that leads to toxicity in unintended tissues. In contrast, if the therapeutic objective is to enhance the therapeutic index by an order of magnitude to permit increased dosing by tenfold than this is something more easily achieved by enriching the pharmacological action at certain tissues. The second challenge of appreciable complexity is the immature nature of the collective knowledge of intracellular biochemistry.

While it is clear that peptide cycling-receptors can internalize a ligand that carries a small molecule pharmacophore it is less clear how to transport the entity to the intracellular site where biological action occurs. The escape of small molecules from the endosome remains an emerging field of study and once liberated facilitated transport to preferred intracellular locations such as the mitochondria, nucleus and other sites largely remains an unknown. Furthermore, once a desired biological effect is achieved the question of its termination stands tall and in particular the danger for reverse extracellular transport to sites that were purposely avoided in peptide-directed tissue targeting. The question is whether the primarily targeted tissues are capable of metabolizing the small molecule drug to something that is innocuous to other tissues once released to general circulation? Finally, there remains the common imbalance between the inherent potency of peptides and small molecules, such that there is a huge deficiency in the transport capacity of the macromolecule relative to the required concentration of the small molecule. In this regard, the assembly of defined macromolecular complexes seems the best hope where large amounts of a single substance or even more than one substance can be packaged for targeted delivery in a nanoparticular or exosome by a peptide-based surface ligand. It requires additional refinement to avoid the endogenous defense mechanisms that are designed for non-specific clearance of macromolecular biological and synthetic entities. The speed in which these fundamental challenges are addressed will to a large degree determine the productivity in this molecular design and the fate of future peptide-drug candidates. Until that point when the molecular design is better defined individual drug candidates will continue to emerge by successfully circumnavigating the current obstacles. We remain sanguine about the amount of research that remains to be performed and its ability to further advance the field.

Author Contributions: R.H.—original draft preparation, B.F., J.P.M., and R.D.D.—review and editing.

Funding: This review received no direct financial support.

Conflicts of Interest: R.H., B.F. and R.D.D. wish to declare their employment association with Novo Nordisk.

Abbreviations

ADCs	Antibody-Drug Conjugates
ADT	Androgen Deprivation Therapy
Ala	Alanine
BBB	Blood–Bain–Barrier
Cit	Citrulline
DAR	Drug-Antibody Ratio
DDI	Drug-Drug Interactions
DIO	Diet-Induced Obese
DOTA	1,4,7,10-Tetraazacyclododeane
DPP4	Dipeptidyl Peptidase 4
DTNP	5,5′-Disulfanediylbis(2-nitrobenzoic acid) or Ellman's reagent
GHIH	Growth Hormone-Inhibiting Hormone
GIP	Gastric Inhibitory Polypeptide
GLP-1	Glucagon-Like Peptide 1
GLP-2	Glucagon-Like Peptide 2
gGlu	gamma glutamic acid
GnRH	Gonadotropin-Releasing Hormone
LHRH	Luteinizing Hormone-Releasing Hormone
LRP1	Low-Density Lipoprotein Receptor-Related Protein 1
NSCLC	Non-Small Cell Lung Cancer
PABC	p-Aminobenzyl Carbamate
PRRT	Peptide Receptor Radionuclide Therapy
PSMA	Prostate Specific Membrane Antigen

PTH	Parathyroid Hormone
SERCA	the Sarco/Endoplasmic Reticulum Calcium ATPase
SSTR	Somatostatin Receptor

References

1. Henninot, A.; Collins, J.C.; Nuss, J.M. The Current State of Peptide Drug Discovery: Back to the Future? *J. Med. Chem.* **2018**, *61*, 1382–1414. [CrossRef]
2. Lau, J.L.; Dunn, M.K. Therapeutic peptides: Historical perspectives, current development trends, and future directions. *Bioorg. Med. Chem.* **2017**. [CrossRef]
3. Fosgerau, K.; Hoffmann, T. Peptide therapeutics: Current status and future directions. *Drug Discov. Today* **2015**, *20*, 122–128. [CrossRef]
4. Kaspar, A.A.; Reichert, J.M. Future directions for peptide therapeutics development. *Drug Discov. Today* **2013**, *18*, 807–817. [CrossRef] [PubMed]
5. Liu, F.; Li, P.; Gelfanov, V.; Mayer, J.; DiMarchi, R. Synthetic Advances in Insulin-like Peptides Enable Novel Bioactivity. *Acc. Chem. Res.* **2017**, *50*, 1855–1865. [CrossRef] [PubMed]
6. Mijalis, A.J.; Thomas, D.A., 3rd; Simon, M.D.; Adamo, A.; Beaumont, R.; Jensen, K.F.; Pentelute, B.L. A fully automated flow-based approach for accelerated peptide synthesis. *Nat. Chem. Biol.* **2017**, *13*, 464–466. [CrossRef] [PubMed]
7. Behrendt, R.; White, P.; Offer, J. Advances in Fmoc solid-phase peptide synthesis. *J. Pept. Sci.* **2016**, *22*, 4–27. [CrossRef]
8. Lau, J.; Bloch, P.; Schaffer, L.; Pettersson, I.; Spetzler, J.; Kofoed, J.; Madsen, K.; Knudsen, L.B.; McGuire, J.; Steensgaard, D.B.; et al. Discovery of the Once-Weekly Glucagon-Like Peptide-1 (GLP-1) Analogue Semaglutide. *J. Med. Chem.* **2015**, *58*, 7370–7380. [CrossRef]
9. Made, V.; Els-Heindl, S.; Beck-Sickinger, A.G. Automated solid-phase peptide synthesis to obtain therapeutic peptides. *Beilstein J. Org. Chem.* **2014**, *10*, 1197–1212. [CrossRef]
10. Mitchell, A.R. Bruce Merrifield and solid-phase peptide synthesis: A historical assessment. *Biopolymers* **2008**, *90*, 175–184. [CrossRef]
11. Baeshen, N.A.; Baeshen, M.N.; Sheikh, A.; Bora, R.S.; Ahmed, M.M.; Ramadan, H.A.; Saini, K.S.; Redwan, E.M. Cell factories for insulin production. *Microb. Cell Fact.* **2014**, *13*, 141. [CrossRef]
12. Meehl, M.A.; Stadheim, T.A. Biopharmaceutical discovery and production in yeast. *Curr. Opin. Biotechnol.* **2014**, *30*, 120–127. [CrossRef] [PubMed]
13. Thayer, A.M. Making Peptides At Large Scale. *Chem. Eng. News* **2011**, *89*, 21–25. [CrossRef]
14. Mayer, J.P.; Zhang, F.; DiMarchi, R.D. Insulin structure and function. *Biopolymers* **2007**, *88*, 687–713. [CrossRef] [PubMed]
15. Blazynski, C. *2016 Completed Clinical Trials: Industry Strategies Revealed and Graded*; Pharma Intelligence: London, UK, 2017.
16. Waring, M.J.; Arrowsmith, J.; Leach, A.R.; Leeson, P.D.; Mandrell, S.; Owen, R.M.; Pairaudeau, G.; Pennie, W.D.; Pickett, S.D.; Wang, J.; et al. An analysis of the attrition of drug candidates from four major pharmaceutical companies. *Nat. Rev. Drug Discov.* **2015**, *14*, 475–486. [CrossRef]
17. Thomas, D.W.; Burns, J.; Audette, J.; Carroll, A.; Dow-Hygelund, C.; Hay, M. *Clinical Development Success Rates 2006–2015*; AMPLION, Biomedtracker, Biotechnology Innovation Organization (BIO): Washington, DC, USA, 2016.
18. Wirtz, V.; Knox, R.; Cao, C.; Mehrtash, H.; Posner, N.W.; McClenathan, J. *Insulin Market Profile*; Health Action International: Amsterdam, The Netherlands, 2016.
19. *Novo Nordisk Annual Report 2017*; Novo Nordisk: Bagsvaerd, Denmark, 2018.
20. Moya-Garcia, A.; Adeyelu, T.; Kruger, F.A.; Dawson, N.L.; Lees, J.G.; Overington, J.P.; Orengo, C.; Ranea, J.A.G. Structural and Functional View of Polypharmacology. *Sci. Rep.* **2017**, *7*, 10102. [CrossRef] [PubMed]
21. Anighoro, A.; Bajorath, J.; Rastelli, G. Polypharmacology: Challenges and opportunities in drug discovery. *J. Med. Chem.* **2014**, *57*, 7874–7887. [CrossRef] [PubMed]
22. Reddy, A.S.; Zhang, S. Polypharmacology: Drug discovery for the future. *Expert Rev. Clin. Pharm.* **2013**, *6*, 41–47. [CrossRef]

23. Tschop, M.; DiMarchi, R. Single-Molecule Combinatorial Therapeutics for Treating Obesity and Diabetes. *Diabetes* **2017**, *66*, 1766–1769. [CrossRef]
24. Khajavi, N.; Biebermann, H.; Tschop, M.; DiMarchi, R. Treatment of Diabetes and Obesity by Rationally Designed Peptide Agonists Functioning at Multiple Metabolic Receptors. *Endocr. Dev.* **2017**, *32*, 165–182. [CrossRef] [PubMed]
25. Sadry, S.A.; Drucker, D.J. Emerging combinatorial hormone therapies for the treatment of obesity and T2DM. *Nat. Rev. Endocrinol.* **2013**, *9*, 425–433. [CrossRef]
26. Finan, B.; Yang, B.; Ottaway, N.; Smiley, D.L.; Ma, T.; Clemmensen, C.; Chabenne, J.; Zhang, L.; Habegger, K.M.; Fischer, K.; et al. A rationally designed monomeric peptide triagonist corrects obesity and diabetes in rodents. *Nat. Med.* **2015**, *21*, 27–36. [CrossRef] [PubMed]
27. Demartis, A.; Lahm, A.; Tomei, L.; Beghetto, E.; Di Biasio, V.; Orvieto, F.; Frattolillo, F.; Carrington, P.E.; Mumick, S.; Hawes, B.; et al. Polypharmacy through Phage Display: Selection of Glucagon and GLP-1 Receptor Co-agonists from a Phage-Displayed Peptide Library. *Sci. Rep.* **2018**, *8*, 585. [CrossRef]
28. Jall, S.; Sachs, S.; Clemmensen, C.; Finan, B.; Neff, F.; DiMarchi, R.D.; Tschop, M.H.; Muller, T.D.; Hofmann, S.M. Monomeric GLP-1/GIP/glucagon triagonism corrects obesity, hepatosteatosis, and dyslipidemia in female mice. *Mol. Metab.* **2017**, *6*, 440–446. [CrossRef]
29. Gault, V.A.; Bhat, V.K.; Irwin, N.; Flatt, P.R. A novel glucagon-like peptide-1 (GLP-1)/glucagon hybrid peptide with triple-acting agonist activity at glucose-dependent insulinotropic polypeptide, GLP-1, and glucagon receptors and therapeutic potential in high fat-fed mice. *J. Biol. Chem.* **2013**, *288*, 35581–35591. [CrossRef]
30. Pocai, A.; Carrington, P.E.; Adams, J.R.; Wright, M.; Eiermann, G.; Zhu, L.; Du, X.; Petrov, A.; Lassman, M.E.; Jiang, G.; et al. Glucagon-like peptide 1/glucagon receptor dual agonism reverses obesity in mice. *Diabetes* **2009**, *58*, 2258–2266. [CrossRef]
31. Day, J.W.; Ottaway, N.; Patterson, J.T.; Gelfanov, V.; Smiley, D.; Gidda, J.; Findeisen, H.; Bruemmer, D.; Drucker, D.J.; Chaudhary, N.; et al. A new glucagon and GLP-1 co-agonist eliminates obesity in rodents. *Nat. Chem. Biol.* **2009**, *5*, 749–757. [CrossRef]
32. Andreassen, K.V.; Feigh, M.; Hjuler, S.T.; Gydesen, S.; Henriksen, J.E.; Beck-Nielsen, H.; Christiansen, C.; Karsdal, M.A.; Henriksen, K. A novel oral dual amylin and calcitonin receptor agonist (KBP-042) exerts antiobesity and antidiabetic effects in rats. *Am. J. Physiol. Endocrinol. Metab.* **2014**, *307*, E24–E33. [CrossRef] [PubMed]
33. Gydesen, S.; Andreassen, K.V.; Hjuler, S.T.; Hellgren, L.I.; Karsdal, M.A.; Henriksen, K. Optimization of tolerability and efficacy of the novel dual amylin and calcitonin receptor agonist KBP-089 through dose escalation and combination with a GLP-1 analog. *Am. J. Physiol. Endocrinol. Metab.* **2017**, *313*, E598–E607. [CrossRef] [PubMed]
34. Gydesen, S.; Hjuler, S.T.; Freving, Z.; Andreassen, K.V.; Sonne, N.; Hellgren, L.I.; Karsdal, M.A.; Henriksen, K. A novel dual amylin and calcitonin receptor agonist, KBP-089, induces weight loss through a reduction in fat, but not lean mass, while improving food preference. *Br. J. Pharm.* **2017**, *174*, 591–602. [CrossRef]
35. Hjuler, S.T.; Gydesen, S.; Andreassen, K.V.; Karsdal, M.A.; Henriksen, K. The Dual Amylin- and Calcitonin-Receptor Agonist KBP-042 Works as Adjunct to Metformin on Fasting Hyperglycemia and HbA1c in a Rat Model of Type 2 Diabetes. *J. Pharm. Exp.* **2017**, *362*, 24–30. [CrossRef] [PubMed]
36. Mullard, A. Bispecific antibody pipeline moves beyond oncology. *Nat. Rev. Drug Discov.* **2017**, *16*, 810. [CrossRef] [PubMed]
37. Clarke, S.C.; Ma, B.; Trinklein, N.D.; Schellenberger, U.; Osborn, M.J.; Ouisse, L.H.; Boudreau, A.; Davison, L.M.; Harris, K.E.; Ugamraj, H.S.; et al. Multispecific Antibody Development Platform Based on Human Heavy Chain Antibodies. *Front. Immunol.* **2018**, *9*, 3037. [CrossRef]
38. Sedykh, S.E.; Prinz, V.V.; Buneva, V.N.; Nevinsky, G.A. Bispecific antibodies: Design, therapy, perspectives. *Drug Des. Dev.* **2018**, *12*, 195–208. [CrossRef]
39. Ma, L.; Wang, C.; He, Z.; Cheng, B.; Zheng, L.; Huang, K. Peptide-Drug Conjugate: A Novel Drug Design Approach. *Curr. Med. Chem.* **2017**, *24*, 3373–3396. [CrossRef]
40. Gilad, Y.; Firer, M.; Gellerman, G. Recent Innovations in Peptide Based Targeted Drug Delivery to Cancer Cells. *Biomedicines* **2016**, *4*, 11. [CrossRef] [PubMed]
41. Firer, M.A.; Gellerman, G. Targeted drug delivery for cancer therapy: The other side of antibodies. *J. Hematol. Oncol.* **2012**, *5*, 70. [CrossRef]

42. Zagorodko, O.; Arroyo-Crespo, J.J.; Nebot, V.J.; Vicent, M.J. Polypeptide-Based Conjugates as Therapeutics: Opportunities and Challenges. *Macromol. Biosci.* **2017**, *17*. [CrossRef] [PubMed]
43. Qi, Y.; Chilkoti, A. Protein-polymer conjugation-moving beyond PEGylation. *Curr. Opin. Chem. Biol.* **2015**, *28*, 181–193. [CrossRef] [PubMed]
44. Vhora, I.; Patil, S.; Bhatt, P.; Misra, A. Protein- and Peptide-drug conjugates: An emerging drug delivery technology. *Adv. Protein Chem. Struct. Biol.* **2015**, *98*, 1–55. [CrossRef] [PubMed]
45. Staderini, M.; Megia-Fernandez, A.; Dhaliwal, K.; Bradley, M. Peptides for optical medical imaging and steps towards therapy. *Bioorg. Med. Chem.* **2017**. [CrossRef]
46. Albada, B.; Metzler-Nolte, N. Highly Potent Antibacterial Organometallic Peptide Conjugates. *Acc. Chem. Res.* **2017**, *50*, 2510–2518. [CrossRef]
47. Santos, R.; Ursu, O.; Gaulton, A.; Bento, A.P.; Donadi, R.S.; Bologa, C.G.; Karlsson, A.; Al-Lazikani, B.; Hersey, A.; Oprea, T.I.; et al. A comprehensive map of molecular drug targets. *Nat. Rev. Drug Discov.* **2017**, *16*, 19–34. [CrossRef] [PubMed]
48. Agarwal, P.; Sanseau, P.; Cardon, L.R. Novelty in the target landscape of the pharmaceutical industry. *Nat. Rev. Drug Discov.* **2013**, *12*, 575–576. [CrossRef]
49. Smietana, K.; Siatkowski, M.; Moller, M. Trends in clinical success rates. *Nat. Rev. Drug Discov.* **2016**, *15*, 379–380. [CrossRef]
50. Bohme, D.; Beck-Sickinger, A.G. Controlling Toxicity of Peptide–Drug Conjugates by Different Chemical Linker Structures. *ChemMedChem.* **2015**, *10*, 804–814. [CrossRef]
51. Diaz, D.; Ford, K.A.; Hartley, D.P.; Harstad, E.B.; Cain, G.R.; Achilles-Poon, K.; Nguyen, T.; Peng, J.; Zheng, Z.; Merchant, M.; et al. Pharmacokinetic drivers of toxicity for basic molecules: Strategy to lower pKa results in decreased tissue exposure and toxicity for a small molecule Met inhibitor. *Toxicol. Appl. Pharm.* **2013**, *266*, 86–94. [CrossRef] [PubMed]
52. Palleria, C.; Di Paolo, A.; Giofre, C.; Caglioti, C.; Leuzzi, G.; Siniscalchi, A.; De Sarro, G.; Gallelli, L. Pharmacokinetic drug-drug interaction and their implication in clinical management. *J. Res. Med. Sci.* **2013**, *18*, 601–610.
53. Ehrlich, P. The relationship existing between chemical constitution, distribution and pharmacological action. In *Collected Studies on Immunity*; Wiley & Sons: Hoboken, NJ, USA, 1906; pp. 441–450.
54. Ehrlich, P. *Chemotherapy. Proceedings of 17th International Congress of Medicine, in Collected Papers of Paul Ehrlich*; Himmelwiet, F., Ed.; Pergamon Press: Oxford, UK, 1913; pp. 505–518.
55. Mathe, G.; Loc, T.B.; Bernard, J.C.C. Effet sur la leucemie L1210 de la souris d'une combinaison par diazotation d'A-methopterine et de gamma-globulines de hamsters porteur de cette leucemie par heterogreffe. *C. R. Acad. Sci.* **1958**, *246*, 1626–1628.
56. Ghose, T.; Cerini, M.; Carter, M.; Nairn, R.C. Immunoradioactive agent against cancer. *Br. Med. J.* **1967**, *1*, 90–93. [CrossRef]
57. Ghose, T.; Nigam, S.P. Antibody as carrier of chlorambucil. *Cancer* **1972**, *29*, 1398–1400. [CrossRef]
58. Rowland, G.F.; O'Neill, G.J.; Davies, D.A. Suppression of tumour growth in mice by a drug-antibody conjugate using a novel approach to linkage. *Nature* **1975**, *255*, 487–488. [CrossRef]
59. Ford, C.H.; Newman, C.E.; Johnson, J.R.; Woodhouse, C.S.; Reeder, T.A.; Rowland, G.F.; Simmonds, R.G. Localisation and toxicity study of a vindesine-anti-CEA conjugate in patients with advanced cancer. *Br. J. Cancer* **1983**, *47*, 35–42. [CrossRef] [PubMed]
60. Beck, A.; Goetsch, L.; Dumontet, C.; Corvaia, N. Strategies and challenges for the next generation of antibody-drug conjugates. *Nat. Rev. Drug Discov.* **2017**, *16*, 315–337. [CrossRef] [PubMed]
61. Perez, H.L.; Cardarelli, P.M.; Deshpande, S.; Gangwar, S.; Schroeder, G.M.; Vite, G.D.; Borzilleri, R.M. Antibody-drug conjugates: Current status and future directions. *Drug Discov. Today* **2014**, *19*, 869–881. [CrossRef] [PubMed]
62. Senter, P.D.; Sievers, E.L. The discovery and development of brentuximab vedotin for use in relapsed Hodgkin lymphoma and systemic anaplastic large cell lymphoma. *Nat. Biotechnol.* **2012**, *30*, 631–637. [CrossRef] [PubMed]
63. Younes, A.; Yasothan, U.; Kirkpatrick, P. Brentuximab vedotin. *Nat. Rev. Drug Discov.* **2012**, *11*, 19–20. [CrossRef] [PubMed]
64. Lambert, J.M.; Chari, R.V. Ado-trastuzumab Emtansine (T-DM1): An antibody-drug conjugate (ADC) for HER2-positive breast cancer. *J. Med. Chem.* **2014**, *57*, 6949–6964. [CrossRef]

65. Available online: https://www.reuters.com/article/us-pfizer-mylotarg/pfizer-pulls-leukemia-drug-from-u-s-market-idUSTRE65K5QG20100621 (accessed on 22 April 2019).
66. Available online: https://www.fda.gov/drugs/informationondrugs/approveddrugs/ucm572133.htm (accessed on 22 April 2019).
67. Available online: https://clinicaltrials.gov/ct2/results?intr=Antibody-Drug+Conjugate&Search=Apply&recrs=b&recrs=a&recrs=f&recrs=d&age_v=&gndr=&type=&rslt=0 (accessed on 22 April 2019).
68. Diamantis, N.; Banerji, U. Antibody-drug conjugates–an emerging class of cancer treatment. *Br. J. Cancer* **2016**, *114*, 362–367. [CrossRef]
69. Bouchard, H.; Viskov, C.; Garcia-Echeverria, C. Antibody-drug conjugates-a new wave of cancer drugs. *Bioorg. Med. Chem. Lett.* **2014**, *24*, 5357–5363. [CrossRef]
70. Sun, X.; Ponte, J.F.; Yoder, N.C.; Laleau, R.; Coccia, J.; Lanieri, L.; Qiu, Q.; Wu, R.; Hong, E.; Bogalhas, M.; et al. Effects of Drug-Antibody Ratio on Pharmacokinetics, Biodistribution, Efficacy, and Tolerability of Antibody-Maytansinoid Conjugates. *Bioconj. Chem.* **2017**, *28*, 1371–1381. [CrossRef]
71. Weckbecker, G.; Lewis, I.; Albert, R.; Schmid, H.A.; Hoyer, D.; Bruns, C. Opportunities in somatostatin research: Biological, chemical and therapeutic aspects. *Nat. Rev. Drug Discov.* **2003**, *2*, 999–1017. [CrossRef]
72. Keskin, O.; Yalcin, S. A review of the use of somatostatin analogs in oncology. *Onco Targets* **2013**, *6*, 471–483. [CrossRef]
73. Spada, F.; Valente, M. Review of recents advances in medical treatment for neuroendocrine neoplasms: Somatostatin analogs and chemotherapy. *J. Cancer Metastasis Treat.* **2016**, *2*, 313–320. [CrossRef]
74. Moller, L.N.; Stidsen, C.E.; Hartmann, B.; Holst, J.J. Somatostatin receptors. *Biochim. Biophys. Acta* **2003**, *1616*, 1–84. [CrossRef]
75. De Jong, M.; Valkema, R.; Jamar, F.; Kvols, L.K.; Kwekkeboom, D.J.; Breeman, W.A.; Bakker, W.H.; Smith, C.; Pauwels, S.; Krenning, E.P. Somatostatin receptor-targeted radionuclide therapy of tumors: Preclinical and clinical findings. *Semin. Nucl. Med.* **2002**, *32*, 133–140. [CrossRef]
76. Pinato, D.J.; Black, J.R.; Ramaswami, R.; Tan, T.M.; Adjogatse, D.; Sharma, R. Peptide receptor radionuclide therapy for metastatic paragangliomas. *Med. Oncol.* **2016**, *33*, 47. [CrossRef]
77. PRRT. Available online: http://www.prrtinfo.org/prrt (accessed on 22 April 2019).
78. Krenning, E.P.; Kooij, P.P.; Bakker, W.H.; Breeman, W.A.; Postema, P.T.; Kwekkeboom, D.J.; Oei, H.Y.; de Jong, M.; Visser, T.J.; Reijs, A.E.; et al. Radiotherapy with a radiolabeled somatostatin analogue, [111In-DTPA-DPhe1]- octreotide: A case history. *Ann. N. Y. Acad. Sci.* **1994**, *733*, 496–506. [CrossRef]
79. Hörsch, D.; Ezziddin, S.; Haug, A.; Gratz, K.F.; Dunkelmann, S.; Miederer, M.; Schreckenberger, M.; Krause, B.J.; Bengel, F.M.; Bartenstein, P.; et al. Effectiveness and side-effects of peptide receptor radionuclide therapy for neuroendocrine neoplasms in Germany: A multi-institutional registry study with prospective follow-up. *Eur. J. Cancer* **2016**, *58*, 41–51. [CrossRef]
80. FDA Approves Lutetium Lu 177 Dotatate for Treatment of GEP-NETS. Available online: https://www.fda.gov/drugs/informationondrugs/approveddrugs/ucm594105.htm (accessed on 22 April 2019).
81. Lutathera. Available online: http://www.ema.europa.eu/ema/index.jsp?curl=pages/medicines/human/medicines/004123/human_med_002163.jsp&mid=WC0b01ac058001d1244 (accessed on 22 April 2019).
82. Emmett, L.; Willowson, K.; Violet, J.; Shin, J.; Blanksby, A.; Lee, J. Lutetium (177) PSMA radionuclide therapy for men with prostate cancer: A review of the current literature and discussion of practical aspects of therapy. *J. Med. Radiat. Sci.* **2017**, *64*, 52–60. [CrossRef]
83. Bodei, L.; Mueller-Brand, J.; Baum, R.P.; Pavel, M.E.; Horsch, D.; O'Dorisio, M.S.; O'Dorisio, T.M.; Howe, J.R.; Cremonesi, M.; Kwekkeboom, D.J.; et al. The joint IAEA, EANM, and SNMMI practical guidance on peptide receptor radionuclide therapy (PRRNT) in neuroendocrine tumours. *Eur. J. Nucl. Med. Mol. Imaging* **2013**, *40*, 800–816. [CrossRef]
84. Van Essen, M.; Krenning, E.P.; De Jong, M.; Valkema, R.; Kwekkeboom, D.J. Peptide Receptor Radionuclide Therapy with radiolabelled somatostatin analogues in patients with receptor positive tumours. *Acta Oncol.* **2007**, *46*, 723–734. [CrossRef]
85. Jamous, M.; Haberkorn, U.; Mier, W. Synthesis of peptide radiopharmaceuticals for the therapy and diagnosis of tumor diseases. *Molecules* **2013**, *18*, 3379–3409. [CrossRef]
86. Reubi, J.C.; Schär, J.C.; Waser, B.; Wenger, S.; Heppeler, A.; Schmitt, J.S.; Mäcke, H.R. Affinity profiles for human somatostatin receptor subtypes SST1-SST5 of somatostatin radiotracers selected for scintigraphic and radiotherapeutic use. *Eur. J. Nucl. Med.* **2000**, *27*, 273–282. [CrossRef]

87. Kwekkeboom, D.J.; de Herder, W.W.; Kam, B.L.; van Eijck, C.H.; van Essen, M.; Kooij, P.P.; Feelders, R.A.; van Aken, M.O.; Krenning, E.P. Treatment with the radiolabeled somatostatin analog [177 Lu-DOTA 0,Tyr3]octreotate: Toxicity, efficacy, and survival. *J. Clin. Oncol.* **2008**, *26*, 2124–2130. [CrossRef]
88. Strosberg, J.; El-Haddad, G.; Wolin, E.; Hendifar, A.; Yao, J.; Chasen, B.; Mittra, E.; Kunz, P.L.; Kulke, M.H.; Jacene, H.; et al. Phase 3 Trial of (177)Lu-Dotatate for Midgut Neuroendocrine Tumors. *N. Engl. J. Med.* **2017**, *376*, 125–135. [CrossRef]
89. Schneider, F.; Tomek, W.; Grundker, C. Gonadotropin-releasing hormone (GnRH) and its natural analogues: A review. *Theriogenology* **2006**, *66*, 691–709. [CrossRef]
90. Millar, R.P.; Lu, Z.L.; Pawson, A.J.; Flanagan, C.A.; Morgan, K.; Maudsley, S.R. Gonadotropin-releasing hormone receptors. *Endocr. Rev.* **2004**, *25*, 235–275. [CrossRef]
91. Madhunapantula, S.V.; Mosca, P.; Robertson, G.P. Steroid hormones drive cancer development. *Cancer Biol.* **2010**, *10*, 765–766. [CrossRef]
92. Capper, C.P.; Rae, J.M.; Auchus, R.J. The Metabolism, Analysis, and Targeting of Steroid Hormones in Breast and Prostate Cancer. *Horm. Cancer* **2016**, *7*, 149–164. [CrossRef]
93. Perrett, R.M.; McArdle, C.A. Molecular mechanisms of gonadotropin-releasing hormone signaling integrating cyclic nucleotides into the network. *Front. Endocrinol. (Lausanne)* **2013**, *4*, 180. [CrossRef]
94. Bolton, E.M.; Lynch, T.H. Are all gonadotropin-releasing hormone agonists equivalent for the treatment of prostate cancer? A systematic review. *BJU Int.* **2018**. [CrossRef]
95. Cheng, C.K.; Leung, P.C. Molecular biology of gonadotropin-releasing hormone (GnRH)-I, GnRH-II, and their receptors in humans. *Endocr. Rev.* **2005**, *26*, 283–306. [CrossRef]
96. Westphalen, S.; Kotulla, G.; Kaiser, F.; Krauss, W.; Werning, G.; Elsasser, H.P.; Nagy, A.; Schulz, K.D.; Grundker, C.; Schally, A.V.; et al. Receptor mediated antiproliferative effects of the cytotoxic LHRH agonist AN-152 in human ovarian and endometrial cancer cell lines. *Int. J. Oncol.* **2000**, *17*, 1063–1069. [CrossRef]
97. Letsch, M.; Schally, A.V.; Szepeshazi, K.; Halmos, G.; Nagy, A. Preclinical evaluation of targeted cytotoxic luteinizing hormone-releasing hormone analogue AN-152 in androgen-sensitive and insensitive prostate cancers. *Clin. Cancer Res.* **2003**, *9*, 4505–4513.
98. Liu, S.V.; Tsao-Wei, D.D.; Xiong, S.; Groshen, S.; Dorff, T.B.; Quinn, D.I.; Tai, Y.C.; Engel, J.; Hawes, D.; Schally, A.V.; et al. Phase I, dose-escalation study of the targeted cytotoxic LHRH analog AEZS-108 in patients with castration- and taxane-resistant prostate cancer. *Clin. Cancer Res.* **2014**, *20*, 6277–6283. [CrossRef]
99. Emons, G.; Kaufmann, M.; Gorchev, G.; Tsekova, V.; Grundker, C.; Gunthert, A.R.; Hanker, L.C.; Velikova, M.; Sindermann, H.; Engel, J.; et al. Dose escalation and pharmacokinetic study of AEZS-108 (AN-152), an LHRH agonist linked to doxorubicin, in women with LHRH receptor-positive tumors. *Gynecol. Oncol.* **2010**, *119*, 457–461. [CrossRef]
100. Engel, J.; Emons, G.; Pinski, J.; Schally, A.V. AEZS-108: A targeted cytotoxic analog of LHRH for the treatment of cancers positive for LHRH receptors. *Expert Opin. Investig. Drugs* **2012**, *21*, 891–899. [CrossRef]
101. Yu, S.S.; Athreya, K.; Liu, S.V.; Schally, A.V.; Tsao-Wei, D.; Groshen, S.; Quinn, D.I.; Dorff, T.B.; Xiong, S.; Engel, J.; et al. A Phase II Trial of AEZS-108 in Castration- and Taxane-Resistant Prostate Cancer. *Clin. Genitourin. Cancer* **2017**, *15*, 742–749. [CrossRef]
102. Emons, G.; Gorchev, G.; Harter, P.; Wimberger, P.; Stahle, A.; Hanker, L.; Hilpert, F.; Beckmann, M.W.; Dall, P.; Grundker, C.; et al. Efficacy and safety of AEZS-108 (LHRH agonist linked to doxorubicin) in women with advanced or recurrent endometrial cancer expressing LHRH receptors: A multicenter phase 2 trial (AGO-GYN5). *Int. J. Gynecol. Cancer* **2014**, *24*, 260–265. [CrossRef]
103. Emons, G.; Gorchev, G.; Sehouli, J.; Wimberger, P.; Stahle, A.; Hanker, L.; Hilpert, F.; Sindermann, H.; Grundker, C.; Harter, P. Efficacy and safety of AEZS-108 (INN: Zoptarelin doxorubicin acetate) an LHRH agonist linked to doxorubicin in women with platinum refractory or resistant ovarian cancer expressing LHRH receptors: A multicenter phase II trial of the ago-study group (AGO GYN 5). *Gynecol. Oncol.* **2014**, *133*, 427–432. [CrossRef] [PubMed]
104. Zoptarelin Doxorubicin Falls Short in Phase III Endometrial Cancer Trial. Available online: https://www.onclive.com/web-exclusives/zoptarelin-doxorubicin-falls-short-in-phase-iii-endometrial-cancer-trial (accessed on 22 April 2019).
105. Hennenfent, K.L.; Govindan, R. Novel formulations of taxanes: A review. Old wine in a new bottle? *Ann. Oncol.* **2006**, *17*, 735–749. [CrossRef]

106. Spencer, C.M.; Faulds, D. Paclitaxel. A review of its pharmacodynamic and pharmacokinetic properties and therapeutic potential in the treatment of cancer. *Drugs* **1994**, *48*, 794–847. [CrossRef] [PubMed]
107. Demeule, M.; Regina, A.; Che, C.; Poirier, J.; Nguyen, T.; Gabathuler, R.; Castaigne, J.P.; Beliveau, R. Identification and design of peptides as a new drug delivery system for the brain. *J. Pharm. Exp.* **2008**, *324*, 1064–1072. [CrossRef]
108. Shao, K.; Huang, R.; Li, J.; Han, L.; Ye, L.; Lou, J.; Jiang, C. Angiopep-2 modified PE-PEG based polymeric micelles for amphotericin B delivery targeted to the brain. *J. Control. Release* **2010**, *147*, 118–126. [CrossRef] [PubMed]
109. Regina, A.; Demeule, M.; Che, C.; Lavallee, I.; Poirier, J.; Gabathuler, R.; Beliveau, R.; Castaigne, J.P. Antitumour activity of ANG1005, a conjugate between paclitaxel and the new brain delivery vector Angiopep-2. *Br. J. Pharm.* **2008**, *155*, 185–197. [CrossRef] [PubMed]
110. Kurzrock, R.; Gabrail, N.; Chandhasin, C.; Moulder, S.; Smith, C.; Brenner, A.; Sankhala, K.; Mita, A.; Elian, K.; Bouchard, D.; et al. Safety, pharmacokinetics, and activity of GRN1005, a novel conjugate of angiopep-2, a peptide facilitating brain penetration, and paclitaxel, in patients with advanced solid tumors. *Mol. Cancer Ther.* **2012**, *11*, 308–316. [CrossRef] [PubMed]
111. Drappatz, J.; Brenner, A.; Wong, E.T.; Eichler, A.; Schiff, D.; Groves, M.D.; Mikkelsen, T.; Rosenfeld, S.; Sarantopoulos, J.; Meyers, C.A.; et al. Phase I study of GRN1005 in recurrent malignant glioma. *Clin. Cancer Res.* **2013**, *19*, 1567–1576. [CrossRef] [PubMed]
112. Bertrand, Y.; Currie, J.C.; Poirier, J.; Demeule, M.; Abulrob, A.; Fatehi, D.; Stanimirovic, D.; Sartelet, H.; Castaigne, J.P.; Beliveau, R. Influence of glioma tumour microenvironment on the transport of ANG1005 via low-density lipoprotein receptor-related protein 1. *Br. J. Cancer* **2011**, *105*, 1697–1707. [CrossRef]
113. Li, F.; Tang, S.C. Targeting metastatic breast cancer with ANG1005, a novel peptide-paclitaxel conjugate that crosses the blood-brain-barrier (BBB). *Genes Dis.* **2017**, *4*, 1–3. [CrossRef]
114. Available online: https://clinicaltrials.gov/ct2/results?term=ANG1005&age_v=&gndr=&type=&rslt=&phase=1&Search=Apply (accessed on 22 April 2019).
115. Angiochem's ANG1005 Received Orphan Drug Designation from FDA for the Treatment of Glioblastoma Multiform. Available online: http://angiochem.com/angiochem%E2%80%99s-ang1005-received-orphan-drug-designation-fda-treatment-glioblastoma-multiform (accessed on 22 April 2019).
116. Available online: https://clinicaltrials.gov/ct2/results?cond=&term=NCT03613181&cntry=&state=&city=&dist= (accessed on 22 April 2019).
117. Quynh Doan, N.T.; Christensen, S.B. Thapsigargin, Origin, Chemistry, Structure-Activity Relationships and Prodrug Development. *Curr. Pharm. Des.* **2015**, *21*, 5501–5517. [CrossRef]
118. Denmeade, S.R.; Isaacs, J.T. Engineering enzymatically activated "molecular grenades" for cancer. *Oncotarget* **2012**, *3*, 666–667. [CrossRef] [PubMed]
119. Denmeade, S.R.; Mhaka, A.M.; Rosen, D.M.; Brennen, W.N.; Dalrymple, S.; Dach, I.; Olesen, C.; Gurel, B.; Demarzo, A.M.; Wilding, G.; et al. Engineering a prostate-specific membrane antigen-activated tumor endothelial cell prodrug for cancer therapy. *Sci. Transl. Med.* **2012**, *4*, 140ra186. [CrossRef]
120. Andersen, T.B.; Lopez, C.Q.; Manczak, T.; Martinez, K.; Simonsen, H.T. Thapsigargin–from Thapsia L. to mipsagargin. *Molecules* **2015**, *20*, 6113–6127. [CrossRef]
121. Silver, D.A.; Pellicer, I.; Fair, W.R.; Heston, W.D.; Cordon-Cardo, C. Prostate-specific membrane antigen expression in normal and malignant human tissues. *Clin. Cancer Res.* **1997**, *3*, 81–85. [PubMed]
122. Kinoshita, Y.; Kuratsukuri, K.; Landas, S.; Imaida, K.; Rovito, P.M., Jr.; Wang, C.Y.; Haas, G.P. Expression of prostate-specific membrane antigen in normal and malignant human tissues. *World J. Surg.* **2006**, *30*, 628–636. [CrossRef] [PubMed]
123. Mahalingam, D.; Wilding, G.; Denmeade, S.; Sarantopoulas, J.; Cosgrove, D.; Cetnar, J.; Azad, N.; Bruce, J.; Kurman, M.; Allgood, V.E.; et al. Mipsagargin, a novel thapsigargin-based PSMA-activated prodrug: Results of a first-in-man phase I clinical trial in patients with refractory, advanced or metastatic solid tumours. *Br. J. Cancer* **2016**, *114*, 986–994. [CrossRef]
124. Available online: https://clinicaltrials.gov/ct2/results?cond=&term=G202&cntry=&state=&city=&dist= (accessed on 22 April 2019).
125. Dissanayake, S.; Denny, W.A.; Gamage, S.; Sarojini, V. Recent developments in anticancer drug delivery using cell penetrating and tumor targeting peptides. *J. Control. Release* **2017**, *250*, 62–76. [CrossRef]

126. Kebebe, D.; Liu, Y.; Wu, Y.; Vilakhamxay, M.; Liu, Z.; Li, J. Tumor-targeting delivery of herb-based drugs with cell-penetrating/tumor-targeting peptide-modified nanocarriers. *Int. J. Nanomed.* **2018**, *13*, 1425–1442. [CrossRef]
127. Timur, S.S.; Bhattarai, P.; Gursoy, R.N.; Vural, I.; Khaw, B.A. Design and In Vitro Evaluation of Bispecific Complexes and Drug Conjugates of Anticancer Peptide, LyP-1 in Human Breast Cancer. *Pharm. Res.* **2017**, *34*, 352–364. [CrossRef]
128. Engel, J.B.; Schally, A.V.; Dietl, J.; Rieger, L.; Honig, A. Targeted therapy of breast and gynecological cancers with cytotoxic analogues of peptide hormones. *Mol. Pharm.* **2007**, *4*, 652–658. [CrossRef]
129. Schally, A.V.; Nagy, A. Cancer chemotherapy based on targeting of cytotoxic peptide conjugates to their receptors on tumors. *Eur. J. Endocrinol.* **1999**, *141*, 1–14. [CrossRef] [PubMed]
130. Nagy, A.; Schally, A.V.; Halmos, G.; Armatis, P.; Cai, R.Z.; Csernus, V.; Kovacs, M.; Koppan, M.; Szepeshazi, K.; Kahan, Z. Synthesis and biological evaluation of cytotoxic analogs of somatostatin containing doxorubicin or its intensely potent derivative, 2-pyrrolinodoxorubicin. *Proc. Natl. Acad. Sci. USA* **1998**, *95*, 1794–1799. [CrossRef] [PubMed]
131. Engel, J.B.; Schally, A.V.; Halmos, G.; Baker, B.; Nagy, A.; Keller, G. Targeted cytotoxic bombesin analog AN-215 effectively inhibits experimental human breast cancers with a low induction of multi-drug resistance proteins. *Endocr. Relat. Cancer* **2005**, *12*, 999–1009. [CrossRef]
132. Nagy, A.; Armatis, P.; Cai, R.Z.; Szepeshazi, K.; Halmos, G.; Schally, A.V. Design, synthesis, and in vitro evaluation of cytotoxic analogs of bombesin-like peptides containing doxorubicin or its intensely potent derivative, 2-pyrrolinodoxorubicin. *Proc. Natl. Acad. Sci. USA* **1997**, *94*, 652–656. [CrossRef]
133. Ibanez-Costa, A.; Lopez-Sanchez, L.M.; Gahete, M.D.; Rivero-Cortes, E.; Vazquez-Borrego, M.C.; Galvez, M.A.; de la Riva, A.; Venegas-Moreno, E.; Jimenez-Reina, L.; Moreno-Carazo, A.; et al. BIM-23A760 influences key functional endpoints in pituitary adenomas and normal pituitaries: Molecular mechanisms underlying the differential response in adenomas. *Sci. Rep.* **2017**, *7*, 42002. [CrossRef] [PubMed]
134. Florio, T.; Barbieri, F.; Spaziante, R.; Zona, G.; Hofland, L.J.; van Koetsveld, P.M.; Feelders, R.A.; Stalla, G.K.; Theodoropoulou, M.; Culler, M.D.; et al. Efficacy of a dopamine-somatostatin chimeric molecule, BIM-23A760, in the control of cell growth from primary cultures of human non-functioning pituitary adenomas: A multi-center study. *Endocr. Relat. Cancer* **2008**, *15*, 583–596. [CrossRef]
135. Jaquet, P.; Gunz, G.; Saveanu, A.; Dufour, H.; Taylor, J.; Dong, J.; Kim, S.; Moreau, J.P.; Enjalbert, A.; Culler, M.D. Efficacy of chimeric molecules directed towards multiple somatostatin and dopamine receptors on inhibition of GH and prolactin secretion from GH-secreting pituitary adenomas classified as partially responsive to somatostatin analog therapy. *Eur. J. Endocrinol.* **2005**, *153*, 135–141. [CrossRef]
136. Bakker, W.H.; Albert, R.; Bruns, C.; Breeman, W.A.; Hofland, L.J.; Marbach, P.; Pless, J.; Pralet, D.; Stolz, B.; Koper, J.W.; et al. [111In-DTPA-D-Phe1]-octreotide, a potential radiopharmaceutical for imaging of somatostatin receptor-positive tumors: Synthesis, radiolabeling and in vitro validation. *Life Sci.* **1991**, *49*, 1583–1591. [CrossRef]
137. Forssell-Aronsson, E.; Bernhardt, P.; Nilsson, O.; Tisell, L.E.; Wangberg, B.; Ahlman, H. Biodistribution data from 100 patients i.v. injected with 111In-DTPA-D-Phe1-octreotide. *Acta Oncol.* **2004**, *43*, 436–442. [CrossRef]
138. Northfelt, D.W.; Allred, J.B.; Liu, H.; Hobday, T.J.; Rodacker, M.W.; Lyss, A.P.; Fitch, T.R.; Perez, E.A.; North Central Cancer Treatment, G. Phase 2 trial of paclitaxel polyglumex with capecitabine for metastatic breast cancer. *Am. J. Clin. Oncol.* **2014**, *37*, 167–171. [CrossRef]
139. Singer, J.W. Paclitaxel poliglumex (XYOTAX, CT-2103): A macromolecular taxane. *J. Control. Release* **2005**, *109*, 120–126. [CrossRef]
140. O'Brien, M.E.; Socinski, M.A.; Popovich, A.Y.; Bondarenko, I.N.; Tomova, A.; Bilynsky, B.T.; Hotko, Y.S.; Ganul, V.L.; Kostinsky, I.Y.; Eisenfeld, A.J.; et al. Randomized phase III trial comparing single-agent paclitaxel Poliglumex (CT-2103, PPX) with single-agent gemcitabine or vinorelbine for the treatment of PS 2 patients with chemotherapy-naive advanced non-small cell lung cancer. *J. Thorac. Oncol.* **2008**, *3*, 728–734. [CrossRef]
141. Langer, C.J.; O'Byrne, K.J.; Socinski, M.A.; Mikhailov, S.M.; Lesniewski-Kmak, K.; Smakal, M.; Ciuleanu, T.E.; Orlov, S.V.; Dediu, M.; Heigener, D.; et al. Phase III trial comparing paclitaxel poliglumex (CT-2103, PPX) in combination with carboplatin versus standard paclitaxel and carboplatin in the treatment of PS 2 patients with chemotherapy-naive advanced non-small cell lung cancer. *J. Thorac. Oncol.* **2008**, *3*, 623–630. [CrossRef]

142. Paz-Ares, L.; Ross, H.; O'Brien, M.; Riviere, A.; Gatzemeier, U.; Von Pawel, J.; Kaukel, E.; Freitag, L.; Digel, W.; Bischoff, H.; et al. Phase III trial comparing paclitaxel poliglumex vs. docetaxel in the second-line treatment of non-small-cell lung cancer. *Br. J. Cancer* **2008**, *98*, 1608–1613. [CrossRef]
143. Curtis, K.K.; Sarantopoulos, J.; Northfelt, D.W.; Weiss, G.J.; Barnhart, K.M.; Whisnant, J.K.; Leuschner, C.; Alila, H.; Borad, M.J.; Ramanathan, R.K. Novel LHRH-receptor-targeted cytolytic peptide, EP-100: First-in-human phase I study in patients with advanced LHRH-receptor-expressing solid tumors. *Cancer Chemother. Pharm.* **2014**, *73*, 931–941. [CrossRef]
144. Leuschner, C.; Coulter, A.; Keener, J.; Alila, H. Targeted Oncolytic Peptide for Treatment of Ovarian Cancers. *Int. J. Cancer Res. Mol. Mech.* **2017**, *3*. [CrossRef]
145. Available online: https://clinicaltrials.gov/ct2/results?cond=&term=NCT01485848&cntry=&state=&city=&dist= (accessed on 22 April 2019).
146. Rothbard, J.B.; Garlington, S.; Lin, Q.; Kirschberg, T.; Kreider, E.; McGrane, P.L.; Wender, P.A.; Khavari, P.A. Conjugation of arginine oligomers to cyclosporin A facilitates topical delivery and inhibition of inflammation. *Nat. Med.* **2000**, *6*, 1253–1257. [CrossRef]
147. Ciclosporin–Cellgate. Available online: https://adisinsight.springer.com/drugs/800018283 (accessed on 18 January 2019).
148. KAI Pharmaceuticals Initiates Phase 1 Trial of KAI-1455 for Ischemic Injury. Available online: https://www.businesswire.com/news/home/20070504005145/en/KAI-Pharmaceuticals-Initiates-Phase-1-Trial-KAI-1455 (accessed on 22 April 2019).
149. Moodie, J.E.; Bisley, E.J.; Huang, S.; Pickthorn, K.; Bell, G. A single-center, randomized, double-blind, active, and placebo-controlled study of KAI-1678, a novel PKC-epsilon inhibitor, in the treatment of acute postoperative orthopedic pain. *Pain Med.* **2013**, *14*, 916–924. [CrossRef]
150. Cousins, M.J.; Pickthorn, K.; Huang, S.; Critchley, L.; Bell, G. The safety and efficacy of KAI-1678- an inhibitor of epsilon protein kinase C (epsilonPKC)-versus lidocaine and placebo for the treatment of postherpetic neuralgia: A crossover study design. *Pain Med.* **2013**, *14*, 533–540. [CrossRef]
151. Available online: https://clinicaltrials.gov/ct2/results?cond=&term=kai-1678&cntry=&state=&city=&dist= (accessed on 18 January 2019).
152. Miyaji, Y.; Walter, S.; Chen, L.; Kurihara, A.; Ishizuka, T.; Saito, M.; Kawai, K.; Okazaki, O. Distribution of KAI-9803, a novel delta-protein kinase C inhibitor, after intravenous administration to rats. *Drug Metab. Dispos.* **2011**, *39*, 1946–1953. [CrossRef]
153. Direct Inhibition of delta-Protein Kinase C Enzyme to Limit Total Infarct Size in Acute Myocardial Infarction (DELTA MI) Investigators; Bates, E.; Bode, C.; Costa, M.; Gibson, C.M.; Granger, C.; Green, C.; Grimes, K.; Harrington, R.; Huber, K.; et al. Intracoronary KAI-9803 as an adjunct to primary percutaneous coronary intervention for acute ST-segment elevation myocardial infarction. *Circulation* **2008**, *117*, 886–896. [CrossRef]
154. Available online: https://clinicaltrials.gov/ct2/results?cond=&term=KAI-9803&cntry=&state=&city=&dist= (accessed on 22 April 2019).
155. Available online: https://clinicaltrials.gov/ct2/results?cond=&term=XG-102&cntry=&state=&city=&dist= (accessed on 22 April 2019).
156. Available online: http://www.xigenpharma.com/clinical-trials (accessed on 22 April 2019).
157. Chiquet, C.; Aptel, F.; Creuzot-Garcher, C.; Berrod, J.P.; Kodjikian, L.; Massin, P.; Deloche, C.; Perino, J.; Kirwan, B.A.; de Brouwer, S.; et al. Postoperative Ocular Inflammation: A Single Subconjunctival Injection of XG-102 Compared to Dexamethasone Drops in a Randomized Trial. *Am. J. Ophthalmol.* **2017**, *174*, 76–84. [CrossRef]
158. Beydoun, T.; Deloche, C.; Perino, J.; Kirwan, B.A.; Combette, J.M.; Behar-Cohen, F. Subconjunctival injection of XG-102, a JNK inhibitor peptide, in patients with intraocular inflammation: A safety and tolerability study. *J. Ocul. Pharm.* **2015**, *31*, 93–99. [CrossRef] [PubMed]
159. Coriat, R.; Faivre, S.J.; Mir, O.; Dreyer, C.; Ropert, S.; Bouattour, M.; Desjardins, R.; Goldwasser, F.; Raymond, E. Pharmacokinetics and safety of DTS-108, a human oligopeptide bound to SN-38 with an esterase-sensitive cross-linker in patients with advanced malignancies: A Phase I study. *Int. J. Nanomed.* **2016**, *11*, 6207–6216. [CrossRef] [PubMed]
160. Meyer-Losic, F.; Nicolazzi, C.; Quinonero, J.; Ribes, F.; Michel, M.; Dubois, V.; de Coupade, C.; Boukaissi, M.; Chene, A.S.; Tranchant, I.; et al. DTS-108, a novel peptidic prodrug of SN38: In vivo efficacy and toxicokinetic studies. *Clin. Cancer Res.* **2008**, *14*, 2145–2153. [CrossRef] [PubMed]

161. Schoffski, P.; Delord, J.P.; Brain, E.; Robert, J.; Dumez, H.; Gasmi, J.; Trouet, A. First-in-man phase I study assessing the safety and pharmacokinetics of a 1-h intravenous infusion of the doxorubicin prodrug DTS-201 every 3 weeks in patients with advanced or metastatic solid tumours. *Eur. J. Cancer* **2017**, *86*, 240–247. [CrossRef] [PubMed]
162. Ravel, D.; Dubois, V.; Quinonero, J.; Meyer-Losic, F.; Delord, J.; Rochaix, P.; Nicolazzi, C.; Ribes, F.; Mazerolles, C.; Assouly, E.; et al. Preclinical toxicity, toxicokinetics, and antitumoral efficacy studies of DTS-201, a tumor-selective peptidic prodrug of doxorubicin. *Clin. Cancer Res.* **2008**, *14*, 1258–1265. [CrossRef]
163. Available online: https://www.clinicaltrialsregister.eu/ctr-search/search?query=DTS-201 (accessed on 22 April 2019).
164. Available online: https://clinicaltrials.gov/ct2/show/NCT03486730 (accessed on 22 April 2019).
165. Available online: https://clinicaltrials.gov/ct2/show/NCT03511664 (accessed on 22 April 2019).
166. Gupte, A.A.; Pownall, H.J.; Hamilton, D.J. Estrogen: An emerging regulator of insulin action and mitochondrial function. *J. Diabetes Res.* **2015**, *2015*, 916585. [CrossRef]
167. Mauvais-Jarvis, F. Estrogen and androgen receptors: Regulators of fuel homeostasis and emerging targets for diabetes and obesity. *Trends Endocrinol. Metab.* **2011**, *22*, 24–33. [CrossRef]
168. Pereira, R.I.; Casey, B.A.; Swibas, T.A.; Erickson, C.B.; Wolfe, P.; Van Pelt, R.E. Timing of Estradiol Treatment After Menopause May Determine Benefit or Harm to Insulin Action. *J. Clin. Endocrinol. Metab.* **2015**, *100*, 4456–4462. [CrossRef] [PubMed]
169. Bonds, D.E.; Lasser, N.; Qi, L.; Brzyski, R.; Caan, B.; Heiss, G.; Limacher, M.C.; Liu, J.H.; Mason, E.; Oberman, A.; et al. The effect of conjugated equine oestrogen on diabetes incidence: The Women's Health Initiative randomised trial. *Diabetologia* **2006**, *49*, 459–468. [CrossRef] [PubMed]
170. Rossouw, J.E.; Anderson, G.L.; Prentice, R.L.; LaCroix, A.Z.; Kooperberg, C.; Stefanick, M.L.; Jackson, R.D.; Beresford, S.A.; Howard, B.V.; Johnson, K.C.; et al. Risks and benefits of estrogen plus progestin in healthy postmenopausal women: Principal results From the Women's Health Initiative randomized controlled trial. *JAMA* **2002**, *288*, 321–333. [PubMed]
171. Kim, J.H.; Meyers, M.S.; Khuder, S.S.; Abdallah, S.L.; Muturi, H.T.; Russo, L.; Tate, C.R.; Hevener, A.L.; Najjar, S.M.; Leloup, C.; et al. Tissue-selective estrogen complexes with bazedoxifene prevent metabolic dysfunction in female mice. *Mol. Metab.* **2014**, *3*, 177–190. [CrossRef]
172. Barrera, J.; Chambliss, K.L.; Ahmed, M.; Tanigaki, K.; Thompson, B.; McDonald, J.G.; Mineo, C.; Shaul, P.W. Bazedoxifene and conjugated estrogen prevent diet-induced obesity, hepatic steatosis, and type 2 diabetes in mice without impacting the reproductive tract. *Am. J. Physiol. Endocrinol. Metab.* **2014**, *307*, E345–E354. [CrossRef] [PubMed]
173. Hansdottir, H. Raloxifene for older women: A review of the literature. *Clin. Interv. Aging* **2008**, *3*, 45–50. [CrossRef]
174. Barrett-Connor, E.; Mosca, L.; Collins, P.; Geiger, M.J.; Grady, D.; Kornitzer, M.; McNabb, M.A.; Wenger, N.K.; Investigators, R.U.f.T.H.R.T. Effects of raloxifene on cardiovascular events and breast cancer in postmenopausal women. *N. Engl. J. Med.* **2006**, *355*, 125–137. [CrossRef]
175. Finan, B.; Yang, B.; Ottaway, N.; Stemmer, K.; Muller, T.D.; Yi, C.X.; Habegger, K.; Schriever, S.C.; Garcia-Caceres, C.; Kabra, D.G.; et al. Targeted estrogen delivery reverses the metabolic syndrome. *Nat. Med.* **2012**, *18*, 1847–1856. [CrossRef]
176. Bullock, B.P.; Heller, R.S.; Habener, J.F. Tissue distribution of messenger ribonucleic acid encoding the rat glucagon-like peptide-1 receptor. *Endocrinology* **1996**, *137*, 2968–2978. [CrossRef]
177. The Human Protein Atlas. Available online: https://www.proteinatlas.org/ENSG00000112164-GLP1R/tissue (accessed on 22 April 2019).
178. Cao, X.; Xu, P.; Oyola, M.G.; Xia, Y.; Yan, X.; Saito, K.; Zou, F.; Wang, C.; Yang, Y.; Hinton, A., Jr.; et al. Estrogens stimulate serotonin neurons to inhibit binge-like eating in mice. *J. Clin. Investig.* **2014**, *124*, 4351–4362. [CrossRef]
179. Vogel, H.; Wolf, S.; Rabasa, C.; Rodriguez-Pacheco, F.; Babaei, C.S.; Stober, F.; Goldschmidt, J.; DiMarchi, R.D.; Finan, B.; Tschop, M.H.; et al. GLP-1 and estrogen conjugate acts in the supramammillary nucleus to reduce food-reward and body weight. *Neuropharmacology* **2016**, *110*, 396–406. [CrossRef]
180. Tiano, J.P.; Tate, C.R.; Yang, B.S.; DiMarchi, R.; Mauvais-Jarvis, F. Effect of targeted estrogen delivery using glucagon-like peptide-1 on insulin secretion, insulin sensitivity and glucose homeostasis. *Sci. Rep.* **2015**, *5*, 10211. [CrossRef]

181. Schwenk, R.W.; Baumeier, C.; Finan, B.; Kluth, O.; Brauer, C.; Joost, H.G.; DiMarchi, R.D.; Tschop, M.H.; Schurmann, A. GLP-1-oestrogen attenuates hyperphagia and protects from beta cell failure in diabetes-prone New Zealand obese (NZO) mice. *Diabetologia* **2015**, *58*, 604–614. [CrossRef]
182. Quarta, C.; Clemmensen, C.; Zhu, Z.; Yang, B.; Joseph, S.S.; Lutter, D.; Yi, C.X.; Graf, E.; Garcia-Caceres, C.; Legutko, B.; et al. Molecular Integration of Incretin and Glucocorticoid Action Reverses Immunometabolic Dysfunction and Obesity. *Cell Metab.* **2017**, *26*, 620–632 e626. [CrossRef] [PubMed]
183. Grozinsky-Glasberg, S.; Fraser, A.; Nahshoni, E.; Weizman, A.; Leibovici, L. Thyroxine-triiodothyronine combination therapy versus thyroxine monotherapy for clinical hypothyroidism: Meta-analysis of randomized controlled trials. *J. Clin. Endocrinol. Metab.* **2006**, *91*, 2592–2599. [CrossRef]
184. Mullur, R.; Liu, Y.Y.; Brent, G.A. Thyroid hormone regulation of metabolism. *Physiol. Rev.* **2014**, *94*, 355–382. [CrossRef] [PubMed]
185. Sinha, R.A.; Singh, B.K.; Yen, P.M. Thyroid hormone regulation of hepatic lipid and carbohydrate metabolism. *Trends Endocrinol. Metab.* **2014**, *25*, 538–545. [CrossRef] [PubMed]
186. Ochs, N.; Auer, R.; Bauer, D.C.; Nanchen, D.; Gussekloo, J.; Cornuz, J.; Rodondi, N. Meta-analysis: Subclinical thyroid dysfunction and the risk for coronary heart disease and mortality. *Ann. Intern. Med.* **2008**, *148*, 832–845. [CrossRef] [PubMed]
187. Baxter, J.D.; Webb, P. Thyroid hormone mimetics: Potential applications in atherosclerosis, obesity and type 2 diabetes. *Nat. Rev. Drug Discov.* **2009**, *8*, 308–320. [CrossRef] [PubMed]
188. Muller, T.D.; Finan, B.; Clemmensen, C.; DiMarchi, R.D.; Tschop, M.H. The New Biology and Pharmacology of Glucagon. *Physiol. Rev.* **2017**, *97*, 721–766. [CrossRef]
189. Finan, B.; Clemmensen, C.; Zhu, Z.; Stemmer, K.; Gauthier, K.; Muller, L.; De Angelis, M.; Moreth, K.; Neff, F.; Perez-Tilve, D.; et al. Chemical Hybridization of Glucagon and Thyroid Hormone Optimizes Therapeutic Impact for Metabolic Disease. *Cell* **2016**, *167*, 843–857 e814. [CrossRef]
190. Cox, D.; Brennan, M.; Moran, N. Integrins as therapeutic targets: Lessons and opportunities. *Nat. Rev. Drug Discov.* **2010**, *9*, 804–820. [CrossRef]
191. Rathinam, R.; Alahari, S.K. Important role of integrins in the cancer biology. *Cancer Metastasis Rev.* **2010**, *29*, 223–237. [CrossRef]
192. Desgrosellier, J.S.; Cheresh, D.A. Integrins in cancer: Biological implications and therapeutic opportunities. *Nat. Rev. Cancer* **2010**, *10*, 9–22. [CrossRef] [PubMed]
193. Ley, K.; Rivera-Nieves, J.; Sandborn, W.J.; Shattil, S. Integrin-based therapeutics: Biological basis, clinical use and new drugs. *Nat. Rev. Drug Discov.* **2016**, *15*, 173–183. [CrossRef] [PubMed]
194. Cox, N.; Kintzing, J.R.; Smith, M.; Grant, G.A.; Cochran, J.R. Integrin-Targeting Knottin Peptide-Drug Conjugates Are Potent Inhibitors of Tumor Cell Proliferation. *Angew. Chem.* **2016**, *55*, 9894–9897. [CrossRef] [PubMed]
195. Toschi, L.; Finocchiaro, G.; Bartolini, S.; Gioia, V.; Cappuzzo, F. Role of gemcitabine in cancer therapy. *Future Oncol.* **2005**, *1*, 7–17. [CrossRef] [PubMed]
196. Noble, S.; Goa, K.L. Gemcitabine. A review of its pharmacology and clinical potential in non-small cell lung cancer and pancreatic cancer. *Drugs* **1997**, *54*, 447–472. [CrossRef]
197. Karampelas, T.; Skavatsou, E.; Argyros, O.; Fokas, D.; Tamvakopoulos, C. Gemcitabine Based Peptide Conjugate with Improved Metabolic Properties and Dual Mode of Efficacy. *Mol. Pharm.* **2017**, *14*, 674–685. [CrossRef]
198. Jain, N.; Smith, S.W.; Ghone, S.; Tomczuk, B. Current ADC Linker Chemistry. *Pharm. Res.* **2015**, *32*, 3526–3540. [CrossRef]
199. Lu, J.; Jiang, F.; Lu, A.; Zhang, G. Linkers Having a Crucial Role in Antibody-Drug Conjugates. *Int. J. Mol. Sci.* **2016**, *17*, 561. [CrossRef]
200. McCombs, J.R.; Owen, S.C. Antibody drug conjugates: Design and selection of linker, payload and conjugation chemistry. *Aaps J.* **2015**, *17*, 339–351. [CrossRef] [PubMed]
201. Gebleux, R.; Casi, G. Antibody-drug conjugates: Current status and future perspectives. *Pharm. Ther.* **2016**, *167*, 48–59. [CrossRef] [PubMed]
202. Kim, E.G.; Kim, K.M. Strategies and Advancement in Antibody-Drug Conjugate Optimization for Targeted Cancer Therapeutics. *Biomol. Ther. (Seoul)* **2015**, *23*, 493–509. [CrossRef] [PubMed]
203. Chari, R.V.; Miller, M.L.; Widdison, W.C. Antibody-drug conjugates: An emerging concept in cancer therapy. *Angew. Chem.* **2014**, *53*, 3796–3827. [CrossRef]

204. Tsuchikama, K.; An, Z. Antibody-drug conjugates: Recent advances in conjugation and linker chemistries. *Protein Cell* **2018**, *9*, 33–46. [CrossRef]
205. Doronina, S.O.; Bovee, T.D.; Meyer, D.W.; Miyamoto, J.B.; Anderson, M.E.; Morris-Tilden, C.A.; Senter, P.D. Novel peptide linkers for highly potent antibody-auristatin conjugate. *Bioconj. Chem.* **2008**, *19*, 1960–1963. [CrossRef] [PubMed]
206. Staben, L.R.; Koenig, S.G.; Lehar, S.M.; Vandlen, R.; Zhang, D.; Chuh, J.; Yu, S.F.; Ng, C.; Guo, J.; Liu, Y.; et al. Targeted drug delivery through the traceless release of tertiary and heteroaryl amines from antibody-drug conjugates. *Nat. Chem.* **2016**, *8*, 1112–1119. [CrossRef]
207. Anami, Y.; Yamazaki, C.M.; Xiong, W.; Gui, X.; Zhang, N.; An, Z.; Tsuchikama, K. Glutamic acid-valine-citrulline linkers ensure stability and efficacy of antibody-drug conjugates in mice. *Nat. Commun.* **2018**, *9*, 2512. [CrossRef]
208. Jeffrey, S.C.; Andreyka, J.B.; Bernhardt, S.X.; Kissler, K.M.; Kline, T.; Lenox, J.S.; Moser, R.F.; Nguyen, M.T.; Okeley, N.M.; Stone, I.J.; et al. Development and properties of beta-glucuronide linkers for monoclonal antibody-drug conjugates. *Bioconj. Chem.* **2006**, *17*, 831–840. [CrossRef]
209. Burke, P.J.; Senter, P.D.; Meyer, D.W.; Miyamoto, J.B.; Anderson, M.; Toki, B.E.; Manikumar, G.; Wani, M.C.; Kroll, D.J.; Jeffrey, S.C. Design, synthesis, and biological evaluation of antibody-drug conjugates comprised of potent camptothecin analogues. *Bioconj. Chem.* **2009**, *20*, 1242–1250. [CrossRef]
210. Gunnoo, S.B.; Madder, A. Chemical Protein Modification through Cysteine. *ChemBioChem* **2016**, *17*, 529–553. [CrossRef]
211. Gunnoo, S.B.; Madder, A. Bioconjugation—Using selective chemistry to enhance the properties of proteins and peptides as therapeutics and carriers. *Org. Biomol. Chem.* **2016**, *14*, 8002–8013. [CrossRef]
212. Su, D.; Kozak, K.R.; Sadowsky, J.; Yu, S.F.; Fourie-O'Donohue, A.; Nelson, C.; Vandlen, R.; Ohri, R.; Liu, L.; Ng, C.; et al. Modulating Antibody-Drug Conjugate Payload Metabolism by Conjugation Site and Linker Modification. *Bioconj. Chem.* **2018**, *29*, 1155–1167. [CrossRef]
213. Spicer, C.D.; Davis, B.G. Selective chemical protein modification. *Nat. Commun.* **2014**, *5*, 4740. [CrossRef]
214. Chudasama, V.; Maruani, A.; Caddick, S. Recent advances in the construction of antibody-drug conjugates. *Nat. Chem.* **2016**, *8*, 114–119. [CrossRef]
215. Schumacher, D.; Hackenberger, C.P.; Leonhardt, H.; Helma, J. Current Status: Site-Specific Antibody Drug Conjugates. *J. Clin. Immunol.* **2016**, *36* (Suppl. 1), 100–107. [CrossRef]
216. Sochaj, A.M.; Swiderska, K.W.; Otlewski, J. Current methods for the synthesis of homogeneous antibody-drug conjugates. *Biotechnol. Adv.* **2015**, *33*, 775–784. [CrossRef]
217. Calce, E.; Leone, M.; Monfregola, L.; De Luca, S. Chemical modifications of peptide sequences via S-alkylation reaction. *Org. Lett.* **2013**, *15*, 5354–5357. [CrossRef]
218. Lu, Y.; Huang, F.; Wang, J.; Xia, J. Affinity-guided covalent conjugation reactions based on PDZ-peptide and SH3-peptide interactions. *Bioconj. Chem.* **2014**, *25*, 989–999. [CrossRef]
219. Calce, E.; Leone, M.; Mercurio, F.A.; Monfregola, L.; De Luca, S. Solid-Phase S-Alkylation Promoted by Molecular Sieves. *Org. Lett.* **2015**, *17*, 5646–5649. [CrossRef]
220. Doan, N.D.; Bourgault, S.; Letourneau, M.; Fournier, A. Effectiveness of the suzuki-miyaura cross-coupling reaction for solid-phase peptide modification. *J. Comb. Chem.* **2008**, *10*, 44–51. [CrossRef]
221. Afonso, A.; Feliu, L.; Planas, M. Solid-phase synthesis of biaryl cyclic peptides by borylation and microwave-assisted intramolecular Suzuki–Miyaura reaction. *Tetrahedron* **2011**, *67*, 2238–2245. [CrossRef]
222. Silvestri, A.P.; Cistrone, P.A.; Dawson, P.E. Adapting the Glaser Reaction for Bioconjugation: Robust Access to Structurally Simple, Rigid Linkers. *Angew. Chem.* **2017**, *56*, 10438–10442. [CrossRef] [PubMed]
223. Pagel, M.; Meier, R.; Braun, K.; Wiessler, M.; Beck-Sickinger, A.G. On-resin Diels-Alder reaction with inverse electron demand: An efficient ligation method for complex peptides with a varying spacer to optimize cell adhesion. *Org. Biomol. Chem.* **2016**, *14*, 4809–4816. [CrossRef] [PubMed]
224. Bartlett, S.; Spring, D.R. C-H activation: Complex peptides made simple. *Nat. Chem.* **2016**, *9*, 9–10. [CrossRef]
225. Oriana, S.; Cai, Y.; Bode, J.W.; Yamakoshi, Y. Synthesis of tri-functionalized MMP2 FRET probes using a chemo-selective and late-stage modification of unprotected peptides. *Org. Biomol. Chem.* **2017**, *15*, 1792–1800. [CrossRef]
226. Decostaire, I.E.; Lelievre, D.; Aucagne, V.; Delmas, A.F. Solid phase oxime ligations for the iterative synthesis of polypeptide conjugates. *Org. Biomol. Chem.* **2014**, *12*, 5536–5543. [CrossRef] [PubMed]

227. VanBrunt, M.P.; Shanebeck, K.; Caldwell, Z.; Johnson, J.; Thompson, P.; Martin, T.; Dong, H.; Li, G.; Xu, H.; D'Hooge, F.; et al. Genetically Encoded Azide Containing Amino Acid in Mammalian Cells Enables Site-Specific Antibody-Drug Conjugates Using Click Cycloaddition Chemistry. *Bioconj. Chem.* **2015**, *26*, 2249–2260. [CrossRef]
228. Presolski, S.I.; Hong, V.P.; Finn, M.G. Copper-Catalyzed Azide-Alkyne Click Chemistry for Bioconjugation. *Curr. Protoc. Chem. Biol.* **2011**, *3*, 153–162. [CrossRef]
229. El-Faham, A.; Albericio, F. Peptide coupling reagents, more than a letter soup. *Chem. Rev.* **2011**, *111*, 6557–6602. [CrossRef]
230. Li, D.; Elbert, D.L. The kinetics of the removal of the N-methyltrityl (Mtt) group during the synthesis of branched peptides. *J. Pept. Res.* **2002**, *60*, 300–303. [CrossRef] [PubMed]
231. Koniev, O.; Wagner, A. Developments and recent advancements in the field of endogenous amino acid selective bond forming reactions for bioconjugation. *Chem. Soc. Rev.* **2015**, *44*, 5495–5551. [CrossRef] [PubMed]
232. Anderson, G.W.; Callahan, F.M.; Zimmerman, J.E. Synthesis of N-hydroxysuccinimide esters of acyl peptides by the mixed anhydride method. *J. Am. Chem. Soc.* **1967**, *89*, 178. [CrossRef] [PubMed]
233. Lapidot, Y.; Rappoport, S.; Wolman, Y. Use of esters of N-hydroxysuccinimide in the synthesis of N-acylamino acids. *J. Lipid Res.* **1967**, *8*, 142–145. [PubMed]
234. Nagy, A.; Schally, A.V.; Armatis, P.; Szepeshazi, K.; Halmos, G.; Kovacs, M.; Zarandi, M.; Groot, K.; Miyazaki, M.; Jungwirth, A.; et al. Cytotoxic analogs of luteinizing hormone-releasing hormone containing doxorubicin or 2-pyrrolinodoxorubicin, a derivative 500–1000 times more potent. *Proc. Natl. Acad. Sci. USA* **1996**, *93*, 7269–7273. [CrossRef]
235. White, C.J.; Yudin, A.K. Contemporary strategies for peptide macrocyclization. *Nat. Chem.* **2011**, *3*, 509–524. [CrossRef] [PubMed]
236. Basle, E.; Joubert, N.; Pucheault, M. Protein chemical modification on endogenous amino acids. *Chem. Biol.* **2010**, *17*, 213–227. [CrossRef]
237. Geng, Q.; Sun, X.; Gong, T.; Zhang, Z.R. Peptide-drug conjugate linked via a disulfide bond for kidney targeted drug delivery. *Bioconj. Chem.* **2012**, *23*, 1200–1210. [CrossRef]
238. Song, Q.; Chuan, X.; Chen, B.; He, B.; Zhang, H.; Dai, W.; Wang, X.; Zhang, Q. A smart tumor targeting peptide-drug conjugate, pHLIP-SS-DOX: Synthesis and cellular uptake on MCF-7 and MCF-7/Adr cells. *Drug Deliv.* **2016**, *23*, 1734–1746. [CrossRef]
239. Witt, D. Recent developments in disulfide bond formation. *Synthesis* **2008**, *16*, 2491–2509. [CrossRef]
240. Mandal, B.; Basu, B. Recent advances in S–S bond formation. *Rsc Adv.* **2014**, *4*, 13854–13881. [CrossRef]
241. Le Guern, F.; Ouk, T.S.; Ouk, C.; Vanderesse, R.; Champavier, Y.; Pinault, E.; Sol, V. Lysine Analogue of Polymyxin B as a Significant Opportunity for Photodynamic Antimicrobial Chemotherapy. *ACS Med. Chem. Lett.* **2018**, *9*, 11–16. [CrossRef] [PubMed]
242. Torres, O.B.; Matyas, G.R.; Rao, M.; Peachman, K.K.; Jalah, R.; Beck, Z.; Michael, N.L.; Rice, K.C.; Jacobson, A.E.; Alving, C.R. Heroin-HIV-1 (H2) vaccine: Induction of dual immunologic effects with a heroin hapten-conjugate and an HIV-1 envelope V2 peptide with liposomal lipid A as an adjuvant. *Npj Vaccines* **2017**, *2*, 13. [CrossRef]
243. Jalah, R.; Torres, O.B.; Mayorov, A.V.; Li, F.; Antoline, J.F.; Jacobson, A.E.; Rice, K.C.; Deschamps, J.R.; Beck, Z.; Alving, C.R.; et al. Efficacy, but not antibody titer or affinity, of a heroin hapten conjugate vaccine correlates with increasing hapten densities on tetanus toxoid, but not on CRM197 carriers. *Bioconj. Chem.* **2015**, *26*, 1041–1053. [CrossRef]
244. Ponte, J.F.; Sun, X.; Yoder, N.C.; Fishkin, N.; Laleau, R.; Coccia, J.; Lanieri, L.; Bogalhas, M.; Wang, L.; Wilhelm, S.; et al. Understanding How the Stability of the Thiol-Maleimide Linkage Impacts the Pharmacokinetics of Lysine-Linked Antibody-Maytansinoid Conjugates. *Bioconj. Chem.* **2016**, *27*, 1588–1598. [CrossRef]
245. Dovgan, I.; Kolodych, S.; Koniev, O.; Wagner, A. 2-(Maleimidomethyl)-1,3-Dioxanes (MD): A Serum-Stable Self-hydrolysable Hydrophilic Alternative to Classical Maleimide Conjugation. *Sci. Rep.* **2016**, *6*, 30835. [CrossRef]
246. Fontaine, S.D.; Reid, R.; Robinson, L.; Ashley, G.W.; Santi, D.V. Long-term stabilization of maleimide-thiol conjugates. *Bioconj. Chem.* **2015**, *26*, 145–152. [CrossRef]

247. Lyon, R.P.; Setter, J.R.; Bovee, T.D.; Doronina, S.O.; Hunter, J.H.; Anderson, M.E.; Balasubramanian, C.L.; Duniho, S.M.; Leiske, C.I.; Li, F.; et al. Self-hydrolyzing maleimides improve the stability and pharmacological properties of antibody-drug conjugates. *Nat. Biotechnol.* **2014**, *32*, 1059–1062. [CrossRef]
248. Schumacher, F.F.; Nunes, J.P.; Maruani, A.; Chudasama, V.; Smith, M.E.; Chester, K.A.; Baker, J.R.; Caddick, S. Next generation maleimides enable the controlled assembly of antibody-drug conjugates via native disulfide bond bridging. *Org. Biomol. Chem.* **2014**, *12*, 7261–7269. [CrossRef]
249. Maruani, A.; Smith, M.E.; Miranda, E.; Chester, K.A.; Chudasama, V.; Caddick, S. A plug-and-play approach to antibody-based therapeutics via a chemoselective dual click strategy. *Nat. Commun.* **2015**, *6*, 6645. [CrossRef]
250. Behrens, C.R.; Ha, E.H.; Chinn, L.L.; Bowers, S.; Probst, G.; Fitch-Bruhns, M.; Monteon, J.; Valdiosera, A.; Bermudez, A.; Liao-Chan, S.; et al. Antibody-Drug Conjugates (ADCs) Derived from Interchain Cysteine Cross-Linking Demonstrate Improved Homogeneity and Other Pharmacological Properties over Conventional Heterogeneous ADCs. *Mol. Pharm.* **2015**, *12*, 3986–3998. [CrossRef]
251. Anderson, R.J.; Li, J.; Kedzierski, L.; Compton, B.J.; Hayman, C.M.; Osmond, T.L.; Tang, C.W.; Farrand, K.J.; Koay, H.F.; Almeida, C.; et al. Augmenting Influenza-Specific T Cell Memory Generation with a Natural Killer T Cell-Dependent Glycolipid-Peptide Vaccine. *ACS Chem. Biol.* **2017**, *12*, 2898–2905. [CrossRef]
252. Speir, M.; Authier-Hall, A.; Brooks, C.R.; Farrand, K.J.; Compton, B.J.; Anderson, R.J.; Heiser, A.; Osmond, T.L.; Tang, C.W.; Berzofsky, J.A.; et al. Glycolipid-peptide conjugate vaccines enhance CD8(+) T cell responses against human viral proteins. *Sci. Rep.* **2017**, *7*, 14273. [CrossRef]
253. Barile, E.; Wang, S.; Das, S.K.; Noberini, R.; Dahl, R.; Stebbins, J.L.; Pasquale, E.B.; Fisher, P.B.; Pellecchia, M. Design, synthesis and bioevaluation of an EphA2 receptor-based targeted delivery system. *ChemMedChem* **2014**, *9*, 1403–1412. [CrossRef]
254. Wang, S.; Placzek, W.J.; Stebbins, J.L.; Mitra, S.; Noberini, R.; Koolpe, M.; Zhang, Z.; Dahl, R.; Pasquale, E.B.; Pellecchia, M. Novel targeted system to deliver chemotherapeutic drugs to EphA2-expressing cancer cells. *J. Med. Chem.* **2012**, *55*, 2427–2436. [CrossRef]
255. Bonaccorso, R.L.; Chepurny, O.G.; Becker-Pauly, C.; Holz, G.G.; Doyle, R.P. Enhanced Peptide Stability Against Protease Digestion Induced by Intrinsic Factor Binding of a Vitamin B12 Conjugate of Exendin-4. *Mol. Pharm.* **2015**, *12*, 3502–3506. [CrossRef]

Sample Availability: To acquire samples of the compounds, please direct attention to primary publications and authors.

MDPI
St. Alban-Anlage 66
4052 Basel
Switzerland
Tel. +41 61 683 77 34
Fax +41 61 302 89 18
www.mdpi.com

Molecules Editorial Office
E-mail: molecules@mdpi.com
www.mdpi.com/journal/molecules

www.ingramcontent.com/pod-product-compliance
Lightning Source LLC
LaVergne TN
LVHW071936080526
838202LV00064B/6614
9783039282883